Angiotensin-converting Enzyme Inhibitors vs. Angiotensin Receptor Blockers

Mukesh Nandave
Editor

Angiotensin-converting Enzyme Inhibitors vs. Angiotensin Receptor Blockers

A Critical Analysis of Antihypertensive Strategies: A Machine-Generated Literature Overview

Springer

Editor
Mukesh Nandave
Department of Pharmacology
Delhi Pharmaceutical Sciences and Research University
New Delhi, Delhi, India

ISBN 978-981-97-7379-4 ISBN 978-981-97-7380-0 (eBook)
https://doi.org/10.1007/978-981-97-7380-0

This Springer imprint is published by the registered company Springer Nature Singapore Pte Ltd.
The registered company address is: 152 Beach Road, #21-01/04 Gateway East, Singapore 189721, Singapore

Foreword

It is with great pleasure that I introduce this comprehensive and meticulously crafted book, *Angiotensin-converting Enzyme Inhibitors vs. Angiotensin Receptor Blockers: A Critical Analysis of Antihypertensive Strategies: A Machine-Generated Literature Overview*, edited by Dr. Mukesh Nandave and published by Springer Nature. As we continue to advance in our understanding of cardiovascular health, the comparative study of ACE inhibitors and ARBs remains pivotal in optimizing hypertensive treatment strategies.

The journey begins with an introduction to the RAAS, setting the stage for the detailed exploration that follows. The authors tried to provide a foundational understanding of the physiological mechanisms that underlie the system, highlighting the pivotal role of RAAS in cardiovascular homeostasis.

In this book, a comparative study is conducted on the impact of ACE inhibitors and ARBs on insulin resistance in hypertensive patients, a vital consideration given the interplay between hypertension and metabolic disorders.

The role of these agents in acute heart failure is meticulously examined with due consideration to evidence-based insights into their efficacy and safety profiles. Of course with availability of ARNI (Angiotensin receptor/neprilysin inhibitor), it has almost replaced ACEI/ARB in management of heart failure. Similarly, this compendium explores the immunomodulatory activities of ACE inhibitors and ARBs, a relatively new and exciting area of research that has significant implications for hypertensive patients.

The therapeutic roles of ACE inhibitors and ARBs in peripheral artery disease, a common comorbidity in hypertensive individuals, are critically analyzed, offering practical guidance for clinicians.

The relevance of ACE inhibitors and ARBs in the context of the COVID-19 pandemic is also addressed. This timely discussion highlights the evolving understanding of how these agents interact with the SARS-CoV-2 virus and their implications for patient management during the pandemic.

Dr. Mukesh Nandave have crafted a text that is not only informative but also thought-provoking. This book is an invaluable resource for clinicians, researchers, and students who seek a deeper understanding of the comparative efficacy and clinical applications of ACE inhibitors and ARBs. I am highly convinced and strongly recommend this critical analysis that it will enrich the reader's knowledge and contribute to improved patient care in the realm of hypertension and cardiovascular disease.

Department of Cardiology, AIIMS, New Delhi, India K. K. Talwar
PGIMER, Chandigarh, India
Cardiology, PSRI Hospital, New Delhi, India

Preface

The management of hypertension remains a critical challenge in contemporary medicine. Over the years, significant advancements have been made in understanding the pathophysiology of hypertension and developing effective therapeutic strategies. Among the myriad of pharmacological interventions, angiotensin-converting enzyme (ACE) inhibitors and angiotensin receptor blockers (ARBs) have emerged as pivotal agents in the management of hypertension. This book, *Angiotensin-Converting Enzyme Inhibitors vs. Angiotensin Receptor Blockers: A Critical Analysis of Antihypertensive Strategies: A Machine-Generated Literature Overview*, edited by Dr. Mukesh Nandave and published by Springer Nature, aims to provide a comprehensive analysis of these two classes of antihypertensive drugs, delving into their mechanisms of action, clinical applications, and emerging trends.

The renin–angiotensin–aldosterone system (RAAS) plays a central role in the regulation of blood pressure and fluid balance. Chapter 1 provides an in-depth introduction to RAAS, setting the foundation for understanding how ACE inhibitors and ARBs exert their antihypertensive effects. This foundational knowledge is crucial for appreciating the subsequent discussions on the role of these agents in various cardiovascular and metabolic disorders.

Chapter 2 explores the role of antihypertensive agents in cardiovascular disorders. Hypertension is a major risk factor for cardiovascular diseases, including coronary artery disease, stroke, and heart failure. This chapter reviews the evidence supporting the use of ACE inhibitors and ARBs in reducing cardiovascular morbidity and mortality, highlighting the clinical trials that have established their efficacy.

In Chap. 3, the focus shifts to comparing ACE inhibitors and ARBs in high-risk patients. ACE inhibitors have long been considered the preferred RAAS inhibitors due to their extensive clinical trial data and proven benefits. However, ARBs offer a viable alternative, particularly in patients who are intolerant to ACE inhibitors. This chapter critically evaluates the evidence supporting the use of each class, providing insights into their relative advantages and disadvantages.

Chapter 4 delves into the transformative role of ACE inhibitors in the renin–angiotensin system. By inhibiting the conversion of angiotensin I to angiotensin II, ACE inhibitors effectively reduce vasoconstriction and aldosterone secretion, leading to decreased blood pressure. This chapter discusses the molecular mechanisms underlying these effects and their clinical implications.

The effect of ACE inhibitors versus ARBs on insulin resistance in hypertensive patients is the focus of Chap. 5. Hypertension and insulin resistance often coexist, contributing to the development of metabolic syndrome and increasing cardiovascular risk. This chapter reviews the impact of ACE inhibitors and ARBs on insulin sensitivity, exploring the potential metabolic benefits of these agents beyond blood pressure control.

Chapter 6 examines the role of ACE inhibitors and ARBs in acute heart failure. Heart failure is a complex clinical syndrome with significant morbidity and mortality. ACE inhibitors and ARBs have demonstrated benefits in reducing hospitalizations and improving survival in patients with heart failure. This chapter reviews the evidence supporting their use in acute settings and discusses their mechanisms of action in heart failure management.

The immunomodulatory activity of ACE inhibitors and ARBs in hypertensive patients is explored in Chap. 7. Emerging evidence suggests that these agents may have anti-inflammatory and immunomodulatory effects, which could contribute to their cardiovascular benefits. This chapter delves into the potential mechanisms and clinical implications of these effects.

Chapter 8 addresses the role of ACE inhibitors and ARBs in peripheral artery disease (PAD). PAD is a common manifestation of systemic atherosclerosis and is associated with increased cardiovascular risk. This chapter reviews the evidence supporting the use of ACE inhibitors and ARBs in improving outcomes in patients with PAD.

The COVID-19 pandemic has brought new challenges to the management of hypertensive patients. Chapter 9 explores the role of ACE inhibitors and angiotensin receptor blockers (ARBs) in COVID-19 patients, addressing both safety concerns and potential therapeutic benefits. Despite initial fears that these medications might worsen COVID-19 outcomes, current evidence suggests they do not increase susceptibility to the virus and may actually confer protective cardiovascular effects. This chapter critically evaluates the latest research and provides guidance on managing hypertensive patients with COVID-19.

Finally, Chap. 10 discusses recent trends in the management of hypertension through RAAS inhibition. This chapter highlights ongoing research, emerging therapeutic strategies, and the future direction of antihypertensive therapy.

This book aims to provide healthcare professionals, researchers, and students with a comprehensive understanding of ACE inhibitors and ARBs, fostering informed decision-making in the management of hypertension and associated conditions. Through critical analysis and evidence-based discussions, we hope to contribute to the ongoing efforts to improve cardiovascular health and patient outcomes.

New Delhi, Delhi, India Mukesh Nandave

Disclaimer

Auto-summaries can be generated by either an abstractive or extractive auto-summarization:

- An extraction-based summarizer identifies the most important sentences of a text and uses the original sentences to create the summary.
- An abstraction-based summarizer creates new text based on deep learning. New phrases are created to summarize the content.

The auto-summaries you will find in this book have been generated via an extractive summarization approach.

Each chapter was carefully edited by Dr. Mukesh Nandave. The editors selected the papers which were then auto-summarized. The editors have not edited the auto-summaries due to the extraction-based approach and have not changed the original sentences. You will find the editors' reviews and guidance on the auto-summaries in their chapter introductions.

In machine-generated books, editors are defined as those who curate the content for the book by selecting the papers to be auto-summarized and by organizing the output into a meaningful order. Next to the thoughtful curation of the papers, editors should guide the readers through the auto-summaries and make transparent why they selected the papers.

The ultimate goal is to provide a current literature review of Springer Nature publications on a given topic in order to support readers in overcoming information overload and to help them dive into a topic faster; to identify interdisciplinary overlaps; and to present papers which might not have been on the readers' radar.

Please note that the selected papers are not used to train a LLM while the auto-summaries are created.

Contents

About the Editor

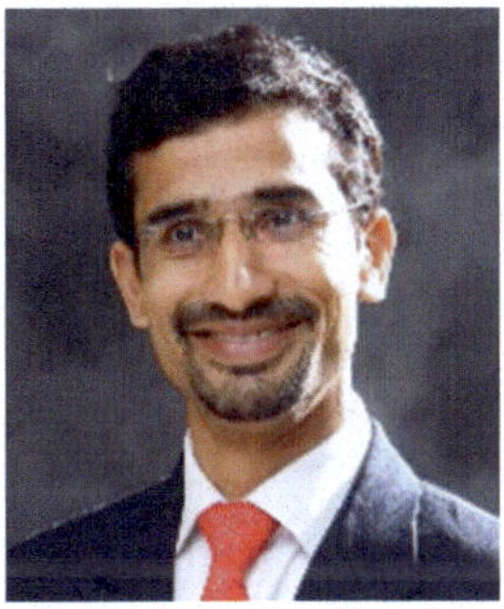

Mukesh Nandave is Associate Dean (Research) and In-charge Director of School of Pharmaceutical Sciences. He is also head of the Department of Pharmacology and Pharmaceutical Biotechnology at the Delhi Pharmaceutical Sciences and Research University, Government of NCT of Delhi, New Delhi, India. He has earlier served as Associate Professor and Head in the Department of Pharmacology at NMIMS University, Mumbai (2010–2017). Dr. Nandave earned his Ph.D. in pharmacology from AIIMS, Delhi, and received his postdoctoral training from the Ohio State University Medical Center, Columbus, USA.

For over 20 years, Dr. Nandave has been actively engaged in investigating the role of nutraceuticals, herbomineral formulations, and phytoconstituents in mitigating myocardial ischemia and reperfusion injury, diabetes, obesity, and pain management. He has published more than 85 papers in peer-reviewed national and international journals. His lab received more than 3.5 crore in total funding from government (DBT, DST, ICMR, and AYUSH) as well as industry (Pharmazz, Dabur, Charak, Madhavbaug, and Sandu).

Dr. Nandave has received numerous awards, including the Distinguished Leadership Award from the International Academy of Cardiovascular Sciences; Prof. S. C. Lahiri Oration and G. Achari Gold Medal from the Indian Pharmacological Society; Young Pharmacy Teacher of the Year Award from the Association of Pharmaceutical Teachers of India (APTI); Early Investigator Award from the International Society for Heart Research; Prof. Duggirala Visweswaram and Prof.

Sreemantula Satyanarayana Prize; Best Research Output of the Year for 2014–2015, 2013–2014, and 2012–2013 Award from SVKM's NMIMS University.

Dr. Nandave is the Secretary General of the India Section of the International Academy of Cardiovascular Sciences (IACS) and Treasurer of the Society for Promotion and Research of Cardiovascular Sciences (SPARCS). He is a life member of various professional bodies, including the International Society for Heart Research (ISHR), International Academy of Cardiovascular Sciences (IACS), Indian Pharmacological Society (IPS), Indian Pharmaceutical Association (IPA), Association of Physiologists and Pharmacologists of India (APPI), Association of Pharmaceutical Teachers of India (APTI), and Society for Ethnopharmacology.

He is also a BOS member at various institutes and expert member in project review panels of ICMR, AYUSH, SERB, and DBT.

Chapter 1
Introduction of Renin-Angiotensin-Aldosterone System (RAAS)

Mukesh Nandave

Introduction by the Editor

The human body is composed of different types of system that are associated with each other. The Renin-Angiotensin-Aldosterone System (RAAS) is one of the most major systems for survival. In 1988, renin was discovered by Tiegerstedt and Bergman, since then extensive research has been carried out to unravel the RAAS and its association with pathophysiology of various diseases. RAAS is responsible for proper functioning of vital organs such as heart and kidney and prevents extreme fluctuations. However, any damage to this system can initiate irregularities in blood pressure that may lead to acute or chronic illness or in severe cases it may result into sudden death. Renin and angiotensin are important components of RAAS, in which renin is secreted by kidney granular cells. Prorenin is a precursor of renin, it is a 406 amino acid protein which gets activated after processing. Prorenin is activated by proteolytical and non-proteolytical processes. Moreover, in proteolytical process, prorenin is activated in kidney with the help of neuroendocrine convertase enzyme 1 or cathepsin. Through non-proteolytical methods, prorenin is activated in various organs by prorenin/renin receptor. Expression of renin is increased by low blood sodium level, low blood pressure, activation of sympathetic nervous system. Renin converts α-2-globulin protein angiotensinogen to angiotensin I by starting the bond between leucine and valine. The level of angiotensinogen in plasma is increased by thyroid hormones, estrogen, corticosteroids. Angiotensin-I is converted to angiotensin II in the capillaries of lungs, kidney epithelial cells and endothelial cells by angiotensin converting enzyme (ACE). Angiotensin II constricts smooth muscles thus it has vasoactive effect on blood vessels. Therefore, it results in increased heart pulse rate, blood pressure. Angiotensin II stimulates plasminogen activator

---

M. Nandave (✉)
Department of Pharmacology, Delhi Pharmaceutical Sciences and Research University, New Delhi, Delhi, India

M. Nandave (ed.), *Angiotensin-converting Enzyme Inhibitors vs. Angiotensin Receptor Blockers*, https://doi.org/10.1007/978-981-97-7380-0_1

inhibitors PAI-1 and PA-2, adrenal cortex to secrete aldosterone. Aldosterone stimulates proximal tubules of kidney to facilitate sodium reabsorption thus regulating sodium-potassium homeostasis [1, 2]. Some factors are responsible for RAAS modulation such as pregnancy, birth control pills, anti-hypertensive agent, vasodilators, hormones (cortisol, thyroid, testosterone, and estrogen), and diuretics. Some tumors such as renin secreting tumors of the juxta-glomerular cell, renal cell carcinoma and Wilms's tumor can raise renin levels [3].

RAAS is a cornerstone for understanding the physiology and pathophysiology of cardiovascular system. RAAS plays a pivotal role in blood pressure regulation and electrolyte balance as well as maintaining vascular homeostasis.

Angiotensin Converting Enzyme and Angiotensin Receptor are two important components of RAAS, and they have emerged as targets for medical treatment in cardiovascular disorders. Angiotensin Converting Enzyme Inhibitors (ACEIs) and Angiotensin Receptor Blockers (ARBs) have brought a transformative shift in the field of cardiovascular medicine. ACEIs and ARBs not only alleviate the symptoms but also prevent the disease progression.

This chapter includes thorough discussion of RAAS and its significant role in cardiovascular health. Dysregulation of RAAS function initiates a series of dysfunction starting from hypertension followed by subsequent chain of events resulting in heart failure.

Moreover, this chapter clarifies the role of angiotensin receptors and angiotensin converting enzymes in coordinating the cardiovascular functions. This chapter explains the remarkable pharmacological effects of ACEs and ARBs in alleviating and slowing down the disease progression thus enhancing patient health. We unravel the mechanism behind the ACEs and ARBs efficacy and explored their clinical applications across the cardiovascular disorders.

Through illuminating the complex association between RAAS and cardiovascular disorders, this chapter aims to provide thorough understanding of RAAS to the clinicians, researchers, and students. This chapter also explains the rationale behind the use of ACEIs and ARBs as the key approach in the treatment of cardiovascular disease. Thus, promoting the development of more effective interventions to enhance patients' well-being (Fig. 1.1).

Machine Generated Summaries

Disclaimer: The summaries in this chapter were generated from Springer Nature publications using extractive AI auto-summarization: An extraction-based summarizer aims to identify the most important sentences of a text using an algorithm and uses those original sentences to create the auto-summary (unlike generative AI). As the constituted sentences are machine selected, they may not fully reflect the body of the work, so we strongly advise that the original content is read and cited. The auto generated summaries were curated by the editor to meet Springer Nature publication standards. To cite this content, please refer to the original papers.

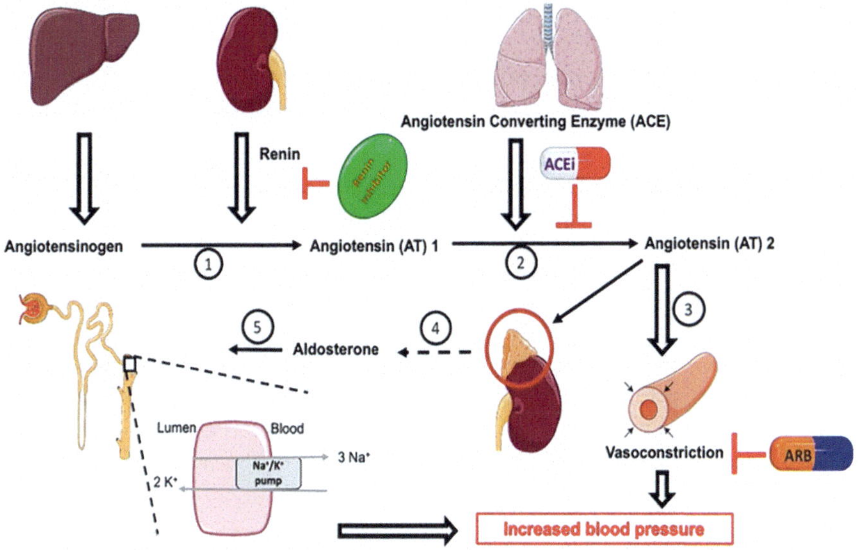

Fig. 1.1 Mechanism of action of angiotensin converting enzyme inhibitors and angiotensin receptor blocker on the renin-angiotensin-aldosterone system (RAAS). The liver secretes angiotensinogen which is then converted to angiotensin 1 via the action of renin (1), which is released by the kidneys. Angiotensin 1 is subsequently converted into its active component (2) angiotensin 2 via the action of angiotensin converting enzyme, which is produced by the pulmonary vasculature. Angiotensin 2 increases blood pressure via two mechanisms: angiotensin 2 by itself is a potent vasoconstrictor (3) which increases systemic blood pressure. Furthermore, angiotensin 2 acts on the adrenal cortex to release aldosterone from the zona glomerulosa (4). Aldosterone acts on the collecting ducts and distal convoluted tubules (DCT) to facilitate sodium ion reabsorption by acting on the sodium-potassium pump (5); water is also reabsorbed in conjunction with sodium ions during this process (not shown). The reabsorption of sodium ions and water increases intravascular volume thereby increasing blood pressure. (Source: Ojha et al. [4])

Machine generated keywords: raas, ang, acei, intake, potassium, aceiarb, combination, atr, angiotensin ang, initial, renin, aldosterone, arb, hfref, serum.

The Renin-Angiotensin-Aldosterone System: A Crossroad from Arterial Hypertension to Heart Failure [5]

This is a machine-generated summary of:

Pugliese, Nicola Riccardo; Masi, Stefano; Taddei, Stefano: The renin-angiotensin-aldosterone system: a crossroad from arterial hypertension to heart failure [5].

Published in: Heart Failure Reviews (2019).

Link to original: https://doi.org/10.1007/s10741-019-09855-5

Copyright of the summarized publication:

If you want to cite the papers, please refer to the original.

For technical reasons we could not place the page where the original quote is coming from.

Abstract-Summary "The RAAS is a crucial therapeutic target for several chronic diseases of the cardiovascular system, spanning from arterial hypertension (AH) to heart failure (HF)."

"AH represents a leading risk factor for the development of symptomatic HF, particularly with left ventricle (LV) preserved ejection fraction (HFpEF)."

"AH develops many years before the diagnosis of overt HF, providing a therapeutic target for preventive strategies."

"The blockers of the RAAS are effective drugs to treat AH and prevent HF with reduced ejection fraction (HFrEF), but the evidence of the potential benefits in patients with HFpEF remains limited."

Introduction

"Although Ang II was initially identified as a potent activator of aldosterone acting at the level of the zona glomerulosa of the adrenal cortex in the adrenal gland, this molecule has now emerged as the most potent active product of the RAAS."

"Sodium and water retention, together with the vasoconstriction caused by activation of RAAS and the sympathetic nervous system, lead to increased ventricular preload and afterload and elevated wall stress which in turn lead to the production of pre-pro B-type natriuretic peptide (BNP) which is cleaved to BNP and N-terminal proBNP (NT-proBNP) [6]."

"CNP is released from endothelial cells and acts in a paracrine fashion on the B-type natriuretic receptor (NPRB); it does not have direct natriuretic activity but is a potent vasodilator with inotropic and chronotropic properties [7]."

The Role of Renin-Angiotensin-Aldosterone System in Arterial Hypertension and Heart Failure

"Ang II receptor type 1 and type 2 (AT1 and AT2, respectively) regulate sodium excretion, but evidence in cross-transplanted kidney suggests that the AT1 receptor has a dominant role in mediating BP responses to Ang II, notably when AGT and renin are overexpressed in the proximal tubules [8, 9]."

"The AT1 and AT2 receptors have also been identified in the brain, where the microinjection of Ang II elicits an increase in BP and sympathetic activation via the AT1 receptor [10]."

"Under high salt intake or treatment with ACE inhibitors, Ang II receptor antagonists or renin inhibitors, the RAAS axis is suppressed; nevertheless, aldosterone receptor blockade is effective in lowering BP [10]."

"They also increase oxidative stress or sensitise the effect of Ang II, thereby activating the paraventricular nucleus to induce sympathetic overactivity [11, 12]."

Arterial Hypertension and Heart Failure

"Pre-onset AH carried a more than twofold increased odds of HFpEF versus HFrEF and, at the onset of HF, a higher systolic BP increased the odds of HFpEF versus HFrEF by 13% for each 10-mmHg increase [13]."

"Ho and others examined the risk profile of HF patients from four longitudinal community-based cohorts, suggesting a poor association between AH and HFrEF, while the relative risk of HFpEF increased by 14% per 20 mmHg systolic BP and by 42% if taking antihypertensive treatment [14]."

"Hypertensive patients can be classified as having stage A HFpEF, according to the American College of Cardiology Foundation/American Heart Association stages of HF [15, 16]."

"LV diastolic dysfunction and cardiac remodelling are the first discernible manifestations of heart disease in patients with AH."

Drugs Inhibiting the Renin-Angiotensin-Aldosterone System in the Management of Arterial Hypertension and Prevention of Heart Failure

"Treatment of AH is based on different classes of drugs; even if all antihypertensive drugs lower BP, there are significant differences in their capacity to prevent the evolution towards HF as well as the occurrence of HF complications."

"Beta-blockers remain a cornerstone in the treatment of HF, but in a large meta-analysis conducted in patients with AH, they did not prove a better preventive effect on HF than do other antihypertensives; this might be related to the limited capacity of beta-blockers to reduce central blood pressure compared with other classes of antihypertensive drugs [17]."

"As regards calcium-channel blockers (CCBs), a meta-analysis demonstrated that CCBs increased the risk of HF events when compared with diuretics, ACE inhibitors and ARBs [18]; therefore, caution should be exercised when using CCBs for prevention of HF in hypertensive patients."

"The blockers of the RAAS are effective drugs to treat AH and prevent HF."

Drugs Inhibiting the Renin-Angiotensin-Aldosterone System in the Management of HFrEF

"The American and European HF Guidelines recommend against the use of all three RAAS inhibiting agents (ACE inhibitors, ARBs and aldosterone antagonists) concomitantly [19, 20]."

"A novel drug has been introduced in HF management: the angiotensin II receptor–neprilysin inhibitor (ARNI) valsartan/sacubitril [19]."

"The first solution to the problem was the adoption of a dual blockade of RAAS and the natriuretic peptide system: the combined ACE and neprilysin inhibitor omapatrilat did not reduce the primary endpoint (death from any cause or HF hospitalisations) in a large randomised controlled trial against enalapril [21]."

"The randomised control trial was conducted in HFrEF outpatients and terminated early due to a sustained and highly significant reduction in the risk of the primary composite endpoint (CV death or HF hospitalisation) and CV mortality in the sacubitril/valsartan group compared with the enalapril group [19]."

Drugs Inhibiting the Renin-Angiotensin-Aldosterone System in the Management of HFpEF

"In the CHARM-Preserved trial, candesartan was compared with placebo in HF patients with an LVEF >40%, demonstrating no difference in the primary outcome of CV death or HF hospitalisation [22]."

"In the TOPCAT trial, HFpEF patients were randomised to spironolactone or placebo: there was no reduction in the incidence of the primary composite outcome of death from cardiovascular causes, aborted cardiac arrest or HF hospitalisation [23]."

"There is little experience with sacubitril/valsartan in HFpEF: in a phase 2 randomised trial of patients with HFpEF, NT-proBNP fell in the sacubitril/valsartan group in comparison with valsartan, along with reductions in NYHA class and left atrial volumes [24]."

"A large multicentre randomised outcome trial of sacubitril/valsartan versus valsartan in HFpEF [25] has been terminated early, and results will be available shortly."

Summary

"Based on current evidence, AH remains the leading cardiovascular risk factor for HF."

"The use of RAAS blockers remains the cornerstone of both AH and HF treatment."

"This drawback might reflect the lack of knowledge on the mechanisms leading the transition from AH to HF and late complications; more studies are needed to fill this gap."

Role of the Renin-Angiotensin-Aldosterone System and Its Pharmacological Inhibitors in Cardiovascular Diseases: Complex and Critical Issues [26]

This is a machine-generated summary of:

Borghi, Claudio; SIIA Task Force, None; Rossi, Francesco; SIF Task Force, None: Role of the Renin-Angiotensin-Aldosterone System and Its Pharmacological Inhibitors in Cardiovascular Diseases: Complex and Critical Issues [26].

Published in: High Blood Pressure & Cardiovascular Prevention (2015).

Link to original: https://doi.org/10.1007/s40292-015-0120-5

If you want to cite the papers, please refer to the original.

For technical reasons we could not place the page where the original quote is coming from.

Abstract-Summary "Hypertension is one of the major risk factor able to promote development and progression of several cardiovascular diseases, including left ventricular hypertrophy and dysfunction, myocardial infarction, stroke, and congestive heart failure."

"Among various regulatory and contra-regulatory systems involved in the pathogenesis of cardiovascular and renal diseases, renin-angiotensin system (RAS) plays a major role."

"These findings suggest that the RAS should be considered to have a central role in the pathogenesis of different cardiovascular diseases, for both therapeutic and preventive purposes, without having to measure its level of activation in each patient."

"The present document will discuss the most critical issues of the pathogenesis of different cardiovascular diseases with a specific focus on RAS blocking agents, including ACE inhibitors and ARBs, in the light of the most recent evidence supporting the use of these drugs in the clinical management of hypertension and hypertension-related cardiovascular diseases."

Introduction

"Pathological activation of tissue RAS in the heart is probably responsible for the initial stages of the hypertension-related heart disease, such as diastolic dysfunction, even in the absence of left ventricular (LV) hypertrophy, which is the first expression of hypertension-induced cardiac organ damage."

"It does, therefore, seem conceivable that hypertension activates tissue RAS, which first leads to the development of LV diastolic dysfunction and then triggers the progression to LV hypertrophy."

"The pathophysiological notions on the RAS have been improved by the results of large, randomized clinical trials, which contributed to better define the role of renin in the clinical practice as a mechanism of transducing both structural and functional damage abnormalities in the presence of vascular atherosclerosis and hypertension."

Hypertension, Heart Failure, and Ischaemic Heart Disease: A Cardiovascular Continuum

"Hypertension is the most relevant risk factor for the development of cardiovascular diseases, including ischemic heart disease and congestive heart failure, and it is usually associated with other cardiovascular risk factors [27]."

"This aspect of treatment is essential not only to obtain clinical response in hypertensive patients, but also to prevent the onset of overt cardiovascular diseases in patients who are asymptomatic."

"Hypertension is a major contributor for development and progression of coronary artery disease."

"Clinical manifestations of coronary artery disease are the result of obstruction of the epicardial arteries by atherosclerotic plaques, microvascular dysfunction and/or dysfunction due to a past myocardial infarct or ischaemic heart disease."

"The recommended treatments at the time of diagnosing coronary artery disease are beta-blockers, calcium-channel blockers and ACE inhibitors or ARBs [28, 29]."

"Coronary artery disease is responsible for over half the cases of heart failure [30]."

Treatment of Hypertension, Heart Failure and Ischaemic Heart Disease

"The main product generated by ACE, and also by alternative pathways, is angiotensin II, which regulates cardiovascular homeostasis by modulating its own effects through binding to specific receptors."

"From a clinical point of view, the most widely used classes of drugs act mainly at four levels: (1) inhibition of renin release (β-blockers, α_2-adrenergic stimulators); (2) inhibition of ACE, which converts angiotensin I into angiotensin II (ACE inhibitors); (3) antagonism of the AT1 receptors of angiotensin II (ARBs); (4) inhibition of renin (direct inhibitors of renin)."

"ACE inhibitors have antimitogenic effects in the heart by inhibiting the action of angiotensin II on cardiac AT1 receptors."

"Since angiotensin II is also implicated in the proliferation of mesangial cells and matrix production, ACE inhibitors have been shown to be effective in inhibiting the growth of these cells, thereby improving renal function and preventing the progression of microalbuminuria to overt proteinuria [31, 32]."

ACE Inhibitors and ARBs

"An all-inclusive meta-analysis involving more than 180 studies and 500,000 patients (31) showed that the ARBs were more effective than the other classes in reducing ischaemic stroke, probably because of the results of the Losartan Intervention For Endpoint reduction in hypertension study (LIFE) study [33], while the ACE inhibitors remain the drugs of first choice for the treatment of ischaemic heart disease and myocardial infarction."

"Both classes of drugs, including ACE inhibitors and ARBs, have been recently demonstrated to be effective in preventing the onset of microalbuminuria [34, 35], thus confirming the primary protective role of RAS blockade in patients with potential or overt kidney disease."

"Treatment with ACE inhibitors or ARBs has been found to be equally effective in reducing atrial fibrillation in patients with heart failure (ACE inhibitors OR: 0.64; 95% CI 19–50%; $p = 0.0003$; ARBs OR: 0.64; 95% CI 22–48%; $p < 0.0001$) [36]."

Appropriateness of the Use of RAS Inhibitors

"It is no longer justifiable to consider only antihypertensive treatment because less than 20% of patients have isolated hypertension, while more than 75% of the hypertensive population have at least one associated risk factor (on average 2 or 3)."

"The RAS inhibitors are used mainly for all states of hypertension associated with any form of heart disease, whether ischaemic or LV dysfunction of variable severity."

"The appropriateness of use of RAS inhibitors also depends on some management aspects, including the patient's preference (nowadays determinant for every drug), the need to ensure temporal stability of successful treatments, periodic estimates of the clinical result and subjective tolerability and the level of loyalty of the patient with regards to a specific product that has been demonstrated, in that case, to be effective."

Conclusions

"When choosing the most appropriate RAS inhibitor, it is essential to consider both the clinical characteristics of the patient and, in particular, the presence of co-morbid conditions, and the pharmacological characteristics of the different compounds with the aim of choosing the drug able to ensure the greatest short and long-term efficacy in terms of cardiovascular prevention."

"A key aspect of this strategy is to promote adherence to treatment which is a concrete aim that can be met easily with RAS inhibitors because of their very good tolerability, provided that the choice focuses on: (a) adequacy of the drug with respect to the patient, (b) intrinsic tolerability of the different compounds, and (c) continuity of effective therapeutic choices."

"The most important drugs that modulate the renin angiotensin system, ACE-inhibitors and ARBs, are effective in systemic hypertension, heart failure and ischaemic heart disease, as demonstrated by experimental findings and many clinical data."

Recent Research Advances in Renin-Angiotensin-Aldosterone System Receptors [37]

This is a machine-generated summary of:

Azushima, Kengo; Morisawa, Norihiko; Tamura, Kouichi; Nishiyama, Akira: Recent Research Advances in Renin-Angiotensin-Aldosterone System Receptors [37].

Published in: Current Hypertension Reports (2020).

Link to original: https://doi.org/10.1007/s11906-020-1028-6

If you want to cite the papers, please refer to the original.

For technical reasons we could not place the page where the original quote is coming from.

Abstract-Summary "Both systemically and locally produced angiotensin II (Ang II) bind to Ang II type 1 receptor (AT1R) and elicit strong biological functions."

"Recent studies have shown that Ang II–induced activation of Ang II type 2 receptor (AT2R) elicits the opposite functions to those of AT1R. However, accumulating evidence has now expanded the components of RAAS, including (pro)renin receptor, angiotensin-converting enzyme 2, angiotensin 1–7, and Mas receptor."

"The signal transductions of AT1R and AT2R are regulated by not only Ang II but also its receptor-associated proteins such as AT1R-associated protein and AT2R-interacting protein."

"Recent studies have indicated that inappropriate activation of local mineralocorticoid receptor contributes to cardiovascular and renal tissue injuries through aldosterone-dependent and -independent mechanisms."

Introduction

"Ang II exerts various physiological and pathophysiological actions such as vasoconstriction, sodium/water retention, inflammation, and fibrosis through activation of Ang II type 1 receptor (AT1R) signaling [38]."

"Ang II type 2 receptor (AT2R) is also a well-known receptor for Ang II, which exerts opposing effects to those of AT1R [39]."

"Accumulating evidence has now expanded the components of RAAS, including (pro)^renin receptor (PPR), ACE2, angiotensin 1–7 [Ang (1–7)], and Mas receptor (MasR), which has complicated our understanding of RAAS signaling pathways [40]."

"This review article focuses on recent research advances in RAAS with an emphasis on its receptor, such as PPR, AT1R, AT2R, MasR, and MR."

(Pro)renin Receptor

"A growing body of evidence has revealed additional roles of PRR, including RAAS-independent activation of mitogen-activated protein kinase kinase (MAPK), as well as its functions as an accessory protein of vacuolar type H^+-ATPase (V-ATPase) and a component of the Wnt/β-catenin signaling pathway [41]."

"PRR might also contribute to the noncanonical Wnt/β-catenin signaling pathway by acting as a planar cell polarity (PCP) core protein that plays an important role in embryonic development [42]."

"Recent studies have shown that PRR expression is significantly increased in many human cancers with an activated Wnt/β-catenin signaling pathway, such as colorectal cancer [43], pancreatic ductal adenocarcinoma (PDAC) [44, 45], glioma [46], breast carcinoma [47], colorectal cancer [48, 49], and aldosterone-producing adenoma [50]."

"These data suggest that PRR-dependent Wnt/β-catenin pathway signaling is a potential diagnostic and therapeutic target for cancer."

"We have developed a specific anti-PRR antibody that inhibits the Wnt/β-catenin signaling pathway, which significantly attenuates the progression of PDAC and colorectal cancer (data not shown)."

Angiotensin II Type 1 Receptor

"To stimulation of Ang II and GPCRs, activation of AT1R signaling has recently been reported to be regulated by other proteins that directly interact with AT1R. The C-terminal cytoplasmic domain of AT1R is an important structure that directly interacts with JAK2 and phospholipase Cγ1 (PLCγ1) to affect the downstream pathways of AT1R, indicating the functional significance of the C-terminal domain in AT1R signaling [51, 52]."

"When these mice are stimulated by Ang II, blood pressure elevation in renal dominant ATRAP-transgenic mice is significantly improved and Ang II–induced hypertension in systemic ATRAP-knockout mice is significantly exacerbated compared with their respective wildtype mice [53, 54]."

"During Ang II–dependent hypertension, ATRAP is likely to influence blood pressure by directly affecting activation of the renal tubular AT1R-ENaC pathway."

"Amiloride, an inhibitor of ENaC, significantly suppresses blood pressure in this transgenic mouse, indicating that ARAP1 influences blood pressure similarly to ATRAP via activating the renal tubular AT1R-ENaC pathway [55]."

Angiotensin II Type 2 Receptor

"Cardiac-specific AT2R-transgenic mice exhibit significant improvement of Ang II–induced perivascular fibrosis, although Ang II–induced myocyte hypertrophy was similar in transgenic and wildtype mice [56]."

"Cardiac-specific AT2R-transgenic mice without any interventions exhibit development of dilated cardiomyopathy and heart failure [57]."

"ATIP/ATBP, a family of at least four members (ATIP1–ATP4), has been reported to cooperate with AT2R to attenuate the transactivation of receptor tyrosine kinases, resulting in the inhibition of ERK2 activities, including DNA synthesis and attenuation of insulin receptor autophosphorylation, in the same manner as AT2R [58]."

"Although systemic ATIP-transgenic mice exhibit no significant difference in blood pressure compared with wildtype mice, these transgenic mice are significantly protected against cuff-induced vascular remodeling along with attenuation of superoxide anion production, proinflammatory cytokine expression, and ERK phosphorylation [59]."

"These findings suggest that ATIP is an agonistic factor of AT2R to exert opposing effects to AT1R, such as organ-protective and anti-inflammatory effects."

Mas Receptor

"Accumulating evidence suggests that Ang (1–7)/MasR signaling mediates the antagonistic effects of Ang II/AT1R signaling, such as vasodilation, and anti-hypertensive and anti-fibrosis effects, in various tissues including kidneys, heart, vasculature, and brain [40, 60]."

"The mechanism of these beneficial effects of Ang (1–7)/MasR signaling are mainly explained by the production of NO."

"Recent reports suggest that Ang (1–7) acts not only on MasR but also on AT2R as a new protective axis of RAAS [61]."

"The protective effect of Ang (1–7) is not blocked by a MasR antagonist but blocked by an AT2R antagonist."

"The beneficial effect of Ang (1–7) treatment in MasR-knockout mice depends on increased AT2R expression [62]."

"Further investigations are required to determine how Ang (1–7)/MasR and Ang (1–7)/AT2R signaling are related to each other and what physiological and pathophysiological effects they have."

Mineralocorticoid Receptor

"It has been considered that inappropriate systemic MR activation induces hypertension via the accumulation of body fluid and sodium [63]."

"Recent studies have indicated that inappropriate MR activation can also result in the development of cardiovascular/renal diseases [63]."

"The regulation of MR activity may be important to prevent not only hypertension but also cardiovascular/renal diseases."

"We have recently shown that glucocorticoid activates MR and induces renal injury that is suppressed by eplerenone, a selective MR antagonist, in high salt–fed adrenalectomized rats treated with hydrocortisone [64]."

"MR is abnormally activated by increased glucocorticoids by lifestyle-related diseases such as obesity, hyperglycemia, and inflammation [63, 65], which may be regulated by eplerenone."

"Rac1-dependent MR activation can lead to and/or worsen cardiovascular/renal diseases."

"Rac1 may mediate MR activation in the myocardium [66]."

Conclusions

"An overview and recent research advantages of RAAS receptors are summarized in this review."

"RAAS is one of the most potent regulators of cardiovascular and renal homeostasis and has been vigorously investigated to date."

"Accumulating evidence has expanded the components of RAAS and further revealed the complexity of this signal transduction system, including direct interactions with other receptors and proteins."

"Because the mechanisms of RAAS signal transduction still remain to be elucidated under physiological and pathophysiological conditions, further investigations are necessary to explore novel molecular mechanisms of the RAAS, which will provide alternative therapeutic agents other than existing RAAS blockers such as direct renin inhibitors, Ang II receptor blockers, ACE inhibitors, and MR antagonists."

Dysregulation of the Renin-Angiotensin System and the Vasopressinergic System Interactions in Cardiovascular Disorders [67]

This is a machine-generated summary of:

Szczepanska-Sadowska, Ewa; Czarzasta, Katarzyna; Cudnoch-Jedrzejewska, Agnieszka: Dysregulation of the Renin-Angiotensin System and the Vasopressinergic System Interactions in Cardiovascular Disorders [67].

Published in: Current Hypertension Reports (2018).

Link to original: https://doi.org/10.1007/s11906-018-0823-9

If you want to cite the papers, please refer to the original.

For technical reasons we could not place the page where the original quote is coming from.

Abstract-Summary "Ang II, acting on AT1 receptors (AT1R), plays a significant role in the release of AVP from vasopressinergic neurons and AVP, stimulating V1a receptors (V1aR), regulates the release of renin in the kidney."

"Ang II and AVP, acting on AT1R and V1aR, respectively, exert vasoconstriction, increase cardiac contractility, stimulate the sympathoadrenal system, and elevate blood pressure."

"The cooperative action of Ang II acting on AT1R and AVP stimulating both V1aR and V2 receptors in the kidney is necessary for the appropriate regulation of renal blood flow and the efficient resorption of sodium and water."

"We (1) point attention to the role of the cooperative action of Ang II and AVP for the regulation of blood pressure and the water-electrolyte balance under physiological conditions, (2) present the subcellular mechanisms underlying interactions of these two peptides, and (3) provide evidence that dysregulation of the cooperative action of Ang II and AVP significantly contributes to the development of disturbances in the regulation of blood pressure and the water-electrolyte balance in cardiovascular diseases."

Introduction

"Both Ang II and AVP directly participate in the regulation of the cardiovascular system."

"The main purpose of the present review is to draw attention to the interactions of Ang II and AVP in the regulation of the water-electrolyte balance and blood pressure in healthy individuals and in patients with cardiovascular diseases."

"We give a description of the regulation and function of the RAS and the VPS and we focus on the mechanisms underlying the interactions of Ang II and AVP in cardiovascular regulation and on disturbances of these interactions in cardiovascular diseases."

Renin-Angiotensin System

"In the cardiovascular system, activation of AT2R exerts opposite effects to those following stimulation of AT1R. After blockade of AT1R, administration of Ang II may result in hypotension, partly mediated by an increased production of BK, NO, and cGMP [68]."

"Ang-(1–7) inhibits the growth of cardiomyocytes and smooth muscle cells, reduces the activity of MAP kinase, inhibits the generation of ROS, reduces Ang II-induced stimulation of ERK1/2 and Rho kinases, causes the downregulation of AT1Rs, and attenuates the unfavorable structural and functional consequences of post-infarct heart failure and cerebral ischemia [69–73]."

"At the cellular level, the central pressor effect of Ang II is mediated by AT1R and is associated with activation of the Rho/Rho-kinase pathway, increased production of O^{*-}generated by NADPH oxidase, enhanced stimulation of P38 MAPK and ERK1/2, and decreased SK current in the PVN neurons projecting to the RVLM [74–76]."

Vasopressin

"The vasoconstrictory effect of AVP is mediated by V1aR. Vasopressin elicits contractile and growth-promoting effects in vascular smooth muscle cells, increases smooth muscle actin and SM22 promoter activities, and stimulates the JNK and p38 MAPK pathways [77]."

"Current evidence indicates that V1aR is the main type of AVP receptors in the adult heart although it appears that, in newborns, V2R are also present and may play an essential role in differentiation of the embryonic stem cells into contracting cells which display cardiac specific transcription factor GATA-4 and ventricle-specific myosin light chain [78]."

"There is significant evidence that centrally acting AVP may evoke both pressor and hypotensive responses [79–82] and that the final effect depends on the stimulation of specific groups of vasopressinergic fibers innervating special sets of cardiovascular neurons and activated by specific stimuli."

Significance of Central and Peripheral Interactions of the RAS and the VPS

"Application of Ang II to the immortalized neuroendocrine rat hypothalamic 4B cell line (the line expressing transcripts of AVP, AT1R, AT1bR, and TRPV4) significantly elevates the expression of TRPV4 and this effect can be abolished by the blockade of AT1R with losartan."

"Several studies have provided evidence that the central pressor action of Ang II can be abolished or significantly reduced by blockade of the brain V1aR and that the combined administration of Ang II and AVP exerts greater changes of blood pressure than those changes observed after the separate application of these peptides."

"Studies on a culture of the area postrema/NTS cells have shown that Ang II and AVP evoke a transient increase in $[Ca^{2+}]$ and that this effect can be abolished by pretreatment with specific antagonists of AT1R or V1R [83, 84]."

"It has been shown that Ang II acting on AT1R stimulates ventilation and increases the metabolic rate during hypercapnia and that this effect is reduced by the simultaneous stimulation of V1aR by vasopressin [85]."

Conclusions and Perspectives

"Precise cooperation of Ang II and AVP is necessary for the efficient regulation of blood pressure and body fluid volume."

"Under physiological conditions, cooperation of Ang II and AVP plays a significant role in the maintenance of cardiovascular homeostasis."

"Excessive stimulation of the RAS and the VPS may have prolonged negative consequences for the cardiovascular system, resulting from the formation of multiple positive feedbacks between renin, angiotensin II, vasopressin, and aldosterone."

"Dysregulation of the interactions between the RAS and vasopressin under pathological conditions may significantly contribute to the generation of disturbances in blood pressure regulation and the development of cardiovascular diseases."

Targeting the Renin–Angiotensin–Aldosterone System in Heart Failure [86]

This is a machine-generated summary of:

Lang, Chim C.; Struthers, Allan D.: Targeting the renin–angiotensin–aldosterone system in heart failure [86].

Published in: Nature Reviews Cardiology (2013).

Link to original: https://doi.org/10.1038/nrcardio.2012.196

If you want to cite the papers, please refer to the original.

For technical reasons we could not place the page where the original quote is coming from.

Abstract-Summary "The renin–angiotensin–aldosterone system (RAAS) is well established as a therapeutic target in patients with heart failure."

Introduction

"No treatment strategy currently exists for patients who have HF with preserved ejection fraction (HFpEF)."

"We believe that improved understanding of the underlying pathophysiology of HF can help to define novel therapeutic strategies."

"An appreciation of the role of the renin–angiotensin–aldosterone system (RAAS) in the pathophysiology of HF, the successful development of angiotensin-converting enzyme (ACE) inhibitors to block the RAAS, and the efficacy of these drugs in treating hypertension and HF illustrate the importance and success of this therapeutic strategy."

"In this Review, we discuss data that highlight the expanding use of existing agents—ACE inhibitors, angiotensin II-receptor blockers (ARBs), and mineralocorticoid-receptor antagonists (MRAs)—and review the evidence for novel pharmacological modulators of the RAAS (such as aliskiren, a direct renin inhibitor, and LCZ696, a combined ARB and neprilysin inhibitor) in patients with HF."

ACE Inhibitors: Novel Indications?

"These drugs have been shown to be effective in the treatment of hypertension, [87] and they reduce both mortality in all grades of HFrEF [88, 89] and left ventricular dysfunction after myocardial infarction."

"[90] Even in patients without known HF or left ventricular dysfunction, ACE inhibitors reduced the rate of death, myocardial infarction, or stroke in high-risk individuals in the HOPE study."

"[91] ACE inhibition has repeatedly been shown in studies to attenuate ventricular remodelling and improve ventricular function in patients with HF and after myocardial infarction."

"Various effects at the cellular level, including on apoptosis, fibrosis, and hypertrophy, have been proposed as potential mechanisms by which ACE inhibitors might inhibit the remodelling process."

"[92] The RAAS has been shown to modulate adverse left ventricular remodelling and myocardial fibrosis caused by increased load resulting from either aortic stenosis or aortic incompetence."

"Adverse left ventricular remodelling might also be induced by right ventricular pacing, and observational studies suggest a beneficial effect of ACE inhibitors in pacing-induced heart disease."

Angiotensin II-Receptor Blockers

"In the HEAAL study, [93] 150 mg daily of losartan significantly reduced the risk of death or hospitalization for HF compared with a dose of 50 mg daily in patients with HF who could not tolerate ACE inhibitors, which emphasizes the importance of incremental inhibition of the RAAS."

"In the CHARM-Added trial, [94] candesartan at a target dose of 32 mg once daily reduced both hospitalization for HF and cardiovascular mortality by 17% and

16%, respectively, compared with placebo in patients with HFrEF who were also treated with an ACE inhibitor."

"[95] Doubts exist regarding dual RAAS blockade with an ACE inhibitor and an ARB, but not with an ACE inhibitor and an MRA—the indication for the latter combination has now been broadened to include potentially all patients with HFrEF."

Mineralocorticoid-Receptor Antagonists

"[96, 97] The first study to show that aldosterone blockade in humans had beneficial cardiac effects when given in addition to ACE inhibitors in patients with HF was published in 1995."

"Trials of MRAs followed a similar pattern to those of ACE inhibitors, beginning in patients with severe HF and gradually progressing to individuals with milder disease."

"Three trials have reported positive results for the use of MRAs in patients with HF resulting from left ventricular systolic dysfunction, and no studies have reported contrary findings."

"Clear data exist that MRAs improve endothelial function in HF by increasing the level of endogenous nitric oxide, which might reduce the incidence of atherothrombotic events."

"In an observational study, Lund and colleagues analysed data from the Swedish Heart Failure registry and reported that the use of ACE inhibitors or ARBs in patients with HF with an ejection fraction >40% was associated with significantly reduced all-cause mortality."

Direct Renin Inhibition

"[98] In the ALOFT study, [99] 322 patients with HF who were receiving an ACE inhibitor and a β-blocker, and who had a plasma BNP level >100 pg/ml, were randomly allocated to 3 months treatment with either aliskiren (150 mg once daily) or placebo."

"[100] MRA status did not affect the efficacy of aliskiren 150 mg, added to standard HF therapy, to lower the levels of BNP, NT-proBNP, plasma renin activity, and urinary aldosterone."

"In ALTITUDE, [101, 102] either aliskiren 300 mg once daily or placebo was added to background ACE-inhibitor or ARB therapy in patients with diabetes and either increased urinary albumin excretion, or both a reduced estimated glomerular filtration rate (30–60 ml/min/1.73 m^2) and established cardiovascular disease."

"The incidence of a doubling of the serum creatinine level and the rate of end-stage renal disease were similar in the two groups, whereas the mean albuminuria level was 14% (95% CI 11–17%) lower in patients treated with aliskiren than with placebo."

Neprilysin and Vasopeptidase Inhibitors

"[103] Subsequently, in the OVERTURE study, [104] which involved 5770 patients with HF, enalapril 10 mg twice daily was compared with omapatrilat 40 mg once daily (mean duration of follow-up 14.5 months)."

"LCZ696 is also being studied in patients with HF."

"A total of 149 patients were randomly allocated to LCZ696 (up to 200 mg twice daily), and 152 patients to valsartan (up to 160 mg twice daily); 134 and 132 patients, respectively, were included in the primary 36-week analysis."

"Plasma NT-proBNP level, the primary end point, dropped by 23% (P = 0.005) over the first 12 weeks, but by only 15% (P = 0.20) after the full 36 weeks, among those receiving LCZ696 compared with valsartan."

"[105] PARADIGM-HF [106] is an ongoing efficacy and safety study of LCZ696 in which enalapril 10 mg twice daily will be compared with LCZ696 200 mg twice daily in patients with chronic HFrEF."

Conclusions

"The most-successful interventions have been ACE inhibitors and MRAs, both of which have consistently produced positive trial results."

"ARBs are an excellent substitute in patients who are intolerant of ACE inhibitors, but might have no other role in HF."

"The RAAS-modulating strategy recommended for patients with HF is a combination of ACE inhibitors and MRAs."

"[107] Whether direct renin inhibitors, combined ARB and neprilysin inhibitors, or both, will alter this recommendation remains to be seen."

The Evolution of Renin-Angiotensin Blockade: Angiotensin-Converting Enzyme Inhibitors as the Starting Point [108]

This is a machine-generated summary of:

Sica, Domenic A.: The Evolution of Renin-Angiotensin Blockade: Angiotensin-Converting Enzyme Inhibitors as the Starting Point [108].

Published in: Current Hypertension Reports (2010).

Link to original: https://doi.org/10.1007/s11906-010-0091-9

If you want to cite the papers, please refer to the original.

For technical reasons we could not place the page where the original quote is coming from.

Abstract-Summary "Several medication classes that block specific aspects of this system have emerged as useful therapies, including angiotensin-converting enzyme inhibitors, angiotensin receptor blockers, and, most recently, direct renin inhibitors."

"There has been scant evidence to favor angiotensin receptor blockers or direct renin inhibitors over angiotensin-converting enzyme inhibitors in treating hypertension or in affording end-organ protection; thus, angiotensin-converting enzyme inhibitors remain the standard of care when renin-angiotensin system blockade is warranted."

Introduction

"The renin-angiotensin system (RAS), however, has been observed to have an important influence on hypertension and end-organ disease and has served as an appealing target for pharmacologic intervention."

"This system can be effectively interrupted at different junctures by angiotensin-converting enzyme (ACE) inhibitors, angiotensin receptor blockers (ARBs), and direct renin inhibitors (DRIs)."

"ACE inhibitors were the first drugs to be used to interrupt the RAS, and 30 years after their introduction, they endure as valuable agents for hypertension management and end-organ protection [109]."

History of ACE Inhibitors

"Following the release of captopril, enalapril, and lisinopril in the early to mid-1980s, the ACE inhibitor field remained relatively quiescent from a developmental perspective until 1991, when four ACE inhibitors (fosinopril, quinapril, benazepril, and ramipril) were released within a span of several months."

"Although it can be speculated that other thiazide-type diuretics, such as chlorthalidone, were considered for combination with an ACE inhibitor, no such fixed-dose combination was ever developed."

"There was a somewhat variable time span for release of any particular fixed-dose ACE inhibitor/HCTZ product into the marketplace, relating to developmental issues as well as a company's perceived need to expand their product's market share."

"Some of the ACE inhibitors were also developed as fixed-dose products in combination with a calcium-channel blocker (CCB), such as enalapril/felodipine (Lexxel; AstraZeneca LP, Wilmington, DE), trandolapril/verapamil (Tarka; Abbott, Abbott Laboratories)."

Pharmacology of Angiotensin-Converting Enzyme Inhibitors

"The in vivo functional inhibition of tissue ACE with an ACE inhibitor corresponds to two properties of a compound: binding affinity and the free inhibitor concentration within a tissue compartment."

"When blood levels of an ACE inhibitor are high (typically in the first half of the dosing period), tissue retention of an ACE inhibitor is not a crucial determinant of functional ACE inhibition."

"During the second half of an ACE inhibitor dosing period, as blood levels drop, two factors appear to be important to prolonging functional ACE inhibition: 1) inhibitor binding affinity for ACE, and 2) tissue retention, which will have a direct impact on the free inhibitor concentration in tissues [110]."

"The positioning for tissue retention is quinaprilat > lisinopril > enalaprilat > captopril, and this ordering reflects both the binding affinity and lipophilicity of specific ACE inhibitors [110]."

Hypertension and ACE Inhibitors

"The enthusiasm for the use of ACE inhibitors is not a matter of effectiveness, because they have a pattern of efficacy comparable to (and no better than) most other drug classes, with response rates ranging from 40% to 70% in Stage I or II hypertension [111]."

"These differences, however, do not translate into different response rates if comparable doses of the individual ACE inhibitors are given."

"Typical confounding variables, which confuse the interpretation of the findings in BP studies with ACE inhibitors, have included differences in study design and methodology, as well as dose frequency and/or amount."

"In head-to-head BP trials comparing ACE inhibitors and either ARBs or DRIs, there is scant difference seen between the drug classes [112, 113]."

"The maximal BP-lowering response to an ACE inhibitor does not occur until several weeks after beginning therapy, which may relate to an incremental effect on BP owing to vascular remodeling [114]."

End-Organ Protection and ACE Inhibitors

"Evidence favors the use of ACE inhibitors and more recently ARBs (on a BP-independent basis) in the diabetic or at-risk cardiac/renal patient with either established atherosclerotic disease or proteinuric renal disease [115–117]."

"These beneficial effects have been observed with several ACE inhibitors, suggesting a class effect for the favorable cardiac outcome benefits with these compounds [115, 118, 119]."

"The Seventh Report of the Joint National Committee (JNC 7) endorses the use of ACE inhibitors in patients with hypertension and chronic kidney disease to both reduce BP and slow the rate of kidney disease progression [120]."

"The renoprotective features of ACE inhibitors should never substitute for tight BP control or other health care measures such as smoking cessation; both are important in managing the hypertensive patient with progressive chronic kidney disease."

Adverse Effects of ACE Inhibitors

"Both physiologic and nonphysiologic adverse effects can be the basis for ACE inhibitor intolerance, but what constitutes true ACE inhibitor intolerance is highly subjective."

"As of now, the available information is less than convincing that ARBs are better tolerated than ACE inhibitors relative to physiologic adverse effects [121]."

"Most ACE inhibitor adverse effects can be viewed as a class effect [122]."

"The concept of an intraclass switch to alleviate an adverse effect has been most commonly applied to the issue of ACE inhibitor-related cough [123, 124]."

"In most instances, a less than rigorous trial design proves to be the unmaking of a claim that one ACE inhibitor is superior to another for less frequent cough, so simply switching from one ACE inhibitor to another will not alleviate the adverse effect."

Conclusions

"If ACE inhibitors offer any particular benefit beyond BP reduction, the mechanism likely relates to positive effects on intermediate end points such as left ventricular hypertrophy, vascular structure, endothelial function, risk biomarkers (indirect), and/or improvement of the metabolic milieu by reducing the risk of new-onset diabetes."

"However, the impact of these drug classes on such intermediate end points is of limited relevance unless meaningful BP reduction has also taken place."

"If and when meaningful BP reduction occurs, intermediate end points are for the most part favorably impacted, and the drug class in use devolves into a secondary consideration."

The Combination of Beta-Blockers and ACE Inhibitors Across the Spectrum of Cardiovascular Diseases [125]

This is a machine-generated summary of:

Strauss, Martin H.; Hall, Alistair S.; Narkiewicz, Krzysztof: The Combination of Beta-Blockers and ACE Inhibitors Across the Spectrum of Cardiovascular Diseases [125].

Published in: Cardiovascular Drugs and Therapy (2021).

Link to original: https://doi.org/10.1007/s10557-021-07248-1

If you want to cite the papers, please refer to the original.

For technical reasons we could not place the page where the original quote is coming from.

Abstract-Summary "Goals are often not met because treatments are not optimized in terms of tailoring therapy to individual patients based on their hypertension subclass and cardiovascular risk profile and initiating early use of adapted-dose, single-pill combinations."

"Beta-blockers in combination with angiotensin-converting enzyme (ACE) inhibitors are of special interest as a result of their complementary actions on the sympathetic nervous system and renin–angiotensin–aldosterone system, two interlinked pathways that influence cardiovascular risk and disease outcomes."

"This paper examines the supporting evidence for beta-blockers and ACE inhibitors in each of the above indications and considers the rationale for combining these agents into a single pill, using data from bisoprolol and perindopril randomized controlled trials as supporting evidence."

"Combining these established antihypertensive agents into a single pill continues to provide effective blood pressure lowering and improved cardiovascular outcomes while allowing a greater proportion of patients to rapidly achieve treatment targets."

Introduction

"The gradual development of atherosclerotic lesions combined with other risk factors leads to the spectrum of cardiovascular diseases, including angina pectoris, myocardial infarction, chronic heart failure, and death."

"Intervention at any point along the continuum can modify CVD progression, but even with a range of evidence-based clinical guidelines and effective interventions, the majority of patients do not achieve sufficient risk factor control [126]."

"This includes a focus on how to optimize treatment by prescribing effective combinations as single pills and tailoring treatment to individual patients based on their cardiovascular risk profile and position in the CVD continuum."

"Two neurohormonal systems, the sympathetic nervous system (SNS) and renin–angiotensin–aldosterone system (RAAS), are intricately involved in the progression of disease throughout the CVD continuum."

Hypertension

"While all hypertension guidelines recommend an initial combination of an ACE inhibitor/ARB with either a CCB or diuretic, beta-blockers may form part of the combination at any stage of treatment when they are specifically indicated, i.e., when a second comorbidity (CAD, symptomatic angina, myocardial infarction, heart failure, atrial fibrillation) is present [127]."

"A meta-analysis of 12 trials found that beta-blocker use for the treatment of hypertension may be associated with an increased risk for new-onset type 2 diabetes, primarily in patients with the metabolic syndrome [128], and their use in these patients would therefore not be recommended unless the benefits outweighed the risks."

"Randomized controlled trials and meta-analyses have demonstrated that when compared with placebo, beta-blockers significantly reduce the risk of stroke, heart failure, and major cardiovascular events in hypertensive patients."

"A recent meta-analysis by Thomopoulos and others [129] concluded that beta-blockers exhibit a substantial risk-reducing ability for all events when prescribed to lower BP and therefore can be used as additional agents in patients with hypertension."

Coronary Artery Disease

"Over a mean follow-up of 4.2 years, the primary endpoint, a composite of cardiovascular death, myocardial infarction, or cardiac arrest, was observed in 8% of patients assigned to perindopril and 10% of patients assigned to placebo (relative risk reduction 20%; 95% CI 9–29%, P = 0.0003) [130]."

"In a further observational study also from Korea, registry data were extracted for 11,288 patients with non-ST-segment elevation myocardial infarction (NSTEMI) who underwent percutaneous coronary intervention with drug-eluting stents and 2-year major clinical outcomes were compared between patients receiving beta-blockers plus ACE inhibitors with those receiving beta-blockers plus ARBs [131]."

"In certain patients with recent myocardial infarction and those with chronic heart failure with reduced ejection fraction, beta-blockers have been associated with a significant reduction in mortality and/or cardiovascular events, but the protective benefit in patients with CAD without prior myocardial infarction or heart failure is less well established and lacks placebo-controlled trials."

Atrial Fibrillation

"Beta-blocker therapy was associated with lower all-cause mortality in AF patients with and without concomitant heart failure; the respective hazard ratios (HR) were 0.75 (95% confidence interval [CI], 0.71–0.79) and 0.73 (95% CI, 0.71–0.76)."

"Similar studies conducted in Asia have found evidence of a lower mortality with beta-blocker therapy in AF patients with concomitant heart failure [132, 133], although not always in patients without heart failure [133]."

"Analysis of a US National Health Insurance Service database in patients with concomitant AF and obstructive lung disease from 2002 to 2015 also revealed that rate control treatment with either cardio-selective or nonselective beta-blockers was associated with a lower risk of mortality (HR 0.84; 95% CI, 0.75–0.94; P = 0.002 and HR 0.85; 95% CI, 0.77–0.95; P = 0.003, respectively) compared with the use of CCBs [134]."

Heart Failure

"A beta-blocker is recommended in addition to an ACE inhibitor for symptomatic patients with HFrEF to reduce the risk of heart failure hospitalization and death [135]; a mineralocorticoid/aldosterone receptor antagonist may be added in those who remain symptomatic despite treatment with a beta-blocker and ACE inhibitor."

"In a recent update from the Heart Failure Association of the ESC, dapagliflozin or empagliflozin is recommended to reduce the risk of heart failure hospitalization and cardiovascular death in HFrEF patients already receiving guideline-directed medical therapy, regardless of the presence of type 2 diabetes [136]."

"The SENIORS (Study of the Effects of Nebivolol Intervention on Outcomes and Rehospitalisation in Seniors with Heart Failure) trial in elderly patients, differed from the above in that it also included patients with HFpEF as well as a primary endpoint that included hospitalization due to cardiovascular causes in addition to all-cause mortality."

Synergistic Neuroendocrine Blockade

"Evidence for the benefits of perindopril in combination with a beta-blocker come from the EUROPA trial, which randomized over 12,000 patients with stable CAD to perindopril or placebo and which included patients with angina or a previous myocardial infarction [130]."

"In these patients, the addition of perindopril to the beta-blocker produced a 24% reduction in relative risk of the combined primary endpoint (cardiovascular death, non-fatal myocardial infarction, and resuscitated cardiac arrest) compared with the beta-blocker/placebo group [137]."

"These data have been extended by a retrospective pooled analysis of patients with vascular disease from three large perindopril outcome trials (EUROPA,

ADVANCE, and PROGRESS) who received perindopril or placebo and were already on beta-blocker therapy."

"Among the 11,418 patients taking a beta-blocker, 5700 were randomized to a perindopril-based regimen and 5718 to placebo [138]."

Single-Pill Delivery of Bisoprolol and Perindopril

"Data supporting the benefits of bisoprolol/perindopril administered as a single-pill combination come from a study completed for 2394 patients, which examined whether heart rate and BP were improved when patients with CAD and hypertension who had previously received bisoprolol were prescribed the fixed-dose combination [139]."

"After 4 weeks of treatment, 84.9% of patients achieved a heart rate ≤70 bpm and 86.9% a BP ≤140/90 mmHg."

"The addition of the same single-pill combination to the treatment regimen of patients after revascularization for an acute coronary syndrome (a very high-risk population) also led to achievement of target BP and heart rate levels within 1 month of starting therapy and stabilization of these hemodynamic values and clinical symptoms by 3 months [140]."

Summary

"There is robust evidence on the benefits of beta-blocker and ACE inhibitor use in patients with hypertension and elevated heart rate, CAD, AF, and heart failure."

"In combination, these two classes provide a comprehensive neuroendocrine blockade targeting both the heart, where beta blockade reduces cardiac output, and the vessels, where ACE inhibition induces vasodilation among other actions."

"The available data suggest that combining these agents into a single pill would provide a valuable treatment option for a number of patient profiles allowing them to more rapidly achieve target heart rate and blood pressure levels at the same time as reducing cardiac events."

A Modern History RAAS Inhibition and Beta Blockade for Heart Failure to Underscore the Non-equivalency of ACEIs and ARBs [141]

This is a machine-generated summary of:

Hyman, Daniel A.; Siebert, Vincent R.; Birnbaum, Gilad D.; Alam, Mahboob; Birnbaum, Yochai: A Modern History RAAS Inhibition and Beta Blockade for Heart Failure to Underscore the Non-equivalency of ACEIs and ARBs [141].

Published in: Cardiovascular Drugs and Therapy (2020).
Link to original: https://doi.org/10.1007/s10557-020-06950-w

If you want to cite the papers, please refer to the original.

For technical reasons we could not place the page where the original quote is coming from.

Abstract-Summary "The seminal BB in HFrEF trials had high prevalence of ACEIs use as ACEIs for HF were standard of care by then, but ARBs as a class were still in their infancy."

"We closely examine the evidence for combinations of BB and ACEIs versus ARBs in HFrEF."

"We demonstrate the lack of evidence for consideration of ARBs to be interchangeable with ACEIs when used in combination with BB and provide evidence that calls in to question the validity of assuming benefits from each drug class are independently cumulative, widening the gap between ACEIs and ARBs when used with BBs."

"Modern guidelines should emphasize this lack of evidence for the combination use of ARB and BB in HFrEF, except for candesartan."

Introduction

"The 2016 European Society of Cardiology (ESC) Guidelines for the management of heart failure give a COR = 1, LOE = a recommendation for an "ACEI… in addition to BB for symptomatic patients with HFrEF" but only a COR = 1, LOE = B recommendation for "ARB…to reduce the risk of HF hospitalization and cardiovascular death in symptomatic patients unable to tolerate an ACEI."".

"The ESC gives a COR = 1 indication for ARB only for HFrEF patients unable to tolerate ACEIs, and gives a COR = II, LOE = B recommendation for the use of ARBs in patients with HF who are symptomatic despite treatment with a BB and unable to tolerate mineralocorticoid receptor antagonists (MRAs) [19]."

[Section 2]

"The 1995 ACC/AHA heart failure guidelines still described BBs in chronic HF as investigational [142, 143]."

"Two seminal trials of BBs in HF were released: the Cardiac Insufficiency Bisoprolol Study-II (CIBIS-II) study [144], the first trial to establish the mortality benefit of bisoprolol in HF, and the Metoprolol CR/XL Randomized Intervention Trial in Congestive Heart Failure (MERIT-HF) trial [145], which established the mortality benefit of metoprolol succinate in heart failure."

"By the 2001 update of the ACC/AHA heart failure guidelines, as well as the 2001 ESC chronic heart failure guidelines, BBs in conjunction with ACEIs were made to be standard of care in heart failure management [146, 147]."

"ACEIs' role in HF management was more immediately pursued and clearly demonstrated by the Cooperative North Scandinavian Enalapril Survival Study (CONSENSUS) [148] (1987) and Studies of Left Ventricular Dysfunction trial (SOLVD) [149] (1991) which were placebo-controlled trials showing significant reduction in HFrEF morbidity and mortality in patients treated with enalapril."

"ACEIs were already accepted as standard of care for HF when BBs and ARBs were being investigated for use in HF."

"Many of the participants in the studies investigating the use of BBs in HF were already on ACEIs."

Review of Evidence

"The 1997 Evaluation of Losartan in the Elderly (ELITE) trial randomized 722 ACEI naïve patients with HF to losartan versus captopril and showed a trend towards a reduction in the composite endpoint of death or HF admission in the ARB arm at 48 weeks (9.4% vs 13.2%, $p = 0.075$); however, this was not statistically significant."

"Among studies that did offer sub-group analysis, the first indication that concomitant BB usage may negate the equivalence of ACEIs and ARBs in HF came with the results of the Losartan Heart Failure Survival Study (ELITE II) (2000) which randomized 3152 HFrEF patients to losartan versus captopril."

"The valsartan group showed a treatment benefit for composite morbidity and mortality; however, subgroup analysis showed evidence of harm in the combined ACEI + ARB + BB ($n = 1610$) group with increased death and a trend towards increased combined morbidity and mortality endpoints."

ARNIs

"It is necessary to note that sacubitril-valsartan, the currently available ARNI, contains an ARB and not an ACEI for concern for unacceptably increased risk of angioedema with ACE inhibition as was seen with omapatrilat, an earlier abandoned agent with neprilysin inhibition properties [150]."

"The 2014 Prospective Comparison of ARNI with ACEI to Determine Impact on Global Mortality and Morbidity in Heart Failure (PARADIGM-HF) trial randomized 8442 HFrEF patients already on an ACEI/ARB and a BB to sacubitril-valsartan versus enalapril."

"A 2.3% absolute risk reduction of death was noted in the ARNI group (HR 0.84%, 95% CI 0.76 to 0.93) [151]."

Shortcomings and Future Steps

"It must be acknowledged that there are significant limitations in the body of evidence that has directly compared HF outcomes in patients on BB with either ACEI or ARB."

"While there is some signal for concurrent BB use attenuating the effect of ARB in HFrEF in post hoc subgroup analyses, subgroup analysis inherently bears increased risk of false-positive findings by virtue of statistical chance."

"For this specific question, at this point, it is unlikely that an RCT primarily comparing ACEI and ARB in HF will ever be performed and definitive evidence will likely remain elusive."

"Given the scant evidence of positive effect and limited evidence for the benefit of BB + ARBs combination in HFrEF, it is plausible that the addition of BB to ARB-containing ARNIs provides no net additional benefit, a significant clinical question heretofore unanswered."

Conclusion

"Current ACC/AHA HF treatment guidelines give both ACEIs and ARBs in conjunction with BBs COR = 1 and LOE = A recommendation status."

"There is not high-quality RCT data demonstrating the equivalence of ARBs to ACEIs when used in conjunction with BBs."

"Preference for ACEI over ARB is implied in recommendations for use of ARBs for ACEI intolerant patients; however, it is not explicit as compared to current ESC heart failure guidelines [19, 152]."

"One may be tempted to write off this subtle distinction as ARNIs as a class begins to demonstrate their potential over ACEIs or ARBs, but for patients who are ARNI intolerant, this distinction remains important."

"For those patients who are on ARBs instead of ACEIs, providers should remain vigilant that an ACEI contraindication or intolerance truly exists."

Impact of Renin–Angiotensin–Aldosterone-System Inhibitor Drugs on Mortality in Patients with Atrial Fibrillation and Hypertension [153]

This is a machine-generated summary of:

Xu, Wei; Yang, Yan-min; Zhu, Jun; Wu, Shuang; Wang, Juan; Zhang, Han; Shao, Xing-hui: Impact of renin–angiotensin–aldosterone-system inhibitor drugs on mortality in patients with atrial fibrillation and hypertension [153].

Published in: BMC Cardiovascular Disorders (2022).

Link to original: https://doi.org/10.1186/s12872-022-02580-2

If you want to cite the papers, please refer to the original.

For technical reasons we could not place the page where the original quote is coming from.

Abstract-Summary "This study aimed to examine the relationship between treatment with ACEIs or ARBs and mortality in emergency department (ED) patients with AF and hypertension."

"Patients were grouped according to whether they were treated with ACEI/ARB or not and completed a 1-year follow-up to evaluate outcomes including all-cause death, cardiovascular death, stroke, and major adverse events (MAEs)."

"Among the 1110 patients with AF and hypertension, 574 (51.7%) received ACEI/ARB treatment."

"According to the multivariate Cox regression analysis, ACEI/ARB therapy was significantly associated with a reduced risk of all-cause death (HR, 0.605; 95% CI 0.431–0.849; P=0.004)."

"ACEI/ARB therapy was independently associated with a reduced risk of cardiovascular death (HR 0.585; 95% CI 0.372–0.921; P=0.020) and MAEs (HR 0.651, 95% CI 0.496–0.855, P=0.002) after adjusting for other risk factors."

"Our results revealed that ACEI/ARB therapy was independently associated with a reduced risk of all-cause death, cardiovascular death, and MAEs in ED patients with AF and hypertension."

Introduction

"The development of AF is characterized by electrical modifications and atrial structural remodeling [154–156]."

"Various animal model studies of AF reiterated that the activation of the renin–angiotensin–aldosterone system (RAAS) leads to fibrosis and myocardial structural remodeling and demonstrated the cardioprotective effects of angiotensin-converting enzyme inhibitors (ACEIs) or angiotensin receptor blockers (ARBs) and anti-inflammatory drugs with antioxidant properties [157, 158]."

"The impact of ACEI/ARB on the mortality of patients with AF remains unclear."

"We performed a study on patients with AF and hypertension with the objective of examining the impact of ACEI/ARB therapy on the mortality of these patients."

Methods

"1110 patients with AF and hypertension were included in the final analysis, who were categorized into two groups based on whether they received ACEI/ARB therapy or not."

"Data of comorbidities were collected at admission regarding history of myocardial infarction, coronary artery disease (CAD), congenital heart disease, diabetes mellitus, heart failure, rheumatic heart disease, left ventricular hypertrophy (LVH), stroke or transient ischemic attack (TIA), sleep apnea, smoking, left ventricular ejection fraction (LVEF) <40%, dementia, hyperthyroidism, chronic obstructive pulmonary disease (COPD), valvular heart disease, and prior major bleeding and the diagnoses were based on physicians' clinical medical records."

"Risk factors adjusted in the multivariable Cox regression models included age, body mass index (BMI), heart rate, heart failure, rheumatic heart disease, significant valvular disease, stroke or transient ischemic attack histories, dementia, COPD, diuretics, warfarin, and $CHADS_2$ score ≥2."

Results

"Patients in the ACEI/ARB group tended to have higher BMI but lower heart rates (all $P < 0.05$) than patients without ACEI/ARB therapy."

"Patients receiving ACEI/ARB therapy were more likely to have myocardial infarction, CAD, and heart failure (all $P < 0.05$)."

"The ACEI/ARB therapy group had a higher percentage of patients with a LVEF <40% and a $CHADS_2$ score ≥ 2 (all $P < 0.05$)."

"Patients receiving ACEI/ARB therapy had a lower incidence of MAEs (19.5% vs. 24.8%, $P = 0.005$) than those not receiving ACEIs/ARBs."

"Cardiovascular death and stroke rates were lower in patients who received ACEI/ARB therapy, but the difference between both groups was not significant."

"The risk of non-cardiovascular death in patients receiving ACEI/ARB therapy was significantly lower than that in the non-ACEI/ARB group ($P = 0.003$)."

Discussion

"The results of this cohort study showed that ED patients with AF and hypertension who received ACEI/ARB therapy had a lower incidence of all-cause death (12.5% vs. 18.1%, P = 0.010) and MAEs (19.5% vs. 24.8%, P = 0.005) than patients who did not receive ACEI/ARBs."

"Similar to the results of the LIFE study, our findings suggested that ACEI/ARB therapy was independently associated with a reduced risk of cardiovascular mortality and MAEs in AF, not limited to LVH."

"In a registry study by Fernandez and others, which included 9365 AF patients aged ≥75 years, ACEI/ARB therapy did not reduce the rates of all-cause deaths and cardiovascular events [159]."

"According to an observational study in patients with hypertension and COVID-19, ACEI/ARB therapy was associated with a lower risk of mortality [160]."

Conclusion

"Our main finding was that ACEI/ARB therapy was associated with a reduced risk of all-cause mortality, cardiovascular mortality, and MAEs in ED patients with AF and hypertension."

"These findings indicate that, in addition to blood pressure control therapy, preventing the activation of the RAAS system might improve prognosis in patients with AF and hypertension."

"These results provide evidence for a tertiary preventive treatment for patients with atrial fibrillation and hypertension."

Effect of Renin Angiotensin Blockers on Angiotensin Converting Enzyme 2 Level in Cardiovascular Patients [161]

This is a machine-generated summary of:

Farid fahmy, Sarah; El Derany, Marwa Omar; Khorshid, Hazem; Saleh, Ayman; El-Demerdash, Ebtehal: Effect of renin angiotensin blockers on angiotensin converting enzyme 2 level in cardiovascular patients [161].

Published in: BMC Pharmacology and Toxicology (2023).

Link to original: https://doi.org/10.1186/s40360-023-00667-w

If you want to cite the papers, please refer to the original.

For technical reasons we could not place the page where the original quote is coming from.

Abstract-Summary "This study aimed to clarify the effect of ACE inhibitors (ACEIs) and angiotensin-receptor blockers (ARBs) on ACE2 and to assess the correlation between ACE2 and several anthropometric and clinic-pathological factors."

"Assessment of serum ACE2 level in different groups showed a significant difference between ACEIs and healthy groups and ACEIs and ARBs group, while there was no difference between ARBs and healthy."

"Multivariate analysis using ACE2 level as constant and age, female sex, ACEIs use and myocardial infarction (MI) showed that there was a significant effect of female sex and ACEIs use on ACE2 level with no effect of age, MI and diabetes."

"It tends to be lower in ACEIs group and there is a strong positive association between ACE2 level and the female sex."

"This needs to be considered in Future studies to further understand the relationship between gender, sex hormones and ACE2 level."

Introduction

"Blockage of renin–angiotensin–aldosterone system (RAAS) by either angiotensin-converting enzyme inhibitors (ACEIs) or angiotensin-receptor blockers (ARBs) is considered the first-choice of drugs for treatment of hypertension, heart failure and chronic kidney diseases [162]."

"The effect of chronic use of RAAS blockers, as in case of treatment of cardiovascular diseases, on the expression of ACE2 is still not well characterized."

"Given the RAAS importance to cardiovascular and kidney physiology, and the association between chronic diseases and COVID-19, could shed light on potential relationships between ACE inhibitor and ARB use and COVID-19 [163], this study aimed to clarify the effect of RAAS blockers on ACE2 and to assess the association between the chronic use of either ACEIs or ARBs on ACE2 level in clinical samples from patients with chronic cardiovascular diseases compared to healthy individuals."

Subjects and Methods

"This prospective case control study included a total of 100 subjects (57 men and 43 women) over a period of 8 months (from June 2021 to February 2022) recruited from Cardiology Department Rehabilitation clinic, Ain Shams University Hospital (ASUH), Cairo, Egypt."

"Only Sixty subjects were being diagnosed with chronic cardiovascular diseases and being treated with either ACEI or ARBs were included in study."

"Laboratory measurement of CBC, liver and kidney function tests were done for all subjects."

"Sample size of 50 participants (25 in Group1 of cardiovascular patients ACEI, 25 patients taking ARBs) and 25 healthy volunteers achieve 100% power to detect a difference of 19.1 between null hypothesis and alternative hypothesis and significance of alpha 0.05 using two sided t test."

"Comparison between 3 groups was done using either analysis of variance (ANOVA) for normally distributed quantitative variables or Kruskal–Wallis test (non-parametric ANOVA) then post-Hoc test" was used for pair-wise comparison based on Kruskal–Wallis distribution."

Results

"Assessment of ACE2 level in different groups showed a significant difference between ACEIs and healthy groups ($p = 0.006$) and ACEIs and ARBs group ($p = 0.001$) using post hoc analysis."

"Concerning the age, there were no differences in ACE2 level between patients in ACEIs or ARBs groups less than 55 years or older age >55 years of age ($p = 0.099$)."

"There was no significant difference regarding ACE2 levels between diabetic and non-diabetic patients ($p = 0.687$) or between hypertensive and non-hypertensive patients ($p = 0.121$)."

"Patients with myocardial infarction showed significant lower ACE2 levels compared to the other patients ($p = 0.002$)."

"Due to the significant effect of sex on ACE2 level ($p < 0.001$) as well as myocardial infarction ($p = 0.002$), multivariate analysis was done using ACE2 level as constant and age, female sex, ACEIs use and MI as variables."

Discussion

"We investigated the serum ACE2 levels in established cardiovascular patients treated with either ACEIs or ARBS and compared them with healthy individuals."

"In an European heart failure study, it was found that the use of neither ACEIs nor ARBs was associated with higher ACE2 levels [164]."

"To further explore the possible association between ACE2 level upon treatment with ACEIs or ARBs and the clinical factors that may play role in COVID severity, we studied the correlation between ACE2 and several clinical factors including age, BMI, sex and diseases such as diabetes, MI, HTN and HF."

"Our results are in contrast to the study of Chirinos and others (2020) who reported an association between lower ACE2 level and older age (above 50 years), male sex and diabetes [165], however, they did not detect any significant difference between the effect of ACEIs and ARBs on the ACE2 level."

Conclusion

"It tends to be lower in ACEIs group and there is a strong positive association between ACE2 level and the female sex."

"This needs to be considered in future studies to further understand the relationship between gender, sex hormones and ACE2 level."

"More studies are needed to examine the implications of these differences in cohorts with ACE2 levels and COVID-19 outcomes."

"More detailed characterization of the different components of RAAS signaling is needed with a focus on absolute quantitative assessment in larger cohort toward establishing normative values, and assessment of their longitudinal changes."

Real-World Use of ACEI/ARB in Diabetic Hypertensive Patients before the Initial Diagnosis of Obstructive Coronary Artery Disease: Patient Characteristics and Long-Term Follow-Up Outcome [166]

This is a machine-generated summary of:

Zhang, Yue; Ding, Xiaosong; Hua, Bing; Liu, Qingbo; Chen, Hui; Zhao, Xue-Qiao; Li, Weiping; Li, Hongwei: Real-world use of ACEI/ARB in diabetic hypertensive patients before the initial diagnosis of obstructive coronary artery disease: patient characteristics and long-term follow-up outcome [166].

Published in: Journal of Translational Medicine (2020).

Link to original: https://doi.org/10.1186/s12967-020-02314-y

If you want to cite the papers, please refer to the original.

For technical reasons we could not place the page where the original quote is coming from.

Abstract-Summary "Current guidelines recommend angiotensin-converting-enzyme inhibitors (ACEI)/angiotensin receptor blockers (ARB) as a first-line therapy in diabetic hypertensive patients and for secondary prevention in patients with obstructive coronary artery disease (OCAD)."

"The effects of using ACEI/ARB before the initial diagnosis of OCAD on major adverse cardiac and cerebral event (MACCE) in diabetic hypertensive patients remain unclear."

"This study investigated whether using ACEI/ARB before the initial diagnosis of OCAD could be associated with improved clinical outcomes in diabetic hypertensive patients."

"Of the 2501 patients, 1300 did not used ACEI/ARB before the initial diagnosis of OCAD [the ACEI/ARB(−) group]; 1201 did [the ACEI/ARB(+) group]."

"Compared with the ACEI/ARB(−) group, the ACEI/ARB(+) group had significantly lower incidence of AMI (22.5% vs. 28.4%, $p < 0.05$), smaller infarct size in patients with AMI (pTNI: 5.7 vs. 6.8 ng/ml, $p < 0.05$; pCKMB: 21.7 vs. 28.7 ng/ml, $p < 0.05$), better heart function (LVEF: 60.0 vs. 58.5%, $p < 0.05$), and lower incidences of non-fatal stroke (2.4% vs. 4.6%, $p < 0.05$) and composite MACCE (23.1% vs. 29.7%, $p < 0.05$)."

"In diabetic hypertensive patients, treatment with ACEI/ARB before the initial diagnosis with OCAD was associated with decreased incidence of AMI, smaller infarct size, improved heart function, and lower incidences of non-fatal stroke and composite MACCE."

Background

"The current guidelines recommend ACEI/ARB as a first-line therapy for diabetic hypertensive patients [167–169] and for secondary prevention in patients with OCAD [170, 171]."

"It has been generally accepted that diabetic hypertensive patients can benefit from ACEI/ARB; however, previous studies have found the ACEI/ARB is underutilized in these patients [172–174]."

"The real-world use of ACEI/ARB in diabetic hypertensive patients in China remains unclear."

"Whether starting ACEI/ARB therapy before the initial diagnosis of OCAD could improve patient outcomes is still unknown."

"We used the Cardiovascular Center Beijing Friendship Hospital Database Bank to evaluate the effectiveness of ACEI/ARB therapy on improving major adverse cardiac and cerebral event (MACCE) outcomes in diabetic hypertensive patients."

Methods

"2501 patients were included in this analysis."

"Patients' demographics, medical and medication history, laboratory test results, echocardiographic and angiographic evaluation results, and clinical outcomes during the hospitalization after the initial diagnosis of OCAD were collected and verified using an electronic medical recording system."

"MACCE included all-cause death, non-fatal myocardial infarction (MI), non-fatal stroke, revascularization, and cardiac rehospitalization (admission because of angina or heart failure)."

"Non-fatal stroke, including ischemic and hemorrhagic stroke, was defined as cerebral dysfunction caused by cerebral vascular obstruction or sudden rupture and was diagnosed based on signs of neurological dysfunction or evidence of brain imaging."

"Baseline variables that were significantly correlated with outcomes by univariate analysis and clinically relevant were used in the multivariate model."

"The included variables for the COX regression were carefully chosen, given the number of events available, to ensure parsimony of the final model."

"1050 ACEI/ARB(+) patients were individually 1:1 matched to 1050 ACEI/ARB(−) controls using nearest available score matching."

Results

"Comparing with the ACEI/ARB (+) group, the ACEI/ARB (−) group showed significantly higher percent of male, lower BMI, higher heart rate, lower percent of dyslipidemia, and significantly less likely to receive antiplatelet therapy, beta-blocker or statins before the hospital admission for OCAD."

"The ACEI/ARB(−) group had significantly higher hsCRP levels than the ACEI/ARB(+) group."

"The ACEI/ARB(−) group had significantly higher incidence of non-fatal stroke than the ACEI/ARB(+) group (Before propensity score matching: 1.6% vs. 0.7%, $p < 0.05$; After propensity score matching:1.7% vs. 0.8%, $p < 0.05$)."

"Non-fatal stroke occurred in 4.0% of the patients in the ACEI/ARB (−) group and 2.4% in the ACEI/ARB (+) group (HR = 1.62, 95%CI 1.03, 2.56, $p < 0.05$)."

Discussion

"The current study was the first to investigate whether ACEI/ARB used before the initial diagnosis of OCAD in diabetic hypertensive patients could be associated with improved clinical outcomes."

"We found that use of ACEI/ARB before the initial diagnosis of OCAD was associated with reduced incidence of AMI, reduced myocardial infarction size, and improved cardiac function, whereas we found no significant correlation between the prior ACEI/ARB therapy and mortality."

"We found that compared with diabetic hypertensive patients who did not use ACEI/ARB before the initial diagnosis of OCAD, those who did had significantly lower incidence of OCAD-associated AMI at the hospital admission and lower incidences of non-fatal stroke and composite MACCE during follow-up."

"The current study found that 52.0% (1300/2501) of patients with diabetic hypertension and diagnosed with OCAD for the first time did not use ACEI/ARB therapy."

Limitations

"This is a single-center study although including a large sample size; thus, generalization of the findings should be cautious."

"This is a retrospective observational study."

"The information on the dosage and duration of ACEI/ARB was limited."

"Prospective cohort studies are required to confirm our findings."

Conclusions

"Use of ACEI/ARB therapy for diabetic hypertensive patients before the initial diagnosis of OCAD was significantly associated with lower incidence of AMI, improved heart function, smaller infarct size, and lower incidences of non-fatal stroke and composite MACCE."

"No prior ACEI/ARB therapy was significantly and independently associated with non-fatal stroke and composite MACCE."

"ACEI/ARB therapy was largely underutilized in diabetic hypertensive patients."

Comparative Efficacy of Angiotensin Converting Enzyme Inhibitors and Angiotensin Receptor Blockers After Coronary Artery Bypass Grafting [175]

This is a machine-generated summary of:

Kim, Jeayoun; Park, Jungchan; Lee, Jong-Hwan; Min, Jeong Jin; Lee, Seung-Hwa; Lee, Young Tak; Kim, Wook Sung; Song, Sanghoon; Yeo, Jung Hyun; Cho, Hyojin: Comparative Efficacy of Angiotensin Converting Enzyme Inhibitors and Angiotensin Receptor Blockers after Coronary Artery Bypass Grafting [175].

Published in: Scientific Reports (2020).

Link to original: https://doi.org/10.1038/s41598-020-58705-0

If you want to cite the papers, please refer to the original.

For technical reasons we could not place the page where the original quote is coming from.

Abstract-Summary "Although angiotensin receptor blockers (ARBs) are considered as an alternative for those with angiotensin converting enzyme inhibitors (ACEi) intolerance, the comparative effectiveness of ARBs and ACEi remains controversial in patients who underwent coronary artery bypass grafting (CABG)."

"We aimed to compare the clinical effects of the two types of renin-angiotensin-aldosterone system (RAAS) inhibitors in patients who underwent CABG."

"ARBs may have comparable protective effects to ACEi and be a reasonable alternative for intolerant patients after CABG."

"The beneficial effects of ARBs depending on follow-up period require further investigation."

Introduction

"There is still a debate on the comparative effects of the two discrete types of RAAS inhibitors (angiotensin converting enzyme inhibitors [ACEi] and angiotensin receptor blockers [ARBs])."

"The effects of the two types of RAAS inhibitors have also not been compared in CABG patients."

"In this study, we aimed to compare the effects of RAAS inhibitors by comparing clinical outcomes after CABG in patients prescribed postoperative ACEi or ARB therapy."

"Our findings might help select the type of RAAS inhibitors in secondary prevention after CABG."

Results

"After excluding patients without a prescription of RAAS inhibitors (N = 4,158) or with concomitant prescription of RAAS inhibitors (N = 23), a total of 1,198 patients were finally left for analysis and were classified into the two groups (ACEi group [N = 900, 75.2%] and ARB group [N = 298, 24.8%])."

"During the first year after CABG, discontinuations of RAAS inhibitors were found in 4 (1.3%) patients of the ARB group and 11 patients (1.2%) of the ACEi group."

"Changes to another type of RAAS inhibitors were found in 2 (0.7%) patients in the ARB group to ACEi and 101 (11.2%) patients in the ACEi group to ARB."

"The median follow-up durations were 61.7 months (interquartile range: 8–107.9) in the ACEi group and 45.3 months (interquartile range: 8.6–86.2) in the ARB group (p = 0.66)."

Discussion

"The main findings of the present study were as follows: (1) postoperative use of ARB after CABG showed a comparable clinical effect to ACEi during median follow-up period of 48 months; (2) the use of ARBs resulted in a significant reduction in adverse events in terms of MACCE during 12 months of follow-up; (3) ARBs showed improved clinical outcomes limited to female patients."

"These findings suggest that in patients who underwent CABG, the effects of the two discrete types of RAAS inhibitors may be comparable, but can differ according to follow-up period or in particular subgroups."

"Postoperative use of ARBs did not result in a different clinical outcome in patients who had undergone CABG relative to those prescribed ACEi during a median follow-up period of 48 months."

Conclusions

"In CABG patients, ARBs may have comparable protective effects to ACEi and be a reasonable alternative for intolerant patients."

"The beneficial effects of ARBs depending on sex and follow-up period require further investigation."

Methods

"We used Clinical Data Warehouse Darwin-C, which is an electric system designed to search for and collect data from electronic medical record systems, to extract all adult CABG patients and their prescriptions at discharge."

"Baseline characteristics were extracted automatically from electronic medical records with the aid of the institutional medical information department and were organized using a standardized form and protocol by a single investigator who was blinded to the prescription at discharge."

"In the propensity-matched population, we compared continuous variables with a paired t-test and categorical variables with a stratified chi-square test."

"We compared HRs for outcomes using univariate Cox's proportion hazard regression models in the matched population with or without Firth's penalized likelihood approach."

"To intention-to-treat analysis, we performed analyses in the population after excluding patients with changes of RAAS inhibitor use during the 12 months after CABG."

Correlation Between Kidney Sodium and Potassium Handling and the Renin-Angiotensin-Aldosterone System in Children with Hypertensive Disorders [176]

This is a machine-generated summary of:

Perrin, Ella C; South, Andrew M: Correlation between kidney sodium and potassium handling and the renin-angiotensin-aldosterone system in children with hypertensive disorders [176].

Published in: Pediatric Nephrology (2021).

Link to original: https://doi.org/10.1007/s00467-021-05204-7

If you want to cite the papers, please refer to the original.

For technical reasons we could not place the page where the original quote is coming from.

Abstract-Summary "Urine sodium and potassium are used as surrogate markers for dietary consumption in adults with hypertension, but their role in youth with hypertension and their association with components of the renin-angiotensin-aldosterone system (RAAS) are incompletely characterized."

"Our objective was to investigate if plasma renin activity and serum aldosterone are associated with urine sodium and potassium in youth referred for hypertensive disorders."

"We recorded urine sodium and potassium concentrations normalized to urine creatinine, plasma renin activity, and serum aldosterone and calculated the sodium/potassium (UNaK) and aldosterone/renin ratios."

"We used multivariable generalized linear models to estimate the associations of renin and aldosterone with urine sodium and potassium."

"Aldosterone was associated inversely with urine sodium/creatinine (β: −0.34, 95% CI −0.62 to −0.06) and UNaK (β: −0.09, 95% CI −0.16 to −0.03), and adjusted for estimated glomerular filtration rate and serum potassium."

"Higher serum aldosterone levels, but not plasma renin activity, were associated with lower urine sodium/creatinine and UNaK at baseline in youth referred for hypertensive disorders."

Introduction

"Urinary sodium and potassium concentrations, and in particular the urine sodium/potassium ratio (UNaK), are considered proxy measures for dietary consumption of sodium relative to potassium; high UNaK has been associated with hypertension and with lower renin-angiotensin-aldosterone system (RAAS) activity in adults [177–180]."

"Evidence suggests that inadequate RAAS suppression in response to high dietary sodium intake may be an important mechanism in hypertension, as the RAAS plays a major role in regulating blood pressure via enhancing sodium retention and subsequently increasing water absorption in the kidneys [181, 182]."

"Further, circulating measurements of RAAS components such as plasma renin activity (PRA) and aldosterone are measured commonly in clinical practice and have been used in adults to define hypertension mechanisms [183]."

"The purpose of this study was to examine the relationship of renin and aldosterone with urine sodium and potassium at baseline in youth referred for hypertensive disorders, with the goal to improve our understanding of the different phenotypes of pediatric hypertension and help guide lifestyle and pharmacological management."

Methods

"We recorded demographic and clinical data from the index date, including self-reported sex, race, ethnicity, insurance status, age, height, weight, hypertensive disorder etiology (primary vs. secondary), and presence and class of antihypertensive medication prescriptions at the time of laboratory sample collection (i.e., whether the participant was already taking an antihypertensive medication at the index date)."

"The final adjustment sets for each model by RAAS component were as follows: (1) PRA: Adjusted for age, sex, body mass index z-score, hypertensive disorder etiology, prescribed antihypertensive medication at the time of blood collection, and PRA laboratory; the urine sodium/creatinine and potassium/creatinine models were adjusted additionally for diastolic blood pressure while the UNaK model was adjusted additionally for systolic blood pressure due to better fit by Akaike information criterion. (2) Aldosterone: Adjusted for estimated glomerular filtration rate and serum potassium. (3) ARR: Adjusted for age, sex, body mass index z-score, hypertensive disorder etiology, prescribed antihypertensive medication at the time of blood collection, and serum potassium; the urine sodium/creatinine and potassium/creatinine models were adjusted additionally for diastolic blood pressure while the UNaK model was adjusted additionally for systolic pressure due to better fit by Akaike information criterion."

Results

"Adjustment for estimated glomerular filtration rate and serum potassium confirmed that a 1-ng/dl higher aldosterone value was associated with lower urine sodium/creatinine (β: −0.34, 95% CI −0.62 to −0.06) and lower UNaK (β: −0.09, 95% CI −0.16 to −0.03)."

"In our sensitivity analyses, we observed that the estimates and 95% CI did not change appreciably when we added hypertensive disorder etiology to the multivariable aldosterone models (urine sodium/creatinine β: −0.35, 95% CI −0.63 to −0.07; UNaK β: −0.09, 95% CI −0.16 to −0.03)."

"The estimates and 95% CI were similar when restricting the multivariable aldosterone model analyses to those participants who had primary etiology ($n = 40$; urine sodium/creatinine β: −0.37, 95% CI −0.67 to −0.07; UNaK β: −0.09, 95% CI −0.16 to −0.02)."

Discussion

"Of youth referred to a Hypertension Clinic for evaluation of hypertensive disorders, we found that higher levels of serum aldosterone at baseline, but not PRA, were associated with lower levels of urine sodium/creatinine and UNaK. Our finding is consistent with the primary role of aldosterone in stimulating renal sodium reabsorption in the collecting ducts to increase circulating volume."

"We did not observe an association between PRA with urine sodium and potassium excretion, which suggests that youth with hypertensive disorders may lack the expected PRA suppression due to high dietary sodium intake."

"Ongoing prospective studies are investigating the associations among formal assessments of dietary sodium intake, both pathways of the RAAS (including angiotensin peptides), renal sodium handling, blood pressure, and target organ damage in youth and young adults with hypertension and those at risk for hypertension [184, 185]."

Should ACE Inhibitors and ARBs be Used in Combination in Children? [186]

This is a machine-generated summary of:

Stotter, Brian R.; Ferguson, Michael A.: Should ACE inhibitors and ARBs be used in combination in children? [186].

Published in: Pediatric Nephrology (2018).

Link to original: https://doi.org/10.1007/s00467-018-4046-8

If you want to cite the papers, please refer to the original.

For technical reasons we could not place the page where the original quote is coming from.

Abstract-Summary "As our understanding of RAAS physiology and the feedback mechanisms of ACE inhibition and angiotensin receptor blockade have improved, questions have been raised as to whether combination ACEI/ARB therapy is warranted in certain patients with incomplete angiotensin blockade on one agent."

"We discuss the rationale for combination ACEI/ARB therapy and summarize the results of key adult studies and the limited pediatric literature that have investigated this therapeutic approach."

"We additionally review novel therapies that have been developed over the past decade as alternative approaches to combination ACEI/ARB therapy, or that may be potentially used in combination with ACEIs or ARBs, in which further adult and pediatric studies are needed."

Introduction

"It was later determined that these extracts could inhibit the conversion of Ang I to Ang II [187], which guided the search for specific pharmacologic inhibitors of RAAS, particularly for hypertension in chronic kidney disease (CKD)."

"Based on the European Union Paediatric Regulation, the Paediatric Committee (PDCO) at the European Medicines Agency (EMA) is tasked with identifying the needs for research of medications for use in children, including ACEIs and ARBs, for CKD, hypertension, and proteinuria [188]."

"Combination angiotensin blockade, such as the use of an ACEI with an ARB, is an appealing option for patients whose hypertension may not be completely controlled with an ACEI or ARB alone, such as those whose hypertension is attributed to upregulation of RAAS."

"In proteinuric kidney diseases, such as primary glomerular disorders or diabetic nephropathy, combination ACEI/ARB therapy has been hypothesized to provide additive effects to reduce proteinuria and delay CKD progression better than with single agent use."

RAAS Physiology

"The renin-angiotensin-aldosterone system is a hormonal system that plays an important role in BP regulation through its effects on vascular tone and sodium homeostasis."

"The next steps of RAAS activation require the sequential cleavage of the glycoprotein angiotensinogen into several active angiotensin peptides that play a role in regulating BP and sodium balance, with Ang II being the major bioactive peptide."

"Ang II-mediated activation of AT_1 in the cardiovascular system induces vasoconstriction and cardiac contractility, whereas activation of AT_1 receptors in the kidney leads to renal vasoconstriction of the afferent and efferent arterioles in the glomerulus and increases sodium reabsorption in the proximal tubule."

"The synergistic effects of Ang II stimulation on AT_1 receptors at multiple tissues act to increase BP and maintain sodium homeostasis."

"The effects of Ang II-mediated stimulation on the AT_2 receptor, though less well understood, are believed to counterbalance AT_1 and include vasodilation (by promoting bradykinin, nitric oxide, and cyclic GMP release), augmenting natriuresis, and inhibiting renin synthesis and release by the JGA [189–191]."

RAAS Breakthrough: A Rationale for Combination ACEI/ARB Therapy?

"Despite the use of an ACEI or ARB as monotherapy in the treatment of hypertension or proteinuria with diabetic or nondiabetic kidney disease, patients may have inadequately controlled BP or proteinuria from suboptimal RAAS blockade and ongoing risk for CKD progression."

"Studies by Cao and others in diabetic spontaneously hypertensive rats showed that ACEI/ARB combination (captopril with either irbesartan or valsartan) produces an additive BP lowering effect and decreases albuminuria more than monotherapy, and is associated with further reduction in cardiac hypertrophy [192, 193]."

"Using diabetic Akita mice with renal proximal tubular cell-specific expression of the rat angiotensinogen transgene, Lo and others demonstrated that combined ACEI/ARB treatment with perindopril and losartan was more effective at preventing hypertension than either agent alone, and also led to a reduction in albuminuria as well as decreased renal tubular cell apoptosis, collagen type IV deposition, and interstitial fibrosis [194]."

Antihypertensive Effects of Combination ACEI/ARB Therapy: Is More Necessarily Better?

"Azizi and others performed the initial studies in normotensive adults comparing combined ACEI/ARB therapy with monotherapy [195, 196]."

"In the CALM study, a randomized controlled trial of the effects of combination ACEI/ARB therapy on hypertension and microalbuminuria in type 2 diabetes, lisinopril plus candesartan reduced diastolic BP by a mean of 8 mmHg more than either medication alone by 24 weeks."

"In a large open-label study of 6465 patients with hypertension, candesartan cilexetil was effective as add-on therapy for patients already receiving monotherapy with an ACEI, diuretic, calcium channel blocker, beta-blocker, or alpha-blocker, with similar systolic and diastolic BP reduction regardless of their background therapy [197]."

"These studies infer that dual ACEI/ARB therapy for hypertension provides at best a modest improvement in short-term BP reduction compared to monotherapy."

ACEI/ARB Combination Therapy for Proteinuria and CKD Progression

"Early cohort and small randomized studies were mostly supportive of the additive effects of dual angiotensin blockade in proteinuria reduction and CKD progression in proteinuric kidney diseases, independent of BP reduction [198–200]."

"One series assessing the antiproteinuric response of dual ACEI/ARB therapy compared to ACEI monotherapy in children with various glomerular diseases showed no significant difference in total proteinuria, but a significant difference in albuminuria reduction with the dual therapy group [201]."

"In a study by Lubrano and others [202], 10 children with CKD of various etiologies who had proteinuria were randomized to ACEI or ARB therapy and then advanced to dual therapy halfway through the study."

"There was a significant reduction in proteinuria using dual therapy compared to single therapy with ACEI or ARB, but no significant difference in GFR at any time point."

Adverse Effects of Dual ACEI/ARB Therapy

"The VA NEPHRON-D study, a large randomized trial comparing ACEI/ARB dual therapy to ARB plus placebo on progression to end-stage renal disease (ESRD) in adults with type 2 diabetes, was terminated early after a mean of 2.2 years of follow-up due to safety concerns in the dual therapy group."

"Few studies have looked at safety in the use of dual ACEI/ARB therapy in patients with ESRD, whose cardiovascular risk is greatest and where the potential cardioprotective effects of dual angiotensin blockade are even more desired."

"Limited to patients on chronic hemodialysis, these studies have shown a higher risk of cardiovascular death with dual ACEI/ARB therapy compared to single therapy with an ACEI, ARB, or other non-ACEI antihypertensive agent [203, 204]."

RAAS Blockade Strategies Beyond Combination ACEI/ARB Therapy

"DRIs have shown comparable effectiveness as other RAAS blockade agents in the treatment of hypertension [205–207] and proteinuria [208–211] in adults with diabetic and nondiabetic kidney disease, combined use of a DRI with an ACEI or ARB has thus far has produced mixed results and concerns for an increased rate of adverse events similar to dual ACEI/ARB therapy."

"One study comparing dual ACE/ARB therapy to dual MRA/ARB therapy in diabetic nephropathy, which had 18 months of follow-up, showed that MRA/ARB was superior in proteinuria reduction independent of BP reduction but GFR decline over the study period was comparable between groups [212]."

"More studies are needed to look at the long-term efficacy of add-on MRA to ACEI or ARB therapy on hard renal outcomes, such as GFR decline and time to dialysis, before such combination therapy can be considered for use in children with CKD."

Conclusion

"The use of ACEIs and ARBs has clear benefits in the treatment of hypertension, proteinuria, and CKD progression in diabetic and nondiabetic kidney diseases for both adults and children."

"This begs the question of whether combining ACEI and ARB therapy provides an additive benefit and improves patient outcomes, or whether it is too much of a good thing."

"Early cohort studies on the short-term use of dual ACEI/ARB therapy in adults with hypertension, with or without diabetic nephropathy, appeared promising."

"Given these concerns, as well as the limited pediatric literature on this topic, we cannot support routine use of combination ACEI/ARB therapy in children at this time; we advise that whenever using ACEI and/or ARB medications in children, the potential risks and benefits should be reviewed with patients and their families by the prescribing physician."

Key Summary Points

"RAAS blockade with ACEI or ARB therapy provides several cardiovascular and renoprotective benefits, including lowering BP, reducing proteinuria, and slowing the progression of CKD."

"Early cohort studies in adults on combination ACEI/ARB therapy for hypertension, proteinuria, and CKD progression were promising, but larger randomized trials have shown no significant difference compared to monotherapy and a higher risk of adverse renal outcomes with dual therapy."

"Pediatric literature on the use of combination ACEI/ARB therapy is limited and, based on the adult data, should be approached with caution."

[Section 10]

"Which of the following mechanisms explains why ACEIs, but not ARBs, are typically associated with cough and angioedema as potential side effects? a)Decreased bradykinin breakdown b) Increased bradykinin production by proteases c) Increased compensatory Ang I production d) Increased local nitric oxide synthesis 4."

"The ONTARGET study found that adults with increased vascular disease risk who took combination ACEI/ARB therapy had a lower risk in which of the following outcomes compared to adults receiving ACEI monotherapy? a) Progression of albuminuria b) Doubling of serum creatinine c) Need for renal replacement therapy d) Mortality 5."

"The VA-NEPHRON study, which compared dual ACEI/ARB therapy to ARB on progression to ESRD in adults with type 2 diabetes, was terminated early due to a higher rate of which of the following in the dual therapy group? a) Doubling of serum creatinine b) Acute kidney injury c) Need for renal replacement therapy d) Cardiovascular mortality."

A Novel Mechanism of ACE Inhibition–Associated Enhanced Platelet Reactivity: Disproof of the ARB-MI Paradox? [213]

This is a machine-generated summary of:

Helten, Carolin; Mourikis, Philipp; Dannenberg, Lisa; M'Pembele, René; Trojovsky, Kajetan; Ayhan, Aysel; Kohlmorgen, Christina; Grandoch, Maria; Levkau, Bodo; Veulemans, Verena; Petzold, Tobias; Hohlfeld, Thomas; Kelm, Malte; Zeus, Tobias; Polzin, Amin: A novel mechanism of ACE inhibition–associated enhanced platelet reactivity: disproof of the ARB-MI paradox? [213].

Published in: European Journal of Clinical Pharmacology (2020).

Link to original: https://doi.org/10.1007/s00228-020-02915-y

If you want to cite the papers, please refer to the original.

For technical reasons we could not place the page where the original quote is coming from.

Abstract-Summary "ACE inhibitors (ACEI) and angiotensin II receptor blockers (ARB) are important drugs in cardiovascular disease."

"Analyses show that the blockade of the renin-angiotensin-aldosterone system (RAAS) influences platelet reactivity."

"We evaluated the effects of ACEI and ARB on platelet reactivity and thrombin generation."

"ACEI treatment significantly increased platelet reactivity already 4 h after initiation of treatment (prior vs. 4 h post ACEI: MoA 41.9 ± 16.2% vs. 55.2 ± 16.7%; p = 0.003)."

"After switching from ACEI to ARB treatment, platelet reactivity decreased significantly (3 months after switching: MoA 34.7 ± 20.9%; p = 0.03)."

"ACEI reduced endogenous thrombin potential significantly from before to 3 months after ACEI (ETP 1527 ± 437 nM × min vs. 1088 ± 631 nM × min; p = 0.025)."

"Platelet thrombin receptor (PAR1) expression increased from 37.38 ± 10.97% before to 49.53 ± 6.04% after ACEI treatment (p = 0.036)."

"The mechanism behind RAAS influencing platelet function seems to be associated with PAR-1 expression."

Introduction

"Antihypertensives such as ACE inhibitors (ACEI) and angiotensin II receptor blockers (ARB) improve outcome in cardiovascular disease [214–218]."

"The "ARB-MI paradox" indicates that despite sufficient blood pressure reduction, none of the major trials observed reduced risk of MI or death in ARB-treated patients [219]."

"Platelet reactivity is a major determinant in pathogenesis of MI [220]."

"We hypothesized that ACEI and ARB treatment could modulate platelet reactivity."

"In certain conditions called high or low on-treatment platelet reactivity, patients have an elevated cardiovascular risk of either ischemia or bleeding [220]."

"Both ACEI and ARB affect the renin-angiotensin-aldosterone system (RAAS)."

"ACEI reduce angiotensin II levels whereas ARB block the AT1 further downstream in the pathway."

"In this study, we evaluated the effects of RAAS inhibition by ACEI and ARB on platelet reactivity."

Methods and Material

"Thrombin generation was measured as endogenous thrombin potential (ETP) via calibrated automated thrombogram."

"The samples were centrifuged in a Heraeus Minifuge RF (Heraeus Holding GmbH, Hanau, Germany) at 260 × g for 10 min to receive PRP and red blood cells."

"The supernatant was again centrifuged at 1600 × g for 10 min to obtain platelet-poor plasma (PPP) which was used to calibrate the aggregometer."

"Platelet aggregation was induced by 500 μM arachidonic acid (NatuTec GmbH, Frankfurt am Main, Germany), 5 μM adenosine diphosphate (ADP), 10 μM thrombin receptor activating peptide 6 (TRAP-6; both Sigma-Aldrich, St. Louis, Missouri, USA) or 10 μg/ml collagen (Collagen Reagens HORM®, NYCOMED Austria GmbH, Linz, Austria)."

"To measure endogenous thrombin potential (ETP), blood samples were centrifuged at 2000 × g for 10 min."

"The supernatant was again centrifuged at 10,000 × g for another 10 min to obtain platelet-free plasma (PFP)."

"Citrate-anticoagulated whole blood was centrifuged at 260 × g for 10 min (room temperature) to generate platelet-rich plasma (PRP)."

Results

"ACEI treatment significantly increased platelet reactivity already 4 h after initiation of treatment (prior vs. 4 h post ACEI: MoA 41.9 ± 16.2% vs. 55.2 ± 16.7%; $p = 0.003$)."

"Platelet reactivity was enhanced during time course at 24 h (MoA 52.3 ± 12.7%; $p = 0.9$) and 3 months of continued medication (MoA 50.3 ± 20.9%; $p = 0.45$)."

"ARB did not affect thrombin potential (ETP 1526 ± 587 nM × min vs. 1369 ± 516 nM × min; $p = 0.3$; data not shown)."

"ARB did not affect PAR1 expression (33.16 ± 11.73% before vs. 32.86 ± 8.99% 3 months after initial ARB treatment; $p = 0.89$; data not shown)."

Discussion

"The major findings of this study are that ACEI increase platelet reactivity by upregulation of platelet thrombin receptors."

"This enhanced platelet reactivity can be abolished by switching to ARB."

"In line with these arguments, we here report that ACE inhibition in contrast to ARB enhances platelet reactivity."

"Thrombin in turn binds to PAR1 on platelets, maintaining a steady state of receptor surface expression and cleavage [221]."

"This in turn enhances PAR1 expression on platelets leading to increased platelet reactivity."

Limitations

"The major limitation of this pilot study was the small number of patients and lack of clinical outcome."

"The sample size was too small to allow reasonable subgroup analysis."

"Blinding and sample size estimation was not conducted beforehand."

"Even though this was an observational study, samples were analysed blindly."

"Possible medication interactions—especially between RAAS blockade and antiplatelet drugs—must be considered and could cause intra-individual pharmacodynamic variances as a bias in our study."

Conclusion

"ACEI significantly increased platelet reactivity by enhanced PAR-1 expression on platelets."

"This represents a translational counterargument to the ARB-MI paradox."

New Therapeutic Approaches for the Treatment of Hyperkalemia in Patients Treated with Renin-Angiotensin-Aldosterone System Inhibitors [222]

This is a machine-generated summary of:

Tamargo, Juan; Caballero, Ricardo; Delpón, Eva: New Therapeutic Approaches for the Treatment of Hyperkalemia in Patients Treated with Renin-Angiotensin-Aldosterone System Inhibitors [222].

Published in: Cardiovascular Drugs and Therapy (2018).

Link to original: https://doi.org/10.1007/s10557-017-6767-5

If you want to cite the papers, please refer to the original.

For technical reasons we could not place the page where the original quote is coming from.

Abstract-Summary "Patients at the highest risk of hyperkalemia are treated with renin-angiotensin-aldosterone system inhibitors (RAASIs) as they improve cardiovascular and renal outcomes and are strongly recommended in clinical guidelines."

"RAASIs cause or increase the risk of hyperkalemia, a key limitation to fully titrate RAASIs in patients who are most likely to benefit from treatment."

"We provide an overview of the mechanisms involved in K^+ homeostasis and the epidemiology and management of hyperkalemia as a complication in cardiovascular patients and, finally, analyze the efficacy and safety of two new polymer-based, non-systemic agents, patiromer calcium and sodium zirconium cyclosilicate (ZS-9), designed to increase fecal K^+ loss and to normalize elevated serum K^+ levels and chronically maintain K^+ homeostasis in hyperkalemic patients treated with RAASIs."

Introduction

"Renal K^+ excretion is dependent on aldosterone secretion and delivery of Na^+ and water to the distal tubule."

"At this level, K^+ secretion involves two steps: active uptake across the basolateral Na^+,K^+-ATPase, followed by electrogenic movement across the luminal membrane through two K^+ channels [ROMK2 (renal outer medullary K^+) and large-conductance Ca^{2+}-activated channel, subfamily M, alpha member 1 (KCNMA1 or BK)] and electroneutral KCl transport [223–226]."

"This increase in flow enhances K^+ excretion via ROMK2 and KCNMA1 channels by diluting luminal K^+ concentration and increases distal Na^+ delivery and reabsorption through ENaC. These mechanisms avoid the development of hyperkalemia."

"High-K^+ intake also stimulates aldosterone release, which, in turn, increases [223–230] (a) the expression and activity of the basolateral Na^+,K^+-ATPase in the principal cells and the transport of K^+ into the collecting principal cells and (b) the density of ENaCs, reducing the intracellular Na^+ concentration."

Hyperkalemia Is a Challenging Clinical Problem

"The prevalence of hyperkalemia increases up to 24.5% of patients with cardiovascular disease receiving antihypertensive drugs, 32.5% in heart failure (HF) patients, and 50–55% of patients with chronic kidney disease (CKD), with 10% of these patients (i.e., up to 1% of hospitalized patients) having s-$K^+ \geq 6$ mEq/L [231–241]."

"Patients with CKD and chronic hyperkalemia can have s-$K^+ > 6.0$ mEq/L without apparent ECG changes [242]."

"When the eGFR decreases from 60–90 to <20 mL/min/1.73 m^2, the prevalence of hyperkalemia (>5 mEq/L) increases from 2 to 42% and to 56.7% in patients with stage 5 CKD, and in hospitalized patients with CKD (eGFR <60 mL/min/1.73 m^2), the prevalence of hyperkalemia ranged from 7.7 to 73%, depending on the studied population, predisposing factors, and the definition of hyperkalemia [237–240, 243–252]."

Hyperkalemia Produced by Renin-Angiotensin-Aldosterone Inhibitors

"Hyperkalemia is an uncommon complication (≤ 2%) of RAASI therapy in patients with normal renal function (mean increase in s-K^+ ~ 0.1–0.2 mEq/L), and in patients with HF and reduced ejection fraction (HFrEF) treated with ACEIs or ARBs, the incidence of s-K^+ ≥ 6 mEq/L is <2% [253]."

"In clinical trials, the risk of hyperkalemia (>5.5 mEq/L) increases up to 5% with dual RAASIs and to 5–10% when dual therapy is administered to patients with CKD, HF, or hypertension [253–255], but severe life-threatening hyperkalemia is uncommon [254–261]."

"The lower incidence of hyperkalemia in controlled trials can be attributed to the exclusion of high-risk patients (i.e., elderly with comorbidities, diabetics, advanced CKD, or HF), differences in comorbidities and concomitant medications, prescribed dosages of RAASIs, and the more frequent and rigorous monitoring of s-K^+ and renal function, so that hyperkalemia is more likely to be reported and appropriately treated [253, 257, 259, 262–266]."

Gap Between Clinical Guideline Recommendations and Real-World Prescribing Patterns

"RAASIs were prescribed at maximum doses in 19–26% and at submaximum doses in 58–65% and were discontinued in 14–16% of patients."

"Cardiorenal adverse event/mortality and mortality occurred in 34.3 and 11.0% of patients who discontinued RAASIs, 24.9 and 8.2% of patients on submaximum doses, and 24.9 and 4.1% of patients on maximum doses, respectively."

"In the BIOSTAT-CHF trial, patients with HFrEF treated with <50% of recommended dose of ACEIs/ARBs seemed to have a greater risk of death and/or HF hospitalization compared with patients reaching ≥100% [267]."

"Because of the limited utility of current options to manage hyperkalemia, clinicians frequently must either stop or discontinue RAASIs or use them at lower than recommended (suboptimal) doses in these high-risk patients who are most likely to benefit most from treatment [229, 268]."

"Patients on submaximum doses or those who discontinue RAASIs have worse outcomes than patients on maximum tolerated doses."

Treatment of Hyperkalemia

"Long-term treatment of mild chronic hyperkalemia includes low-K^+ diet (<2.4 g/day in stage 3–5 CKD), reduced dietary intake, reduction or discontinuation of K^+ supplements and drugs that compromise renal function and increase s-K^+, treatment of modifiable risk factors, and increase of K^+ excretion with loop or thiazide diuretics [231, 232, 235, 241, 257, 269–274]."

"These drugs provide a temporary benefit (1–4 h), but a rebound can occur after 2 h. Intravenous sodium bicarbonate also facilitates K^+ shift into the cells, but it does not lower s-K^+ in the absence of metabolic acidosis, is less effective in patients with advanced CKD, produces Na^+ retention and volume overload, and requires multiple dose adjustments. (1) Prevent and treat life-threatening cardiac arrhythmias by administering intravenous Ca^{2+} salts (chloride and gluconate) that stabilize the cardiac resting membrane potential and reduce cardiac excitability. (2) Remove K^+ from the body by increasing its renal and fecal excretion, using loop and thiazide diuretics, fludrocortisone, hemodialysis (in advanced CKD), or cation-exchange resins."

New Approaches in the Treatment of Hyperkalemia

"Two new orally active K^+ binders, patiromer sorbitex calcium (Veltassa®, RLY5016) and sodium zirconium cyclosilicate (ZS-9) were approved by the European Medicines Agency, but its approval by the FDA has been delayed by manufacturing process concerns."

"In randomized clinical trials, these drugs normalize s-K^+, maintain s-K^+ within the therapeutic range, and prevent recurrences of hyperkalemia in patients treated with RAASIs."

"They have been approved for the treatment of hyperkalemia in adult patients."

Patiromer Sorbitex Calcium

"In a phase 1 open-label study in 25 patients with hyperkalemia (5.5 to <6.5 mEq/L) and CKD (eGFR 15 to <60 mL/min) receiving a controlled K^+ diet and taking at least one RAASI, patiromer (8.4 g BID) reduced s-K^+ 0.20 and 0.75 mEq/L at 7 and 48 h, respectively, and 20% of patients achieved s-$K^+ \leq 5.5$ mEq/L after 7 h [275]."

"Patiromer decreased s-K^+ 0.65 and 1.23 mEq/L in patients with mild and moderate-to-severe hyperkalemia, respectively, and 76% of patients achieved normokalemia."

"In 102 patients from the OPAL-HK trial with hyperkalemia and HF, patiromer decreased s-K^+ at week 4 by 1.06 mEq/L (0.74 and 1.26 mEq/L in patients with mild and with moderate-to-severe hyperkalemia, respectively) and 76% of patients achieved normokalemia [276]."

Sodium Zirconium Cyclosilicate

"In the acute phase, patients were randomized to ZS-9 or placebo TID for 48 h. Then, patients who achieved normokalemia (3.5–4.9 mEq/L) were re-randomized to the same dose of ZS-9 or placebo QD; patients previously assigned to the placebo group were randomized to 1.25 or 2.5 g ZS-9 QD for 12 additional days."

"In 45 patients from the ZS-003 and HAMONIZE trials with a mean s-K^+ of 6.3 mEq/L (≥6.1–7.2 mEq/L), a single 10 g dose of ZS-9 produced a rapid and significant reduction in s-K^+ which averaged 0.4, 0.6, and 0.7 mEq/L at 1, 2, and 4 h, respectively."

"Despite doses of RAASIs were kept constant, patients on 5, 10, and 15 g ZS-9 maintained a lower s-K^+ (4.7, 4.5, and 4.4 mEq/L, respectively) than the placebo group (5.2 mEq/L) and more patients on ZS-9 maintained normokalemia (83, 89, and 92 vs. 40% with placebo)."

Gaps in Knowledge

"Hyperkalemia increases cardiovascular morbidity and mortality and complicates the management of patients with CKD, HF, diabetes, or hypertension treated with RAASIs."

"Patiromer and ZS-9 produce a dose-dependent and sustained reduction in s-K^+ and prevent the recurrence of hyperkalemia in these patients with an acceptable safety profile."

"They represent a promising therapeutic approach for lowering the risk of hyperkalemia associated with RAASIs and may allow the maintenance and titration of these drugs to the maximum guideline-recommended doses in high-risk patients previously ineligible for treatment, so that they might benefit most from their cardio- and nephroprotective effects."

"Trials are needed to confirm whether patiromer and ZS-9 may improve clinical outcomes in patients at high risk of hyperkalemia by allowing the titration of RAASIs to the optimal doses and their long-term efficacy and tolerability need to be evaluated in those patients with comorbidities and polymedicated and excluded from randomized clinical trials."

Bibliography

1. Thatcher SE (2017) A brief introduction into the renin-angiotensin-aldosterone system: new and old techniques. Methods Mol Biol 1614:1–19
2. Borghi F, Sevá-Pessôa B, Grassi-Kassisse DM (2016) The adipose tissue and the involvement of the renin-angiotensin-aldosterone system in cardiometabolic syndrome. Cell Tissue Res 366(3):543–548
3. Patel S, Rauf A, Khan H, Abu-Izneid T (2017) Renin-angiotensin-aldosterone (RAAS): the ubiquitous system for homeostasis and pathologies. Biomed Pharmacother 94:317–325
4. Ojha U, Ruddaraju S, Sabapathy N et al (2022) Current and emerging classes of pharmacological agents for the management of hypertension. Am J Cardiovasc Drugs 22:271–285
5. Pugliese NR, Masi S, Taddei S (2019) The renin-angiotensin-aldosterone system: a crossroad from arterial hypertension to heart failure. Heart Fail Rev 25:31–42. https://doi.org/10.1007/s10741-019-09855-5
6. Jhund PS, McMurray JJV (2016) The neprilysin pathway in heart failure: a review and guide on the use of sacubitril/valsartan. Heart 102:1342–1347

7. Daniels LB, Maisel AS (2007) Natriuretic peptides. J Am Coll Cardiol 50:2357–2368. https://doi.org/10.1016/j.jacc.2007.09.021
8. Lavoie JL, Lake-Bruse KD, Sigmund CD (2004) Increased blood pressure in transgenic mice expressing both human renin and angiotensinogen in the renal proximal tubule. Am J Physiol Physiol 286:F965–F971. https://doi.org/10.1152/ajprenal.00402.2003
9. Crowley SD, Gurley SB, Herrera MJ, Ruiz P, Griffiths R, Kumar AP, Kim HS, Smithies O, Le TH, Coffman TM (2006) Angiotensin II causes hypertension and cardiac hypertrophy through its receptors in the kidney. Proc Natl Acad Sci 103:17985–17990. https://doi.org/10.1073/pnas.0605545103
10. Shimosawa T (2013) Salt, the renin–angiotensin–aldosterone system and resistant hypertension. Hypertens Res 36:657–660. https://doi.org/10.1038/hr.2013.69
11. Xue B, Zhang Z, Roncari CF et al (2012) Aldosterone acting through the central nervous system sensitizes angiotensin II-induced hypertension. Hypertension 60:1023–1030. https://doi.org/10.1161/HYPERTENSIONAHA.112.196576
12. Nakagaki T, Hirooka Y, Matsukawa R et al (2012) Activation of mineralocorticoid receptors in the rostral ventrolateral medulla is involved in hypertensive mechanisms in stroke-prone spontaneously hypertensive rats. Hypertens Res 35:470–476. https://doi.org/10.1038/hr.2011.220
13. Lee DS, Gona P, Vasan RS, Larson MG, Benjamin EJ, Wang TJ, Tu JV, Levy D (2009) Relation of disease pathogenesis and risk factors to heart failure with preserved or reduced ejection fraction. Circulation 119:3070–3077. https://doi.org/10.1161/CIRCULATIONAHA.108.815944
14. Ho JE, Enserro D, Brouwers FP, Kizer JR, Shah SJ, Psaty BM, Bartz TM, Santhanakrishnan R, Lee DS, Chan C, Liu K, Blaha MJ, Hillege HL, van der Harst P, van Gilst WH, Kop WJ, Gansevoort RT, Vasan RS, Gardin JM, Levy D, Gottdiener JS, de Boer RA, Larson MG (2016) Predicting heart failure with preserved and reduced ejection fraction. Circ Hear Fail 9. https://doi.org/10.1161/CIRCHEARTFAILURE.115.003116
15. Teo LYL, Chan LL, Lam CSP (2016) Heart failure with preserved ejection fraction in hypertension. Curr Opin Cardiol 31:410–416. https://doi.org/10.1097/HCO.0000000000000292
16. Yancy CW, Jessup M, Chair V et al (2013) 2013 ACCF/AHA guideline for the management of heart failure: executive summary: a report of the American College of Cardiology Foundation/American Heart Association Task Force on practice guidelines. JAC 62:1495–1539. https://doi.org/10.1016/j.jacc.2013.05.020
17. Williams B, Lacy PS, Thom SM et al (2006) Differential impact of blood pressure–lowering drugs on central aortic pressure and clinical outcomes. Circulation 113:1213–1225. https://doi.org/10.1161/CIRCULATIONAHA.105.595496
18. Zhou M, Chen N, Yang M et al (2009) Calcium channel blockers versus other classes of drugs for hypertension. Cochrane Database Syst Rev. https://doi.org/10.1002/14651858.CD003654.pub3
19. Ponikowski P, Voors AA, Anker SD, Bueno H, Cleland JGF, Coats AJS, Falk V, González-Juanatey JR, Harjola VP, Jankowska EA, Jessup M, Linde C, Nihoyannopoulos P, Parissis JT, Pieske B, Riley JP, Rosano GMC, Ruilope LM, Ruschitzka F, Rutten FH, van der Meer P (2016) 2016 ESC guidelines for the diagnosis and treatment of acute and chronic heart failure. Eur Heart J 37:2129–2200. https://doi.org/10.1093/eurheartj/ehw128
20. Yancy CW, Jessup M, Bozkurt B, Butler J, Casey DE Jr, Colvin MM, Drazner MH, Filippatos GS, Fonarow GC, Givertz MM, Hollenberg SM, Lindenfeld JA, Masoudi FA, McBride PE, Peterson PN, Stevenson LW, Westlake C (2017) 2017 ACC/AHA/HFSA focused update of the 2013 ACCF/AHA guideline for the management of heart failure. J Am Coll Cardiol 70:776–803. https://doi.org/10.1016/j.jacc.2017.04.025
21. Packer M, Califf RM, Konstam MA, Krum H, McMurray JJ, Rouleau JL, Swedberg K (2002) Comparison of omapatrilat and enalapril in patients with chronic heart failure. Circulation 106:920–926. https://doi.org/10.1161/01.cir.0000029801.86489.50
22. Yusuf S, Pfeffer MA, Swedberg K, Granger CB, Held P, McMurray JJV, Michelson EL, Olofsson B, Östergren J (2003) Effects of candesartan in patients with chronic heart fail-

ure and preserved left-ventricular ejection fraction: the CHARM-preserved trial. Lancet 362:777–781. https://doi.org/10.1016/S0140-6736(03)14285-7
23. Pitt B, Pfeffer MA, Assmann SF, Boineau R, Anand IS, Claggett B, Clausell N, Desai AS, Diaz R, Fleg JL, Gordeev I, Harty B, Heitner JF, Kenwood CT, Lewis EF, O'Meara E, Probstfield JL, Shaburishvili T, Shah SJ, Solomon SD, Sweitzer NK, Yang S, McKinlay SM (2014) Spironolactone for heart failure with preserved ejection fraction. N Engl J Med 370:1383–1392
24. Solomon SD, Zile M, Pieske B, Voors A, Shah A, Kraigher-Krainer E, Shi V, Bransford T, Takeuchi M, Gong J, Lefkowitz M, Packer M, McMurray JJV (2012) The angiotensin receptor neprilysin inhibitor LCZ696 in heart failure with preserved ejection fraction: a phase 2 double-blind randomised controlled trial. Lancet 380:1387–1395. https://doi.org/10.1016/S0140-6736(12)61227-6
25. Solomon SD, Rizkala AR, Gong J, Wang W, Anand IS, Ge J, Lam CSP, Maggioni AP, Martinez F, Packer M, Pfeffer MA, Pieske B, Redfield MM, Rouleau JL, van Veldhuisen DJ, Zannad F, Zile MR, Desai AS, Shi VC, Lefkowitz MP, McMurray JJV (2017) Angiotensin receptor neprilysin inhibition in heart failure with preserved ejection fraction: rationale and design of the PARAGON-HF trial. JACC Hear Fail 5:471–482
26. Borghi C, SIIA Task Force, Rossi F, SIF Task Force (2015) Role of the renin-angiotensin-aldosterone system and its pharmacological inhibitors in cardiovascular diseases: complex and critical issues. High Blood Press Cardiovasc Prev 22:429–444. https://doi.org/10.1007/s40292-015-0120-5
27. Mancia G, Fagard R, Narkiewicz K, Redon J, Zanchetti A, Bohm M et al (2013) 2013 ESH/ESC guidelines for the management of arterial hypertension: the Task Force for the Management of Arterial Hypertension of the European Society of Hypertension (ESH) and of the European Society of Cardiology (ESC). Eur Heart J 34(28):2159–2219
28. Task Force on the management of STseamiotESoC, Steg PG, James SK, Atar D, Badano LP, Blomstrom-Lundqvist C et al (2012) ESC guidelines for the management of acute myocardial infarction in patients presenting with ST-segment elevation. Eur Heart J 33(20):2569–2619
29. Task Force M, Montalescot G, Sechtem U, Achenbach S, Andreotti F, Arden C et al (2013) 2013 ESC guidelines on the management of stable coronary artery disease: the Task Force on the management of stable coronary artery disease of the European Society of Cardiology. Eur Heart J 34(38):2949–3003
30. Ackerman MJ, Priori SG, Willems S, Berul C, Brugada R, Calkins H et al (2011) HRS/EHRA expert consensus statement on the state of genetic testing for the channelopathies and cardiomyopathies this document was developed as a partnership between the Heart Rhythm Society (HRS) and the European Heart Rhythm Association (EHRA). Heart Rhythm 8(8):1308–1339
31. Ohsawa M, Tamura K, Kanaoka T, Wakui H, Maeda A, Dejima T et al (2013) Addition of aliskiren to angiotensin receptor blocker improves ambulatory blood pressure profile and cardiorenal function better than addition of benazepril in chronic kidney disease. Int J Mol Sci 14(8):15361–15375
32. Kanaoka T, Tamura K, Ohsawa M, Wakui H, Maeda A, Dejima T et al (2012) Effects of aliskiren-based therapy on ambulatory blood pressure profile, central hemodynamics, and arterial stiffness in nondiabetic mild to moderate hypertensive patients. J Clin Hypertens (Greenwich) 14(8):522–529
33. Dahlof B, Devereux RB, Kjeldsen SE, Julius S, Beevers G, de Faire U et al (2002) Cardiovascular morbidity and mortality in the Losartan Intervention For Endpoint reduction in hypertension study (LIFE): a randomised trial against atenolol. Lancet 359(9311):995–1003
34. Castro Hevia J, Antzelevitch C, Tornes Barzaga F, Dorantes Sanchez M, Dorticos Balea F, Zayas Molina R et al (2006) Tpeak-Tend and Tpeak-Tend dispersion as risk factors for ventricular tachycardia/ventricular fibrillation in patients with the Brugada syndrome. J Am Coll Cardiol 47(9):1828–1834
35. Haller H, Ito S, Izzo JL Jr, Januszewicz A, Katayama S, Menne J et al (2011) Olmesartan for the delay or prevention of microalbuminuria in type 2 diabetes. N Engl J Med 364(10):907–917

36. Schneider MP, Hua TA, Bohm M, Wachtell K, Kjeldsen SE, Schmieder RE (2010) Prevention of atrial fibrillation by renin-angiotensin system inhibition a meta-analysis. J Am Coll Cardiol 55(21):2299–2307
37. Azushima K, Morisawa N, Tamura K, Nishiyama A (2020) Recent research advances in renin-angiotensin-aldosterone system receptors. Curr Hypertens Rep 22. https://doi.org/10.1007/s11906-020-1028-6
38. de Gasparo M, Catt KJ, Inagami T, Wright JW, Unger T (2000) International union of pharmacology. XXIII. The angiotensin II receptors. Pharmacol Rev 52(3):415–472
39. Padia SH, Carey RM (2013) AT2 receptors: beneficial counter-regulatory role in cardiovascular and renal function. Arch Eur J Physiol 465(1):99–110. https://doi.org/10.1007/s00424-012-1146-3
40. Forrester SJ, Booz GW, Sigmund CD, Coffman TM, Kawai T, Rizzo V et al (2018) Angiotensin II signal transduction: an update on mechanisms of physiology and pathophysiology. Physiol Rev 98(3):1627–1738. https://doi.org/10.1152/physrev.00038.2017. This paper summarizes detailed mechanisms of the angiotensin II signal transduction in various tissues
41. Ichihara A, Yatabe MS (2019) The (pro)renin receptor in health and disease. Nat Rev Nephrol 15:693–712. https://doi.org/10.1038/s41581-019-0160-5
42. Hermle T, Guida MC, Beck S, Helmstadter S, Simons M (2013) Drosophila ATP6AP2/VhaPRR functions both as a novel planar cell polarity core protein and a regulator of endosomal trafficking. EMBO J 32(2):245–259. https://doi.org/10.1038/emboj.2012.323
43. Forgac M (2007) Vacuolar ATPases: rotary proton pumps in physiology and pathophysiology. Nat Rev Mol Cell Biol 8(11):917–929. https://doi.org/10.1038/nrm2272
44. Shibayama Y, Fujimori T, Nguyen G, Hirose T, Totsune K, Ichihara A et al (2015) (Pro) renin receptor is crucial for Wnt/beta-catenin-dependent genesis of pancreatic ductal adenocarcinoma. Sci Rep 5:8854. https://doi.org/10.1038/srep08854. In this paper, the authors identified aberrant expression of PRR in pancreatic ductal adenocarcinoma (PDAC) tissues. Furthermore, plasma soluble PRR levels were significantly increased in patients with PDAC. Further molecular studies revealed new critical aspects that strongly indicate a potential role of (P)RR in Wnt/β-catenin signaling-dependent genesis of PDAC
45. Arundhathi A, Chuang WH, Chen JK, Wang SE, Shyr YM, Chen JY et al (2016) Prorenin receptor acts as a potential molecular target for pancreatic ductal adenocarcinoma diagnosis. Oncotarget 7(34):55437–55448. https://doi.org/10.18632/oncotarget.10583
46. Kouchi M, Shibayama Y, Ogawa D, Miyake K, Nishiyama A, Tamiya T (2017) (Pro)renin receptor is crucial for glioma development via the Wnt/beta-catenin signaling pathway. J Neurosurg 127(4):819–828. https://doi.org/10.3171/2016.9.JNS16431
47. Ohba K, Suzuki T, Nishiyama H, Kaneko K, Hirose T, Totsune K et al (2014) Expression of (pro)renin receptor in breast cancers and its effect on cancercell proliferation. Biomed Res 35(2):117–126
48. Beitia M, Solano-Iturri JD, Errarte P, Calvete-Candenas J, Loizate A, Etxezarraga MC et al (2019) (Pro)renin receptor expression increases throughout the colorectal adenoma-adenocarcinoma sequence and it is associated with worse colorectal cancer prognosis. Cancers (Basel) 11(6):881. https://doi.org/10.3390/cancers11060881
49. Wang J, Shibayama Y, Zhang A, Ohsaki H, Asano E, Suzuki Y et al (2019) (Pro)renin receptor promotes colorectal cancer through the Wnt/beta-catenin signalling pathway despite constitutive pathway component mutations. Br J Cancer 120(2):229–237. https://doi.org/10.1038/s41416-018-0350-0
50. Yamamoto H, Kaneko K, Ohba K, Morimoto R, Hirose T, Satoh F et al (2013) Increased expression of (pro)renin receptor in aldosterone-producing adenomas. Peptides 49:68–73. https://doi.org/10.1016/j.peptides.2013.08.022
51. Ali MS, Sayeski PP, Dirksen LB, Hayzer DJ, Marrero MB, Bernstein KE (1997) Dependence on the motif YIPP for the physical association of Jak2 kinase with the intracellular carboxyl tail of the angiotensin II AT1 receptor. J Biol Chem 272(37):23382–23388. https://doi.org/10.1074/jbc.272.37.23382

52. Venema RC, Ju H, Venema VJ, Schieffer B, Harp JB, Ling BN et al (1998) Angiotensin II-induced association of phospholipase Cgamma1 with the G-protein-coupled AT1 receptor. J Biol Chem 273(13):7703–7708. https://doi.org/10.1074/jbc.273.13.7703
53. Wakui H, Tamura K, Masuda S, Tsurumi-Ikeya Y, Fujita M, Maeda A et al (2013) Enhanced angiotensin receptor-associated protein in renal tubule suppresses angiotensin-dependent hypertension. Hypertension 61(6):1203–1210. https://doi.org/10.1161/HYPERTENSIONAHA.111.00572
54. Ohsawa M, Tamura K, Wakui H, Maeda A, Dejima T, Kanaoka T et al (2014) Deletion of the angiotensin II type 1 receptor-associated protein enhances renal sodium reabsorption and exacerbates angiotensin II-mediated hypertension. Kidney Int 86(3):570–581. https://doi.org/10.1038/ki.2014.95
55. Guo DF, Chenier I, Lavoie JL, Chan JS, Hamet P, Tremblay J et al (2006) Development of hypertension and kidney hypertrophy in transgenic mice overexpressing ARAP1 gene in the kidney. Hypertension 48(3):453–459. https://doi.org/10.1161/01.HYP.0000230664.32874.52
56. Kurisu S, Ozono R, Oshima T, Kambe M, Ishida T, Sugino H et al (2003) Cardiac angiotensin II type 2 receptor activates the kinin/NO system and inhibits fibrosis. Hypertension 41(1):99–107. https://doi.org/10.1161/01.hyp.0000050101.90932.14
57. Yan X, Price RL, Nakayama M, Ito K, Schuldt AJ, Manning WJ et al (2003) Ventricular-specific expression of angiotensin II type 2 receptors causes dilated cardiomyopathy and heart failure in transgenic mice. Am J Physiol Heart Circ Physiol 285(5):H2179–H2187. https://doi.org/10.1152/ajpheart.00361.2003
58. Nouet S, Amzallag N, Li JM, Louis S, Seitz I, Cui TX et al (2004) Trans-inactivation of receptor tyrosine kinases by novel angiotensin II AT2 receptor-interacting protein, ATIP. J Biol Chem 279(28):28989–28997. https://doi.org/10.1074/jbc.M403880200
59. Fujita T, Mogi M, Min LJ, Iwanami J, Tsukuda K, Sakata A et al (2009) Attenuation of cuff-induced neointimal formation by overexpression of angiotensin II type 2 receptor-interacting protein 1. Hypertension 53(4):688–693. https://doi.org/10.1161/HYPERTENSIONAHA.108.128140
60. Passos-Silva DG, Verano-Braga T, Santos RA (2013) Angiotensin-(1-7): beyond the cardio-renal actions. Clin Sci 124(7):443–456. https://doi.org/10.1042/CS20120461
61. Karnik SS, Singh KD, Tirupula K, Unal H (2017) Significance of angiotensin 1-7 coupling with MAS1 receptor and other GPCRs to the renin-angiotensin system: IUPHAR review 22. Br J Pharmacol 174(9):737–753. https://doi.org/10.1111/bph.13742
62. Ohshima K, Mogi M, Nakaoka H, Iwanami J, Min LJ, Kanno H et al (2014) Possible role of angiotensin-converting enzyme 2 and activation of angiotensin II type 2 receptor by angiotensin-(1-7) in improvement of vascular remodeling by angiotensin II type 1 receptor blockade. Hypertension 63(3):e53–e59. https://doi.org/10.1161/HYPERTENSIONAHA.113.02426
63. Nishiyama A (2019) Pathophysiological mechanisms of mineralocorticoid receptor-dependent cardiovascular and chronic kidney disease. Hypertens Res 42(3):293–300. https://doi.org/10.1038/s41440-018-0158-6
64. Rafiq K, Nakano D, Ihara G, Hitomi H, Fujisawa Y, Ohashi N et al (2011) Effects of mineralocorticoid receptor blockade on glucocorticoid-induced renal injury in adrenalectomized rats. J Hypertens 29(2):290–298
65. Vitellius G, Trabado S, Bouligand J, Delemer B, Lombes M (2018) Pathophysiology of glucocorticoid signaling. Ann Endocrinol 79(3):98–106. https://doi.org/10.1016/j.ando.2018.03.001
66. Ayuzawa N, Nagase M, Ueda K, Nishimoto M, Kawarazaki W, Marumo T et al (2016) Rac1-mediated activation of mineralocorticoid receptor in pressure overload-induced cardiac injury. Hypertension 67(1):99–106. https://doi.org/10.1161/HYPERTENSIONAHA.115.06054
67. Szczepanska-Sadowska E, Czarzasta K, Cudnoch-Jedrzejewska A (2018) Dysregulation of the renin-angiotensin system and the vasopressinergic system interactions in cardiovascular disorders. Curr Hypertens Rep 20:19. https://doi.org/10.1007/s11906-018-0823-9

68. Siragy HM, Inagami T, Carey RM (2007) NO and cGMP mediate angiotensin AT 2 receptor-induced renal renin inhibition in young rats. Am J Physiol Regul Integr Comp Physiol 293(4):R1461–R1467
69. Clark MA, Diz DI, Tallant EA (2001) Angiotensin-(1-7) downregulates the angiotensin II type 1 receptor in vascular smooth muscle cells. Hypertension 37(4):1141–1146
70. Santos RA, Ferreira AJ, Simões e Silva AC. (2008) Recent advances in the angiotensin-converting enzyme 2-angiotensin (1-7)-Mas axis. Exp Physiol 93(5):519–527
71. Ferreira AJ, Jacoby BA, Araújo CA, Macedo FA, Silva GA, Almeida AP et al (2007) The nonpeptide angiotensin-(1–7) receptor Mas agonist AVE-0991 attenuates heart failure induced by myocardial infarction. Am J Physiol Heart Circ Physiol 292(2):H1113–H1119
72. Giani JF, Gironacci MM, Muñoz MC, Turyn D, Dominici FP (2008) Angiotensin-(1–7) has a dual role on growth-promoting signalling pathways in rat heart in vivo by stimulating STAT3 and STAT5a/b phosphorylation and inhibiting angiotensin II-stimulated ERK1/2 and Rho kinase activity. Exp Physiol 93(5):570–578
73. Tallant EA, Ferrario CM, Gallagher PE (2005) Angiotensin-(1–7) inhibits growth of cardiac myocytes through activation of the Mas receptor. Am J Physiol Heart Circ Physiol 289(4):H1560–H1566
74. Chan SH, Hsu KS, Huang CC, Wang LL, Ou CC, Chan JY (2005) NADPH oxidase-derived superoxide anion mediates angiotensin II-induced pressor effect via activation of p38 mitogen-activated protein kinase in the rostral ventrolateral medulla. Circ Res 97(8):772–780. https://doi.org/10.1161/01.res.0000185804.79157.c0
75. DiBona GF (1999) Central sympathoexcitatory actions of angiotensin II: role of type 1 angiotensin II receptors. J Am Soc Nephrol 10(Suppl 11):S90–S94
76. Sagara Y, Hirooka Y, Nozoe M, Ito K, Kimura Y, Sunagawa K (2007) Pressor response induced by central angiotensin II is mediated by activation of Rho/Rho-kinase pathway via AT1 receptors. J Hypertens 25(2):399–406
77. Kaplan-Albuquerque N, Garat C, Van Putten V, Nemenoff RA (2003) Regulation of SM22α expression by arginine vasopressin and PDGF-BB in vascular smooth muscle cells. Am J Physiol Heart Circ Physiol 285(4):H1444–H1452
78. Gutkowska J, Miszkurka M, Danalache B, Gassanov N, Wang D, Jankowski M (2007) Functional arginine vasopressin system in early heart maturation. Am J Physiol Heart Circ Physiol 293(4):H2262–H2270
79. Lon S, Szczepanska-Sadowska E, Szczypaczewska M (1996) Evidence that centrally released arginine vasopressin is involved in central pressor action of angiotensin II. Am J Physiol Heart Circ Physiol 270(1):H167–H173
80. Szczepanska-Sadowska E, Paczwa P, Lon S, Ganten D (1998) Increased pressor function of central vasopressinergic system in hypertensive renin transgenic rats. J Hypertens 16(10):1505–1514
81. Martin S, Malkinson T, Veale W, Pittman Q (1985) The action of centrally administered arginine vasopres-sin on blood pressure in the conscious rabbit. Brain Res 348(1):137–145
82. Noszczyk B, Łon S, Szczepańska-Sadowska E (1993) Central cardiovascular effects of AVP and AVP analogs with V 1, V 2 and 'V 3'agonistic or anatagonistic properties in conscious dog. Brain Res 610(1):115–126
83. Consolim-Colombo FM, Hay M, Smith TC, Elizondo-Fournier M, Bishop VS (1996) Subcellular mecha-nisms of angiotensin II and arginine vasopressin activation of area postrema neurons. Am J Physiol Regul Integr Comp Physiol 271(1):R34–R41
84. Hay M, Edwards G, Lindsley K, Murphy S, Sharma R, Bhalla R et al (1993) Increases in cytosolic Ca^{2+} in rat area postrema/mNTS neurons produced by angiotensin II and arginine-vasopressin. Neurosci Lett 151(2):121–125
85. Walker J, Jennings DB (1995) During acute hypercapnia vasopressin inhibits an angiotensin drive to ventilation in conscious dogs. J Appl Physiol 79(3):786–794
86. Lang CC, Struthers AD (2013) Targeting the renin–angiotensin–aldosterone system in heart failure. Nat Rev Cardiol 10:125–134. https://doi.org/10.1038/nrcardio.2012.196

87. van Vark LC et al (2012) Angiotensin-converting enzyme inhibitors reduce mortality in hypertension: a meta-analysis of randomized clinical trials of renin-angiotensin-aldosterone system inhibitors involving 158,998 patients. Eur Heart J 33:2088–2097
88. SOLVD Investigators (1991) Effect of enalapril on survival in patients with reduced left ventricular ejection fractions and congestive heart failure. N Engl J Med 325:293–302
89. The Consensus Trial Study Group (1987) Effects of enalapril on mortality in severe congestive heart failure. N Engl J Med 316:1429–1435
90. Pfeffer MA et al (1992) Effect of captopril on mortality and morbidity in patients with left ventricular dysfunction after myocardial infarction. N Engl J Med 327:669–677
91. Weber KT (1997) Extracellular matrix remodeling in heart failure. A role for de novo angiotensin II generation. Circulation 96:4065–4082
92. Elder DH, McAlpine-Scott J, Choy AM, Struthers AD, Lang CC. Aortic valvular heart disease—is there a place for angiotensin-converting enzyme?. Expert Rev Cardiovasc Ther (in press)
93. Konstam MA et al (2009) Effects of high-dose versus low-dose losartan on clinical outcomes in patients with heart failure (HEAAL study): a randomised, double-blind trial. Lancet 374:1840–1848
94. McMurray JJV et al (2003) Effects of candesartan in patients with chronic heart failure and reduced left-ventricular systolic function taking angiotensin-converting-enzyme inhibitors: the CHARM-Added trial. Lancet 362:767–771
95. Lakhdar R, Al-Mallah MH, Lanfear DE (2008) Safety and tolerability of angiotensin-converting enzyme inhibitor versus the combination of angiotensin-converting enzyme inhibitor and angiotensin receptor blocker in patients with left ventricular dysfunction: a systematic review and meta-analysis of randomized controlled trials. J Card Fail 14:181–188
96. Brilla CG, Weber KT (1992) Reactive and reparative myocardial fibrosis in arterial hypertension in the rat. Cardiovasc Res 26:671–677
97. Brilla CG, Zhou G, Matsubara L, Weber KT (1994) Collagen metabolism in cultured adult rat cardiac fibroblasts: response to angiotensin II and aldosterone. J Mol Cell Cardiol 26:809–820
98. Seed A et al (2007) Neurohumoral effects of the new orally active renin inhibitor, aliskiren, in chronic heart failure. Eur J Heart Fail 9:1120–1127
99. McMurray JJV et al (2008) Effects of the oral direct renin inhibitor aliskiren in patients with symptomatic heart failure. Circ Heart Fail 1:17–24
100. Pitt B et al (2011) Neurohumoral effects of aliskiren in patients with symptomatic heart failure receiving a mineralocorticoid receptor antagonist: the Aliskiren Observation of Heart Failure Treatment study. Eur J Heart Fail 13:755–764
101. Parving HH et al (2009) Aliskiren Trial in Type 2 Diabetes Using Cardio-Renal Endpoints (ALTITUDE): rationale and study design. Nephrol Dial Transplant 24:1663–1671
102. Parving HH et al (2012) Cardiorenal end points in a trial of aliskiren for type 2 diabetes. N Engl J Med 367:2204–2213
103. Rouleau JL et al (2000) Comparison of vasopeptidase inhibitor, omapatrilat, and lisinopril on exercise tolerance and morbidity in patients with heart failure: IMPRESS randomised trial. Lancet 356:615–620
104. Packer M et al (2002) Comparison of omapatrilat and enalapril in patients with chronic heart failure: the Omapatrilat Versus Enalapril Randomized Trial of Utility in Reducing Events (OVERTURE). Circulation 106:920–926
105. Solomon SD et al (2012) The angiotensin receptor neprilysin inhibitor LCZ696 in heart failure with preserved ejection fraction: a phase 2 double-blind randomised controlled trial. Lancet 380:1387–1395
106. US National Library of Medicine. ClinicalTrial.gov [online] (2012)
107. McMurray JJV et al (2012) ESC guidelines for the diagnosis and treatment of acute and chronic heart failure 2012: the Task Force for the Diagnosis and Treatment of Acute and Chronic Heart Failure 2012 of the European Society of Cardiology: developed in collaboration with the Heart Failure Association (HFA) of the ESC. Eur J Heart Fail 14:803–869

108. Sica DA (2010) The evolution of renin-angiotensin blockade: angiotensin-converting enzyme inhibitors as the starting point. Curr Hypertens Rep 12:67–73. https://doi.org/10.1007/s11906-010-0091-9
109. Sica D, Gehr TW (2005) Angiotensin converting enzyme inhibitors. In: Oparil S, Weber M (eds) Hypertension, a companion to the kidney, 2nd edn. WB Saunders, Philadelphia, pp 669–682
110. Dzau VJ, Bernstein K, Celermajer D et al (2001) The relevance of tissue angiotensin-converting enzyme: manifestations in mechanistic and endpoint data. Am J Cardiol 88(Suppl 9):1L–20L
111. Materson BJ, Reda DJ, Cushman WC et al (1993) Single-drug therapy for hypertension in men. A comparison of six antihypertensive agents with placebo. N Engl J Med 328:914–921
112. Elliott WJ (2000) Therapeutic trials comparing angiotensin converting enzyme inhibitors and angiotensin II receptor blockers. Curr Hypertens Rep 2:402–411
113. Andersen K, Weinberger MH, Egan B et al (2008) Comparative efficacy and safety of aliskiren, an oral direct renin inhibitor, and ramipril in hypertension: a 6-month, randomized, double-blind trial. J Hypertens 26:589–599. This was one of the first trials published comparing an ACE inhibitor and a direct renin inhibitor as to comparative blood pressure reduction
114. Schiffrin EL (2001) Effects of antihypertensive drugs on vascular remodeling: do they predict outcome in response to antihypertensive therapy? Curr Opin Nephrol Hypertens 10:617–624
115. Yusuf S, Sleight P, Pogue J et al (2000) Effects of an angiotensin-converting enzyme inhibitor, ramipril, on cardiovascular events in high-risk patients. The Heart Outcomes Prevention Evaluation Study Investigators. N Engl J Med 342:145–153
116. Brenner BM, Cooper ME, de Zeeuw D et al (2001) Effects of losartan on renal and cardiovascular outcomes in patients with type 2 diabetes and nephropathy. N Engl J Med 345:861–869
117. Halkin A, Keren G (2002) Potential indications for angiotensin-converting enzyme inhibitors in atherosclerotic vascular disease. Am J Med 112:126–134
118. ALLHAT Officers and Coordinators for the ALLHAT Collaborative Research Group (2002) The Antihypertensive and Lipid-Lowering Treatment to Prevent Heart Attack Trial: major outcomes in high-risk hypertensive patients randomized to angiotensin converting enzyme inhibitor or calcium channel blocker vs diuretic. JAMA 288:1981–1997
119. Wing LM, Reid CM, Ryan P et al (2002) A comparison of outcomes with angiotensin-converting enzyme inhibitors and diuretics for hypertension in the elderly. N Engl J Med 348:583–592
120. Chobanian AV, Bakris GL, Black HR et al (2003) The seventh report of the Joint National Committee on Prevention, Detection, Evaluation, and Treatment of High Blood Pressure: the JNC 7 report. JAMA 289:2560–2572
121. Granger CB, McMurray JJ, Yusuf S et al (2003) Effects of candesartan in patients with chronic heart failure and reduced left-ventricular systolic function intolerant to angiotensin-converting-enzyme inhibitors: the CHARM-Alternative trial. Lancet 362:772–776
122. Sica DA (2001) The Heart Outcomes Prevention Evaluation study: angiotensin-converting enzyme inhibitors: are their benefits a class effect or do individual agents differ? Curr Opin Nephrol Hypertens 10:597–601
123. David D, Jallad N, Germino FW et al (1995) A comparison of the cough profile of fosinopril and enalapril in hypertensive patients with a history of ACE Inhibitor-associated cough. Am J Ther 2:806–813
124. Sharif MN, Evans BL, Pylypchuk GB (1994) Cough induced by quinapril with resolution after changing to fosinopril. Ann Pharmacother 28:720–722
125. Strauss MH, Hall AS, Narkiewicz K (2021) The combination of beta-blockers and ACE inhibitors across the spectrum of cardiovascular diseases. Cardiovasc Drugs Ther 37:757–770. https://doi.org/10.1007/s10557-021-07248-1
126. GBD 2015 Risk Factors Collaborators (2016) Global, regional, and national comparative risk assessment of 79 behavioural, environmental and occupational, and metabolic risks or

clusters of risks, 1990–2015: a systematic analysis for the Global Burden of Disease Study 2015. Lancet 388(10053):1659–1724
127. Williams B, Mancia G, Spiering W, ESC Scientific Document Group et al (2018) ESC/ESH guidelines for the management of arterial hypertension. Eur Heart J 39(33):3021–3104
128. Bangalore S, Parkar S, Grossman E, Messerli FH (2007) A meta-analysis of 94,492 patients with hypertension treated with beta blockers to determine the risk of new-onset diabetes mellitus. Am J Cardiol 100(8):1254–1262
129. Thomopoulos C, Bazoukis G, Tsioufis C, Mancia G (2020) Beta-blockers in hypertension: overview and meta-analysis of randomized outcome trials. J Hypertens 38(9):1669–1681
130. Fox KM (2003) For The EURopean trial On reduction of cardiac events with perindopril in stable coronary artery disease Investigators. Efficacy of perindopril in reduction of cardiovascular events among patients with stable coronary artery disease: randomised, double-blind, placebo-controlled, multicentre trial (the EUROPA study). Lancet 362:782–788
131. Kim YH, Her AY, Shin ES, Jeong MH (2019) Long-term clinical outcome between beta-blocker with ACEI or ARB in patients with NSTEMI who underwent PCI with drug-eluting stents. J Geriatr Cardiol 16(3):280–290
132. Chao TF, Liu CJ, Tuan TC, Chen SJ, Wang KL, Lin YJ, Chang SL, Lo LW, Hu YF, Chen TJ, Chiang CE, Chen SA (2015) Rate-control treatment and mortality in atrial fibrillation. Circulation 132(17):1604–1612
133. Yu HT, Yang PS, Lee H, You SC, Kim TH, Uhm JS, Kim JY, Pak HN, Lee MH, Joung B (2018) Outcomes of rate-control treatment in patients with atrial fibrillation and heart failure—a nationwide cohort study. Circ J 82(3):652–658
134. You SC, An MH, Yoon D, Ban GY, Yang PS, Yu HT, Park RW, Joung B (2018) Rate control and clinical outcomes in patients with atrial fibrillation and obstructive lung disease. Heart Rhythm 15(12):1825–1832
135. Ponikowski P, Voors AA, Anker SD et al (2016) For the Task Force for the diagnosis and treatment of acute and chronic heart failure of the European Society of Cardiology (ESC). 2016 ESC guidelines for the diagnosis and treatment of acute and chronic heart failure. Eur Heart J 37:2129–2200
136. Seferović PM, Fragasso G, Petrie M et al (2020) Heart Failure Association of the European Society of Cardiology update on sodium–glucose co-transporter 2 inhibitors in heart failure (an update on the sodium–glucose co-transporter 2 inhibitors in heart failure: beyond glycaemic control. A position paper of the Heart Failure Association of the European Society of Cardiology). Eur J Heart Fail 22(11):1984–1986
137. Bertrand ME, Ferrari R, Remme WJ, Simoons ML, Fox KM (2015) Perindopril and β-blocker for the prevention of cardiac events and mortality in stable coronary artery disease patients: a EUropean trial on Reduction Of cardiac events with Perindopril in stable coronary Artery disease (EUROPA) subanalysis. Am Heart J 170(6):1092–1098
138. Brugts JJ, Bertrand M, Remme W, Ferrari R, Fox K, MacMahon S et al (2017) The treatment effect of an ACE-inhibitor based regimen with perindopril in relation to beta-blocker use in 29,463 patients with vascular disease: a combined analysis of individual data of ADVANCE, EUROPA and PROGRESS trials. Cardiovasc Drugs Ther 31(4):391–400
139. Lutai MI, Golikova IP (2019) The effectiveness of treatment of patients with stable coronary heart disease and concomitant arterial hypertension: the results of a multicenter study PRESTOL. Ukrainian J Cardiol 1:19–30
140. Korennova OY, Turusheva EA, Podolnaya SP et al (2019) Efficacy and tolerability of a fixed combination of bisoprolol and perindopril in the treatment of hypertensive patients after revascularization. Arterial Hypertens 25:295–306
141. Hyman DA, Siebert VR, Birnbaum GD, Alam M, Birnbaum Y (2020) A modern history RAAS inhibition and beta blockade for heart failure to underscore the non-equivalency of ACEIs and ARBs. Cardiovasc Drugs Ther 34:215–221. https://doi.org/10.1007/s10557-020-06950-w

142. Waagstein F, Hjalmarson F, Varnauskas E, Wallentin I (1975) Effect of chronic beta-adrenergic receptor blockade in congestive cardiomyopathy. Heart 37:1022–1036. https://doi.org/10.1136/hrt.37.10.1022
143. Williams J, Bristow R, Fowler MB et al (1995) Guidelines for the evaluation and management of heart failure. Circulation 92(9):2764–2784. https://doi.org/10.1161/01.CIR.92.9.2764
144. CIBIS-II Investigators and Committees (1999) The Cardiac Insufficiency Bisoprolol Study II (CIBIS-II): a randomised trial. Lancet 353(9146):9–13
145. MERIT-HF Study Group (1999) Effect of metoprolol CR/XL in chronic heart failure: metoprolol CR/XL randomised intervention trial in congestive heart failure (MERIT-HF). Lancet 353:2001–2007
146. Hunt SA, Baker DW, Chin MH et al (2001) ACC/AHA guidelines for the evaluation and management of chronic heart failure in the adult: executive summary a report of the American College of Cardiology/American Heart Association Task Force on practice guidelines (Committee to revise the 1995 guidelines for the evaluation and management of heart failure). Circulation 104:2996–3007. https://doi.org/10.1161/hc4901.102568
147. Remme W (2001) Guidelines for the diagnosis and treatment of chronic heart failure. Eur Heart J 22(17):1527–1560. https://doi.org/10.1053/euhj.2001.2783
148. Swedberg K, Idanpaan-Heikkila U, Remes J (1987) Effects of enalapril on mortality in severe congestive heart failure. Results of the Cooperative North Scandinavian Enalapril Survival Study (CONSENSUS). N Engl J Med 316(23):1429–1435. https://doi.org/10.1056/NEJM198706043162301
149. Yusuf S, Pitt B, Davis CE, Hood WB, Cohn JN (1991) Effect of enalapril on survival in patients with reduced left ventricular ejection fractions and congestive heart failure. N Engl J Med 325(5):293–302. https://doi.org/10.1056/NEJM199108013250501
150. Shi V, Senni M, Streefkerk H, Modgill V, Zhou W, Kaplan A (2018) Angioedema in heart failure patients treated with sacubitril/valsartan (LCZ696) or enalapril in the PARADIGM-HF study. Int J Cardiol 264:118–123. https://doi.org/10.1016/j.ijcard.2018.03.121
151. McMurray JJV, Packer M, Desai AS et al (2014) Angiotensin–neprilysin inhibition versus enalapril in heart failure. N Engl J Med 371:993–1004. https://doi.org/10.1056/NEJMoa1409077
152. Yancy CW, Mariell Jessup C, Chair Biykem Bozkurt V et al (2017) Writing Group Members* 2017 ACC/AHA/HFSA focused update of the 2013 ACCF/AHA guideline for the management of heart failure ACC/AHA/HFSA focused update Yancy et al. Selection of Writing Committee members evidence review and evidence review committees class of recommendation and level of evidence. Circulation 136:137–161. https://doi.org/10.1161/CIR.0000000000000509
153. Xu W, Yang Y-M, Zhu J, Wu S, Wang J, Zhang H, Shao X-H (2022) Impact of renin–angiotensin–aldosterone-system inhibitor drugs on mortality in patients with atrial fibrillation and hypertension. BMC Cardiovasc Disord 22:141. https://doi.org/10.1186/s12872-022-02580-2
154. Wijffels MC, Kirchhof CJ, Dorland R, Allessie MA (1995) Atrial fibrillation begets atrial fibrillation. A study in awake chronically instrumented goats. Circulation 92(7):1954–1968
155. Allessie M, Ausma J, Schotten U (2002) Electrical, contractile and structural remodeling during atrial fibrillation. Cardiovasc Res 54(2):230–246
156. Nattel S, Li D (2000) Ionic remodeling in the heart: pathophysiological significance and new therapeutic opportunities for atrial fibrillation. Circ Res 87(6):440–447
157. Jalife J (2014) Mechanisms of persistent atrial fibrillation. Curr Opin Cardiol 29(1):20–27
158. Savelieva I, Kakouros N, Kourliouros A, Camm AJ (2011) Upstream therapies for management of atrial fibrillation: review of clinical evidence and implications for European Society of Cardiology guidelines. Part II: secondary prevention. Europace: European pacing, arrhythmias, and cardiac electrophysiology: journal of the working groups on cardiac pacing, arrhythmias, and cardiac cellular electrophysiology of the European Society of Cardiology. Eurospace 13(5):610–625

159. Cespón-Fernández M, Raposeiras-Roubín S, Abu-Assi E, Melendo-Viu M, García-Campo E, Íñiguez-Romo A (2021) Renin-angiotensin system inhibitors prognostic benefit in older patients with atrial fibrillation. J Am Med Direct Assoc 22:2190–2195
160. Zhang P, Zhu L, Cai J, Lei F, Qin JJ, Xie J, Liu YM, Zhao YC, Huang X, Lin L et al (2020) Association of inpatient use of angiotensin-converting enzyme inhibitors and angiotensin II receptor blockers with mortality among patients with hypertension hospitalized with COVID-19. Circ Res 126(12):1671–1681
161. Farid fahmy S, El Derany MO, Khorshid H, Saleh A, El-Demerdash E (2023) Effect of renin angiotensin blockers on angiotensin converting enzyme 2 level in cardiovascular patients. BMC Pharmacol Toxicol 24. https://doi.org/10.1186/s40360-023-00667-w
162. Ma TK, Kam KK, Yan BP, Lam YY (2010) Renin-angiotensin-aldosterone system blockade for cardiovascular diseases: current status. Br J Pharmacol 160(6):1273–1292. https://doi.org/10.1111/j.476-5381.2010.00750.x. PMID: 20590619; PMCID: PMC2938800
163. Wang JJ, Edin ML, Zeldin DC, Li C, Wang DW, Chen C (2020) Good or bad: application of RAAS inhibitors in COVID-19 patients with cardiovascular comorbidities. Pharmacol Ther 215:107628
164. Sama IE, Ravera A, Santema BT, van Goor H, Ter Maaten JM, Cleland JGF et al (2020) Circulating plasma concentrations of angiotensin-converting enzyme 2 in men and women with heart failure and effects of renin-angiotensin-aldosterone inhibitors. Eur Heart J 41(19):1810–1817
165. Chirinos JA, Cohen JB, Zhao L, Hanff T, Sweitzer N, Fang J et al (2020) Clinical and proteomic correlates of plasma ACE2 (angiotensin-converting enzyme 2) in human heart failure. Hypertension 76(5):1526–1536
166. Zhang Y, Ding X, Hua B, Liu Q, Chen H, Zhao X-Q, Li W, Li H (2020) Real-world use of ACEI/ARB in diabetic hypertensive patients before the initial diagnosis of obstructive coronary artery disease: patient characteristics and long-term follow-up outcome. J Transl Med 18:150. https://doi.org/10.1186/s12967-020-02314-y
167. American Diabetes Association (2013) Standards of medical care in diabetes-2013. Diab Care 36(Suppl 1):11–66
168. Williams B, Mancia G, Spiering W, Agabiti Rosei E, Azizi M, Burnier M, Clement DL, Coca A, de Simone G, Dominiczak A, Kahan T, Mahfoud F, Redon J, Ruilope L, Zanchetti A, Kerins M, Kjeldsen SE, Kreutz R, Laurent S, Lip GYH, McManus R, Narkiewicz K, Ruschitzka F, Schmieder RE, Shlyakhto E, Tsioufis C, Aboyans V, Desormais I, ESC Scientific Document Group, de Backer G, Heagerty AM, Agewall S, Bochud M, Borghi C, Boutouyrie P, Brguljan J, Bueno H, Caiani EG, Carlberg B, Chapman N, Cífková R, Cleland JGF, Collet JP, Coman IM, de Leeuw PW, Delgado V, Dendale P, Diener HC, Dorobantu M, Fagard R, Farsang C, Ferrini M, Graham IM, Grassi G, Haller H, Hobbs FDR, Jelakovic B, Jennings C, Katus HA, Kroon AA, Leclercq C, Lovic D, Lurbe E, Manolis AJ, McDonagh TA, Messerli F, Muiesan ML, Nixdorff U, Olsen MH, Parati G, Perk J, Piepoli MF, Polonia J, Ponikowski P, Richter DJ, Rimoldi SF, Roffi M, Sattar N, Seferovic PM, Simpson IA, Sousa-Uva M, Stanton AV, van de Borne P, Vardas P, Volpe M, Wassmann S, Windecker S, Zamorano JL, Windecker S, Aboyans V, Agewall S, Barbato E, Bueno H, Coca A, Collet JP, Coman IM, Dean V, Delgado V, Fitzsimons D, Gaemperli O, Hindricks G, Iung B, Jüni P, Katus HA, Knuuti J, Lancellotti P, Leclercq C, McDonagh TA, Piepoli MF, Ponikowski P, Richter DJ, Roffi M, Shlyakhto E, Simpson IA, Sousa-Uva M, Zamorano JL, Tsioufis C, Lurbe E, Kreutz R, Bochud M, Rosei EA, Jelakovic B, Azizi M, Januszewics A, Kahan T, Polonia J, van de Borne P, Williams B, Borghi C, Mancia G, Parati G, Clement DL, Coca A, Manolis A, Lovic D, Benkhedda S, Zelveian P, Siostrzonek P, Najafov R, Pavlova O, de Pauw M, Dizdarevic-Hudic L, Raev D, Karpettas N, Linhart A, Olsen MH, Shaker AF, Viigimaa M, Metsärinne K, Vavlukis M, Halimi JM, Pagava Z, Schunkert H, Thomopoulos C, Páll D, Andersen K, Shechter M, Mercuro G, Bajraktari G, Romanova T, Trušinskis K, Saade GA, Sakalyte G, Noppe S, DeMarco DC, Caraus A, Wittekoek J, Aksnes TA, Jankowski P, Polonia J, Vinereanu D, Baranova EI, Foscoli M, Dikic AD, Filipova S, Fras Z, Bertomeu-Martínez

V, Carlberg B, Burkard T, Sdiri W, Aydogdu S, Sirenko Y, Brady A, Weber T, Lazareva I, Backer TD, Sokolovic S, Jelakovic B, Widimsky J, Viigimaa M, Pörsti I, Denolle T, Krämer BK, Stergiou GS, Parati G, Trušinskis K, Miglinas M, Gerdts E, Tykarski A, de Carvalho Rodrigues M, Dorobantu M, Chazova I, Lovic D, Filipova S, Brguljan J, Segura J, Gottsäter A, Pechère-Bertschi A, Erdine S, Sirenko Y, Brady A (2018) 2018 ESC/ESH guidelines for the management of arterial hypertension. Eur Heart J 39:3021–3104
169. James PA, Oparil S, Carter BL et al (2014) 2014 evidence-based guideline for the management of high blood pressure in adults: report from the panel members appointed to the Eighth Joint National Committee (JNC 8). JAMA 311(5):507–520
170. Amsterdam EA, Wenger NK, Brindis RG et al (2014) 2014 AHA/ACC guideline for the management of patients with non-ST-elevation acute coronary syndromes: a report of the American College of Cardiology/American Heart Association Task Force on practice guidelines. J Am Coll Cardiol 64(24):e139–e228
171. Roffi M, Patrono C, Collet JP et al (2016) 2015 ESC guidelines for the management of acute coronary syndromes in patients presenting without persistent ST-segment elevation: task force for the management of acute coronary syndromes in patients presenting without persistent ST-segment elevation of the European Society of Cardiology (ESC). Eur Heart J 37(3):267–315
172. Yang Y, Thumula V, Pace PF, Banahan BF, Wilkin NE, Lobb WB (2010) Nonadherence to angiotensin-converting enzyme inhibitors and/or angiotensin II receptor blockers among high-risk patients with diabetes in medicare part D programs. J Am Pharm Assoc 50(4):527–531
173. Aparasu RR, Aparasu A (2008) Hypertension management in outpatient visits by diabetic patients. Res Social Adm Pharm 4(3):284–291
174. Johnson ML, Singh H (2005) Patterns of antihypertensive therapy among patients with diabetes. J Gen Intern Med 20(9):842–846
175. Kim J, Park J, Lee J-H, Min JJ, Lee S-H, Lee YT, Kim WS, Song S, Yeo JH, Cho H (2020) Comparative efficacy of angiotensin converting enzyme inhibitors and angiotensin receptor blockers after coronary artery bypass grafting. Sci Rep 10. https://doi.org/10.1038/s41598-020-58705-0
176. Perrin EC, South AM (2021) Correlation between kidney sodium and potassium handling and the renin-angiotensin-aldosterone system in children with hypertensive disorders. Pediatr Nephrol 37:633–641. https://doi.org/10.1007/s00467-021-05204-7
177. Frisancho AR, Leonard WR, Bollettino LA (1984) Blood pressure in blacks and whites and its relationship to dietary sodium and potassium intake. J Chronic Dis 37:515–519. https://doi.org/10.1016/0021-9681(84)90002-X
178. Ganguli M (1997) Higher education and income are related to a better Na:K ratio in Blacks baseline results of the Treatment of Mild Hypertension Study (TOMHS) data. Am J Hypertens 10:979–984. https://doi.org/10.1016/S0895-7061(97)00162-3
179. Walker WG, Whelton PK, Saito H, Russell RP et al (1979) Relation between blood pressure and renin, renin substrate, angiotensin II, aldosterone and urinary sodium and potassium in 574 ambulatory subjects. Hypertension 1:287–291. https://doi.org/10.1161/01.HYP.1.3.287
180. Lee S-G, Lee W, Kwon OH, Kim J-H (2013) Association of urinary sodium/creatinine ratio and urinary sodium/specific gravity unit ratio with blood pressure and hypertension: KNHANES 2009–2010. Clin Chim Acta 424:168–173. https://doi.org/10.1016/j.cca.2013.05.027
181. Flynn J (2013) The changing face of pediatric hypertension in the era of the childhood obesity epidemic. Pediatr Nephrol 28:1059–1066. https://doi.org/10.1007/s00467-012-2344-0
182. South AM, Arguelles L, Finer G, Langman CB (2017) Race, obesity, and the renin-angiotensin-aldosterone system: treatment response in children with primary hypertension. Pediatr Nephrol 32:1585–1594. https://doi.org/10.1007/s00467-017-3665-9
183. Ibrahim MM (2006) RAS inhibition in hypertension. J Hum Hypertens 20:101–108. https://doi.org/10.1038/sj.jhh.1001960
184. (2021) Pediatric Hypertension and the Renin-Angiotensin SystEm (PHRASE). https://clinicaltrials.gov/ct2/show/NCT04752293. Accessed 12 Feb 2021

185. (2019) Uric acid, klotho and salt sensitivity in young adults born preterm (PEPC3). https://clinicaltrials.gov/ct2/show/NCT04026776. Accessed 2 Nov 2020
186. Stotter BR, Ferguson MA (2018) Should ACE inhibitors and ARBs be used in combination in children? Pediatr Nephrol 34:1521–1532. https://doi.org/10.1007/s00467-018-4046-8
187. Ondetti MA, Williams NJ, Sabo EF, Pluscec J, Weaver ER, Kocy O (1971) Angiotensin-converting enzyme inhibitors from the venom of Bothrops jararaca. Isolation, elucidation of structure, and synthesis. Biochemistry 10(22):4033–4039
188. European Medicines Agency (2014) Inventory of paediatric therapeutic needs: nephro-urology. http://www.ema.europa.eu/docs/en_GB/document_library/Other/2014/09/WC500172596.pdf
189. Crowley SD, Gurley SB, Coffman TM (2007) AT(1) receptors and control of blood pressure: the kidney and more…. Trends Cardiovasc Med 17(1):30–34. https://doi.org/10.1016/j.tcm.2006.11.002
190. Siragy HM (2004) AT1 and AT2 receptor in the kidney: role in health and disease. Semin Nephrol 24(2):93–100. https://doi.org/10.1016/j.semnephrol.2003.11.009
191. Carey RM, Padia SH (2008) Angiotensin AT2 receptors: control of renal sodium excretion and blood pressure. Trends Endocrinol Metab 19(3):84–87. https://doi.org/10.1016/j.tem.2008.01.003
192. Cao Z, Bonnet F, Davis B, Allen TJ, Cooper ME (2001) Additive hypotensive and anti-albuminuric effects of angiotensin-converting enzyme inhibition and angiotensin receptor antagonism in diabetic spontaneously hypertensive rats. Clin Sci 100(6):591–599. https://doi.org/10.1042/cs1000591
193. Lassila M, Davis BJ, Allen TJ, Burrell LM, Cooper ME, Cao Z (2003) Cardiovascular hypertrophy in diabetic spontaneously hypertensive rats: optimizing blockade of the renin-angiotensin system. Clin Sci 104(4):341–347. https://doi.org/10.1042/cs1040341
194. Lo CS, Liu F, Shi Y, Maachi H, Chenier I, Godin N, Filep JG, Ingelfinger JR, Zhang SL, Chan JS (2012) Dual RAS blockade normalizes angiotensin-converting enzyme-2 expression and prevents hypertension and tubular apoptosis in Akita angiotensinogen-transgenic mice. Am J Physiol Renal Physiol 302(7):F840–F852. https://doi.org/10.1152/ajprenal.00340.2011
195. Azizi M, Chatellier G, Guyene TT, Murieta-Geoffroy D, Ménard J (1995) Additive effects of combined angiotensin-converting enzyme inhibition and angiotensin II antagonism on blood pressure and renin release in sodium-depleted normotensives. Circulation 92(4):825–834. https://doi.org/10.1161/01.CIR.92.4.825
196. Azizi M, Guyene TT, Chatellier G, Wargon M, Ménard J (1997) Additive effects of losartan and enalapril on blood pressure and plasma active renin. Hypertension 29(2):634–640. https://doi.org/10.1161/01.HYP.29.2.634
197. Weir MR, Weber MA, Neutel JM, Vendetti J, Michelson EL, Wang RY (2001) Efficacy of candesartan cilexetil as add-on therapy in hypertensive patients uncontrolled on background therapy: a clinical experience trial. ACTION study investigators. Am J Hypertens 14(6 Pt 1):567–572. https://doi.org/10.1016/S0895-7061(00)01304-2
198. Russo D, Pisani A, Balletta MM, De Nicola L, Savino FA, Andreucci M, Minutolo R (1999) Additive antiproteinuric effect of converting enzyme inhibitor and losartan in normotensive patients with IgA nephropathy. Am J Kidney Dis 33(5):851–856. https://doi.org/10.1016/S0272-6386(99)70416-6
199. Luño J, Barrio V, Goicoechea MA, González C, de Vinuesa SG, Gómez F, Bernis C, Espinosa M, Ahijado F, Gómez J, Escalada P (2002) Effects of dual blockade of the renin-angiotensin system in primary proteinuric nephropathies. Kidney Int Supp 82:S47–S52. https://doi.org/10.1046/j.1523-1755.62.s82.10.x
200. Kanno Y, Takenaka T, Nakamura T, Suzuki H (2006) Add-on angiotensin receptor blocker in patients who have proteinuric chronic kidney diseases and are treated with angiotensin-converting enzyme inhibitors. Clin J Am Soc Nephrol 1(4):730–737. https://doi.org/10.2215/CJN.01110905

201. Chandar J, Abitbol C, Montané B, Zilleruelo G (2007) Angiotensin blockade as sole treatment for proteinuric kidney disease in children. Nephrol Dial Transplant 22(5):1332–1337. https://doi.org/10.1093/ndt/gfl839
202. Lubrano R, Soscia F, Elli M, Ventriglia F, Raggi C, Travasso E, Scateni S, Di Maio V, Versacci P, Masciangelo R, Romero S (2006) Renal and cardiovascular effects of angiotensin-converting enzyme inhibitor plus angiotensin II receptor antagonist therapy in children with proteinuria. Pediatrics 118(3):e833–e838. https://doi.org/10.1542/peds.2005-2053
203. Chan KE, Ikazler TA, Gamboa JL, Yu C, Hakim RM, Brown NJ (2011) Combined angiotensin-converting enzyme inhibition and receptor blockade associate with increased risk of cardiovascular death in hemodialysis patients. Kidney Int 80(9):978–985. https://doi.org/10.1038/ki.2011.228
204. Kido R, Akizawa T, Fukagawa M, Onishi Y, Yamaguchi T, Fukuhara S (2017) Interactive effectiveness of angiotensin-converting enzyme inhibitors and angiotensin receptor blockers or their combination on survival of hemodialysis patients. Am J Nephrol 46(6):439–447. https://doi.org/10.1159/000482013
205. Verdecchia P, Angeli F, Mazzotta G, Martire P, Garofoli M, Gentile G, Reboldi G (2010) Aliskiren versus ramipril in hypertension. Ther Adv Cardiovasc Dis 4(3):193–200. https://doi.org/10.1177/1753944710369682
206. Pool JL, Schmieder RE, Azizi M, Aldigier JC, Januszewicz A, Zidek W, Chiang Y, Satlin A (2007) Aliskiren, an orally effective renin inhibitor, provides antihypertensive efficacy alone and in combination with valsartan. Am J Hypertens 20(1):11–20. https://doi.org/10.1016/j.amjhyper.2006.06.003
207. Solomon SD, Appelbaum E, Manning WJ, Verma A, Berglund T, Lukashevich V, Cherif Papst C, Smith BA, Dahlöf B, Aliskiren in Left Ventricular Hypertrophy (ALLAY) Trial Investigators (2009) Effect of the direct renin inhibitor aliskiren, the angiotensin receptor blocker losartan, or both on left ventricular mass in patients with hypertension and left ventricular hypertrophy. Circulation 119(4):530–537. https://doi.org/10.1161/CIRCULATIONAHA.108.826214
208. Parving HH, Persson F, Lewis JB, Lewis EJ, Hollenberg NK, AVOID Study Investigators (2008) Aliskiren combined with losartan in type 2 diabetes and nephropathy. N Engl J Med 358(23):2433–2446. https://doi.org/10.1056/NEJMoa0708379
209. Uzu T, Araki SI, Kashiwagi A, Haneda M, Koya D, Yokoyama H, Kida Y, Ikebuchi M, Nakamura T, Nishimura M, Takahara N, Obata T, Omichi N, Sakamoto K, Shingu R, Taki H, Nagai Y, Tokuda H, Kitada M, Misawa M, Nishiyama A, Kobori H, Maegawa H, Shiga Committee for Preventing Diabetic Nephropathy (2016) Comparative effects of direct renin inhibitor and angiotensin receptor blocker on albuminuria in hypertensive patients with type 2 diabetes—a randomized controlled trial. PLoS One 11(12):e0165936. https://doi.org/10.1371/journal.pone.0164936
210. Soji K, Doi S, Nakashima A, Sasaki K, Kawai T, Aoki A, Kyuden Y, Fujiwara K, Yokoyama Y, Masaki T (2015) Efficacy of add-on therapy of aliskiren to an angiotensin II receptor blocker on renal outcomes in advanced-stage chronic kidney disease: a prospective, randomized, open-label study. Clin Exp Nephrol 19(4):631–638. https://doi.org/10.1007/s10157-014-1044-4
211. Li SY, Chen YT, Yang WC, Tarng DC, Lin CC, Yang CY, Liu WS (2012) Effect of add-on direct renin inhibitor aliskiren in patients with non-diabetes related chronic kidney disease. BMC Nephrol 13:89. https://doi.org/10.1186/1471-2369-13-89
212. Esteghamati A, Noshad S, Jarrah S, Mousavizadeh M, Khoee SH, Nakhjavani M (2013) Long-term effects of addition of mineralocorticoid receptor antagonist to angiotensin II receptor blocker in patients with diabetic nephropathy: a randomized clinical trial. Nephrol Dial Transplant 28(11):2823–2833. https://doi.org/10.1093/ndt/gft281
213. Helten C, Mourikis P, Dannenberg L, M'Pembele R, Trojovsky K, Ayhan A, Kohlmorgen C, Grandoch M, Levkau B, Veulemans V, Petzold T, Hohlfeld T, Kelm M, Zeus T, Polzin A (2020) A novel mechanism of ACE inhibition–associated enhanced platelet reactivity: dis-

proof of the ARB-MI paradox? Eur J Clin Pharmacol 76:1245–1251. https://doi.org/10.1007/s00228-020-02915-y
214. Messerli FH, Bangalore S (2017) Angiotensin receptor blockers reduce cardiovascular events, including the risk of myocardial infarction. Circulation 135:2085–2087. https://doi.org/10.1161/CIRCULATIONAHA.116.025950
215. van Vark LC, Bertrand M, Akkerhuis KM, Brugts JJ, Fox K, Mourad JJ, Boersma E (2012) Angiotensin-converting enzyme inhibitors reduce mortality in hypertension: a meta-analysis of randomized clinical trials of renin-angiotensin-aldosterone system inhibitors involving 158,998 patients. Eur Heart J 33:2088–2097
216. Reboldi G, Angeli F, Cavallini C, Gentile G, Mancia G, Verdecchia P (2008) Comparison between angiotensin-converting enzyme inhibitors and angiotensin receptor blockers on the risk of myocardial infarction, stroke and death: a meta-analysis. J Hypertens 26:1282–1289
217. Ettehad D, Emdin CA, Kiran A, Anderson SG, Callender T, Emberson J, Chalmers J, Rodgers A, Rahimi K (2016) Blood pressure lowering for prevention of cardiovascular disease and death: a systematic review and meta-analysis. Lancet 387:957–967
218. Messerli FH, Bangalore S, Bavishi C, Rimoldi SF (2018) Angiotensin-converting enzyme inhibitors in hypertension: to use or not to use? J Am Coll Cardiol 71(13):1474–1482. https://doi.org/10.1016/j.jacc.2018.01.058
219. Strauss MH, Hall AS (2006) Angiotensin receptor blockers may increase risk of myocardial infarction: unraveling the ARB-MI paradox. Circulation 114(8):838–854
220. Tantry US, Bonello L, Aradi D, Price MJ, Jeong YH, Angiolillo DJ, Stone GW, Curzen N, Geisler T, Ten Berg J, Kirtane A, Siller-Matula J, Mahla E, Becker RC, Bhatt DL, Waksman R, Rao SV, Alexopoulos D, Marcucci R, Reny JL, Trenk D, Sibbing D, Gurbel PA, Working Group on On-Treatment Platelet R (2013) Consensus and update on the definition of on-treatment platelet reactivity to adenosine diphosphate associated with ischemia and bleeding. J Am Coll Cardiol 62:2261–2273
221. Antoniak S, Cardenas JC, Buczek LJ, Church FC, Mackman N, Pawlinski R (2017) Protease-activated receptor 1 contributes to angiotensin ii-induced cardiovascular remodeling and inflammation. Cardiology 136:258–268
222. Tamargo J, Caballero R, Delpón E (2018) New therapeutic approaches for the treatment of hyperkalemia in patients treated with renin-angiotensin-aldosterone system inhibitors. Cardiovasc Drugs Ther 32:99–119. https://doi.org/10.1007/s10557-017-6767-5
223. Palmer BF (2015) Regulation of potassium homeostasis. Clin J Am Soc Nephrol 10:1050–1060
224. McCormick JA, Ellison DH (2015) Distal convoluted tubule. Compr Physiol 5:45–98
225. Ellison DH, Terker AS, Gamba G (2016) Potassium and its discontents: new insight, new treatments. J Am Soc Nephrol 27:981–989
226. Welling PA (2016) Roles and regulation of renal K channels. Annu Rev Physiol 78(1):415–435
227. Youn JH, McDonough AA (2009) Recent advances in understanding integrative control of potassium homeostasis. Annu Rev Physiol 71:381–401
228. Gumz ML, Rabinowitz L, Wingo C (2015) An integrated view of potassium homeostasis. N Engl J Med 373:60–72
229. Epstein M, Lifschitz MD (2016) The unappreciated role of extrarenal and gut sensors in modulating renal potassium handling: implications for diagnosis of dyskalemias and interpreting clinical trials. Kidney Int Rep 1(1):43–56
230. Wang W (2004) Regulation of renal K transport by dietary K intake. Annu Rev Physiol 66:547–569
231. Nyirenda MJ, Tang JI, Padfield PL, Seckl JR (2009) Hyperkalaemia. BMJ 339:b4114
232. Kovedsky CP (2017) Updates in hyperkalemia: outcomes and therapeutic strategies. Rev Endocr Metab Disord 18:41–47
233. Phillips BM, Milner S, Zouwail S, Roberts G, Cowan M, Riley SG et al (2014) Severe hyperkalaemia: demographics and outcome. Clin Kidney J 7:127–133
234. Paice B, Gray JM, McBride D, Donnelly T, Lawson DH (1983) Hyperkalaemia in patients in hospital. Br Med J (Clin Res Ed) 286:1189–1192

235. Acker CG, Johnson JP, Palevsky PM, Greenberg A (1998) Hyperkalemia in hospitalized patients: causes, adequacy of treatment, and results of an attempt to improve physician compliance with published therapy guidelines. Arch Intern Med 158(8):917–924
236. Stevens MS, Dunlay RW (2000) Hyperkalemia in hospitalized patients. Int Urol Nephrol 32:177–180
237. An JN, Lee JP, Jeon HJ, Kim DH, Oh YK, Kim YS et al (2012) Severe hyperkalemia requiring hospitalization: predictors of mortality. Crit Care 16:R225
238. McMahon GM, Mendu ML, Gibbons FK, Christopher KB (2012) Association between hyperkalemia at critical care initiation and mortality. Intensive Care Med 38:1834–1842
239. Khanagavi J, Gupta T, Aronow WS, Shah T, Garg J, Ahn C et al (2014) Hyperkalemia among hospitalized patients and association between duration of hyperkalemia and outcomes. Arch Med Sci 2:251–257
240. Dunn JD, Benton WW, Orozco-Torrentera E, Adamson RT (2015) The burden of hyperkalemia in patients with cardiovascular and renal disease. Am J Manag Care 21(15 Suppl):s307–s301
241. Alfonzo A, Soar J, MacTier R, Fox J, Shillday I, Nolan J et al. Clinical practical guidelines. Treatment of acute hyperkalaemia in adults. http://www.renal.org/docs/default-source/default-document-library/hyperkalaemia-guideline%2D%2D-march-2014.pdf. Accessed 1 Sept 2017
242. Aslam S, Friedman EA, Ifudu O (2002) Electrocardiography is unreliable in detecting potentially lethal hyperkalaemia in haemodialysis patients. Nephrol Dial Transplant 17:1639–1642
243. Einhorn LM, Zhan M, Hsu VD, Walker LD, Moen MF, Seliger SL et al (2009) The frequency of hyperkalemia and its significance in chronic kidney disease. Arch Intern Med 169(12):1156–1162
244. Go AS, Chertow GM, Fan D, McCulloch CE, Hsu CY (2004) Chronic kidney disease and the risks of death, cardiovascular events, and hospitalization. N Engl J Med 351:1296–1305
245. Ahn SY, Ryu J, Baek SH, Kim S, Na KY, Kim KW et al (2013) Incident chronic kidney disease and newly developed complications related to renal dysfunction in an elderly population during 5 years: a community-based elderly population cohort study. PLoS One 8(12):e84467
246. Kidney Disease: Improving Global Outcomes (KDIGO) CKD Work Group (2013) KDIGO 2012 clinical practice guideline for the evaluation and management of chronic kidney disease. Kidney Int 3:S1–S150
247. National Institute for Health and Care Excellence (NICE). Chronic kidney disease: early identification and management of chronic kidney disease in adults in primary and secondary care. National Institute for Health and Care Excellence website. http://www.nice.org.uk/guidance/cg182. Accessed 4 Sept 2017
248. Weinberg JM, Appel LJ, Bakris G, Gassman JJ, Greene T, Kendrick CA et al (2009) Risk of hyperkalemia in nondiabetic patients with chronic kidney disease receiving antihypertensive therapy. Arch Intern Med 169:1587–1594
249. Moranne O, Froissart M, Rossert J, Gauci C, Boffa JJ, Haymann JP et al (2009) Timing of onset of CKD-related metabolic complications. J Am Soc Nephrol 20:164–171
250. Sarafidis PA, Blacklock R, Wood E, Rumjon A, Simmonds S, Fletcher-Rogers J et al (2012) Prevalence and factors associated with hyperkalemia in predialysis patients followed in a low-clearance clinic. Clin J Am Soc Nephrol 7(8):1234–1241
251. Drawz PE, Babineau DC, Rahman M (2012) Metabolic complications in elderly adults with chronic kidney disease. J Am Geriatr Soc 60(2):310–315
252. Kidney Disease Outcomes Quality Initiative (K/DOQI) (2004) K/DOQI clinical practice guidelines on hypertension and antihypertensive agents in chronic kidney disease. Am J Kidney Dis 43(5 Suppl 1):S1–S290
253. Weir MR, Rolfe M (2010) Potassium homeostasis and renin-angiotensin-aldosterone system inhibitors. Clin J Am Soc Nephrol 5(3):531–538
254. Desai A (2008) Hyperkalemia associated with inhibitors of the renin-angiotensin-aldosterone system: balancing risk and benefit. Circulation 118(16):1609–1611

255. Maddirala S, Khan A, Vincent A, Lau K (2008) Effect of angiotensin converting enzyme inhibitors and angiotensin receptor blockers on serum potassium levels and renal function in ambulatory outpatients: risk factors analysis. Am J Med Sci 336:330–335
256. Ramadan FH, Masoodi N, El-Solh AA (2005) Clinical factors associate with hyperkalemia in patients with congestive heart failure. J Clin Pharm Ther 30(3):233–239
257. Palmer BF (2004) Managing hyperkalemia caused by inhibitors of the renin–angiotensin–aldosterone system. N Engl J Med 351:585–592
258. Sarwar CM, Papadimitriou L, Pitt B, Piña I, Zannad F, Anker SD et al (2016) Hyperkalemia in heart failure. J Am Coll Cardiol 68:1575–1589
259. Raebel MA (2012) Hyperkalemia associated with use of angiotensin-converting enzyme inhibitors and angiotensin receptor blockers. Cardiovasc Ther 30:e156–e166
260. Pitt B, Remme W, Zannad F, Neaton J, Martinez F, Roniker B et al (2003) Eplerenone, a selective aldosterone blocker, in patients with left ventricular dysfunction after myocardial infarction. N Engl J Med 348(14):1309–1321
261. de Denus S, Tardif J-C, White M, Bourassa MG, Racine N, Levesque S et al (2006) Quantification of the risk and predictors of hyperkalemia in patients with left ventricular dysfunction: a retrospective analysis of the Studies of Left Ventricular Dysfunction (SOLVD) trials. Am Heart J 152(4):705–712
262. Navaneethan SD, Nigwekar SU, Sehgal AR, Strippoli GF (2009) Aldosterone antagonists for preventing the progression of chronic kidney disease: a systematic review and meta-analysis. Clin J Am Soc Nephrol 4:542–551
263. Raebel MA, Ross C, Xu S, Roblin DW, Cheetham C, Blanchette CM et al (2010) Diabetes and drug-associated hyperkalemia: effect of potassium monitoring. J Gen Intern Med 25(4):326–333
264. MacKinnon M, Shurraw S, Akbari A, Knoll GA, Jaffey J, Clark HD (2006) Combination therapy with an angiotensin receptor blocker and an ACE inhibitor in proteinuric renal disease: a systematic review of the efficacy and safety data. Am J Kidney Dis 48:8–20
265. Shah KB, Rao K, Sawyer R, Gottlieb SS (2005) The adequacy of laboratory monitoring in patients treated with spironolactone for congestive heart failure. J Am Coll Cardiol 46(5):845–849
266. Raebel MA, McClure DL, Simon SR et al (2007) Laboratory monitoring of potassium and creatinine in ambulatory patients receiving angiotensin converting enzyme inhibitors and angiotensin receptor blockers. Pharmacoepidemiol Drug Saf 16:55–64
267. Ouwerkerk W, Voors AA, Anker SD, Cleland JG, Dickstein K, Filippatos G et al (2017) Determinants and clinical outcome of uptitration of ACE-inhibitors and beta-blockers in patients with heart failure: a prospective European study. Eur Heart J 38(24):1883–1890
268. Epstein M, Alvarez PJ, Reaven NL, Funk SE, McGaughey KJ, Brenner MS et al (2016) Evaluation of clinical outcomes and costs based on prescribed dose level of renin-angiotensin-aldosterone system inhibitors. Am J Manag Care 22(11 Suppl):s311–s324
269. Weisberg LS (2008) Management of severe hyperkalemia. Crit Care Med 36:3246–3251
270. Elliott MJ, Ronksley PE, Clase CM, Ahmed SB, Hemmelgarn BR (2010) Management of patients with acute hyperkalemia. CMAJ 182:1631–1635
271. Kovesdy CP (2015) Management of hyperkalemia: an update for the internist. Am J Med 128:1281–1287
272. Pitt B, Bakris GL (2015) New potassium binders for the treatment of hyperkalemia: current data and opportunities for the future. Hypertension 66:731–738
273. Fordjour KN, Walton T, Doran JJ (2014) Management of hyperkalemia in hospitalized patients. Am J Med Sci 347:93–100
274. Rossignol P, Legrand M, Kosiborod M, Hollenberg SM, Peacock WF, Emmett M et al (2016) Emergency management of severe hyperkalemia: guideline for best practice and opportunities for the future. Pharmacol Res 113:585–591

275. Bushinsky DA, Williams GH, Pitt B, Weir MR, Freeman MW, Garza D et al (2015) Patiromer induces rapid and sustained potassium lowering in patients with chronic kidney disease and hyperkalemia. Kidney Int 88(6):1427–1433
276. Pitt B, Bakris GL, Bushinsky DA, Garza D, Mayo MR, Stasiv Y et al (2015) Effect of patiromer on reducing serum potassium and preventing recurrent hyperkalaemia in patients with heart failure and chronic kidney disease on RAAS inhibitors. Eur J Heart Fail 17:1057–1065

Chapter 2
Role of Anti-hypertensive Agents in Cardiovascular Disorders

Mukesh Nandave

Introduction by the Editor

Hypertension is one of the major causes of cardiovascular complications and its global prevalence continues to rise. Globally, over half of the hypertensive patients have greater than 140 mmHg (systolic) and 80 mmHg (diastolic) blood pressure. In different parts of Asia, prevalence of hypertension lies between 15% and 35%. Hypertension management is poorer in Asia majorly in China and India [1]. The rising prevalence of hypertension is associated with ageing, population growth, excessive use of alcohol, unhealthy diet, sedentary life style, obesity, and continuous exposure to stress. Hypertension leads to reduced life expectancy and increases the risk of early development of cardiovascular events. With ageing systolic blood pressure increases progressively in both genders. However, it is reported that blood pressure is significantly high in men in comparison to women in their early adulthood [2].

Hypertension can lead to retinopathy, cognitive impairment, vascular stiffness, microalbuminuria, and other disorders. Hypertension is one of the major factors that contribute to cardiovascular complications. Hypertension leads to structural and functional modifications including diastolic dysfunction, endothelial dysfunction, dysrhythmias. Adherence to anti-hypertensive agents plays a crucial role in hypertension management. Treatment with anti-hypertensive agents is necessary to decrease the relative risk of stroke and other cardiovascular disease. However, adherence to anti-hypertensive agents is still a challenge among the patients due to its asymptomatic nature and indefinite duration of treatment. Therefore, successful rate of treatment depends on adherence to therapy [3]. According to the reports,

M. Nandave (✉)
Department of Pharmacology, Delhi Pharmaceutical Sciences and Research University, New Delhi, Delhi, India

M. Nandave (ed.), *Angiotensin-converting Enzyme Inhibitors vs. Angiotensin Receptor Blockers*, https://doi.org/10.1007/978-981-97-7380-0_2

patients who have high adherence to the anti-hypertensive therapies are more likely to have controlled blood pressure than patients who have medium or low adherence to anti-hypertensive agents. According to the World Health Organization (WHO) medicine adherence is "the extent to which a person's behavior-taking medications, following a diet, and/or executing lifestyle changes corresponds with agreed recommendations from a healthcare provider."

Anti-hypertensive agents improve endothelial dysfunction which in turn is essential for proper blood vessel functioning. Thus, reducing risk of atherosclerosis [4]. Anti-hypertensive agents are administered as primary prevention to prevent the risk of cardiovascular events in hypertensive patients and as secondary prevention to prevent the risk of subsequent cardiovascular events.

Anti-hypertensive agents, especially Angiotensin Converting Enzyme (ACE) Inhibitors, Angiotensin Receptor Blockers (ARBs) and beta blockers slow down the progression of heart failure. Moreover, these agents improve symptoms, reduce hospitalization and mortality in heart failure patients. However, ACEI and ARBs not only showed efficacy in the treatment of cardiovascular complications but also found to be reno-protective [5]. Long term therapy of ACE inhibitors reduces the risk of left ventricular hypertrophy, improving endothelial function. ACE inhibitors and ARBs were found to improve renal function as well. Thus, anti-hypertensive agents play a pivotal role in the management and treatment of cardiovascular disorders.

This chapter explores the significant role of anti-hypertensive agents, specifically ACE) Inhibitors and ARBs in the treatment of cardiovascular disorders. ACE inhibitors and ARBs are characterized by their specific action on Renin-Angiotensin-Aldosterone System (RAAS), these interventions have transformed the process of hypertension management and its complications. This chapter discusses the association between ACE levels and different cardiovascular complications, targeting these enzymes with anti-hypertensive agents is one of the most effective ways to treat and manage cardiovascular disorders. This chapter also explains the complex mechanism of ACE inhibitors and ARBs in the management and treatment of several cardiovascular complications by targeting specifically RAAS. This chapter provides a deeper understanding of the significant role of ACE inhibitors and ARBs as anti-hypertensive agents and in the treatment of cardiovascular complications to the clinician, researchers, and students (Fig. 2.1).

Machine Generated Summaries

Disclaimer: The summaries in this chapter were generated from Springer Nature publications using extractive AI auto-summarization: An extraction-based summarizer aims to identify the most important sentences of a text using an algorithm and

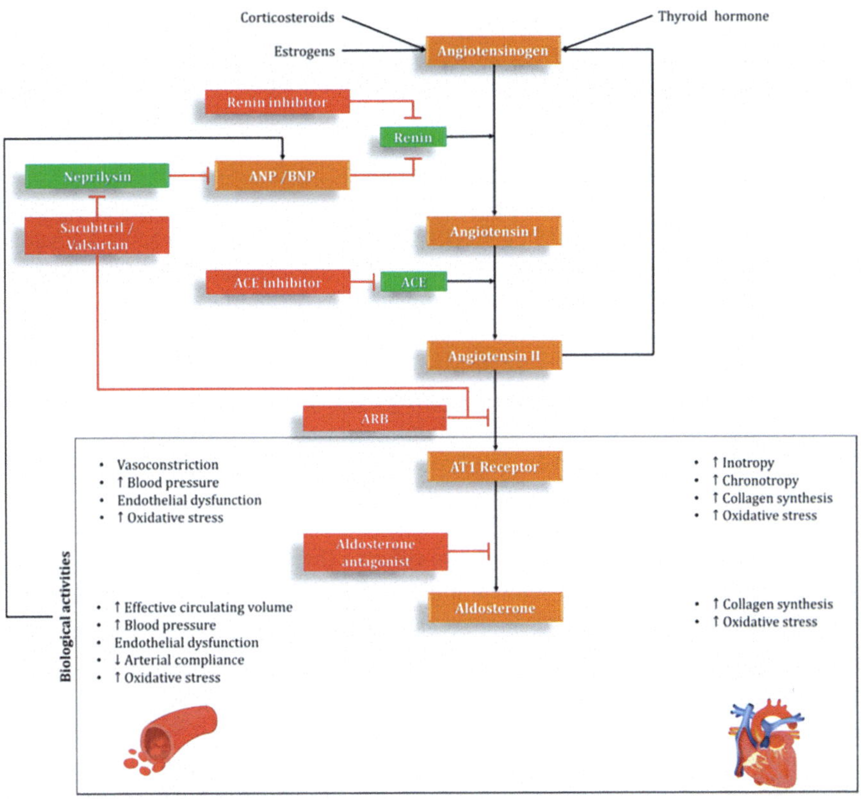

Fig. 2.1 Simplified flowchart of the renin-angiotensin-aldosterone system(RAAS) showing the site of actions of RAAS blockers and the biological effects of the RAAS active products on the heart and blood vessels. Orange boxes represent endogenous substrates/peptides, green boxes endogenous enzymes and red boxes drugs. *ACE* angiotensin converting enzyme, *ANP* atrial natriuretic peptide, *ARB* angiotensin II receptor blockers, *AT1 receptor* angiotensin II receptor type 1, *BNP* brain natriuretic peptide. (Source: Pugliese et al. [6])

uses those original sentences to create the auto-summary (unlike generative AI). As the constituted sentences are machine selected, they may not fully reflect the body of the work, so we strongly advise that the original content is read and cited. The auto generated summaries were curated by the editor to meet Springer Nature publication standards. To cite this content, please refer to the original papers.

Machine generated keywords: soluble, rct, vascular, antihypertensive drug, hypertensive patient, safety, pool, modulation, adverse event, followup, antihypertensive, hypertensive, arb, plasma, ace.

Soluble Angiotensin-Converting Enzyme Levels in Heart Failure or Acute Coronary Syndrome: Revisiting Its Modulation and Prognosis Value [7]

This is a machine-generated summary of:

Almengló, Cristina; Couselo-Seijas, Marinela; Agra, Rosa M.; Varela-Román, Alfonso; García-Acuña, José M.; González-Peteiro, Mercedes; González-Juanatey, José R.; Eiras, Sonia; Álvarez, Ezequiel: Soluble angiotensin-converting enzyme levels in heart failure or acute coronary syndrome: revisiting its modulation and prognosis value [7].

Published in: Journal of Molecular Medicine (2021).

Link to original: https://doi.org/10.1007/s00109-021-02129-4

If you want to cite the papers, please refer to the original.

For technical reasons we could not place the page where the original quote is coming from.

Abstract-Summary "The main objective was to compare the meaning of soluble angiotensin-converting enzyme-2 (sACE2) plasma levels modulation on the prognosis of two cohorts of heart failure (HF) and acute coronary syndrome (ACS)."

"We conducted an observational clinical study where sACE2 was measured in two cohorts of HF or ACS (102 patients each), matched by age and gender."

"The levels of sACE2 were significantly higher in the HF than ACS cohort."

"The levels of sACE2 were related to long-term prognosis and confirmed as a non-independent predictor in the HF cohort."

"Plasma levels of sACE2 were higher in HF than in ACS, independently of age and gender, and were related to long-term cardiac death in the HF cohort."

"Losartan and metoprolol, but not enalapril, upregulated ACE expression in endothelial cells, accordingly with higher levels of sACE2 in patients using these drugs."

Highlights

"Soluble ACE2 levels are elevated in heart failure in comparison with the acute coronary syndrome."

"Soluble ACE2 is related to the long-term prognosis of death in heart failure."

"Levels of soluble ACE2 could be affected by angiotensin receptor blockers and ß-blockers."

Introduction

"Despite the beneficial effects of ACE2, its elevated circulating levels and activity have been related to poor prognosis in patients with cardiovascular diseases."

"It has been recently reported that increased plasma ACE2 levels are associated with an increased risk of major cardiovascular events in the general population [8]."

"Although there is no consensus, drugs targeting RAAS as renin inhibitors, ACE inhibitors (ACEI), angiotensin receptor type I blockers (ARB) and aldosterone antagonists and the cardiovascular disease itself could modulate ACE2 expression and/or ACE2 activity."

"High levels of ACE2 expression have been reported in patients with HF [9], where high levels of soluble ACE2 (sACE2) were correlated with the severity of the disease independently of other disease states and medication used [10]."

"The apparent paradox between the beneficial effects of ACE2 activity and its relationship with poor prognosis or cardiovascular risk is also translated to the case of novel infectious coronavirus disease 2019 (COVID-19)."

"ACE2 activity counteracts the balance of the RAAS, which participates in the progression of cardiovascular diseases of patients suffering from COVID-19 [11–13]."

Materials and Methods

"In the cohort of HF, patients with acute coronary syndrome and/or who had undergone myocardial revascularisation in the previous 3 months were also excluded to avoid the influence of concomitant coronary artery disease at the moment of inclusion."

"In the cohort of ACS, patients with previous myocardial infarction, a history of HF, cardiomyopathy or moderate/severe valvular heart disease, prior stroke, arterial or venous thromboembolic disease or peripheral artery disease were excluded to avoid simultaneity of HF and previously established symptomatic ischemic disease."

"Human umbilical vein endothelial cells (HUVEC) were isolated from freshly obtained human umbilical cords donated under informed consent from mothers, following the method previously described [14] and detailed in the Supplementary Material."

"The student t-test was used to compare continuous variables between groups of patients (two tail distribution and equal variances between samples) when variables fulfilled the condition of normality, whereas the Mann–Whitney U test was used when not."

Results

"We found higher levels of sACE2 in patients under treatment with β-blockers, although the percentage of use of these drugs in each cohort is quite different (86% in HF, 9% in ACS)."

"Patients with events in the HF cohort showed more incidence of reduced LVEF and GFR and higher NTproBNP and sACE2 levels."

"In the ACS cohort, more patients presented reduced LVEF, were diabetic and presented higher glycated haemoglobin levels and lower body mass index, but no differences were observed in sACE2 levels."

"Although sACE2 levels, considered a continuous variable, showed a significant value for predicting secondary events ($p = 0.030$) and the combination of MACE ($p = 0.030$) by the univariate Cox regression tests in the HF cohort, they did not reach statistical significance in the multivariate regression models for long-term prognosis adjusted by age, gender, diabetes mellitus, reduced GFR and reduced LVEF."

Discussion

"Pharmacotherapy with ACEI did not influence sACE2 plasma levels in both cohorts, but ARB or β-blockers could enhance ACE2 expression in the endothelium and blood."

"In our in vitro experiments, a direct correlation between the expression levels of ACE2 at the mRNA level, protein level and sACE2 were observed, but angiotensin II did not increase sACE2."

"We did not observe an increase in sACE2 levels in the ACS cohort, whereas the elevation of sACE2 activity was reported in patients with an acute myocardial infarction after 7 days [15]."

"The sACE2 plasma levels were higher in patients on β-blockers."

"In the case of metoprolol, the increased levels of sACE2 observed in patients treated with β-blockers agree with the increased expression of all forms of ACE2 at the cellular level."

Conclusions

"Higher levels of sACE2 were observed in patients with HF than in those with ACS, independently of age and gender."

"No such associations were observed in the ACS cohort, where sACE2 levels were only related to age and glycaemic parameters."

"ARB and β-blockers were associated with higher levels of sACE2, and both types of drugs enhanced ACE2 and sACE2 expression on human endothelial cells in vitro."

Determinants of Soluble Angiotensin-Converting Enzyme 2 Concentrations in Adult Patients with Complex Congenital Heart Disease [16]

This is a machine-generated summary of:

Raedle-Hurst, Tanja; Wissing, Sarah; Mackenstein, Nils; Obeid, Rima; Geisel, Juergen; Wagenpfeil, Stefan; Abdul-Khaliq, Hashim: Determinants of soluble angiotensin-converting enzyme 2 concentrations in adult patients with complex congenital heart disease [16].

Published in: Clinical Research in Cardiology (2020).

Link to original: https://doi.org/10.1007/s00392-020-01782-y

If you want to cite the papers, please refer to the original.

For technical reasons we could not place the page where the original quote is coming from.

Abstract-Summary "SACE2 concentrations were significantly elevated in patients with a higher NYHA class ≥III (1856.2 pg/ml vs 714.5 pg/ml in patients with NYHA class I/II, $p < 0.001$)."

"Using linear regression analysis, higher sACE2 levels were associated with a higher NYHA class ≥III, more severe CHD, a morphological left systemic ventricle, higher creatinine and the use of mineralocorticoid receptor antagonists (MRA) in the univariable model."

"The use of ACE inhibitors or angiotensin receptor blockers (ARB) was associated with lower sACE2 levels."

"In the multivariable model, higher sACE2 levels were independently associated with a higher NYHA class ≥III ($p = 0.002$) and lower sACE2 levels with the use of ACE inhibitors or ARB ($p = 0.001$)."

"Soluble ACE2 concentrations were significantly increased in all types of complex CHD with highest levels found in patients with NYHA class ≥III."

"A higher NYHA class ≥III was the most significant determinant that was independently associated with elevated sACE2 concentrations."

Introduction

"Several epidemiological studies have also shown the severity of the SARS-CoV-2 disease (COVID-19) in older patients and particularly those with cardiovascular rather than pulmonary predisposing risk factors [17–19]."

"SACE2 concentrations were found to be elevated in men and older patients with different cardiovascular morbidities, such as hypertension, diabetes, coronary heart disease and heart failure [18, 20–24]."

"These interactions of ACE2 may explain the higher vulnerability and predisposition of such patients to have a severe or fatal outcome after SARS-CoV-2 infection [25–27]."

"An increased vulnerability of older and male patients with cardiovascular disease or heart failure can be seen that could also be related to increased sACE2 levels [20–22, 28]."

"In adult patients with complex CHD who often present with altered myocardial function or even symptomatic heart failure, data on sACE2 levels are lacking."

Methods

"In our outpatient clinic for adults with CHD, several prospective studies for the evaluation of different biomarkers in serum as well as micro-RNA signatures in whole blood had been performed in the past [29–31]."

"To assess sACE2 concentrations, existing serum samples of these patients frozen at -80° C representing the pre-COVID-19 era were used for analysis."

"Serum samples of 182 consecutive patients with complex CHD ≥18 years of age who were regularly seen in our outpatient clinic between 22/01/2015 and 02/12/2019 were analyzed in the present study."

"Mean age was 30.1 ± 10.5 years (range 18–62 years) and 103 patients were male (56.6%)."

"All patients and healthy controls gave written informed consent before enrollment."

"In the patient group, routine laboratory tests, such as liver function tests and creatinine measurements, were performed using standard laboratory techniques."

"All biochemical analyses were performed by investigators blinded to the clinical and echocardiographic data of the patients."

Results

"In patients with complex CHD, sACE2 levels ranged from 55.0 to 4526.1 pg/ml with a median of 761.9 pg/ml (419.2–1277.7 pg/ml) and were significantly elevated as compared to healthy controls showing a median sACE2 level of 365.2 pg/ml (237.7–656.3 pg/ml; $p < 0.001$)."

"Patients with a systemic morphological left ventricle displayed higher sACE2 levels than those with a systemic morphological right ventricle (median 841.7 pg/ml vs 633.9 pg/ml, $p = 0.026$)."

"In the multivariable model, however, the most significant factor independently associated with higher levels of sACE2 was found to be a higher NYHA class ≥ III ($p = 0.002$) whereas the use of ACEI or ARB was the most significant factor associated with lower levels of sACE2 ($p = 0.001$)."

Discussion

"Significantly higher sACE2 serum levels were found in adult patients with complex CHD in comparison to healthy controls indicating the relationship of ACE2 expression to cardiovascular disease."

"Our results are consistent with a previous study illustrating increasing plasma sACE2 concentrations according to NYHA class in heart failure patients with highest levels found in the acute setting [10]."

"SACE2 levels were also significantly higher in patients with multi-vessel than single-vessel disease in that study."

"Our results are in accordance with a previous study investigating two independent cohorts of patients with left heart failure illustrating that ACEI or ARB uses were independent predictors of lower sACE2 concentrations whereas the use of MRA was an independent predictor of higher sACE2 concentrations [28]."

"Further studies are warranted to evaluate the direct relationship of sACE2 concentrations and the susceptibility or course of COVID-19 disease in adult patients with complex CHD."

Conclusion

"Soluble ACE2 concentrations were significantly elevated in adults with various types of complex CHD as compared to healthy controls with highest levels found in those with Eisenmenger physiology or a higher NYHA-class ≥ III reflecting advanced heart failure."

"A higher NYHA class ≥ III was the most significant determinant that was independently associated with increased sACE2 levels."

Effects of ACE Inhibition on Circulating Endothelial Progenitor Cells, Vascular Damage, and Oxidative Stress in Hypertensive Patients [32]

This is a machine-generated summary of:

Cacciatore, Francesco; Bruzzese, Giuseppe; Vitale, Dino Franco; Liguori, Antonio; de Nigris, Filomena; Fiorito, Carmela; Infante, Teresa; Donatelli, Francesco; Minucci, Pellegrino Biagio; Ignarro, Louis Joseph; Napoli, Claudio: Effects of ACE inhibition on circulating endothelial progenitor cells, vascular damage, and oxidative stress in hypertensive patients [32].

Published in: European Journal of Clinical Pharmacology (2011).

Link to original: https://doi.org/10.1007/s00228-011-1029-0

If you want to cite the papers, please refer to the original.

For technical reasons we could not place the page where the original quote is coming from.

Abstract-Summary "The pathogenic role of angiotensin-converting enzyme (ACE) inhibition in hypertensive patients regarding endothelial progenitor-cell (EPC) function is still poorly understood."

"The aim of the study was to evaluate EPC number, function, and relationship to carotid intima media thickness (IMT) progression."

"EPC number increased during the follow-up, with no statistical differences between treatment groups."

"There was an inverse correlation between circulating EPCs and IMT increase over time."

"Multiple linear regression model demonstrated that carotid IMT was significantly inversely correlated with EPC but not with migratory cells after adjusting for confounders."

"The study demonstrated that EPC levels increased during the follow-up in both groups of newly diagnosed hypertensive patients treated with ACE inhibitors."

"These drugs prevented progression of vascular damage, with an inverse correlation between circulating EPC levels and IMT values."

Introduction

"The pathobiology of EPC is an emerging field in the clinical setting of cardiovascular diseases."

"Some preclinical studies suggest that angiotensin-converting enzyme (ACE) inhibition may have potential effects on EPC [33, 34]."

"As ACE inhibitors are widely used in cardiovascular therapy, this promoted further investigation into the effects of such compounds on circulating EPC and their role in vascular healing, repair, and postnatal neovascularization."

"We used a previous clinical trial [35] on ACE inhibition and vascular damage to study EPC number, function, and relation to carotid intima media thickness (IMT) progression over time."

Methods

"All carotid ultrasonography measurements were made by two investigators (GB and AL) to eliminate interobserver variability and who were blinded to treatment randomization, as previously described [35]."

"Carotid artery IMT was measured by high-resolution B-mode ultrasonography with a 7.5-MHz high-resolution transducer (Sonos-5500 system; Philips Medical Systems, Andover, MA, USA), as described previously [36, 37]."

"We measured IMT of the common carotid arteries bilaterally at three points (1, 2, and 3 cm proximal to the carotid bifurcation); the averaged value was taken as the carotid IMT."

"Systolic and diastolic BPs (mmHg) were defined according to Korotkoff sounds I and V. All BP measurements were done by a physician blinded to patients' profiles and treatment assignments just before carotid ultrasound measurements and after drug administration."

"Cells migrating into the lower chamber were counted manually in several random microscopic fields [38]. Measurements were blinded to treatment randomization".

Statistical Analysis

"Analysis of variance (ANOVA) for repeated measures was used to test the effect of treatment (enalapril vs zofenopril) over time (baseline, 1 year, 5 years) on systolic and diastolic BP, IMT, EPCs, migratory cells, NOx, and PGF2-α and showed statistical significance for treatment effect, time effect, and interaction between treatment and time."

"To assess the association between IMT vs EPC and/or migratory cells controlling for confounder effect of treatment, time, and other variables, we used linear regression analysis with robust variance estimation clustering for each patient to compensate for the correlation between repeated measures [39]."

"Analysis was performed using STATA 10 software."

Results

"EPCs increased during the follow-up, with no statistical differences between treatment groups."

"Migrating capacity of EPCs did not change during the study, and no differences were evident between treatment groups."

"Plasma NOx decreased significantly, whereas no differences were evident between the treatment groups."

"IMT increased, and this effect was more evident in the group of patients treated with enalapril, even though this difference did not reach statistical significance when compared with the zofenopril-treated group."

Discussion

"The major findings of our study are: (1) an EPC increase during the follow-up in both groups of patients treated with enalapril and zofenopril, (2) an inverse correlation between circulating EPCs and IMT increase over time, (3) a plasma NOx decrease without evident differences between treatment groups, and (4) 8-iso-PGF2-α decrease more evidently in zofenopril-treated patients."

"They also found an inverse correlation with EPC number ($r = -0.349$) but with no statistical significance ($p = 0.063$), demonstrating an age-related decrease in EPC function and a possible effect on vascular remodelling [40]. Another study [41] demonstrated that a significantly higher carotid mean maximum IMT, prevalence of carotid plaque, and a lower number of circulating $CD34^+/KDR^+$ EPCs was found in stroke patients compared with controls."

"Our study demonstrated that EPC levels increased during treatment in both groups of patients treated with ACE inhibitors, indicating that these drugs prevent vascular damage in newly hypertensive patients, not only by reducing BP but also acting on circulating EPCs."

The Effects of Angiotensin-Converting Enzyme-Inhibitory Peptide LAP on the Left Common Carotid Artery Remodeling in Spontaneously Hypertensive Rats [42]

This is a machine-generated summary of:

Hong, F.; Junling, H.; Yi, S.; Chi, L.; Huan, Z.; Yu qing, D.; Lingxia, L.; Yang, G.; Ming, L.: The effects of angiotensin-converting enzyme-inhibitory peptide LAP on the left common carotid artery remodeling in spontaneously hypertensive rats [42].

Published in: Irish Journal of Medical Science (2013).

Link to original: https://doi.org/10.1007/s11845-013-0963-5

Copyright of the summarized publication:

If you want to cite the papers, please refer to the original.

For technical reasons we could not place the page where the original quote is coming from.

Abstract-Summary "To investigate the protective effect of angiotensin-converting enzyme (ACE)-inhibitory peptide LAP on the left common carotid artery remodeling in spontaneously hypertensive rats (SHRs)."

"It was observed that the vascular medial thickness, media thickness/lumen diameter, medial cross-sectional area and mean nuclear area of smooth muscle cells of the left common carotid artery in the LAP group or enalapril group were significantly lower than those in the pseudo-experimental group, while there was no significant difference in these parameters observed between the LAP group and enalapril group."

"The vascular area percentage of collagen fibers of the left common carotid artery in the LAP group and enalapril group was significantly lower than that of the pseudo-experimental group."

Introduction

"Vascular remodeling is not only an important pathological change in hypertension, but also the structural basis leading to hypertension worsening."

"Vascular remodeling is defined as any enduring change in size or composition of blood vessels in response to altered blood flow, mechanical load, or after vascular injury."

"Vascular remodeling is a response of the vessel to hemodynamic changes or injury."

"It is presently clear that hypertension is a major risk factor for vascular remodeling."

"Angiotensin II has been regarded as a pleiotropic local mediator capable of modulating cell growth, apoptosis, migration of vascular smooth muscle cells, and extracellular matrix modulation, all of which are biologic mechanisms of vascular remodeling and intimal formation."

"The left common carotid artery was studied and the effect of angiotensin-converting enzyme-inhibitory peptide LAP on vascular remodeling was investigated."

Methods

"The body weight of rats used was between 220 and 260 g. SHRs were assigned to three groups (10 rats in each group): the blank group (no drugs was given), enalapril group (enalapril was given), ACE-inhibitory peptide LAP group (LAP was given)."

"The effects of ACE-inhibitory peptide LAP on the blood pressure of SHRs were determined by intraperitoneal injection of LAP into the SHRs."

"Intraperitoneal injection of LAP into SHRs were performed at 0, 1, 2, 3, 4, 5, 6, 7, and 8 weeks."

"The blood pressure during the experimental period was measured at the desired intervals (2, 4, 8, 12, 20 weeks) after injection by the tail-cuff method."

"Acclimation to the mouse holders and tail-cuff apparatus was initiated and continued daily 4 days prior to data acquisition using an MK-2000 blood pressure system."

Pathophysiological Investigations

"The left cervical total artery was further dissected, and the fixed transverse sections of the tissues were embedded in paraffin (LEICA EG 1160 Embedding Center)."

"The media thickness (M) and luminal radius (L) were traced manually on digitized images using a computer-assisted image analysis system (Image-Pro Plus, Version: 4.5)."

"The media transversal area = external elastic membranes in group area—internal elastic membranes in group area."

"The nuclear areas of media cells were measured with computer-assisted image analysis system."

"The mean value is the average nuclear area of the media cells [43]."

"The area percentage of collagen fibers in the left common carotid artery of rat media was measured with computer-assisted image analysis system [43, 44]."

Results

"After LAP or enalapril administration for 2 weeks, the blood pressure in the LAP and enalapril group began to decrease until the end of the experiment."

"When therapy was completed, the vascular medial thickness, media thickness/lumen diameter, cross-sectional medial area in LAP and enalapril group all decreased."

"At the end of treatment, the vascular area percentage of collagen fibers in the left common carotid artery of the LAP group and enalapril group was significantly lower than that of the blank group [left common carotid artery: [(24.74 ± 0.97) vs. (32.53 ± 1.46), (24.30 ± 0.978) vs. (32.53 ± 1.46), $P < 0.001$]."

Discussion

"Many kinds of animal experiments and clinical study have demonstrated that ACEI could improve vascular remodeling [45, 46]."

"ACE inhibitors play an extremely important role in vascular remodeling of hypertensive target organ damage."

"In the East and the West, there have been a number of animal experiments and clinical studies confirmed that angiotensin converting enzyme inhibitors can effectively improve the hypertensive vascular remodeling, and ACEI in the treatment of hypertension with a class effect, ACEI drugs provides a strong evidence-based medical evidence [47, 48]."

"The antihypertensive effect of chemical synthesis in ACEI drugs is clearly, and hypertensive vascular remodeling to be improved or even reverse the role."

"Structural changes of left common carotid artery in the hypertensive process were improved by angiotensin converting enzyme inhibitory peptide LAP."

Conclusion

"The decrease of blood pressure in SHRs by ACE-inhibitory peptide LAP was safe and effective, and the antihypertensive effect was similar to that of enalapril."

"The inhibition of smooth muscle cell hypertrophy and reduction of the proliferation of collagen fibers by LAP were also similar to that of enalapril."

"The ACE-inhibitory peptide LAP derived from lactoferrin hydrolysates would be useful for the development of new antihypertensive agent and/or new ACE inhibitor."

Limitation

"Whether LAP improves vascular remolding for long-term outcomes still remains to be investigated."

"The underlying molecular mechanism has not been completely elucidated."

"More studies are required to clarify the detailed mechanism of this action, both in animal and human subjects in the future."

Choice of Generic Antihypertensive Drugs for the Primary Prevention of Cardiovascular Disease—A Cost-Effectiveness Analysis [49]

This is a machine-generated summary of:

Wisløff, Torbjørn; Selmer, Randi M; Halvorsen, Sigrun; Fretheim, Atle; Norheim, Ole F; Kristiansen, Ivar Sønbø: Choice of generic antihypertensive drugs for the primary prevention of cardiovascular disease—A cost-effectiveness analysis [49].

Published in: BMC Cardiovascular Disorders (2012).

Link to original: https://doi.org/10.1186/1471-2261-12-26

If you want to cite the papers, please refer to the original.

For technical reasons we could not place the page where the original quote is coming from.

Abstract-Summary "The objective of this study was to explore the cost-effectiveness of different generic antihypertensive drugs as first, second and third choice for primary prevention of cardiovascular disease."

"In single-drug treatment, all antihypertensives are cost-effective compared to no drug treatment."

"In the base-case analysis, the first, second and third choice of antihypertensive were calcium channel blocker, thiazide and angiotensin-converting enzyme inhibitor."

"The sensitivity and scenario analyses indicated considerable uncertainty in that angiotensin receptor blockers as well as, angiotensin-converting enzyme inhibitors, beta blockers and thiazides could be the most cost-effective antihypertensive drugs."

"Generic antihypertensives are cost-effective in a wide range of risk groups."

"There is considerable uncertainty, however, regarding which drug is the most cost-effective."

Background

"This implies that health authorities issue guidelines for choice of drugs and may even deny reimbursement of drugs that are too expensive in relation to the effectiveness."

"The National Institute of Health and Clinical Excellence (NICE) in the UK may recommend against reimbursement of drugs when the cost per quality adjusted life year (QALY) exceeds £30,000 [50]."

"Cost-effectiveness analyses have been widely used for some types of therapies such as cholesterol lowering drugs."

"A recent project funded by Norwegian health authorities offered a basis for developing guidelines for choice of antihypertensive drugs."

"The aim of this study was to explore the life-time cost-effectiveness of various generic antihypertensive drugs in order to propose first-line therapy of hypertension and later add-ons for patients who need more than one drug."

Methods

"The effectiveness of antihypertensive drugs was modelled by reducing the risk of primary CVD events based on meta-analyses from a recent systematic review [51]."

"We did not include any impact of antihypertensives on the risk of heart failure and angina as primary events in the base case analyses because these outcomes are "softer" and more difficult to measure uniformly in trials."

"The final result of the analysis has been expressed as an incremental cost-effectiveness ratio (ICER): In order to maximize health (e.g. life years) within a given budget, decision makers ought to prioritize treatments with the lowest ICER's until the budget is exploited."

"The INHB has the following definition: If for example a treatment on average generates 1.3 life years per patient, have lifetime costs of €31,000 (including off-sets from avoided events) and T is €62,000, then INHB = 1.3 – 31,000/62,000 = 0.8. "

Results

"The difference in (discounted) costs was also highest for the oldest age groups, which implies that INHB was highest for 70 year olds (0.42 and 0.39 for women and men respectively), and lower for the other age groups."

"These analyses indicate that CCB may be the most cost-effective for all age groups (both men and women)."

"We also included other combinations of three drugs and none of these were more cost-effective than the combination of thiazide, CCB and ACE-inhibitors in any age group."

"When we included heart failure and angina in the model, ARB was more likely than CCB to be the most cost-effective first-line treatment for hypertension (36% and 24% respectively)(data not shown)."

"In analyses of the combination of three drugs; all combinations seems almost equally likely of being the most cost-effective alternative if this more comprehensive model is used (results not shown)."

Discussion

"For 40, 50, 60 and 70 year old men and women, generic CCB, thiazide, ACE inhibitor, ARB and beta blocker are all cost-effective and even cost-saving antihypertensives, even when two or all three are used in combination when this is indicated."

"Because benefits from antihypertensives in terms of life years gained occur at a late stage in life, discounting leads to lower incremental health benefit in the younger compared to the older age groups."

"We assume that our results would not be substantially different if they were based on other meta-analyses of antihypertensive drug trials."

"We have not incorporated side effects into our model, mainly because we use life years gained as measure of effectiveness and then possible fatal side effects will be captured in the clinical trials."

"However, that side effects in terms of mortality is captured in the model because we used intention-to-treat data from trials."

Conclusions

"CCB, ARB, thiazide, ACE inhibitor and beta blocker all represent cost-effective antihypertensives either alone or in combination."

"Based on our findings, new clinical practice guidelines for antihypertensive treatment may do well in recommending more than one drug class as first choice."

Angiotensin-Converting Enzyme Inhibitors Versus Angiotensin Receptor Blockers in Hypertensive Patients with Myocardial Infarction or Heart Failure: A Systematic Review and Meta-Analysis [52]

This is a machine-generated summary of:

Ohtsubo, Toshio; Shibata, Rei; Kai, Hisashi; Okamoto, Ryuji; Kumagai, Eita; Kawano, Hiroaki; Fujiwara, Akira; Kitazono, Takanari; Murohara, Toyoaki; Arima, Hisatomi: Angiotensin-converting enzyme inhibitors versus angiotensin receptor blockers in hypertensive patients with myocardial infarction or heart failure: a systematic review and meta-analysis [52].

Published in: Hypertension Research (2019).

Link to original: https://doi.org/10.1038/s41440-018-0167-5

If you want to cite the papers, please refer to the original.

For technical reasons we could not place the page where the original quote is coming from.

Abstract-Summary "It is unclear whether ACEIs or ARBs are more appropriate first-line drugs in hypertensive patients with MI or heart failure (HF)."

"The present study aimed to compare the effects of ACEIs and those of ARBs in these patients."

"Sixty randomized controlled trails (RCTs) that compared the effects of ACEIs and ARBs in patients with MI or HF were extracted by searching PubMed/

MEDLINE, Cochrane Database, and the Medical Central Journal database according to the PRISMA guidelines."

"There were no significant differences between ACEIs and ARBs for all outcomes, except adverse events."

"Study discontinuation owing to adverse events was significantly more common with ACEIs than with ARBs."

"Among hypertensive patients with MI or HF, it appears desirable to select the most appropriate drugs, ACEIs or ARBs, in each case by considering the function level, patient background, comorbidity presence, blood pressure target, drug price and other such factors comprehensively in addition to considering tolerability."

Introduction

"In the VALIANT study that targeted patients with MI or HFrEF, there were no significant differences in total or cardiovascular death, MI recurrence, and hospitalization for HF between the ARB valsartan and the ACEI captopril [53]."

"It is unclear which of ACEIs or ARBs are more appropriate in hypertensive patients with MI or HF."

"With respect to the effects of ARBs on HFrEF, the rates of cardiovascular death and hospitalization for HF were lower with candesartan than with placebo among patients who could not tolerate ACEIs in the CHARM-Alternative trial [54]."

"In the VALIANT trial of patients with HFrEF after acute MI and in the ELITE II trial of elderly HF patients, the number of adverse events was lower with ARBs than with ACEIs; however, ARBs had no advantage with regard to the suppression of cardiovascular events [53, 55]."

"It is important to clarify which of ACEIs or ARBs should be used preferentially in hypertensive patients with MI or HF."

Methods

"This systematic review and meta-analysis adhered to the Preferred Reporting Items for Systematic Reviews and Meta-Analyses (PRISMA) guidelines [56]."

"We also checked the studies included in previous systematic review articles to find other eligible trials [57–59]."

"The literature search, data extraction and quality assessment were conducted independently by two systematic reviewers (TO and RS)."

"We searched PubMed/MEDLINE (1966 to July 2017), Cochrane Database of Systematic Reviews (third quarter of 2017), and the Medical Central Journal database (1981 to July 2017)."

"Inclusion criteria was: (A) RCTs that compared the effects of ACEIs and ARBs, (B) participants involve patients with MI/HF and hypertension, and (C) outcomes reported involve (1) recurrence or new onset of MI, (2) hospitalization for HF, (3) cardiovascular or total mortality, (4) cardiovascular events or stroke, (5) adverse events, (6) renal impairment or proteinuria, and/or (7) atrial fibrillation."

Results

"The rates of recurrence or new onset of MI in all patients with MI or HF were 6.25% (n = 836/13,374) among those treated with ACEIs and 6.49% (n = 866/13,336) among those treated with ARBs."

"The rates of cardiovascular or total mortality in all patients with MI or HF were 20.7% (n = 3783/18,283) among those treated with ACEIs and 21.0% (n = 3831/18,245) among those treated with ARBs."

"The rates of cardiovascular events or stroke in all patients with MI or HF were 19.3% (n = 2579/13,374) among those treated with ACEIs and 19.4% (n = 2590/13,336) among those treated with ARBs."

"The rates of adverse events in all patients with MI or HF were 21.1% (n = 4644/18,253) among those treated with ACEIs and 18.3% (n = 3867/18,245) among those treated with ARBs."

Discussion

"The present study found no significant difference in the effectiveness of ACEIs and ARBs with regard to recurrence or new onset of MI in hypertensive patients with MI or HF."

"The main limitation of this study is the indirect assessment of hypertensive patients with MI or HF owing to the absence of RCTs that directly compared the effects of ARBs and ACEIs in hypertensive patients with MI or HF."

"The findings of the effects of ACEIs and ARBs on recurrence or new onset of MI, hospitalization for HF, cardiovascular or total mortality, and cardiovascular disease or stroke in patients with MI or HF were not different from the results of previous systematic reviews and meta-analyses identified in this study."

Azilsartan Compared to ACE Inhibitors in Anti-hypertensive Therapy: One-Year Outcomes of the Observational EARLY Registry [60]

This is a machine-generated summary of:

Gitt, Anselm K.; Bramlage, Peter; Potthoff, Sebastian A.; Baumgart, Peter; Mahfoud, Felix; Buhck, Hartmut; Ehmen, Martina; Ouarrak, Taoufik; Senges, Jochen; Schmieder, Roland E.; for the EARLY Registry Group, None: Azilsartan compared to ACE inhibitors in anti-hypertensive therapy: one-year outcomes of the observational EARLY registry [60].

Published in: BMC Cardiovascular Disorders (2016).

Link to original: https://doi.org/10.1186/s12872-016-0222-6

If you want to cite the papers, please refer to the original.

For technical reasons we could not place the page where the original quote is coming from.

Abstract-Summary "We aimed to compare the efficacy, safety, and tolerability of AZL-M with that of ACE-inhibitors in a real life clinical setting."

"Patients who initiated monotherapy at baseline comprising either AZL-M or an ACE-inhibitor were included at a ratio of seven to three."

"Results demonstrated that a blood pressure target of <140/90 mmHg was achieved by a significantly greater proportion of patients in the AZL-M group (61.1%) compared with the ACE-inhibitor group (56.4%; $p < 0.05$; OR, 1.21; 95% CI, 1.03–1.42), with this finding maintained after adjusting for differences in baseline characteristics."

"AZL-M appeared to have an equivalent safety profile to the ACE-inhibitors, with a similar incidence of adverse events in the two patient groups ($p = 0.73$)."

Background

"Despite the availability of many safe and effective antihypertensive drugs, target blood pressure (BP) is only obtained in approximately 20% of hypertensive patients in Germany [61]."

"ARBs have demonstrated similar or improved efficacy for reducing BP but appear to be more tolerable, with fewer side effects such as coughing reported [62], although no significant differences in the occurrence of drug-related adverse events (AEs) have been noted [59, 63]."

"This comparison is particularly valuable as ramipril is considered to be a benchmark antihypertensive drug that has been shown to be highly effective in lowering BP [64, 65]."

"In a randomized clinical trial AZL-M was found to be more effective in lowering BP in comparison to ramipril; furthermore, patients in the ARB group experienced fewer AEs leading to discontinuation of treatment [66]."

"The EARLY "Treatment with Azilsartan Compared to ACE-Inhibitors in Anti-Hypertensive Therapy" registry was designed to document BP control and its impact on cardiovascular and renal events during a 12 month follow-up period in patients administered either AZL-M or an ACE-inhibitor at baseline [67]."

Methods

"Establishment of the registry had two primary objectives: 1) documentation of the achievement of target BP values set according to recent national and international guidelines [68], and 2) description of the safety profile of AZL-M. Further secondary objectives are listed in the protocol published previously [67] and include the 1) absolute and relative BP reduction with antihypertensive treatment over the duration of one year 2) documentation of the adherence to guidelines for the diagnosis and treatment of hypertension in ambulatory care 3) persistence understood as the mean duration of monotherapy and/or AZL-M based combination therapy during follow-up 4) documentation of adverse events 5) prospective documentation of cardiovascular and renal events."

"Patients over 18 years of age with essential arterial hypertension were included on a consecutive basis [68], given that they had provided written informed consent and fulfilled the following two criteria: 1) they had either no antihypertensive treatment prior to inclusion or were on a non-RAS based antihypertensive monotherapy, and 2) monotherapy consisting of AZL-M or an ACE-inhibitor was initiated at baseline."

Results

"There were fewer newly diagnosed patients in the AZL-M group (34.2% vs. 43.9%), and those with established hypertension had a longer mean time since diagnosis in comparison to the ACE-inhibitor group (67.2 ± 65.3 months vs. 57.7 ± 60.9 months; $p < 0.001$)."

"Using raw unadjusted data for patients who completed the 12 month follow-up, mean reductions in SBP and DBP in the AZL-M group (25.9 and 13.0 mmHg, respectively) were greater than those recorded for the ACE-inhibitor group (22.6 and 11.4 mmHg, respectively; $p < 0.0001$ and <0.001, respectively)."

"Following adjustment for baseline SBP/DBP (model 1), and for baseline SBP/DBP, newly diagnosed or established hypertension, age, gender, and the presence of diabetes (model 2), compared with ACE-inhibitor treatment, AZL-M treatment was still associated with statistically significant reductions in SBP ($p < 0.05$ and 0.01 for the two respective models) and DBP ($p < 0.05$ for both models)."

Discussion

"The key finding was that after 12 months of treatment, both reductions in SBP and DBP, and the percentage of patients who attained target BP levels, were significantly greater with AZL-M treatment compared to that with an ACE-inhibitor."

"On analysis of the raw data, it was seen that the mean reductions in SBP and DBP were greater in the AZL-M group (Δ25.9 mmHg) relative to the ACE-inhibitor group (Δ22.6 mmHg), with an additional 4.7% of patients reaching the target level of BP control."

"In the present registry, no difference in the rate of target BP achievement was found in the gender and BMI subgroups; however, patients with newly diagnosed hypertension, those aged 50–69 years, and those without diabetes were more likely to reach the target value if treated with AZL-M rather than an ACE-inhibitor."

Conclusions

"Data from this study may help to inform clinical decisions as to which is the most appropriate RAS-targeted antihypertensive agent."

"The relative impact of ACE-inhibitors versus ARBs on the rate of specific cardiovascular events and other clinically relevant endpoints is yet to be resolved."

"This study adds to the body of literature suggesting that when BP is taken as the sole measure of the efficacy of these drugs, AZL-M is more effective than ACE-inhibitors."

"This study indicates that data from clinical trials of AZL-M may be extrapolated to real life clinical practice."

Assessing the Risk of Angiotensin Receptor Blockers on Major Cardiovascular Events: A Systematic Review and Meta-Analysis of Randomized Controlled Trials [69]

This is a machine-generated summary of:

Wanas, Yara; Bashir, Rim; Islam, Nazmul; Furuya-Kanamori, Luis: Assessing the risk of angiotensin receptor blockers on major cardiovascular events: a systematic review and meta-analysis of randomized controlled trials [69].

Published in: BMC Cardiovascular Disorders (2020).

Link to original: https://doi.org/10.1186/s12872-020-01466-5

If you want to cite the papers, please refer to the original.

For technical reasons we could not place the page where the original quote is coming from.

Abstract-Summary "The VALUE trial found an increased risk of myocardial infarction in participants receiving ARBs compared to other antihypertensive."

"The aim of the meta-analysis was to synthetize the available evidence of randomised controlled trials (RCTs) and elucidate if ARBs increase the risk of cardiovascular events."

"Multiple sensitivity analyses were conducted to assess the effect of ARBs by restricting the analysis to different participants' characteristics."

"The pooled estimates revealed that ARBs do not increase the risk of all-cause mortality (RR 1.00; 95%CI 0.97–1.04), myocardial infarction (RR 1.01; 95%CI 0.96–1.06), and stroke (RR 0.92; 95%CI 0.83–1.01)."

"The sensitivity analysis did not yield a particular group of patients at increased risk of cardiovascular events with ARBs."

"Risk of all-cause mortality and stroke decreased with ARB when the proportion of smokers in a population was <25% (RR 0.91; 95%CI 0.84–0.98) and in females (RR 0.76; 95%CI 0.68–0.84), respectively."

"ARBs do not increase the risk of major cardiovascular events and are safe for use in patients."

Background

"The risk of major cardiovascular events can be reduced by a wide spectrum of antihypertensive drugs including angiotensin receptor blockers (ARBs) [70]."

"The VALUE trial found that ARBs (valsartan) increased the risk of myocardial infarction (fatal and non-fatal) by 19% compared with calcium channel blockers (amlodipine) [71]."

"The point estimate of the CHARM-alternative trial suggests a 36% increase in myocardial infarction with candesartan (versus placebo) regardless of the reduction in blood pressure [54]."

"It was unclear the mechanism that could explain an increase in risk of myocardial infarction with ARBs."

"Due to the wide use of ARBs for many CVDs and the contradictory results, we decided to conduct a systematic review and meta-analysis of randomised controlled trials (RCTs) to elucidate the cardiovascular safety profile of ARBs."

Methods

"The inclusion of studies was restricted to human studies; RCTs comparing ARBs versus a control (either a placebo or another antihypertensive medication); follow-up of at least 12 months; and reported all-cause mortality, myocardial infarction, and stroke as outcomes."

"Recurrent myocardial infarction and stroke were also considered if the study only included patients that have had recently experienced myocardial infarction or stroke."

"The number of participants and the number events (i.e. all-cause mortality, myocardial infarction, and stroke) in each intervention group (ARBs [active] and non-ARBs [control]) were extracted."

"The Cochrane Collaboration's tool for assessing risk of bias in randomized trials [72] was used to assess the risk of bias of the included studies."

"The outcomes of interest were the relative risks (RRs) of all-cause mortality, myocardial infarction, and stroke with ARBs compared to the control group."

"Sensitivity analyses were conducted to identify potential scenarios where ARBs increase the risk of all-cause mortality, myocardial infarction, and stroke."

Result

"The publication by Chaturvedi and others [73] reported findings from two RCTs, the DIRECT-Prevent 1 and DIRECT-Protect 1 studies."

"Only two RCTs, DIRECT-Prevent 1 and DIRECT-Protect 1 enrolled participants with a median age <50 years."

"All-cause mortality, myocardial infarction, and stroke were assessed in 39, 37, and 36 RCTs."

"The Doi plots revealed minor asymmetry for all-cause mortality (LFK index = −1.24) and myocardial infarction (LFK index = −1.33) for RCTs reporting favourable results for ARBs."

Discussion

"Bangalore and others [74] conducted a meta-analysis on ARBs and the risk of myocardial infarction and found that ARBs do not increase the risk of cardiovascular events."

"Multiple RCTs have been published; in our meta-analysis we pooled the most updated evidence (45 RCTs comprising of 170,794 participants – 8 RCTs and 23,000 more participants that Bangalore and others) and corroborated that ARBs are safe medications as they do not increase the risk of all-cause mortality, myocardial infarction, or stroke."

"It is worth pointing out that our meta-analysis (in line with previous studies [74, 75]) also found that ARBs do not reduce the risk of all-cause mortality and myocardial infarction when compared to placebo."

"In none of the cases, ARBs were found to increase the risk of all-cause mortality, myocardial infarction, and stroke."

Bibliography

1. Mahmood S, Jalal Z, Hadi MA, Khan TM, Haque MS, Shah KU (2021) Prevalence of non-adherence to antihypertensive medication in Asia: a systematic review and meta-analysis. Int J Clin Pharm 43(3):486–501
2. Di Giosia P, Giorgini P, Stamerra CA, Petrarca M, Ferri C, Sahebkar A (2018) Gender differences in epidemiology, pathophysiology, and Treatment of hypertension. Curr Atheroscler Rep 20(3):13. Published 2018 Feb 14
3. Asgedom SW, Atey TM, Desse TA (2018) Antihypertensive medication adherence and associated factors among adult hypertensive patients at Jimma University Specialized Hospital, southwest Ethiopia [published correction appears in BMC Res Notes. 2018 Aug 16;11(1):592]. BMC Res Notes 11(1):27
4. Honda A, Tahara N, Tahara A et al (2023) Effects of olmesartan and amlodipine on blood pressure, endothelial function, and vascular inflammation. J Nucl Cardiol 30:1613–1626. https://doi.org/10.1007/s12350-023-03200-y
5. Vejakama P, Thakkinstian A, Lertrattananon D, Ingsathit A, Ngarmukos C, Attia J (2012) Reno-protective effects of renin-angiotensin system blockade in type 2 diabetic patients: a systematic review and network meta-analysis. Diabetologia 55(3):566–578. https://doi.org/10.1007/s00125-011-2398-8
6. Pugliese NR, Masi S, Taddei S (2020) The renin-angiotensin-aldosterone system: a crossroad from arterial hypertension to heart failure. Heart Fail Rev 25:31–42. https://doi.org/10.1007/s10741-019-09855-5
7. Almengló C, Couselo-Seijas M, Agra RM, Varela-Román A, García-Acuña JM, González-Peteiro M, González-Juanatey JR, Eiras S, Álvarez E (2021) Soluble angiotensin-converting enzyme levels in heart failure or acute coronary syndrome: revisiting its modulation and prognosis value. J Mol Med 99:1741–1753. https://doi.org/10.1007/s00109-021-02129-4
8. Narula S, Yusuf S, Chong M, Ramasundarahettige C, Rangarajan S, Bangdiwala SI, van Eikels M, Leineweber K, Wu A, Pigeyre M, Pare G (2020) Plasma ACE2 and risk of death or cardiometabolic diseases: a case-cohort analysis. Lancet 396:968–976. https://doi.org/10.1016/S0140-6736(20)31964-4
9. Oudit GY, Liu GC, Zhong J, Basu R, Chow FL, Zhou J, Loibner H, Janzek E, Schuster M, Penninger JM, Herzenberg AM, Kassiri Z, Scholey JW (2010) Human recombinant ACE2 reduces the progression of diabetic nephropathy. Diabetes 59:529–538. https://doi.org/10.2337/db09-1218
10. Epelman S, Tang WH, Chen SY, Van Lente F, Francis GS, Sen S (2008) Detection of soluble angiotensin-converting enzyme 2 in heart failure: insights into the endogenous counter-regulatory pathway of the reninangiotensin-aldosterone system. J Am Coll Cardiol 52:750–754. https://doi.org/10.1016/j.jacc.2008.02.088

11. Behl T, Kaur I, Bungau S, Kumar A, Uddin MS, Kumar C, Pal G, Sahil SK, Zengin G, Arora S (2020) The dual impact of ACE2 in COVID-19 and ironical actions in geriatrics and pediatrics with possible therapeutic solutions. Life Sci 257:118075. https://doi.org/10.1016/j.lfs.2020.118075
12. Sharma RK, Li J, Krishnan S, Richards EM, Raizada MK, Mohandas R (2021) Angiotensin-converting enzyme 2 and COVID-19 in cardiorenal diseases. Clin Sci (Lond) 135:1–17. https://doi.org/10.1042/CS20200482
13. Danser AHJ, Epstein M, Batlle D (2020) Renin-angiotensin system blockers and the COVID-19 pandemic: at present there is no evidence to abandon renin-angiotensin system blockers. Hypertension 75:1382–1385. https://doi.org/10.1161/HYPERTENSIONAHA.120.15082
14. Paradela-Dobarro B, Rodiño-Janeiro BK, Alonso J, Raposeiras-Roubín S, González-Peteiro M, González-Juanatey JR, Álvarez E (2016) Key structural and functional differences between early and advanced glycation products. J Mol Endocrinol 56:23–37. https://doi.org/10.1530/JME-15-0031
15. Ortiz-Pérez JT, Riera M, Bosch X, De Caralt TM, Perea RJ, Pascual J et al (2013) Role of circulating angiotensin converting enzyme 2 in left ventricular remodeling following myocardial infarction: a prospective controlled study. PLoS One 8(4):e61695. https://doi.org/10.1371/journal.pone.0061695. PMID: 23630610; PMCID
16. Raedle-Hurst T, Wissing S, Mackenstein N, Obeid R, Geisel J, Wagenpfeil S, Abdul-Khaliq H (2020) Determinants of soluble angiotensin-converting enzyme 2 concentrations in adult patients with complex congenital heart disease. Clin Res Cardiol 111:154–162. https://doi.org/10.1007/s00392-020-01782-y
17. Huang C, Wang Y, Li X, Ren L, Zhao J, Hu Y, Zhang L, Fan G, Xu J, Gu X, Cheng Z, Yu T, Xia J, Wei Y, Wu W, Xie X, Yin W, Li H, Liu M, Xiao Y, Gao H, Guo L, Xie J, Wang G, Jiang R, Gao Z, Jin Q, Wang J, Cao B (2020) Clinical features of patients infected with 2019 novel coronavirus in Wuhan, China. Lancet 395:497–506. https://doi.org/10.1016/s0140-6736(20)30183-5
18. Zhou F, Yu T, Du R, Fan G, Liu Y, Liu Z, Xiang J, Wang Y, Song B, Gu X, Guan L, Wei Y, Li H, Wu X, Xu J, Tu S, Zhang Y, Chen H, Cao B (2020) Clinical course and risk factors for mortality of adult inpatients with COVID-19 in Wuhan, China: a retrospective cohort study. Lancet 395:1054–1062. https://doi.org/10.1016/s0140-6736(20)30566-3
19. Li X, Molina-Molina M, Abdul-Hafez A, Uhal V, Xaubet A, Uhal BD (2008) Angiotensin converting enzyme-2 is protective but downregulated in human and experimental lung fibrosis. Am J Physiol Lung Cell Mol Physiol 295:L178–L185. https://doi.org/10.1152/ajplung.00009.2008
20. Diaz JH (2020) Hypothesis: angiotensin-converting enzyme inhibitors and angiotensin receptor blockers may increase the risk of severe COVID-19. J Travel Med 27(3):taaa041. https://doi.org/10.1093/jtm/taaa041
21. Kuster GM, Pfister O, Burkard T, Zhou Q, Twerenbold R, Haaf P, Widmer AF, Osswald S (2020) SARS-CoV2: should inhibitors of the renin-angiotensin system be withdrawn in patients with COVID-19? Eur Heart J 41:1801–1803. https://doi.org/10.1093/eurheartj/ehaa235
22. Goulter AB, Goddard MJ, Allen JC, Clark KL (2004) ACE2 gene expression is up-regulated in the human failing heart. BMC Med 2:19. https://doi.org/10.1186/1741-7015-2-19
23. Culebras E, Hernández F (2020) ACE2 is on the X chromosome: could this explain COVID-19 gender differences? Eur Heart J 41:3095. https://doi.org/10.1093/eurheartj/ehaa521
24. Li S, Wang Z, Yang X, Hu B, Huang Y, Fan S (2017) Association between circulating angiotensin-converting enzyme 2 and cardiac remodeling in hypertensive patients. Peptides 90:63–68. https://doi.org/10.1016/j.peptides.2017.02.007
25. Karlberg J, Chong DS, Lai WY (2004) Do men have a higher case fatality rate of severe acute respiratory syndrome than women do? Am J Epidemiol 159:229–231. https://doi.org/10.1093/aje/kwh056
26. Onder G, Rezza G, Brusaferro S (2020) Case-fatality rate and characteristics of patients dying in relation to COVID-19 in Italy. JAMA 323:1775–1776. https://doi.org/10.1001/jama.2020.4683

27. Palmieri L, Vanacore N, Donfrancesco C, Lo Noce C, Canevelli M, Punzo O, Raparelli V, Pezzotti P, Riccardo F, Bella A, Fabiani M, D'Ancona FP, Vaianella L, Tiple D, Colaizzo E, Palmer K, Rezza G, Piccioli A, Brusaferro S, Onder G (2020) Clinical characteristics of hospitalized individuals dying with COVID-19 by age group in Italy. J Gerontol A Biol Sci Med Sci 75:1796–1800. https://doi.org/10.1093/gerona/glaa146
28. Sama IE, Ravera A, Santema BT, van Goor H, Ter Maaten JM, Cleland JGF et al (2020) Circulating plasma concentrations of angiotensin-converting enzyme 2 in men and women with heart failure and effects of renin-angiotensin-aldosterone inhibitors. Eur Heart J 41(19):1810–1817
29. Laqqan M, Schwaighofer C, Graeber S, Raedle-Hurst T (2018) Predictive value of soluble ST2 in adolescent and adult patients with complex congenital heart disease. PLoS One 13:e0202406. https://doi.org/10.1371/journal.pone.0202406
30. Abu-Halima M, Meese E, Saleh MA, Keller A, Abdul-Khaliq H, Raedle-Hurst T (2019) Micro-RNA 150–5p predicts overt heart failure in patients with univentricular hearts. PLoS One 14:e0223606. https://doi.org/10.1371/journal.pone.0223606
31. Abu-Halima M, Meese E, Keller A, Abdul-Khaliq H, Radle-Hurst T (2017) Analysis of circulating microRNAs in patients with repaired tetralogy of Fallot with and without heart failure. J Transl Med 15:156. https://doi.org/10.1186/s12967-017-1255-z
32. Cacciatore F, Bruzzese G, Vitale DF, Liguori A, de Nigris F, Fiorito C, Infante T, Donatelli F, Minucci PB, Ignarro LJ, Napoli C (2011) Effects of ACE inhibition on circulating endothelial progenitor cells, vascular damage, and oxidative stress in hypertensive patients. Eur J Clin Pharmacol 67:877–883. https://doi.org/10.1007/s00228-011-1029-0
33. You D, Cochain C, Loinard C et al (2008) Combination of the angiotensin-converting enzyme inhibitor perindropil and diuretic indapamide activate postnatal vasculogenesis in spontaneously hypertensive rats. J Pharmacol Exp Ther 325:766–773
34. Muller P, Kazalov A, Jagoda P, Semenov A, Bohm M, Laufs U (2009) ACE inhibition promotes upregulation of endothelial progenitor cells and neoangiogenesis in cardiac pressure overload. Cardiovasc Res 83:106–114
35. Napoli C, Bruzzese G, Ignarro LJ et al (2008) Long-term treatment with sulfhydryl angiotensin-converting enzyme inhibition reduces carotid intima-media thickening and improbe the nitric oxide/oxidative stress pathways in newly diagnosed patients with mild to moderate primary hypertension. Am Heart J 156:1154–1162
36. Napoli C, Lerman LO, de Nigris F, Gossl M, Balestrieri ML, Lerman A (2006) Rethinking primary prevention of atherosclerosis-related diseases. Circulation 114:2517–2527
37. Napoli C, Liguori A, Sorice P et al (1996) Relations between vasoactive hormones and diastolic function in hypertensive uraemic patients. J Intern Med 240:389–394
38. Casamassimi A, Balestrieri ML, Fiorito C et al (2007) Comparison between total endothelial progenitor cell isolation versus enriched Cd133+ culture. J Biochem 141:503–511
39. Williams RL (2000) A note on robust variance estimation for cluster-correlated data. Biometrics 56:645–646
40. Keymel S, Kalka C, Rassaf T, Yeghiazarians Y, Kelm M, Heiss C (2008) Impaired endothelial progenitor cell function predicts age-dependent carotid intimal thickening. Basic Res Cardiol 103:582–586
41. Lau KK, Chan YH, Yiu KH et al (2007) Burden of carotid atherosclerosis in patients with stroke: relationships with circulating endothelial progenitor cells and hypertension. J Hum Hypertens 21:445–451
42. Hong F, Junling H, Yi S, Chi L, Huan Z, Yu qing D, Lingxia L, Yang G, Ming L (2013) The effects of angiotensin-converting enzyme-inhibitory peptide LAP on the left common carotid artery remodeling in spontaneously hypertensive rats. Ir J Med Sci 182(4):711–718. https://doi.org/10.1007/s11845-013-0963-5
43. Levy BI, Michel JB, Salzmann JL (1989) Effects of chronic converting enzyme inhibition on the structure and function of large arteries in the rat. Clin Exp Hypertens A 11(Suppl 2):487–498

44. Nehme J, Mercier N, Labat C, Benetos A, Safar ME, Delcayre C, Lacolley P (2006) Differences between cardiac and arterial fibrosis and stiffness in aldosterone-salt rats: effect of eplerenone. J Renin-Angiotensin-Aldosterone Syst 7(1):31–39
45. Dupuis F, Vincent JM, Limiñana P et al (2010) Effects of suboptimal doses of the AT1 receptor blocker, telmisartan, with the angiotensin-converting enzyme inhibitor, ramipril, on cerebral arterioles in spontaneously hypertensive rat. J Hypertens 28(7):1566–1573
46. Dendorfer A, Dominiak P, Schunkert H (2005) ACE inhibitors and angiotensin II receptor antagonists. Handb Exp Pharmacol 170:407–442
47. Hong F, Min L, Yi S et al (2008) The antihypertensive effect of peptides: a novel alternative to drugs? Peptides 29(6):1062–1071
48. Pandey R, Quan WY, Hong F et al (2009) Vaccine for hypertension: modulating the renin–angiotensin system. Int J Cardiol 134(2):16016–16018
49. Wisløff T, Selmer RM, Halvorsen S, Fretheim A, Norheim OF, Kristiansen IS (2012) Choice of generic antihypertensive drugs for the primary prevention of cardiovascular disease—a cost-effectiveness analysis. BMC Cardiovasc Disord 12:26. https://doi.org/10.1186/1471-2261-12-26
50. McCabe C, Claxton K, Culyer AJ (2008) The NICE cost-effectiveness threshold: what it is and what that means. PharmacoEconomics 26:733–744. https://doi.org/10.2165/00019053-200826090-00004
51. Håheim LL, Fretheim A, Brørs O, Kjeldsen SE, Kristiansen IS, Madsen S, Njølstad I, Norheim OF, Ose L, Svilaas A et al (2008) Primærforebygging av hjerte- og karsykdom, med hovedvekt på medikamentelle tiltak. https://www.fhi.no/publ/eldre/primarforebygging-av-hjerte--og-karsykdom--med-hovedvekt-pa-medikamentelle-/
52. Ohtsubo T, Shibata R, Kai H, Okamoto R, Kumagai E, Kawano H, Fujiwara A, Kitazono T, Murohara T, Arima H (2019) Angiotensin-converting enzyme inhibitors versus angiotensin receptor blockers in hypertensive patients with myocardial infarction or heart failure: a systematic review and meta-analysis. Hypertens Res 42(5):641–649. https://doi.org/10.1038/s41440-018-0167-5
53. Pfeffer MA, McMurray JJV, Velazquez EJ et al (2003) Valsartan, captopril, or both in myocardial infarction complicated by heart failure, left ventricular dysfunction, or both. N Engl J Med 349:1893–1906. https://doi.org/10.1056/NEJMoa032292
54. Granger CB, McMurray JJ, Yusuf S et al (2003) Effects of candesartan in patients with chronic heart failure and reduced left-ventricular systolic function intolerant to angiotensin-converting-enzyme inhibitors: the CHARM-Alternative trial. Lancet 362:772–776
55. Pitt B, Poole-Wilson PA, Segal R, Martinez FA, Dickstein K, Camm AJ et al (2000) Effect of losartan compared with captopril on mortality in patients with symptomatic heart failure: randomised trial—the Losartan Heart Failure Survival Study ELITE II. Lancet 355(9215):1582–1587
56. Moher D, Liberati A, Tetzlaff J, Altman DG, PRISMA Group (2009) Preferred reporting items for systematic reviewes and meta-analyses: the PRISMA statement. J Clin Epidemiol 62:1006–1012
57. Blood Pressure Lowering Treatment Trialists' Collaboration, Turnbull F, Neal B et al (2007) Blood pressure-dependent and independent effects of agents that inhibit the renin-angiotensin system. J Hypertens 25:951–958. This is an insightful review into the issue of blood pressure-independent effects of agents inhibiting the renin-angiotensin system
58. Heran BS, Musini VM, Bassett K, Taylor RS, Wright JM (2012) Angiotensin receptor blockers for heart failure. Cochrane Database Syst Rev 4:CD003040
59. Li EC, Heran BS, Wright JM (2014) Angiotensin converting enzyme (ACE) inhibitors versus angiotensin receptor blockers for primary hypertension. Cochrane Database Syst Rev 8:CD009096
60. Gitt AK, Bramlage P, Potthoff SA, Baumgart P, Mahfoud F, Buhck H, Ehmen M, Ouarrak T, Senges J, Schmieder RE, For the EARLY Registry Group (2016) None Azilsartan compared to

ACE inhibitors in anti-hypertensive therapy: one-year outcomes of the observational EARLY registry. BMC Cardiovasc Disord. 16:56. https://doi.org/10.1186/s12872-016-0222-6
61. Sharma AM, Wittchen HU, Kirch W, Pittrow D, Ritz E, Goke B et al (2004) High prevalence and poor control of hypertension in primary care: cross-sectional study. J Hypertens 22(3):479–486
62. Appel GB, Appel AS (2004) Angiotensin II receptor antagonists: role in hypertension, cardiovascular disease, and renoprotection. Prog Cardiovasc Dis 47(2):105–115
63. Roy J, Shah NR, Wood GC, Townsend R, Hennessy S (2012) Comparative effectiveness of angiotensin-converting enzyme inhibitors and angiotensin receptor blockers for hypertension on clinical end points: a cohort study. J Clin Hypertens (Greenwich) 14(7):407–414
64. Anderson VR, Perry CM, Robinson DM (2006) Ramipril: a review of its use in preventing cardiovascular outcomes in high-risk patients. Am J Cardiovasc Drugs 6(6):417–432
65. Yusuf S, Sleight P, Pogue J et al (2000) Effects of an angiotensin-converting enzyme inhibitor, ramipril, on cardiovascular events in high-risk patients. The Heart Outcomes Prevention Evaluation Study Investigators. N Engl J Med 342:145–153
66. Bonner G, Bakris GL, Sica D, Weber MA, White WB, Perez A et al (2013) Antihypertensive efficacy of the angiotensin receptor blocker azilsartan medoxomil compared with the angiotensin-converting enzyme inhibitor ramipril. J Hum Hypertens 27(8):479–486
67. Gitt AK, Baumgart P, Bramlage P, Mahfoud F, Potthoff SA, Senges J et al (2013) EARLY Treatment with azilsartan compared to ACE-inhibitors in anti-hypertensive therapy--rationale and design of the EARLY hypertension registry. BMC Cardiovasc Disord 13:46
68. Mancia G, Fagard R, Narkiewicz K, Redon J, Zanchetti A, Bohm M et al (2013) 2013 ESH/ESC guidelines for the management of arterial hypertension: the Task Force for the Management of Arterial Hypertension of the European Society of Hypertension (ESH) and of the European Society of Cardiology (ESC). Eur Heart J 34(28):2159–2219
69. Wanas Y, Bashir R, Islam N, Furuya-Kanamori L (2020) Assessing the risk of angiotensin receptor blockers on major cardiovascular events: a systematic review and meta-analysis of randomized controlled trials. BMC Cardiovasc Disord 20:188. https://doi.org/10.1186/s12872-020-01466-5
70. Suzanne Oparil RES (2015) New approaches in the treatment of hypertension. Circ Res 116(6):1075
71. Julius S, Kjeldsen SE, Weber M, Brunner HR, Ekman S, Hansson L et al (2004) Outcomes in hypertensive patients at high cardiovascular risk treated with regimens based on valsartan or amlodipine: the VALUE randomised trial. Lancet 363(9426):2022–2031
72. Higgins JP, Altman DG, Gotzsche PC, Juni P, Moher D, Oxman AD et al (2011) The Cochrane Collaboration's tool for assessing risk of bias in randomised trials. BMJ 343:d5928
73. Chaturvedi N, Porta M, Klein R, Orchard T, Fuller J, Parving HH et al (2008) Effect of candesartan on prevention (DIRECT-prevent 1) and progression (DIRECT-protect 1) of retinopathy in type 1 diabetes: randomised, placebo-controlled trials. Lancet 372(9647):1394–1402
74. Bangalore S, Kumar S, Wetterslev J, Messerli FH (2011) Angiotensin receptor blockers and risk of myocardial infarction: meta-analyses and trial sequential analyses of 147,020 patients from randomised trials. BMJ 342:d2234
75. Strauss MH, Hall AS (2017) Angiotensin receptor blockers do not reduce risk of myocardial infarction, cardiovascular death, or total, mortality: further evidence for the ARB-MI paradox. Circulation 135(22):2088–2090
76. Larouche-Lebel É, Loughran KA, Oyama MA (2019) Plasma and tissue angiotensin-converting enzyme 2 activity and plasma equilibrium concentrations of angiotensin peptides in dogs with heart disease. J Vet Intern Med 33:1571–1584. https://doi.org/10.1111/jvim.15548
77. Lambert DW, Yarski M, Warner FJ, Thornhill P, Parkin ET, Smith AI, Hooper NM, Turner AJ (2005) Tumor necrosis factor-alpha convertase (ADAM17) mediates regulated ectodomain shedding of the severe-acute respiratory syndrome-coronavirus (SARS-CoV) recep-

tor, angiotensin-converting enzyme-2 (ACE2). J Biol Chem 280:30113–30119. https://doi.org/10.1074/jbc.M505111200
78. Patel VB, Clarke N, Wang Z, Fan D, Parajuli N, Basu R, Putko B, Kassiri Z, Turner AJ, Oudit GY (2014) Angiotensin II induced proteolytic cleavage of myocardial ACE2 is mediated by TACE/ADAM-17: a positive feedback mechanism in the RAS. J Mol Cell Cardiol 66:167–176. https://doi.org/10.1016/j.yjmcc.2013.11.017
79. Laurent S (2017) Antihypertensive drugs. Pharmacol Res 124:116–125

Chapter 3
ACE Inhibitors: Preferred RAAS Inhibitor in High-Risk Patients as Compared to ARBs

Mukesh Nandave

Introduction by the Editor

In the treatment of cardiovascular disorder, targeting the Renin-Angiotensin-Aldosterone System (RAAS) plays a significant approach. Angiotensin receptor blockers (ARBs) and Angiotensin converting enzyme (ACE) inhibitors are recommended as first line therapy in management of hypertension as they effectively lower blood pressure by RAAS inhibition. Among the available options for RAAS inhibition, ACE inhibitors are preferred over ARBs especially in high-risk patients. ACE inhibitors are the first RAAS inhibitors that are introduced to be administered in humans. In 1981, captopril is the ACE inhibitor to be approved by FDA. After the FDA approval, several ACE inhibitors were synthesized and are being used till date. Over a decade, angiotensin receptor blockers (ARB) were discovered. In 1995, US-FDA approved the first ARB, losartan. From then on, ACE inhibitors and ARBs have been used as anti-hypertensive medicines for several diseases including hypertension, congestive heart failure, chronic kidney disease and coronary heart disease. ACE inhibitors inhibits angiotensin converting enzyme that converts angiotensin I to angiotensin II. Moreover, the inhibition of this enzyme prevents the breakdown of bradykinin thus promoting vasodilation via kinin-kallikrein-bradykinin system. On the other hand, ARBs displace angiotensin II from the AT1 receptor. This displacement can stimulate the AT2 receptor, resulting invasodilation and increased sodium excretion. However, the autocrine cascade associated to ARBs involving nitric oxide, bradykinin and vasoactive prostaglandins is less clinically significant in comparison to that observed with ACE inhibitors [1].

M. Nandave (✉)
Department of Pharmacology, Delhi Pharmaceutical Sciences and Research University, New Delhi, Delhi, India

M. Nandave (ed.), *Angiotensin-converting Enzyme Inhibitors vs. Angiotensin Receptor Blockers*, https://doi.org/10.1007/978-981-97-7380-0_3

ACE inhibitors are generally prescribed for the patients with non-complicated hypertension as well as they are used in hypertension with concomitant chronic kidney disease, coronary artery disease, arterial fibrillation, heart failure with reduced ejection fraction and diabetes. The UK National Institute for Health and Care Excellence (NICE) suggests the usage of ACE inhibitors as first line treatment in hypertensive patients with type 2 diabetes mellitus while recommends usage of angiotensin receptor blockers (ARBs) in patients who have low tolerance to ACE inhibitors. ACE inhibitors not only reduce blood pressure but also found to be effective in high-risk patients with coronary artery disease. ACE inhibitors prevent degradation of bradykinin as a result it facilitates nitric oxide induced ischemic preconditioning, fibrinolysis, and endothelial function. Vasoconstriction results in thrombosis, increased oxidative stress and inflammation, however these could be prevented with the administration of ACE inhibitors. In a study involving elderly (≥60 age) acute myocardial infarction patients without hypertension history who underwent percutaneous coronary intervention (PCI) with drug-eluting stents (DES), reduced risk of stroke and rehospitalization due to heart failure was observed associated with ACE inhibitors as compared to ARBs. According to the reports it is suggested that ACE inhibitors significantly reduce the risk of heart disease, stroke, and mortality than ARBs. These effects should be considered prior to opting ARBs over ACE inhibitors [2, 3].

This chapter discusses the ACE inhibitors as the preferred choice over ARBs in high-risk patients. The evidence collected from clinical trials, meta-analysis, systematic reviews suggests that ACE inhibitors provides better outcomes in relation with morality and cardiovascular events especially in patients with diabetes, heart failure and chronic kidney disease. Despite ACE inhibitors associated with most common adverse events such as angioedema and dry cough their efficacy makes them a preferred option especially in vulnerable populations. However, treatment decisions must be based on individual patient factors, and further research is needed to understand the controversial data between ACE inhibitors and ARBs.

This chapter delves into prominent characteristics of ACE inhibitors required for the treatment of cardiovascular disorders by targeting RAAS. This chapter not only explored the significant role of ACE inhibitors but also discussed the comparative effectiveness of ACE inhibitors and ARBs. Through illuminating distinctive characteristics, we aim to provide diverse knowledge to healthcare professionals so that they can make well informed decisions to deliver the best possible healthcare to the patients (Fig. 3.1).

Machine Generated Summaries

Disclaimer: The summaries in this chapter were generated from Springer Nature publications using extractive AI auto-summarization: An extraction-based summarizer aims to identify the most important sentences of a text using an algorithm and

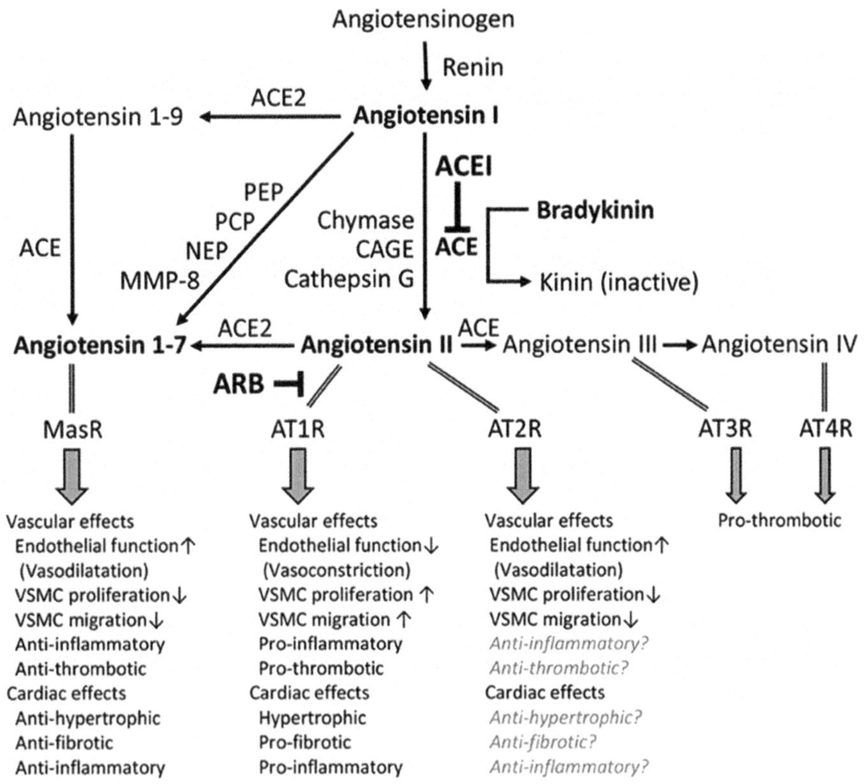

Fig. 3.1 RAAS blockade with ACE and ARBS. There are controversies about the effects of AT2R signaling, which are indicated in *gray italic*. *ARB* angiotensin receptor blocker, *AT1R* angiotensin type one receptor, *AT2R* angiotensin type two receptor, *AT3R* angiotensin type three receptor, *AT4R* angiotensin type four receptor, *CAGE* chymostatin-sensitive angiotensin-II-generating enzyme, *MasR* Mas receptor, *MMP-8* matrix metalloproteinase-8, *NEP* neutral endopeptidase, *PCP* prolyl carboxypeptidase, *PEP* prolyl endopeptidase, *RAS* renin-angiotensin system, *VSMC* vascular smooth muscle cell. (Source: Borghi and Omboni [4])

uses those original sentences to create the auto-summary (unlike generative AI). As the constituted sentences are machine selected, they may not fully reflect the body of the work, so we strongly advise that the original content is read and cited. The auto generated summaries were curated by the editor to meet Springer Nature publication standards. To cite this content, please refer to the original papers.

Machine generated keywords: remodeling, ami, acei, pci, acei arb, day, fibrosis, rat, ang, raas, infarction ami, atherosclerosis, atherosclerotic, coronary heart, patient treat.

The Impact of Dose of the Angiotensin-Receptor Blocker Valsartan on the Post-Myocardial Infarction Ventricular Remodeling: Study Protocol for a Randomized Controlled Trial [5]

This is a machine-generated summary of:

Cho, Young-Rak; Kim, Young-Dae; Park, Tae-Ho; Park, Kyungil; Park, Jong-Sung; Baek, Heekyung; Choi, Sun-Young; Kim, Kee-Sik; Hong, Taek-Jong; Yang, Tae-Hyun; Hwang, Jin-Yong; Park, Jong-Seon; Hur, Seung-Ho; Lee, Sang-Gon: The impact of dose of the angiotensin-receptor blocker valsartan on the post-myocardial infarction ventricular remodeling: study protocol for a randomized controlled trial [5].

Published in: Trials (2011).

Link to original: https://doi.org/10.1186/1745-6215-12-247

If you want to cite the papers, please refer to the original.

For technical reasons we could not place the page where the original quote is coming from.

Abstract-Summary “Valsartan in post-MI remodeling (VALID) is a randomized, open-label, single-blinded multicenter study designed to compare the efficacy of different clinical dose of valsartan on the post-MI ventricular remodeling.”

“This study also aims to assess neurohormone change and clinical parameters of patients during the post-infarct period.”

“A total of 1116 patients with left ventricular dysfunction following the first episode of acute ST-elevation MI are to be enrolled and randomized to a maximal tolerable dose (up to 320 mg/day) or usual dose (80 mg/day) of valsartan for 12 months in 2:1 ratio.”

“Echocardiographic analysis for quantifying post-MI ventricular remodeling is to be conducted in central core laboratory.”

“VALID is a multicenter collaborative study to evaluate the impact of dose of valsartan on the post-MI ventricular remodeling.”

“The results of the study provide information about optimal dosing of the drug in the management of patients after MI.”

Background

"Although administration of higher dose of angiotensin-converting enzyme (ACE) inhibitor was more beneficial than lower dose in animal model of post-MI remodeling [6], results of clinical studies were not confirmatory."

"The question of whether submaximal dose of ARB, which are lower than those in major pivotal trials but typically used in clinical practice, can offer similar benefit in post-MI ventricular remodeling remains to be solved."

"The primary objective of the VALsartan in post-mI remoDeling (VALID) study is to address this issue in Korean patients who suffered their first acute ST-elevation MI by comparing the impact of different doses of valsartan, an ARB demonstrated as effective as ACE inhibitor in post-MI patients [7], on echocardiographic variables of left ventricular remodeling during the follow-up period of 1 year."

Methods and Design

"In the VALIANT Echo study, [8] a sample size of 600 patients was determined necessary to detect, with a 90% power, a 7.6 mL difference in end-diastolic volume between the treatment groups."

"Because the present study enrolls more patients with mild degree (EF < 50%) LV dysfunction, we anticipate that the difference of ventricular volume between treatment groups will be smaller than the previous study."

"Detection of 3.8 mL difference, with a two-sided level of significance $\alpha = 5\%$ and a power of $1 - \beta = 90\%$, in end-diastolic volume between treatment groups would require a sample size of 279 patients in a usual dose of valsartan group and 558 patients in a high dose valsartan group."

"Assessments for the change of neurohormone and other echocardiographic indices will be compared between treatment groups at 12-month follow-up using 2-sample t tests."

Discussion

"Despite the accepted roles of ACE inhibitors and the ARB agent valsartan in the treatment of post-MI LV dysfunction [7–9], the appropriate dose remains unclear."

"Although the recent HEAAL study demonstrated a superiority of higher dose over low dose losartan in ACE intolerant patients with heart failure, the evidence is still lacking for the setting of post-MI LV dysfunction and for general population."

"The VALID study has been designed to address the issue of optimal dosing of ARB valsartan in the post-MI patients by comparing the major echocardiographic outcome of post-MI LV remodeling, which is the LV volume index."

Conclusions

"As the proportion of elderly population among the patients with acute MI is increasing, the pattern of post-MI remodeling may exhibit a different picture."

"Elderly patients seem to undergo LV remodeling more commonly than younger patients, even after smaller size acute MI."

"In the PREAMI study [10], ACE inhibitor (8 mg/day of perindopril) could reduce progressive LV remodeling in elderly patients who had a relatively preserved LV function with EF ≥40%."

"The increasing proportion of elderly population in acute MI cases in Korea [11] can make it feasible to examine the effect of ARB agent on post-MI remodeling in the presence of moderate LV dysfunction for the VALID study."

Angiotensin-Converting Enzyme Inhibitors and Angiotensin Receptor Blockers in Acute Coronary Syndrome: Implications for Platelet Reactivity? [12]

This is a machine-generated summary of:

Tscharre, Maximilian; Wadowski, Patricia P.; Weikert, Constantin; Pultar, Joseph; Eichelberger, Beate; Panzer, Simon; Gremmel, Thomas: Angiotensin-Converting Enzyme Inhibitors and Angiotensin Receptor Blockers in Acute Coronary Syndrome: Implications for Platelet Reactivity? [12].

Published in: Cardiovascular Drugs and Therapy (2020).

Link to original: https://doi.org/10.1007/s10557-020-07128-0

If you want to cite the papers, please refer to the original.

For technical reasons we could not place the page where the original quote is coming from.

Abstract-Summary "In a recent pilot study, treatment with ACE inhibitors was associated with increased platelet reactivity compared to ARBs."

"We sought to investigate the impact of renin-angiotensin-aldosterone system (RAAS) blockade with ACE inhibitors and ARBs on platelet aggregation in patients with ACS undergoing percutaneous coronary intervention."

"On-treatment residual AA- and ADP-inducible platelet reactivity was significantly higher in patients with ACE inhibitors (both $p < 0.05$)."

"SFLLRN was significantly higher in patients with ACE inhibitors ($p = 0.036$) and there was a trend for higher AYPGKF- and collagen-inducible platelet reactivity ($p = 0.053$ and $p = 0.082$)."

"The incidence of high on-treatment residual platelet reactivity AA was significantly higher in patients with ACE inhibitors (52 [31.5%] vs. 3 [9.4%] patients; $p = 0.019$)."

"ACE inhibitors are associated with increased on-treatment residual platelet reactivity in ACS patients with potent DAPT."

Introduction

"According to current guidelines, renin-angiotensin-aldosterone system (RAAS) blockade with an angiotensin-converting enzyme (ACE) inhibitor or an angiotensin receptor blocker (ARB) should be considered in all patients presenting with ST-elevation myocardial infarction (STEMI) and is recommended for all ACS patients suffering from either arterial hypertension, chronic kidney disease, diabetes, or reduced left-ventricular ejection fraction [13, 14]."

"In a recent pilot-analysis by Helten and others including patients with an indication for RAAS blockade (arterial hypertension or heart failure), ACE inhibitors were associated with increased platelet surface expression of protease-activated receptor-1 (PAR-1) and enhanced SFLLRN (=thrombin receptor activating peptide [TRAP])-inducible platelet reactivity compared to ARBs [15]."

"Considering these recent data, we sought to assess the impact of RAAS blockade with ACE inhibitors or ARBs on platelet aggregation in ACS patients receiving either prasugrel or ticagrelor following acute PCI."

Methods

"Blood sampling was performed 72 h after acute PCI with stent implantation."

"Due to the short half-life of unfractionated heparin, all patients were free of heparin from PCI at the time of blood sampling [16]."

"To avoid procedural deviations, blood sampling was performed by the same physician applying a light tourniquet, which was immediately released, and the samples were mixed by gently inverting the tubes."

"Blood was drawn into hirudin-coated tubes (Roche Diagnostics, Mannheim, Germany) for multiple electrode aggregometry (MEA)."

"Whole blood impedance aggregometry was performed using the Multiplate analyzer (Roche Diagnostics) as previously described [17]."

"Titration experiments were carried out, increasing the dosages of SFLLRN and AYPGKF, respectively, until both agonists induced platelet aggregation >60 aggregation units (AU) by MEA, but less than maximal response in healthy Caucasian individuals (n = 30)."

"χ^2 test or Fisher's exact test was performed for comparison of categorical variables, as appropriate."

Results

"In multivariable linear regression analysis, ACE inhibitor therapy remained significantly associated with increased AA- and ADP-inducible platelet reactivity (both $p < 0.05$), whereas after adjustment, no association with SFLLRN-, AYPGKF-, and collagen-induced platelet reactivity was detectable (all $p > 0.05$)."

"After adjustment, ACE inhibitors no longer were associated with agonist-inducible residual platelet reactivity in patients treated with prasugrel (all $p > 0.05$)."

"In patients on ticagrelor, residual AA-inducible platelet reactivity was numerically but not statistically and ADP-inducible reactivity significantly higher in patients with ACE inhibitors."

"In multivariable regression analysis, ACE inhibitors remained associated with ADP-inducible platelet reactivity ($p = 0.002$) but were not associated with AA-, SFLLRN-, AYPGKF-, and collagen-inducible residual platelet reactivity in patients on ticagrelor (all $p > 0.05$)."

Discussion

"This is the first study investigating the association of ACE inhibitors and ARBs with on-treatment residual platelet reactivity in ACS patients on potent DAPT undergoing PCI."

"Our main finding was that agonist-inducible platelet reactivity as assessed by MEA was higher in patients receiving ACE inhibitors as compared to patients receiving ARBs."

"In a randomized controlled study including aspirin-treated patients with coronary artery disease (CAD; defined as <50% stenosis in coronary angiography) comparing the impact RAAS blockade on platelet aggregation, irbesartan (an ARB) significantly reduced TXA2-induced platelet aggregation, whereas enalapril (an ACE inhibitor) had no effect on TXA2-induced platelet aggregation assessed by turbidometry [18]."

"In our cohort, we detected higher on-treatment residual AA- and ADP-inducible platelet reactivity by MEA in patients with ACE inhibitor therapy."

"Our data indicate a benefit of ARBs over ACE inhibitors with respect to on-treatment residual platelet reactivity in ACS patients with potent DAPT."

Limitations

"The present investigation should be interpreted with the following limitations in mind: Our study is not powered nor intended to provide clinical outcome data."

"We measured platelet aggregation at only one time point using a single test system."

"MEA is a highly standardized platelet function test ensuring a good comparability of the obtained results with other laboratories, and platelet aggregation by MEA has repeatedly been linked to cardiovascular outcomes following PCI [19, 20]."

Conclusion

"ACE inhibitors are associated with increased on-treatment residual platelet reactivity in ACS patients on potent DAPT."

"Further clinical trials are needed to elucidate the role of RAAS blockade with ACE inhibitors and ARBs in ACS patients treated according to modern standards."

Angiotensin-Converting-Enzyme Inhibitor Prevents Skeletal Muscle Fibrosis in Myocardial Infarction Mice [21]

This is a machine-generated summary of:

Kakutani, Naoya; Takada, Shingo; Nambu, Hideo; Matsumoto, Junichi; Furihata, Takaaki; Yokota, Takashi; Fukushima, Arata; Kinugawa, Shintaro: Angiotensin-converting-enzyme inhibitor prevents skeletal muscle fibrosis in myocardial infarction mice [21].

Published in: Skeletal Muscle (2020).

Link to original: https://doi.org/10.1186/s13395-020-00230-9

If you want to cite the papers, please refer to the original.

For technical reasons we could not place the page where the original quote is coming from.

Abstract-Summary "We found higher skeletal muscle fibrosis in MI mice compared with control mice, and we investigated the mechanisms involved therein."

"We administered an inhibitor based on the above mechanism and investigated its preventive effects on skeletal muscle fibrosis."

"The time course of skeletal muscle fibrosis post-MI was analyzed by picrosirius-red staining (days 1, 3, 7, and 14)."

"Mice were then divided into 3 groups: sham + vehicle (Sham + Veh), MI + Veh, and MI + lisinopril (an angiotensin-converting enzyme [ACE] inhibitor, 20 mg/kg body weight/day in drinking water; MI + Lis)."

"Skeletal muscle fibrosis was significantly increased in MI mice compared with sham mice from 3 to 14 days postsurgery."

"Skeletal muscle fibrosis and hydroxyproline (a key marker of collagen content) were significantly increased in MI + Veh mice compared with the Sham + Veh mice."

"Consistent with these results, protein expression of TGF-β and phosphorylated Smad2/3 in the skeletal muscle during the early time points after surgery (days 1–7 postsurgery) and blood angiotensin II at 14 days postsurgery was increased in MI mice compared with sham mice."

"These impairments were improved in MI + Lis mice, without any effects on spontaneous physical activity, muscle strength, muscle weight, and blood pressure."

"ACE inhibitor administration prevents increased skeletal muscle fibrosis during the early phase after MI."

Background

"Fibrosis is associated with an impairment of various organs, including the heart, kidney, lung, and skeletal muscle, and has become a major cause of death in the developed world [22, 23]."

"Skeletal muscle fibrosis has been reported to be caused by several diseases (e.g., chronic kidney disease and Duchenne muscular dystrophy) [24, 25], or in response to injury [26] and immobilization [27]."

"It is unclear whether skeletal muscle fibrosis is induced by the induction of MI by surgery."

"In this study, we first sought to determine whether skeletal muscle fibrosis is present in mice with MI."

"We further analyzed whether skeletal muscle fibrosis in MI mice can be prevented by administration of an inhibitor of angiotensin-converting enzyme (ACE)."

Methods

"Echocardiography measurements were performed 1, 3, 7, and 14 days postsurgery, and then, mice were sacrificed, and their skeletal muscles were excised."

"There was no difference in skeletal muscle fibrosis area between the Sham + Veh and Sham + Lis mice (Sham 3.9% ± 0.3% vs. Sham + Lis 3.4% ± 0.3%, n = 5, respectively) at 14 days postsurgery."

"To clarify the effects of Lis on skeletal muscle fibrosis in MI mice, Sham mice (n = 24) were randomly assigned to 4 groups after the surgery for sacrifice on days 1, 3, 7, and 14 (n = 6 each)."

"The Sham + Veh and the MI + Lis mice were analyzed by echocardiography at 1, 3, 7, and 14 days postsurgery, and then, they were sacrificed, and their skeletal muscles were excised (n = 6 each)."

Results

"Skeletal muscle fibrosis was significantly increased in the MI mice from 3 to 14 days postsurgery compared with sham mice."

"Heart weight/BW was significantly increased in the MI and MI + Lis mice compared with the sham mice."

"LV end-diastolic diameter was significantly increased, and fractional shortening and anterior wall thickness (AWT) were significantly decreased in MI + Veh and MI + Lis mice compared with Sham mice, but there was no difference in the function of and the AWT of the LV between the MI groups."

"We next analyzed whether an ACE inhibitor, which has been shown to exert secondary anti-fibrotic effects [28], prevents the increase in skeletal muscle fibrosis of MI mice."

Discussion

"We next analyzed whether a mouse model with MI-induced skeletal muscle fibrosis improves by administration of an ACE inhibitor."

"Our series of results suggest that factors other than Ang II may also be important for the increase of skeletal muscle fibrosis in MI model mice, but this could not be clarified in the present study."

"To our knowledge, there is no treatment for fibrosis to date, but preventive or early administration of an ACE inhibitor in MI mice may suppress the increase in skeletal muscle fibrosis [29–31]."

"Abramowitz and others reported that skeletal muscle fibrosis was increased in patients with chronic kidney disease and negatively correlates with physical fitness levels [32]."

"The prevention of skeletal muscle fibrosis using early and continuous ACE inhibitor treatment in heart disease patients may play a role in muscle function."

Conclusions

"ACE inhibitor administration prevents the increase in skeletal muscle fibrosis during the early phase after MI."

"Our findings may provide a new therapeutic target to skeletal muscle abnormalities in heart diseases."

"Future studies are required to clarify whether skeletal muscle fibrosis is also directly linked to physical fitness."

Beta-Blockers and Renin-Angiotensin System Inhibitors in Acute Myocardial Infarction Managed with Inhospital Coronary Revascularization [33]

This is a machine-generated summary of:

Sim, Hui Wen; Zheng, Huili; Richards, A. Mark; Chen, Ruth W.; Sahlen, Anders; Yeo, Khung-Keong; Tan, Jack W.; Chua, Terrance; Tan, Huay Cheem; Yeo, Tiong Cheng; Ho, Hee Hwa; Liew, Boon-Wah; Foo, Ling Li; Lee, Chi-Hang; Hausenloy, Derek J.; Chan, Mark Y.: Beta-blockers and renin-angiotensin system inhibitors in acute myocardial infarction managed with inhospital coronary revascularization [33].

Published in: Scientific Reports (2020).

Link to original: https://doi.org/10.1038/s41598-020-72232-y

If you want to cite the papers, please refer to the original.

For technical reasons we could not place the page where the original quote is coming from.

Abstract-Summary "At 12 months, BB was significantly associated with a lower incidence of major adverse cardiovascular events (MACE, adjusted HR 0.80, 95% CI 0.70–0.93) and all-cause mortality (adjusted HR 0.69, 95% CI 0.55–0.88), while ACEI/ARB was significantly associated with lower all-cause mortality (adjusted HR 0.80, 95% CI 0.66–0.98) and heart failure (HF) hospitalization (adjusted HR 0.80, 95% CI 0.68–0.95)."

"Combined BB and ACEI/ARB use was associated with the lowest incidence of MACE (adjusted HR 0.70, 95% CI 0.57–0.86), all-cause mortality (adjusted HR 0.55, 95% CI 0.40–0.77) and HF hospitalization (adjusted HR 0.64, 95% CI 0.48–0.86)."

"In AMI managed with revascularization, both BB and ACEI/ARB were associated with a lower incidence of 12-month all-cause mortality."

"Combined BB and ACEI/ARB was associated with the lowest incidence of all-cause mortality and HF hospitalization."

Introduction

"Beta-blockers (BB) and angiotensin-converting enzyme inhibitors/angiotensin receptor blockers (ACEI/ARB) have been the cornerstone of treatment for acute myocardial infarction (AMI) due to their salutary effects on short- and long-term mortality."

"ACEI/ARB have been shown to reduce mortality in AMI but a class I recommendation is only assigned to patients with anterior myocardial infarction (MI), heart failure (HF) and/or reduced LVEF [7–11, 13–20, 22–32, 34–42]."

"There is a need to reassess the role of BB and ACEI/ARB in this contemporary treatment era of routine early revascularization for AMI."

"We evaluated the association of BB and ACEI/ARB with 12-month mortality, HF hospitalization and MI in patients with AMI who had undergone inhospital coronary revascularization."

Methods

"Multivariable Cox proportional hazard regression models were constructed to estimate the hazard ratio (HR) and 95% confidence interval (CI) for the risk of composite endpoint, all-cause mortality, MI and HF hospitalization, for patients who were given (1) BB and those who were not given (reference group) and (2) ACEI/ARB compared to those who were not given these medications (reference group)."

"Included in the multivariable models were age, gender, ethnicity, hypertension, diabetes, hyperlipidemia, history of MI/PCI/CABG, smoking status, Killip class on admission, creatinine level on admission and in-hospital LVEF <50%."

"Secondary subgroup analysis examined clinical outcomes stratified by the following categories: types of AMI (STEMI or NSTEMI), age (<65 years old or ≥65 years old), sex (male or female), history of diabetes, history of hypertension, Killip class on presentation (I/II or III/III), LVEF during hospitalization (<50% or ≥50%), PCI during hospitalization and CABG during hospitalization."

Results

"BB use at discharge was associated with a lower incidence of the combined MACE endpoint (adjusted HR 0.80, 95% CI 0.70–0.93) and all-cause mortality (adjusted HR 0.69, 95% CI 0.55–0.88) while ACEI/ARB use at discharge was associated with lower all-cause mortality (adjusted HR 0.80, 95% CI 0.66–0.98) and lower hospitalization for HF (adjusted HR 0.80, 95% CI 0.68–0.95)."

"The BB + ACEI/ARB group had the lowest incidence of MACE (adjusted HR 0.70, 95% CI 0.57–0.86), all-cause mortality (adjusted HR 0.55, 95% CI 0.40–0.77) and hospitalization for HF (adjusted HR 0.64, 95% CI 0.48–0.86) among all four groups."

"In patients who receive ACEI/ARB, the risk of mortality, HF and MI hospitalization were consistently higher in the subgroup who underwent revascularization with CABG as compared to PCI."

Discussion

"In this contemporary cohort of patients with AMI undergoing inhospital revascularization, we observed that prescription of either BB or ACEI/ARB at discharge was associated with a lower incidence of 12-month all-cause mortality compared with patients who received neither drug at discharge, even after adjusting for relevant confounding variables."

"Several contemporary observational studies have found no reduction in mortality or hospitalization for HF associated with ACEI/ARB among patients with AMI and preserved LVEF [10, 43]."

"One other observational study that looked at AMI patients who underwent PCI in South Korea (N = 33,390) found no significant differences in the adjusted risk of all-cause mortality for patients treated with BB + ACEI/ARB, BB-only, ACEI/ARB-only as compared to non-treatment [44]."

"Forth, the subgroup analysis showed that in patients prescribed with BB or ACEI/ARB at discharge, risk of adverse clinical outcomes (except HF hospitalization in BB) was higher in the group who underwent revascularization with CABG as compared to PCI."

Conclusion

"Among patients with AMI who are managed with inhospital revascularization and who are receiving high levels of dual antiplatelet and lipid-lowering therapy, either BB or ACEI/ARB use was associated with a lower incidence of 12-month all-cause mortality than if neither drug was prescribed at discharge."

"Our study findings conflict with that of other contemporary observation studies, highlighting continuing knowledge gaps in the appropriate use of BB and ACEI/ARB among patients with AMI in the current treatment era."

"While randomized trials of BB are ongoing in contemporarily-managed AMI populations, we propose that the role ACEI/ARB treatment also be re-examined in randomized trials of patients with AMI who undergo early revascularization and are already receiving high levels of dual antiplatelet and lipid-lowering therapy."

Recent Developments in Imaging of Myocardial Angiotensin Receptors [45]

This is a machine-generated summary of:

Lautamäki, Riikka; Knuuti, Juhani; Saraste, Antti: Recent Developments in Imaging of Myocardial Angiotensin Receptors [45].

Published in: Current Cardiovascular Imaging Reports (2013).

Link to original: https://doi.org/10.1007/s12410-013-9245-x

If you want to cite the papers, please refer to the original.

For technical reasons we could not place the page where the original quote is coming from.

Abstract-Summary "Upregulation of the systemic and myocardial renin-angiotensin system (RAS) plays a role in adverse left ventricle (LV) remodeling and development of heart failure in various cardiac diseases."

"Molecular imaging of increased myocardial angiotensin converting enzyme (ACE) activity or angiotensin II type 1 –receptor (AT1R) upregulation might identify patients at risk of developing heart failure or optimize treatment of heart failure."

"The recent advances and new tracers for molecular imaging of myocardial RAS activation are reviewed together with the discussion on patophysiology and the potential clinical implications."

Introduction

"The underlying etiology in heart failure is coronary artery disease and myocardial infarction in the majority of the patients [46]."

"Myocardial remodeling is a common mechanism of the development and the progression of heart failure caused by different etiologies [47]."

"Numerous investigations have demonstrated that the remodeling is associated with poor outcome in patients with heart failure or previous myocardial infarction [47]."

"Molecular imaging of the biological processes involved in myocardial remodeling can provide new biomarkers for the early detection, the evaluation of therapy response and the risk stratification of heart failure [48, 49]."

"Numerous clinical studies have shown the beneficial effects of ACE inhibitors or ATR1 blockers for prevention of myocardial remodeling and improving survival of patients with heart failure [50]."

"The molecular imaging of increased myocardial ACE activity or AT1R upregulation might identify the patients at risk of developing heart failure or optimize the treatment of heart failure."

Renin-Angiotensin System in Myocardial Remodeling

"Angiotensin II stimulates AT1R and type 2 receptors."

"Local renin-angiotensin system with the trophic effects to modify gene expression may be more important for the remodeling than systemic RAS [51]."

"Increased amount of prorenin, renin, ACE and the density of AT1R may be observed in the patients with heart failure [52]."

"The local RAS system is activated by serine proteases causing activation of the angiotensinogen gene expression and ACE action, and eventually increased angiotensin II production, which causes the remodeling of the LV [53]."

"Recent advances in molecular imaging may provide new tools for evaluating the level of RAS activation in heart failure and, thus, enable timely and dose-optimized targeted therapies for the reverse remodeling pathways."

Molecular Imaging of the Renin-Angiotensin System in the Heart

"These studies with highly specific binding of the tracer with a close correlation with ex vivo findings provide rationale for further testing in the experimental setting. [^{11}C]MK-996 and [^{11}C]L-159884 were the first tracers for AT1R imaging [54, 55]."

"Technetium-99 m-labeled losartan showed significant uptake of the tracer in the infarct regions in a mouse model of myocardial infarction as seen with SPECT imaging [56]."

"These early studies proved the feasibility of the tracer for PET imaging in general and due to the observed high myocardial uptake, these studies suggested that the tracer could be used for the evaluation of the RAS in heart."

"This experimental study shows highly specific binding of AT1R of the tracer and similarities of the binding pattern between human and pig myocardium were observed, however, further testing is needed for its use in imaging of human disease."

Conclusions

"The current experimental data have shown the feasibility of in vivo imaging of the activation of the myocardial RAS with AT1R targeted radiolabeled tracers after myocardial infarction."

"The relatively modest, two to three fold tracer uptake indicates that probes with improved targeting characteristics could be useful for improving the sensitivity of the imaging."

"Whether the technique is sensitive enough to monitor the therapies in patients remain to be studied."

"The proof of concept is clear and the methods show a significant potential, however, further studies will determine its role in clinical medicine."

Influence of On-Going Treatment with Angiotensin-Converting Enzyme Inhibitor or Angiotensin Receptor Blocker on the Outcome of Patients Treated with Intravenous rt-PA for Ischemic Stroke [57]

This is a machine-generated summary of:

Gilliot, Sixtine; Sibon, Igor; Mas, Jean-Louis; Moulin, Thierry; Béjot, Yannick; Cordonnier, Charlotte; Giroud, Maurice; Odou, Pascal; Bordet, Régis; Vivien, Denis; Leys, Didier; The OPHELIE Investigators, None: Influence of on-going treatment with angiotensin-converting enzyme inhibitor or angiotensin receptor blocker on the outcome of patients treated with intravenous rt-PA for ischemic stroke [57].

Published in: Journal of Neurology (2018).

Link to original: https://doi.org/10.1007/s00415-018-8827-6

If you want to cite the papers, please refer to the original.

For technical reasons we could not place the page where the original quote is coming from.

Abstract-Summary "Many patients who receive intravenous (i.v.) recombinant tissue-plasminogen activator (rt-PA) for acute cerebral ischemia were under angiotensin-converting enzyme inhibitors (ACE-Is) or angiotensin receptor blockers (ARBs) at stroke onset."

"We compared outcomes between patients with and without ACE-Is/ARBs according to the modified Rankin scale (mRS) at month 3, using logistic regression analyses adjusted on propensity scores, and propensity-matched analyses."

"Of 1803 patients, 455 (25.2%) were under ACE-Is (259), ARBs (188) or both (8)."

"At 3 months, patients under ACE-Is or ARBs were more likely to have an mRS 0–1, but did not differ for mRS 0–2, s-ICH and death."

"After adjustment on propensity scores, the association between ACE-Is/ARBs and mRS 0–1 disappeared."

"The propensity-matched analysis, performed in 397 pairs of patients, found no difference in outcomes between patients with and without ACE-Is or ARBs."

"In patients treated by intravenous thrombolytic therapy for ischemic stroke, on-going treatment with ACE-Is or ARBs does not influence on outcomes after adjustment on baseline characteristics and propensity scores."

Introduction

"Many patients who receive intravenous (i.v.) recombinant tissue plasminogen activator (rt-PA) for acute cerebral ischemia are under angiotensin-converting enzyme inhibitors (ACE-Is) or angiotensin receptor blockers (ARBs) for arterial hypertension, diabetes mellitus with micro-albuminuria, or congestive heart failure."

"In clinical practice, pre-stroke inhibition of the renin–angiotensin–aldosterone system might be associated with a lower severity of stroke and a better outcome: a large Danish nationwide study conducted in 83,736 patients with ischemic stroke showed that those under ACE-Is or ARBs had lower case-fatality rates [58]."

"No study has evaluated the effect of previous chronic administration of ACE-Is or ARBs in a cohort of patients who underwent a recanalization procedure with rt-PA, mechanical thrombectomy, or both."

"rt-PA for cerebral ischemia in clinical practice was influenced by on-going therapy with ACE-Is/ARBs."

Method

"The Lille stroke thrombolysis registry includes prospectively all consecutive patients treated with i.v."

"We classified as being treated by ACE-I/ARBS patients with on-going therapy with ACE-Is or ARBs at stroke onset, not those who stopped the treatment before."

"We calculated adjusted p values for the association between outcomes and on-going treatment with ACE-Is/ARBs, with forward logistic regression analyses [59], including the outcome (mRS 0–1, mRS 0–2, s-ICH and death) classified 1 when present and 0 when absent as a dependent variable."

"Variables for the propensity score were variables present before stroke, included step-by-step using an alpha value of 0.10: age, arterial hypertension, diabetes mellitus, previous stroke, smoking, on-going anticoagulation therapy, on-going antiplatelet therapy, cardio-embolic source, and other defined causes of stroke."

Results

"Patients under ACE-Is/ARBs were more likely to have had a previous stroke, arterial hypertension, diabetes mellitus, and a cardio-embolic cause of stroke, to be under antiplatelet agent, to have had MRI as baseline imaging procedure and mechanical thrombectomy, and less likely to have an mRS 0–1 before stroke, to be smokers, to have a known onset-to-needle time, and to have an unknown cause of stroke."

"Patients under ACE-Is/ARBs did not significantly differ for any of the 4 outcome measures."

"After adjustment on potential confounders, patients under ACE-Is/ARBs were more likely to have an mRS 0–1 at 3 months, but did not differ for mRS 0–2, s-ICH and death."

"After adjustment on propensity scores, the association between ACE-Is/ARBs and mRS 0–1 disappeared."

"The propensity-matched analysis was possible in 397 pairs of patients with and without ACE-Is/ARBs."

Discussion

"We did not evaluate the influence of ACE-Is/ARBs on the risk of orolingual angioedema because (1) OLAE was not recorded in the OPHELIE database, (2) this has already been studied in patients from the Lille database [60], and (3) this was out of the scope of our study."

"Our study did not find a difference in baseline stroke severity: in case of neuroprotective effect, we could have expected a slightly lower NIHSS score in patients under ACE-Is/ARBs."

"We cannot exclude that a neuroprotective effect exists, but (i) is too small to be identified in a cohort of less than 2000 patients, or (ii) is masked by the presence of more vascular risk factors in patients treated with ACE-Is/ARBs, especially those on which we could not adjust for."

"The decision to use ACE-Is/ARBs in patients at risk for stroke should therefore not be influenced by a possible neuroprotective or deleterious effect in case of treatment by thrombolytic therapy."

Angiotensin II Receptor Blocker Irbesartan Attenuates Cardiac Dysfunction Induced by Myocardial Infarction in the Presence of Renal Failure [61]

This is a machine-generated summary of:

Watanabe, Ryo; Suzuki, Jun-ichi; Wakayama, Kouji; Kumagai, Hidetoshi; Ikeda, Yuichi; Akazawa, Hiroshi; Komuro, Issei; Isobe, Mitsuaki: Angiotensin II receptor blocker irbesartan attenuates cardiac dysfunction induced by myocardial infarction in the presence of renal failure [61].

Published in: Hypertension Research (2015).
Link to original: https://doi.org/10.1038/hr.2015.141

If you want to cite the papers, please refer to the original.

For technical reasons we could not place the page where the original quote is coming from.

Abstract-Summary "Irbesartan, an angiotensin II receptor blocker, has non-hemodynamic cardiovascular and renal protective effects."

"The effect of irbesartan on heart failure complicated by renal failure has not yet been elucidated."

"The purpose of this study was to evaluate the effect of irbesartan on the pathophysiology of cardiorenal syndrome in a rat model."

"MI with NTX model rats showed an impaired post-MI survival rate and enhanced cardiac inflammation in comparison to MI without NTX rats."

"Although irbesartan treatment did not improve the survival rate, it suppressed cardiac inflammation, left ventricular function decline, cardiac fibrosis, hypertrophy of cardiomyocytes and renal fibrosis in MI with NTX rats."

"Increases in protein expression levels related to oxidative stress and inflammation (NADPH oxidase 4, phospho-nuclear factor-κB and phospho-c-Jun) observed in the hearts of non-treated MI with NTX rats were attenuated by irbesartan treatment."

"We conclude that irbesartan has a cardioprotective effect after MI when renal dysfunction is present."

Introduction

"The activity of the renin–angiotensin system (RAS) is known to be a key factor in the development of heart failure and renal failure."

"[62–66] Myocardial infarction (MI) is a common antecedent event that predisposes a patient to congestive heart failure."

"A previous study reported that renal injury deteriorates remodeling after MI through excessive RAS activation."

"Many chronic kidney disease patients are more likely to die of cardiovascular disease than end-stage renal disease and dialysis."

"[67] Furthermore, it has been reported that MI is more likely to develop in end-stage renal disease patients within 2 years after initiating dialysis therapy, and the mortality in these patients is high."

"[68] Thus we investigated whether irbesartan has a treatment effect on adverse myocardial remodeling after MI with renal failure."

Methods

"Measurement of the serum creatinine level on Days 0 and 35 was performed before the operation."

"Formaldehyde-fixed paraffin-embedded sections from the midventricular-level heart slices of each group of rats were stained with the Mallory method and the silver impregnation method."

"The content of collagen in the cardiac and renal tissue sections was measured using a Sirius Red/Fast Green Collagen Staining Kit (Chondrex, Redmond, WA, USA) according to the manufacturer's instruction."

"To extract cardiac protein, frozen peri-infarct zone tissues from apex-level heart slices harvested on Day 63 were homogenized in lysis buffer (50 mm Tris–HCl (pH 7.5), 150 mM NaCl, 1% Triton X-100, 1% sodium deoxycholate, 1% sodium dodecyl sulfate (SDS)) containing a protease inhibitor cocktail tablet (Roche Diagnostic, Basel, Switzerland) and a phosphatase inhibitor tablet (Roche Diagnostic)."

Results

"In the post-MI survival curve, the post-MI survival rate of the MI and MI+irbesartan groups were both 100%."

"We measured the collagen level in heart slices from each group to examine the severity of cardiac fibrosis."

"We analyzed the infarct size, compensatory hypertrophy of the non-infarct area and cardiac inflammation to examine the effect of irbesartan treatment on the progression of post-MI remodeling."

"[69, 70] Therefore, we measured the protein expression of NOX4, c-Jun (the component of activator protein-1 (AP-1)) and NF-κB p65 to examine the mechanisms of the treatment effect of irbesartan."

"We measured the serum creatinine and renal collagen levels as markers of renal damage to examine the effect of irbesartan treatment on renal dysfunction in cardiorenal syndrome."

Discussion

"Enhanced inflammation in the NTX-MI model was significantly attenuated by irbesartan treatment."

"Although the treatment effect of irbesartan did not improve the survival rate, our results suggest the possibility that the anti-inflammatory effect of irbesartan in the early phase of post-MI remodeling improves the prognosis after MI in the presence of renal dysfunction."

"Cardiac function decline after MI was significantly attenuated with irbesartan treatment in the surviving NTX-MI model animals."

"These results suggest that irbesartan treatment prevented the progression of cardiac remodeling and improved the pathophysiology after MI in the presence of renal dysfunction."

"[71] An increase in the renal collagen level in the NTX-MI model was significantly suppressed by irbesartan treatment."

"Although a sufficient treatment effect in the kidney was not observed, our data showed that low-dose irbesartan, which did not affect the blood pressure, suppressed cardiac remodeling after MI in the presence of renal dysfunction."

Efficacy of Angiotensin-Converting Enzyme Inhibitors and Angiotensin-Receptor Blockers in Coronary Artery Disease Without Heart Failure in the Modern Statin Era: A Meta-Analysis of Randomized-Controlled Trials [72]

This is a machine-generated summary of:

Hoang, Vu; Alam, Mahboob; Addison, Daniel; Macedo, Francisco; Virani, Salim; Birnbaum, Yochai: Efficacy of Angiotensin-Converting Enzyme Inhibitors and Angiotensin-Receptor Blockers in Coronary Artery Disease without Heart Failure in the Modern Statin Era: a Meta-Analysis of Randomized-Controlled Trials [72].

Published in: Cardiovascular Drugs and Therapy (2016).

Link to original: https://doi.org/10.1007/s10557-016-6652-7

If you want to cite the papers, please refer to the original.

For technical reasons we could not place the page where the original quote is coming from.

Abstract-Summary "Current practice guidelines support the use of angiotensin-converting enzyme inhibitors (ACEi) and angiotensin-receptor blockers (ARBs) in patients with coronary artery disease (CAD) without heart failure (HF)."

"Our objective was to evaluate the effectiveness of ACEi and ARBs in reducing cardiovascular events as well as the impact of statin therapy."

"We searched the MEDLINE and EMBASE databases for randomized-controlled trials (1/1/1980 – 8/31/2015) with ACEi or ARBs as the single intervention for patients with CAD without HF."

"Treatment with ACEi was associated with decreased non-fatal MI (RR 0.83; 95% CI 0.75–0.91), stroke (RR 0.76; 95% CI 0.68–0.86), cardiovascular mortality (RR 0.83; 95% CI 0.72–0.95), and all-cause mortality (RR 0.86; 95% CI 0.80–0.93)."

"When adjusted for statin use, there was a trend towards an attenuated effect of ACEi in reducing cardiovascular mortality with increased use of statins (p-value = 0.063)."

"In CAD patients without HF, ACEi, but not ARBs decreases the risk of non-fatal MI, cardiovascular mortality and all-cause mortality, while both ACEi and ARBs decrease the risk of stroke."

Introduction

"These findings led to further examination of the role of ACEi and ARBs in patients with stable coronary artery disease (CAD) and no evidence of heart failure (HF)."

"Results from two large RCTs, the Heart Outcomes Prevention Evaluation (HOPE) and the European Trial on Reduction of Cardiac Events with Perindopril in Patients with Stable Coronary Artery Disease Study (EUROPA) studies, showed benefit from the addition of ACEi in patients with stable CAD or at high-risk for CV disease without HF."

"As it is plausible that concomitant use of statins could attenuate the beneficial effects of ACEi and ARBs therapy, the present analysis was undertaken to clarify whether the potential benefit of ACEi and/or ARBs in patients with stable CAD or at risk for CAD would persist when accounting for the increasing use of statin therapy in the past two decades."

Methods

"The publications were filtered for randomized-controlled trials, multicenter studies, controlled clinical trials, and adult human subjects, focusing on patients with CAD and CAD risk factors."

"We wanted to perform an inclusive analysis of most major ACEi and ARB trials."

"Baseline statin use (percentage reported) was extracted from all trials that met the inclusion criteria, where data is available."

"To investigate observed heterogeneity, the random effects meta-regression of the RCT results was performed against the percentage of reported statin use."

"The relationship between endpoints across the included trials and the percentage of patients on statin in each trial (with available data) was evaluated using the regression analysis."

"Covariates for this analysis included percentage of beta-blockers, statins, calcium channel blockers, diuretics, and aspirin as reported in the included ACEi trials."

Results

"In the ten ACEi trials, treatment was also associated with a statistically significant reduction in non-fatal MI (RR 0.83; 95% CI 0.75–0.91)."

"Taking the nine ACEi trials with available statin data, the percentage of patients on statin therapy exhibited no significant relationship with the reduction in outcomes due to ACEi therapy."

"Of the three ARB trials with statin data, no statistical significance was found in terms of outcome and percentage of patients on statin therapy."

"Performing multivariate regression model including aspirin, statin, beta-blocker, calcium channel blockers and diuretic use, we found that increasing percentage of aspirin use was associated with a significant reduction in CV mortality in the background of ACEi therapy, as evidence by the reduction in odds ratio for CV mortality ($p = 0.029$)."

Discussion

"The fact that the magnitude of the effect of ACEi in the HOPE trial could not be reproduced in the subsequent studies also further questioned the utility of ACEi in patients with CAD."

"This is an ARB study in the HF population, and current guidelines for HF do recommend a combination of beta-blockers and ACEi or ARBs in ACEi-intolerant patients with HF [73]."

"There appears to be a synergistic effect with increasing aspirin therapy in the background of ACEi therapy in improving outcomes for patients with CAD without HF."

"The mitigating effects of statin therapy on the potential benefits of ACEi and ARBs may be affected by whether the patients were also receiving high or low dose statin (data related to statin dose and potency were not available in the trials)."

Conclusion

"This systematic meta-analysis of randomized-controlled trials demonstrates that the treatment with ACEi reduces all-cause mortality, CV mortality, non-fatal MI, and stroke in all CAD patients without HF."

"The treatment with ARBs is associated with a significant reduction only in stroke events."

"These benefits also appear to be extended to patients at high risk for CAD."

"There is a trend that the additive benefits of ACEi in reducing CV mortality is attenuated in patients on statin therapy, however the effect is not statistically significant."

Relationship Between Circulating Levels of Angiotensin-Converting Enzyme 2-Angiotensin-(1–7)-MAS Axis and Coronary Heart Disease [74]

This is a machine-generated summary of:

Zhou, Xiaomin; Zhang, Ping; Liang, Tao; Chen, Yongyue; Liu, Dan; Yu, Huimin: Relationship between circulating levels of angiotensin-converting enzyme 2-angiotensin-(1–7)-MAS axis and coronary heart disease [74].

Published in: Heart and Vessels (2019).

Link to original: https://doi.org/10.1007/s00380-019-01478-y

If you want to cite the papers, please refer to the original.

For technical reasons we could not place the page where the original quote is coming from.

Abstract-Summary "The link between circulating levels of ACE2-Ang-(1–7)-Mas axis and coronary atherosclerosis in humans is not determined."

"The object of present study was to investigate the association of circulating levels of ACE2, Ang-(1–7) and Ang-(1–9) with coronary heart disease (CHD) defined by coronary angiography (CAG)."

"In females, circulating ACE2 levels were higher in the CHD group than in the non-CHD group (5617.16 ± 5206.67 vs. 3124.06 ± 3005.36 pg/ml, P = 0.009), and subgroup analysis showed the significant differences in ACE2 levels between the two groups only exist in patients with multi-vessel lesions (P = 0.009)."

"Circulating Ang-(1–7) and Ang-(1–9) levels had no significant differences between the two groups."

"In males, there were no significant differences in the levels of ACE2-Ang-(1–7)-MAS axis between two groups."

" Circulating ACE2 levels, but not Ang-(1–7) and Ang-(1–9) levels, significantly increased in female CHD group when compared with non-CHD group, increased ACE2 was independently associated with CHD in female and in patients with multi-vessel lesions even after adjusting for the confounding factors, indicating that ACE2 may participate as a compensatory mechanism in CHD."

Introduction

"Several lines of evidence have showed the role of ACE2-Ang-(1–7)-Mas axis in atherosclerosis."

"ACE2 overexpression significantly inhibits early atherosclerotic lesions development both in human endothelial cells in vitro and in apoE-deficient mice in vivo [75]."

"Similar to ACE2, the atheroprotection of Ang-(1–7) has been shown in many previous studies."

"Ang-(1–7) dose dependently inhibited early atherosclerotic lesions via suppressing vascular smooth muscle cells proliferation and migration, and a large dose of Ang-(1–7) enhanced plaque stability via inhibiting plaque inflammation [76]."

"As is mentioned above, the role of ACE2-Ang-(1–7)-Mas axis in the pathogenesis of atherosclerosis has been investigated with use of various animal models, but most of the studies have focused on ACE2, not much is known regarding the role of Ang-(1–7) and Ang-(1–9) in coronary atherosclerosis, there have been no clinical studies to confirm the link between circulating levels of ACE2-Ang-(1–7)-Mas axis and coronary atherosclerosis in humans."

Materials and Methods

"275 consecutive patients who underwent CAG for the evaluation of suspected CHD in the Cardiology Department of Guangdong Provincial People's Hospital were enrolled in the present study."

"CHD was defined as significant coronary stenosis (≥50%) in at least one major coronary artery following the World Health Organization (WHO) criteria, it was assessed using CAG or if a subject showed prior percutaneous or surgical coronary revascularization."

"According to this, all subjects were divided into two groups: CHD group (diameter narrowing ≥50%, n = 218) and non-CHD group (diameter narrowing <50%, n = 57)."

"Major exclusion criteria included: congestive heart failure; clinically important cardiac arrhythmia; valvular heart disease; ongoing systemic inflammatory diseases; renal or hepatic dysfunction; malignant disease; the use of drugs that may influence RAS hormone levels, such as direct renin inhibitors (DRIs), ACE inhibitors (ACEIs), Ang II receptor blockers (ARBs), or aldosterone antagonists (AAs); pregnancy or lactation in women; patient's unwillingness to participate in the survey."

Angiographic Analysis

"The severity of CHD was assessed by the number of stenotic coronary vessels."

"Single-vessel disease was defined as a ≥50% stenosis in only one major epicardial artery or an important branch of a major epicardial coronary artery."

"Multi-vessel coronary disease means the presence of a ≥50% stenosis in two or more major epicardial arteries or left main coronary artery."

Clinical and Laboratory Assessments

"Biochemical parameters such as serum potassium, sodium, chloride, creatinine, blood urea nitrogen (BUN), FBG, total cholesterol (TC), triglyceride (TG), high-density lipoprotein cholesterol (HDL-C), and low-density lipoprotein cholesterol (LDL-C) were measured using standard procedures in the hospital clinical laboratory."

"The circulating levels of ACE2-Ang-(1–7)-MAS axis were measured using commercial enzyme-linked immunosorbent assay (ELISA) kits (Cloud-Clone Corp, Houston)."

"The ELISA for measurement of ACE2 employed the sandwich enzyme immunoassay technique and the ELISA for measurement of Ang-(1–7) and Ang-(1–9) employed the competitive inhibition enzyme immunoassay."

"The content of ACE2, Ang-(1–7) and Ang-(1–9) were calculated in accordance with the standard curve (for plasma measurement, blood was collected within 48 h)."

"Chi square test and a standard one-way analysis of variance (ANOVA) test were used for comparisons of categorical and continuous variables, respectively."

"Univariable and multivariate logistic regression analyses were performed to determine factors associated with CHD."

Results

"The serum sodium, HDL-C levels of CHD patients were lower than that of non-CHD patients."

"The quartiles of ACE2 were significantly associated with CHD in female (P for trend = 0.025), compared with the people in the lowest ACE2 quartile, those in the highest quartile had an OR of 4.33 (95% CI 1.20–15.61) for the CHD."

"After adjustment for age, diabetes, SBP, sodium, FBG, HDL-C (model 3), the OR was 5.94 (95% CI 1.08–32.51) for the third ACE2 quartile and 9.58 (95% CI 1.61–56.95) for the highest ACE2 quartile (P for trend = 0.022)."

"The study subjects were divided into three groups according to the number of diseased coronary arteries (non-CHD, single vessel and multi-vessels), then stratified into three groups based on SYNTAX score (low score ≤ 22, intermediate score 23–32, and high score ≥33) [77, 78]."

Discussion

"We first examine the influence of gender on circulating levels of Ang-(1–7) in patients with and without CHD, and our results showed the levels of Ang-(1–7) in men are higher than that in women, the higher levels of Ang-(1–7) in men might be linked to increases in ACE2 which could promote Ang-(1–7) formation from Ang II."

"This is one of the first studies to demonstrate the levels of Ang-(1–7) and Ang-(1–9) are not parallel with the increase of serum ACE2 levels in patients suspected with CHD, suggesting increased ACE2 activity might directly affect atherosclerosis progress rather than induce more conversion from Ang II to Ang-(1–7) or Ang I to Ang-(1–9)."

"Curating ACE2 levels, but not Ang-(1–7) and Ang-(1–9) levels, significantly increased in female CHD group compared with non-CHD group, with subgroup analysis showing that the significant difference only exists in patients with multi-vessel lesions."

Arg^{972} Insulin Receptor Substrate-1 Is Associated with Decreased Serum Angiotensin-Converting Enzyme 2 Levels in Acute Myocardial Infarction Patients: In Vivo and In Vitro Evidence [79]

This is a machine-generated summary of:

Liu, Wei; Zhou, Xinmin; Yu, Fenglei; Hu, Jianguo; Hu, Wen: Arg^{972} Insulin receptor substrate-1 is associated with decreased serum angiotensin-converting enzyme 2 levels in acute myocardial infarction patients: in vivo and in vitro evidence [79].

Published in: Cardiovascular Diabetology (2013).

Link to original: https://doi.org/10.1186/1475-2840-12-151

If you want to cite the papers, please refer to the original.

For technical reasons we could not place the page where the original quote is coming from.

Abstract-Summary "Both angiotensin-converting enzyme 2 (ACE2) and insulin/insulin receptor substrate-1 (IRS-1) show cardioprotective effects after acute MI."

"We explored the association among Arg^{972} IRS-1, acute MI, and serum levels of ACE2."

"Serum levels of ACE2 and MI severity scores were determined."

"Primary human cardiomyocytes with overexpression of wild type IRS-1 or Arg^{972} IRS-1 or knockdown of endogenous IRS-1 were exposed to normoxia and hypoxia, and the expression levels of ACE2 were determined."

"The serum ACE2 level was significantly increased in acute MI patients compared with that of non-MI controls."

"Compared with wild type IRS-1 carriers, Arg^{972} IRS-1 carriers exhibited decreased serum ACE2 levels and increased MI severity scores after MI."

"Our in vitro data demonstrate that impairment of insulin/IRS-1/PI3K signaling by overexpression of Arg^{972}-IRS-1, knockdown of endogenous IRS-1, or PI3K inhibitor can abolish hypoxia-induced IRS-1-associated PI3K activity and ACE2 expression in human cardiomyocytes, which suggests a causal relationship between Arg^{972}-IRS-1 and decreased serum ACE2 levels in acute MI patients."

Background

"RAS blockade with angiotensin-converting enzyme (ACE) inhibitors improves cardiac remodeling and outcomes in both experimental models of MI as well as in humans [80]."

"After MI, there is significant activation of cardiac ACE2 in rats and humans, which acts to combat the adverse effects of an activated cardiac RAS [81]."

"It has been reported that ACE2 serum activity rises during the first week following acute MI and that ACE2 activation may be a compensatory mechanism in advanced heart failure [82]."

"Results from one of our pilot studies suggested that the Arg^{972} IRS-1 polymorphism might be associated with ACE2 activation in MI patients."

"We explored the association among Arg^{972} IRS-1, acute MI, and serum levels of ACE2 in a relatively large sample of acute MI patients, with an aim to identify potential interaction between insulin/IRS-1 signaling and RAS in the pathophysiology of acute MI."

Methods

"Between July 2010 and October 2012, 351 subjects with first-time acute MI (mean age 62.7 ± 15.9 years; range, 27–78 years) were recruited to this study at the Second Xiangya Hospital of Central South University."

"A fragment of human genomic DNA containing the entire coding sequence of IRS-1 was cloned and ligated into pcDNA3.1 expression vector (pcDNA-WT-IRS-1) as previously described [83]."

"IRS-1 (sc-29376-V) short hairpin RNA (shRNA) lentiviral particles, control shRNA lentiviral particles-A (sc-108080), and anti-ACE2 (sc-73668) antibody were purchased from Santa Cruz Biotechnology (Santa Cruz, CA, USA)."

"ACE2 (human) ELISA Kit (AG-45A-0022EK-KI01) was purchased from Adipogen (San Diego, CA, USA)."

"Comparison of serum ACE2 levels before and after acute MI in the same genotype group was performed with paired t-tests."

"Comparison of serum ACE2 levels after acute MI between two genotype groups was performed with analysis of covariance using serum ACE2 levels before acute MI as a covariate."

Results

"In the acute MI subjects, the GA+AA genotype group had significantly lower serum ACE2 levels and higher MI severity scores than the GG genotype group ($p < 0.05$)."

"The Arg^{972} IRS-1 genotype and acute MI showed significant interaction ($p=0.00$) that contributes to the variance of serum ACE2 levels."

"The results suggest that after acute MI, Arg^{972} IRS-1 carriers tend to have decreased serum ACE2 levels than wild type IRS-1 carriers."

"After the occurrence of acute MI, the GA+AA genotype group had significantly lower serum ACE2 levels than the GG genotype group ($p < 0.05$)."

"The results indicate that the presence of Arg^{972} IRS-1 leads to significantly reduced serum ACE2 levels and more severe MI in acute MI patients independent of gender."

"To explore the potential causal relationship between Arg^{972} IRS-1 and serum ACE2 levels in acute MI subjects, we performed in vitro experiments using human cardiomyocytes treated with hypoxia."

Discussion

"When the IRS-1-associated PI3K activity and the need for wild type IRS-1 were significantly increased by hypoxia in cardiomyocytes, however, the competition of overexpressed Arg^{972} IRS-1 would manifest significant inhibitory effect on insulin/IRS-1/PI3K signaling and thereby ACE2 expression."

"It would be interesting in future studies to explore the effects of insulin/IRS-1 signaling on ACE2 expression in other cell types. (2) There are many other pathophysiological factors involved in acute MI besides hypoxia."

"Our findings suggest that insulin/IRS-1/PI3K signaling exerts cardioprotective effects after acute MI at least partially through increased ACE2 expression; in agreement with this, Arg^{972} IRS-1 impairs insulin/IRS-1 signaling and results in decreased ACE2 expression after acute MI, which leads to more severe MI."

"Our in vitro data demonstrate that impairment of insulin/IRS-1/PI3K signaling by overexpression of Arg^{972}-IRS-1, knockdown of endogenous IRS-1, or PI3K inhibitor can abolish hypoxia-induced IRS-1-associated PI3K activity and ACE2 expression in human cardiomyocytes, which suggests a causal relationship between Arg^{972}-IRS-1 and decreased serum ACE2 levels in acute MI patients."

The Impact of Angiotensin-Converting-Enzyme Inhibitors Versus Angiotensin Receptor Blockers on 3-Year Clinical Outcomes in Elderly (≥65) Patients with Acute Myocardial Infarction Without Hypertension [84]

This is a machine-generated summary of:

Ahn, Woo Jin; Rha, Seung-Woon; Choi, Byoung Geol; Jeong, Myung Ho: The impact of angiotensin-converting-enzyme inhibitors versus angiotensin receptor blockers on 3-year clinical outcomes in elderly (≥65) patients with acute myocardial infarction without hypertension [84].

Published in: Heart and Vessels (2023).

Link to original: https://doi.org/10.1007/s00380-023-02244-x

If you want to cite the papers, please refer to the original.

For technical reasons we could not place the page where the original quote is coming from.

Abstract-Summary "This study aimed to investigate the impact of angiotensin-converting-enzyme inhibitors (ACEI) and angiotensin II type 1 receptor blockers (ARB) on 3-year clinical outcomes in elderly (≥65) acute myocardial infarction (AMI) patients without a history of hypertension who underwent successful percutaneous coronary intervention (PCI) with drug-eluting stents (DES)."

"To adjust baseline potential confounders, an inverse probability weighting (IPTW) analysis was performed."

"After IPTW matching, baseline characteristics were balanced."

"Incidence of stroke (hazard ratio [HR], 0.375; 95% confidence interval [CI], 0.166–0.846; $p = 0.018$) and re-hospitalization due to heart failure (HF) (HR, 0.528; 95% CI, 0.289–0.965; $p = 0.038$) in the ACEI group were significantly lower than in the ARB group."

"In elderly AMI patients who underwent PCI with DES without a history of hypertension, the use of ACEI was significantly associated with reduced incidences of stroke, and re-hospitalization due to HF than those with the use of ARB."

Introduction

"In a meta-analysis of several randomized controlled trials, significant risk reduction of cardiovascular events (odds ratio [OR], 0.89; 95% confidence interval [CI], 0.85–0.93) was demonstrated among patients with history of cardiovascular disease without hypertension treated with ACEI or ARB [85], additional to the well-known benefits of ACEI or ARB in high risk patients with hypertension demonstrated in many previous studies [7, 86–88]."

"Although unprevented cardiovascular events would have larger negative impact on quality of life of the elderly population (≥65), hence making optimal choices of medication even more important, there are limited data on the relative superiority of the effects of ACEI and ARB on the long-term clinical outcomes in these patients."

"This study aims to evaluate the effect of ACEI and ARB on 3-year clinical outcomes in elderly AMI patients without hypertension who underwent successful percutaneous coronary intervention (PCI) with drug-eluting stents (DES)."

Materials and Methods

"A total of 13,104 patients were enrolled, through November 2011 to December 2015, from KAMIR-National Institutes of Health (NIH) registry."

"The secondary endpoints include all-cause death, recurrent MI, any repeat revascularization, target lesion failure, target lesion revascularization (TLR), target vessel revascularization (TVR), stent thrombosis, stroke, and re-hospitalization due to HF."

"Repeated PCI within the index procedure stent or 5 mm edge was defined as TLR and repeated PCI or CABG of any segment in target vessel was defined as TVR."

"Target lesion failure was defined as the composite of TLR, recurrent MI, and cardiac death associated with the target vessel."

"All patients were encouraged to visit after a month and then every six months after the PCI procedure."

"Other medications (e.g., aspirin, anti-platelets, CCB, BB, and statins), and PCI procedural characteristics (e.g., target vessel, lesion type and DES type) were also considered."

Results

"The average left ventricle (LV) ejection fraction was more preserved in the ARB group (52.4 ± 11.0 vs. 49.9 ± 10.3%; $p < 0.001$) and the incidence of STEMI at final diagnosis was higher in the ACEI group (54.9 vs. 48.2%; $p = 0.016$)."

"Without IPTW adjustment, the cumulative incidence of stroke was significantly higher in the ARB group (3.0 vs. 1.4%; $p = 0.041$)."

"Stroke and re-hospitalization due to HF were significantly lower in the ACEI group (stroke: 1.2 vs. 2.9%; $p = 0.001$, re-hospitalization due to HF: 2.6 vs. 4.5%; $p = 0.006$) after the adjustment."

"Compared to the ARB group, the risks for total death in patients with eGFR-MDRD ≥ 90 were lower in the ACEI group (HR 0.52, 95% CI, 0.30–0.90; $p = 0.020$)."

Discussion

"The main findings of this study are as follows: in elderly AMI patients without hypertension, (1) ACEI shows more benefit in risk reduction for stroke and re-hospitalization due to HF; (2) these benefits of ACEI could be maximized when prescribed to patients with LVEF ≥ 40% or NT-pro BNP ≥400 pg/mL; (3) the relative superiority of ACEI is maintained throughout a wide range of renal function (eGFR-MDRD ≥30); (4) there were no significant differences in cumulative incidences of MACE, target lesion failure, all-cause death, recurrent MI, any repeat revascularization, and stent thrombosis between two groups."

"Korean national registry data suggested use of ACEI was associated with reduced cumulative incidences of MACE, any repeat vascularization, stroke, and re-hospitalization due to HF at 3 years compared to ARB in patients with AMI without hypertension [89]."

"Despite these current situations, direct comparison trial of ACEI and ARB in elderly AMI patients without hypertension is very limited, thus making our findings in the present study particularly more meaningful."

Effect of Angiotensin-Converting Enzyme Inhibitors and Angiotensin Receptor Antagonists in Atherosclerosis Prevention [90]

This is a machine-generated summary of:

Patarroyo Aponte, Maria M.; Francis, Gary S.: Effect of Angiotensin-Converting Enzyme Inhibitors and Angiotensin Receptor Antagonists in Atherosclerosis Prevention [90].

Published in: Current Cardiology Reports (2012).

Link to original: https://doi.org/10.1007/s11886-012-0275-9

If you want to cite the papers, please refer to the original.

For technical reasons we could not place the page where the original quote is coming from.

Abstract-Summary "Endothelial dysfunction is the first step in the development of atherosclerosis."

"The renin-angiotensin-aldosterone system (RAAS) plays an important role in the development of endothelial dysfunction and atherosclerosis."

"These findings suggest that ACEIs and ARBs can play an important role in prevention of atherosclerosis and in the delay of its progression."

"We focus on the importance of RAAS blockade to prevent or delay progression of atherosclerosis and its impact on reduction of cardiovascular events."

Introduction

"Dysfunction of the endothelium can be a consequence of many factors including inflammation, atherosclerosis, diabetes mellitus, hypertension, renal disease, smoking, and oxidative stress."

"Although the endothelium is under the control of many humoral factors, it is clear that the renin-angiotensin-aldosterone system (RAAS) is one of the most important drivers in the development of atherosclerosis [91]."

"This is almost certainly the case, as treatment of atherosclerotic vascular and heart disease with drugs designed to block the RAAS, such as angiotensin-converting enzyme inhibitors (ACEI) and angiotensin receptor blockers (ARBs), has repeatedly demonstrated a reduction in cardiovascular events."

"We focus on the importance of blocking the RAAS to prevent the development of atherosclerosis or in some cases inhibit its progression, and thereby reduce the clinical burden of cardiovascular events."

Endothelial Dysfunction and Atherosclerosis

"It is responsible for maintaining smooth muscle vascular tone, altering abnormal shear stress, and very importantly releasing multiple inflammatory cytokines [92]."

"This dysfunction is characterized by an increase in the release of inflammatory cytokines such as interleukin-6 (IL-6), tumor necrosis factor-α (TNF-α), chemoattractant substances such as monocyte chemoattractant protein-1 (MCP-1), and growth factors such as macrophage colony-stimulating factor-1."

"Endothelium also releases transforming growth factor (TGF)-α and TGF-β in response to various conditions, and these factors are known to increase activation and proliferation of macrophages in the subendothelial space."

"Expression of these molecules by the endothelium leads to platelet aggregation and further activation of the coagulation cascade with abnormal vascular tone."

Role of RAAS in Endothelial Dysfunction and Atherosclerosis

"Angiotensin II has been found to play an important role in the atherosclerotic process, with profound effects on endothelial function."

"Angiotensin II Has Proinflammatory Effects Mediated by an Increase in Oxidative Stress."

"These positive effects of increased tissue bradykinin tend to reverse vascular smooth cell proliferation and inhibit platelet adhesion by release of tissue plasminogen activator (tPA), both of which tend to facilitate and restore the fibrinolytic balance [93]."

"It has been suggested that blocking ACE by ACEIs reduces the formation of angiotensin II and diminishes degradation of bradykinin, thus improving vasodilation and diminishing myocardial and perhaps vascular remodeling."

"Losartan, an ARB, also increases angiotensin$_{1\text{-}7,}$ which has favorable effects on vascular biology. This effect is related to in vitro reduction in LDL oxidation, MCP-1 levels, and circulating monocyte CD11b expression."

"Enalapril and perindopril reduce ACE activity in aortic tissue, decrease angiotensin II levels, and prevent extension of atherosclerotic plaque."

Clinical Studies

"EUROPA (European Trial on Reduction of Cardiac Events with Perindopril in Stable Coronary Artery Disease) studied the ACEI perindopril and found it to have a significant effect on cardiovascular mortality, nonfatal MI, and resuscitated cardiac arrest when compared with placebo (RRR 20%) [94]."

"Nakamura and others [95] studied the effect of enalaprilat on endothelial-dependent vasodilation and demonstrated a significant increase in forearm blood flow after use of acetylcholine in patients with mild heart failure and in normal controls."

"These effects were also more durable with ACEIs relative to other therapies [96, 97]. The TREND (Trial on Reversing Endothelial Dysfunction) study randomized 105 normotensive patients with established CAD to quinapril 40 mg versus placebo."

"Patients demonstrated an increase in number of regenerative endothelial progenitor cells, a reduction in number of atherosclerotic plaques, an improvement in vascular compliance, a decrease in central aortic pressure, and a reduction in wall-to-lumen ratio of resistance arteries [92, 98]."

Conclusions

"We have made tremendous strides in the management of patients with cardiovascular disease."

"There is absolutely no doubt that ACEIs and ARBs reduce cardiovascular events in patients with underlying cardiovascular disease or with multiple cardiovascular risk factors."

"The striking reduction in cardiovascular events when ACEIs or ARBs are used in patients with underlying cardiovascular disease or excessive risk factors is undoubtedly further magnified when they are used in conjunction with statins and aspirin."

Genetic Variation in the Renin–Angiotensin–Aldosterone System Is Associated with Cardiovascular Risk Factors and Early Mortality in Established Coronary Heart Disease [99]

This is a machine-generated summary of:

Ellis, K L; Palmer, B R; Frampton, C M; Troughton, R W; Doughty, R N; Whalley, G A; Ellis, C J; Pilbrow, A P; Skelton, L; Yandle, T G; Richards, A M; Cameron, V A: Genetic variation in the renin–angiotensin–aldosterone system is associated with cardiovascular risk factors and early mortality in established coronary heart disease [99].

Published in: Journal of Human Hypertension (2012).

Link to original: https://doi.org/10.1038/jhh.2012.24

If you want to cite the papers, please refer to the original.

For technical reasons we could not place the page where the original quote is coming from.

Abstract-Summary "The AGT M235T 'T' allele was associated with a younger age of clinical coronary disease onset (P = 0.006), and the AGT rs2478545 minor allele was associated with lower circulating natriuretic peptides (P = 0.0001–P = 0.001) and E/E[1] (P = 0.018)."

"Minor alleles of AGT SNPs rs1926723 and rs11122576 were associated with more frequent history of renal disease ($P \leq 0.04$) and type-2 diabetes ($P \leq 0.02$), higher body mass index ($P \leq 0.02$) and greater mortality ($P \leq 0.007$)."

"AGT rs11568054 minor allele carriers had more frequent history of renal disease (P = 0.04) and higher plasma creatinine (P = 0.033)."

"AGT rs6687360 minor allele carriers exhibited worse survival (P = 0.02)."

"ACE rs4267385 was associated with older clinical coronary disease onset (P = 0.008) and hypertension (P = 0.013) onset, increased plasma creatinine (P = 0.01), yet greater mortality (P = 0.044)."

"Less history of hypertension was observed with the AGTR1 rs12685977 minor allele (P = 0.039)."

Introduction

"The renin–angiotensin–aldosterone (RAAS) system has a central role in the regulation of renal sodium and water absorption, blood pressure, the control of thirst, cardiac function and cellular growth, [100] and has been established as one of the most important systems in the pathogenesis of coronary heart disease."

"[101] Numerous RAAS gene linkage and gene association studies have reported associations with cardiovascular diseases, including hypertension."

"[102] Within the AGT gene, the coding M235T and T174M polymorphisms have been particularly well studied, as have the ACE insertion/deletion and angiotensin-II type-1 receptor (AGTR1) A1166C gene variants."

"We have screened polymorphisms in genes encoding AGT, ACE, AGTR1 and CYP11B2, selected either because of previous associations with CAD risk or as key tagging single-nucleotide polymorphisms (SNPs) in these genes, for association with cardiovascular risk factors and outcomes in a prospective cohort of patients with established coronary heart disease."

Methods

"Associations between genotype and baseline patient characteristics were tested using an additive genetic model, except for those SNPs where the minor genotype occurred at a frequency of <10%."

"Before undertaking statistical analyses to investigate the association between SNPs and baseline characteristics, associations between genotype and ethnicity were assessed."

"For SNPs where a significant difference in genotype frequency was observed, subsequent analyses were performed on each ethnic subgroup separately as well as on the cohort as a whole."

"Cox-proportional hazard analysis was performed to establish independent associations with outcome by adjusting for established predictors of increased risk; age of disease onset, gender, ethnicity, history of myocardial infarction, history of hypertension, β-blocker treatment, plasma creatinine, left ventricular ejection fraction and NT-proBNP."

"Cox-proportional hazards modeling was performed if the association between SNP and outcome was $P < 0.1$ in Kaplan–Meier analyses."

Results

"AGT rs2478545 minor allele carriers (n=373) had lower levels of circulating ANP ($P = 0.00017$; $b = -1.16$; 95% CI = −1.25 to −1.07), NT-proANP ($P=0.00012$; $b = -1.15$; 95% CI = −1.23 to −1.07), BNP ($P = 0.00025$; $b = -1.23$; 95%

CI = −1.37 to −1.10), NT-proBNP ($P = 0.00049$; $b = -1.24$; 95% CI = −1.39 to −1.10), CNP ($P = 0.001$; $b = -1.10$; 95% CI = −1.17 to −1.04) and cGMP ($P = 0.013$; $b = -1.09$; 95% CI = −1.16 to −1.02) after adjustment for potential confounders age, gender, ethnicity and BMI."

"The association between the 235 'T' allele and a younger age of clinical coronary disease onset was present in the other/unknown ethnic groups only ($P < 0.043$)."

"Minor alleles of rs2933249, rs931490, rs1492103 and rs1492099 occurred at a lower frequency in European patients when compared with individuals of other/unknown ethnicity ($P < 0.05$; European minor allele frequency = 0.176–0.241, other/unknown minor allele frequency = 0.268–0.328)."

Discussion

"An intriguing association was observed between the minor allele of the AGT tag SNP rs2478545 and circulating levels of natriuretic peptides."

"Two AGT variants (rs1926723 and rs11122576), were associated with increased BMI, type-2 diabetes and renal disease."

"We also identified an association between the minor allele of the tag SNP rs4267385 and a 3 year older age of onset of clinical coronary disease and onset of hypertension, but also a greater mortality independent of age and other prognostic markers."

"Associations were observed between the minor allele of AGT rs2478545 and lower levels of plasma natriuretic peptides, and between the AGT M235T 'T' allele and an earlier age of clinical coronary disease onset."

Comparative Effectiveness of Angiotensin II Receptor Blockers and Angiotensin-Converting Enzyme Inhibitors in Older Nursing Home Residents After Myocardial Infarction: A Retrospective Cohort Study [103]

This is a machine-generated summary of:

Zullo, Andrew R.; Riester, Melissa R.; Erqou, Sebhat; Wu, Wen-Chih; Rudolph, James L.; Steinman, Michael A.: Comparative Effectiveness of Angiotensin II Receptor Blockers and Angiotensin-Converting Enzyme Inhibitors in Older Nursing Home Residents After Myocardial Infarction: A Retrospective Cohort Study [103].

Published in: Drugs & Aging (2020).

Link to original: https://doi.org/10.1007/s40266-020-00791-w

Copyright of the summarized publication:

If you want to cite the papers, please refer to the original.

For technical reasons we could not place the page where the original quote is coming from.

Abstract-Summary "Evidence regarding differences in outcomes between angiotensin II receptor blockers (ARBs) and angiotensin-converting enzyme inhibitors (ACEIs) among older nursing home (NH) residents after acute myocardial infarction (AMI) is limited."

"The purpose of our study was to estimate the post-AMI effects of ARBs versus ACEIs on mortality, rehospitalization, and functional decline outcomes in this important population."

"We compared 90-day mortality, rehospitalization, and functional decline outcomes between ARB and ACEI users with inverse-probability-of-treatment-weighted binomial and multinomial logistic regression models."

"Of the 2765 NH residents, 270 (9.8%) used ARBs and 2495 (90.2%) used ACEIs."

"No marked differences existed between ARB and ACEI users for mortality [odds ratio (OR) 1.18; 95% confidence interval (CI) 0.78–1.79], rehospitalization (OR 1.22; 95% CI 0.90–1.65), or functional decline (OR 1.23; 95% CI 0.88–1.74)."

"Our findings align with prior data and suggest that clinicians can prescribe either ARBs or ACEIs post-AMI for secondary prevention in NH residents, although the subgroup findings merit further scrutiny and replication."

Introduction

"Data from randomized controlled trials (RCTs) and observational studies support a mortality benefit from using either ARBs or ACEIs after AMI in older adults aged ≥65 years [9, 104–110]."

"If differences were to exist between ARBs and ACEIs, especially for key subgroups, information on the comparative effectiveness of the two classes in older NH residents would be necessary to systematically optimize health outcomes after AMI."

"We compared the effectiveness of ARB and ACEI use on 90-day mortality, rehospitalization, and functional decline among older NH residents after AMI."

"We anticipated that, if this hypothesis were correct, our results would help to emphasize that the selection between ARBs and ACEIs for older NH residents post-AMI should be based on other important factors such as patient preferences, known adverse effects (e.g., ACEI-induced cough and angioedema), drug costs, and drug availability given increasingly common drug shortages."

Methods

"The three outcomes were 90-day mortality, all-cause rehospitalization, and functional decline."

"Functional decline was defined as an increase of 3 points on the validated 28-point MDS Morris scale of independence in ADL between the prehospital baseline assessment and the first available assessment after hospitalization up to 3 months after discharge [111]."

"For the functional decline outcome, at the end of the 90-day follow-up period, participants were classified as alive without functional decline, having had functional decline documented on an MDS assessment in that period, or having died without evidence of functional decline on the MDS."

"We estimated odds ratios (ORs) with 95% confidence intervals (CIs) using IPTW multinomial logistic regression models to compare new ARB users and ACEI users for rehospitalization and functional decline."

"We conducted stability analyses for 180-day and 365-day post-AMI mortality, rehospitalization, and functional decline outcomes to provide confidence in the validity of the main findings."

Results

"Prior to IPTW, the mean ± standard deviation age of the study cohort was 82.3 ± 9.1 years in the ARB group and 82.7 ± 8.2 years in the ACEI group."

"We observed that 37.8% of the ARB group versus 49.3% of the ACEI group had moderate to severe cognitive impairment prior to the AMI hospitalization, and 24.4 versus 30.5% had extensive impairment in their physical functioning."

"The median [interquartile range (IQR)] pre-AMI length of NH stay was 147 (60–753) days for the ARB group and 396 (90–1120) days for the ACEI group."

"The IPTW estimate for functional decline attenuated toward the null (IPTW adjusted OR 1.23; 95% CI 0.88–1.74), suggesting no marked difference between ARB and ACEI users."

Discussion

"In this national retrospective cohort study, we found that 90-day mortality, rehospitalization, and functional decline outcomes did not markedly differ between older ARB and ACEI users residing in NHs after AMI."

"Data on the comparative effectiveness of ARBs and ACEIs among older NH residents are scarce, both after AMI and in general."

"Both studies observed no difference in all-cause mortality between ARB and ACEI users."

"One such study used 1994–2004 Medicare Parts A and B claims linked to prescription drug data for New Jersey and Pennsylvania residents to examine 1-year all-cause mortality between ARB and ACEI users post-AMI [110]."

"Related to the cognitive impairment subgroup findings, several studies have examined the effects of RAAS agents on cognition and dementia, but few have directly compared how the effects of ARBs and ACEIs differ or whether cognitive status might modify effects [112–115]."

Conclusion

"Use of an ARB or ACEI was associated with similar 90-day mortality, rehospitalization, and functional decline outcomes in older NH residents post-AMI."

"Our findings align with prior data and suggest that clinicians can reasonably prescribe either an ARB or ACEI after AMI for secondary prevention."

"Carefully designed RCTs could be considered to further evaluate whether cognitive status truly modifies the effects of ARBs versus ACEIs on rehospitalization and mortality outcomes."

"Providers, patients, and their caregivers should consider other factors such as patient preferences, known adverse events specific to one of the two medication classes or individual drugs within them, and drug costs to guide their selection of ARBs or ACEIs."

Bibliography

1. Turner JM, Kodali R (2020) Should angiotensin-converting enzyme inhibitors ever be used for the management of hypertension? Curr Cardiol Rep 22(9):95
2. Strauss MH, Hall AS, Narkiewicz K (2023) The combination of beta-blockers and ACE inhibitors across the spectrum of cardiovascular diseases. Cardiovasc Drugs Ther 37(4):757–770. https://doi.org/10.1007/s10557-021-07248-1
3. Ahn WJ, Rha SW, Choi BG, Jeong MH, Other Korea Acute Myocardial Infarction Registry (KAMIR)-National Institutes of Health (NIH) Investigators (2023) The impact of angiotensin-converting-enzyme inhibitors versus angiotensin receptor blockers on 3-year clinical outcomes in elderly (≥65) patients with acute myocardial infarction without hypertension. Heart Vessels 38(7):898–908
4. Borghi C, Omboni S (2020) Angiotensin-converting enzyme inhibition: beyond blood pressure control—the role of zofenopril. Adv Ther 37:4068–4085. https://doi.org/10.1007/s12325-020-01455-2
5. Cho Y-R, Kim Y-D, Park T-H, Park K, Park J-S, Baek H, Choi S-Y, Kim K-S, Hong T-J, Yang T-H, Hwang J-Y, Park J-S, Hur S-H, Lee S-G (2011) The impact of dose of the angiotensin-receptor blocker valsartan on the post-myocardial infarction ventricular remodeling: study protocol for a randomized controlled trial. Trials 12:247. https://doi.org/10.1186/1745-6215-12-247
6. Yang Y, Zhang P, Song L, Ruan Y, Xu X, Li Y, Zhou Y, Tian Y, Xu Y, Chen Z (2002) Comparision of the doses of enalapril in preventing left ventricular remodeling after acute myocardial infarction in the rat. Chin Med J (Engl) 115:347–351

7. Pfeffer MA, McMurray JJV, Velazquez EJ et al (2003) Valsartan, captopril, or both in myocardial infarction complicated by heart failure, left ventricular dysfunction, or both. N Engl J Med 349:1893–1906. https://doi.org/10.1056/NEJMoa032292
8. Solomon SD, Skali H, Anavekar NS, Bourgoun M, Barvik S, Ghali JK, Warnica W, Khrakovskaya M, Arnold MO, Schwarz Y, Velazquez EJ, Califf RM, McMurray JV, Pfeffer MA (2005) Changes in ventricular size and function in patients treated with valsartan, captopril or both after myocardial infarction. Circulation 111:3411–3419. https://doi.org/10.1161/CIRCULATIONAHA.104.508093
9. Pfeffer MA, Braunwald E, Moyé LA et al (1992) Effect of captopril on mortality and morbidity in patients with left ventricular dysfunction after myocardial infarction: results of the survival and ventricular enlargement trial. N Engl J Med 327(10):669–677. https://doi.org/10.1056/NEJM199209033271001
10. The PREAMI Investigators (2006) Effect of angiotensin-converting enzyme inhibition with perindopril on left ventricular remodeling and clinical outcome. Results of the Randomized Perindopril and Remodeling in Elderly with Acute Myocardial Infarction (PREAMI) study. Arch Intern Med 166:659–666
11. Moon HK, Kim YD, Yang DG, Kim SG, Cha KS, Kim MH, Kim JS, Cha TJ, Joo SJ, Lee JW, Hong TJ, Shin YW, Kim DI, Kim DS, Park JS, Shin DG, Kim YJ (2003) Age and gender distribution of patients with acute myocardial infarction admitted to university hospitals during the period of 1990–1999. Korean Circul J 33:92–96
12. Tscharre M, Wadowski PP, Weikert C, Pultar J, Eichelberger B, Panzer S, Gremmel T (2020) Angiotensin-converting enzyme inhibitors and angiotensin receptor blockers in acute coronary syndrome: implications for platelet reactivity? Cardiovasc Drugs Ther 35(6):1183–1190. https://doi.org/10.1007/s10557-020-07128-0
13. Collet J-P, Thiele H, Barbato E, Barthélémy O, Bauersachs J, Bhatt DL et al (2020) ESC Guidelines for the management of acute coronary syndromes in patients presenting without persistent ST-segment elevation: the Task Force for the management of acute coronary syndromes in patients presenting without persistent ST-segment elevation. Eur Heart J 42(14):1289–1367. https://doi.org/10.1093/eurheartj/ehaa575
14. Ibanez B, James S, Agewall S, Antunes MJ, Bucciarelli-Ducci C, Bueno H et al (2018) 2017 ESC Guidelines for the management of acute myocardial infarction in patients presenting with ST-segment elevation. Eur Heart J 39:119–177
15. Helten C, Mourikis P, Dannenberg L, M'Pembele R, Trojovsky K, Ayhan A et al (2020) A novel mechanism of ACE inhibition–associated enhanced platelet reactivity: disproof of the ARB-MI paradox? Eur J Clin Pharmacol 76:1245–1251
16. Verstraete M (1990) Pharmacotherapeutic aspects of unfractionated and low molecular weight heparins. Drugs 40:498–530
17. Badr Eslam R, Lang IM, Koppensteiner R, Calatzis A, Panzer S, Gremmel T (2013) Residual platelet activation through protease-activated receptors (PAR)-1 and -4 in patients on P2Y12 inhibitors. Int J Cardiol 168:403–406
18. Schieffer B, Bünte C, Witte J, Hoeper K, Böger RH, Schwedhelm E et al (2004) Comparative effects of AT1-antagonism and angiotensin-converting enzyme inhibition on markers of inflammation and platelet aggregation in patients with coronary artery disease. J Am Coll Cardiol 44:362–368
19. Mayer K, Bernlochner I, Braun S, Schulz S, Orban M, Morath T et al (2014) Aspirin treatment and outcomes after percutaneous coronary intervention. J Am Coll Cardiol 64:863–871
20. Sibbing D, Braun S, Morath T, Mehilli J, Vogt W, Schömig A et al (2009) Platelet reactivity after clopidogrel treatment assessed with point-of-care analysis and early drug-eluting stent thrombosis. J Am Coll Cardiol 53:849–856
21. Kakutani N, Takada S, Nambu H, Matsumoto J, Furihata T, Yokota T, Fukushima A, Kinugawa S (2020) Angiotensin-converting-enzyme inhibitor prevents skeletal muscle fibrosis in myocardial infarction mice. Skeletal Muscle. 10(1):11. https://doi.org/10.1186/s13395-020-00230-9

22. Rockey DC, Bell PD, Hill JA (2015) Fibrosis—a common pathway to organ injury and failure. N Engl J Med 372:1138–1149
23. Wynn TA (2007) Common and unique mechanisms regulate fibrosis in various fibroproliferative diseases. J Clin Invest 117:524–529
24. Dong J, Dong Y, Chen Z, Mitch WE, Zhang L (2017) The pathway to muscle fibrosis depends on myostatin stimulating the differentiation of fibro/adipogenic progenitor cells in chronic kidney disease. Kidney Int 91:119–128
25. Jin Q et al (2019) A GDF11/myostatin inhibitor, GDF11 propeptide-Fc, increases skeletal muscle mass and improves muscle strength in dystrophic mdx mice. Skelet Muscle 9:16
26. Billin AN et al (2018) HIF prolyl hydroxylase inhibition protects skeletal muscle from eccentric contraction-induced injury. Skelet Muscle 8:35
27. Rebolledo DL et al (2019) Denervation-induced skeletal muscle fibrosis is mediated by CTGF/CCN2 independently of TGF-beta. Matrix Biol 82:20–37
28. Morales MG et al (2013) Inhibition of the angiotensin-converting enzyme decreases skeletal muscle fibrosis in dystrophic mice by a diminution in the expression and activity of connective tissue growth factor (CTGF/CCN-2). Cell Tissue Res 353:173–187
29. Mueller AA, van Velthoven CT, Fukumoto KD, Cheung TH, Rando TA (2016) Intronic polyadenylation of PDGFRalpha in resident stem cells attenuates muscle fibrosis. Nature 540:276–279
30. Wang Z et al (2018) Cardiac fibrosis can be attenuated by blocking the activity of transglutaminase 2 using a selective small-molecule inhibitor. Cell Death Dis 9:613
31. Nakamura J et al (2019) Myofibroblasts acquire retinoic acid-producing ability during fibroblast-to-myofibroblast transition following kidney injury. Kidney Int 95:526–539
32. Abramowitz MK et al (2018) Skeletal muscle fibrosis is associated with decreased muscle inflammation and weakness in patients with chronic kidney disease. Am J Physiol Renal Physiol 315:F1658–F1F69
33. Sim HW, Zheng H, Richards AM, Chen RW, Sahlen A, Yeo K-K, Tan JW, Chua T, Tan HC, Yeo TC, Ho HH, Liew B-W, Foo LL, Lee C-H, Hausenloy DJ, Chan MY (2020) Beta-blockers and renin-angiotensin system inhibitors in acute myocardial infarction managed with inhospital coronary revascularization. Sci Rep. 10(1):15184. https://doi.org/10.1038/s41598-020-72232-y
34. Bangalore S, Fakheri R, Toklu B, Ogedegbe G, Weintraub H, Messerli FH (2016) Angiotensin-converting enzyme inhibitors or angiotensin receptor blockers in patients without heart failure? Insights from 254,301 patients from randomized trials. Mayo Clin Proc 91:51–60. https://doi.org/10.1016/J.MAYOCP.2015.10.019
35. Yang JH et al (2014) Angiotensin receptor blocker in patients with ST segment elevation myocardial infarction with preserved left ventricular systolic function: prospective cohort study. BMJ 349:g6650. https://doi.org/10.1136/bmj.g6650
36. Nakaya M et al (2012) Induction of cardiac fibrosis by beta-blocker in G protein-independent and G protein-coupled receptor kinase 5/beta-arrestin2-dependent signaling pathways. J Biol Chem 287:35669–35677
37. Kadoguchi T et al (2015) Angiotensin II can directly induce mitochondrial dysfunction, decrease oxidative fibre number and induce atrophy in mouse hindlimb skeletal muscle. Exp Physiol 100:312–322
38. The Acute Infarction Ramipril Efficacy (AIRE) Study Investigators (1993) Effect of ramipril myocardial infarction with clinical evidence of heart failure. Lancet 342:821–828
39. Flather MD, Yusuf S, Kober L, Pfeffer M, Hall A, Murray G et al (2000) Long-term ACE-inhibitor therapy in patients with heart failure or left-ventricular dysfunction: a systematic overview of data from individual patients. ACE-Inhibitor Myocardial Infarction Collaborative Group. Lancet 355:1575–1581
40. Dickstein K, Kjekshus J (2002) Effects of losartan and captopril on mortality and morbidity in high-risk patients after acute myocardial infarction: the OPTIMAAL randomised trial. Lancet 360(9335):752–760. https://doi.org/10.1016/S0140-6736(02)09895-1

41. Amsterdam EA et al (2014) 2014 AHA/ACC guideline for the management of patients with non-ST-elevation acute coronary syndromes: executive summary. Circulation 130:2354–2394
42. O'Gara PT et al (2012) 2013 ACCF/AHA guideline for the management of ST-elevation myocardial infarction: executive summary. Circulation 127:529–555
43. Cespón-Fernández M et al (2019) Renin-angiotensin system blockade and risk of heart failure after myocardial infarction based on left ventricular ejection fraction: a retrospective cohort study. Am J Cardiovasc Drugs 19(5):487–495. https://doi.org/10.1007/s40256-019-00343-7
44. Lee PH et al (2016) Effect of beta blockers and renin—angiotensin system inhibitors on survival in patients with acute myocardial infarction undergoing percutaneous coronary intervention. Medicine (Baltimore) 95:1–7
45. Lautamäki R, Knuuti J, Saraste A (2013) Recent developments in imaging of myocardial angiotensin receptors. Curr Cardiovasc Imaging Rep 7:9245. https://doi.org/10.1007/s12410-013-9245-x
46. Gheorghiade M, Bonow RO (1998) Chronic heart failure in the United States: a manifestation of coronary artery disease. Circulation 97:282–289
47. Konstam MA, Kramer DG, Patel AR, Maron MS, Udelson JE (2011) Left ventricular remodeling in heart failure: current concepts in clinical significance and assessment. JACC Cardiovasc Imaging 4:98–108
48. Nahrendorf M, Sosnovik DE, French BA, Swirski FK, Bengel F, Sadeghi MM et al (2009) Multimodality cardiovascular molecular imaging, Part II. Circ Cardiovasc Imaging 2:56–70
49. Saraste A, Nekolla SG, Schwaiger M (2009) Cardiovascular molecular imaging: an overview. Cardiovasc Res 83:643–652
50. McMurray JJ, Pfeffer MA (2005) Heart failure. Lancet 365:1877–1889
51. Re RN (2001) The clinical implication of tissue renin angiotensin systems. Curr Opin Cardiol 16:317–327
52. Swedberg K, Eneroth P, Kjekshus J, Wilhelmsen L (1990) Hormones regulating cardiovascular function in patients with severe congestive heart failure and their relation to mortality. CONSENSUS Trial Study Group. Circulation 82:1730–1736
53. Sutton MG, Sharpe N (2000) Left ventricular remodeling after myocardial infarction: pathophysiology and therapy. Circulation 101:2981–2988
54. Mathews WB, Burns D, Dannals RF, Ravert HT, Naylor EM (1995) Carbon-11 labeling of a potent, nonpeptide, at1-selective angiotensin-II receptor antagonist: MK-996. J Label Compd Radiopharm 36:729–737
55. Hamill TG, Burns HD, Dannals RF, Mathews WB, Musachio JL, Ravert HT et al (1996) Development of [11C]L-159,884: a radiolabelled, nonpeptide angiotensin II antagonist that is useful for angiotensin II, AT1 receptor imaging. Appl Radiat Isot 47:211–218
56. Verjans JW, Lovhaug D, Narula N, Petrov AD, Indrevoll B, Bjurgert E et al (2008) Noninvasive imaging of angiotensin receptors after myocardial infarction. JACC Cardiovasc Imaging 1:354–362
57. Gilliot S, Sibon I, Mas J-L, Moulin T, Béjot Y, Cordonnier C, Giroud M, Odou P, Bordet R, Vivien D, Leys D, The OPHELIE Investigators (2018) Influence of on-going treatment with angiotensin-converting enzyme inhibitor or angiotensin receptor blocker on the outcome of patients treated with intravenous rt-PA for ischemic stroke. J Neurol 265:1166–1173. https://doi.org/10.1007/s00415-018-8827-6
58. Sundbøll J, Schmidt M, Horváth-Puhó E et al (2015) Preadmission use of ACE inhibitors or angiotensin receptor blockers and short-term mortality after stroke. J Neurol Neurosurg Psychiatry 86:748–754
59. Bendel RB, Afifi AA (1977) Comparison of stopping rules in forward regression. J Am Stat Assoc 72:46–53
60. Myslimi F, Caparros F, Dequatre-Ponchelle N et al (2016) Orolingual angioedema during or after thrombolysis for cerebral ischemia. Stroke 47:1825–1830
61. Watanabe R, Suzuki J, Wakayama K, Kumagai H, Ikeda Y, Akazawa H, Komuro I, Isobe M (2015) Angiotensin II receptor blocker irbesartan attenuates cardiac dysfunction induced by

myocardial infarction in the presence of renal failure. Hypertens Res. 39(4):237–244. https://doi.org/10.1038/hr.2015.141
62. Siragy HM, Carey RM (2010) Role of the intrarenal renin-angiotensin-aldosterone system in chronic kidney disease. Am J Nephrol 31:541–550
63. Sun Y (2010) Intracardiac renin-angiotensin system and myocardial repair/remodeling following infarction. J Mol Cell Cardiol 48:483–489
64. Kim S, Iwao H (2000) Molecular and cellular mechanisms of angiotensin II-mediated cardiovascular and renal diseases. Pharmacol Rev 52:11–34
65. Zhang Y, Shao L, Ma A, Guan G, Wang J, Wang Y, Tian G (2014) Telmisartan delays myocardial fibrosis in rats with hypertensive left ventricular hypertrophy by TGF-beta1/Smad signal pathway. Hypertens Res 37:43–49
66. Zouein FA, Zgheib C, Hamza S, Fuseler JW, Hall JE, Soljancic A, Lopez-Ruiz A, Kurdi M, Booz GW (2013) Role of stat3 in angiotensin II-induced hypertension and cardiac remodeling revealed by mice lacking stat3 serine 727 phosphorylation. Hypertens Res 36:496–503
67. Bongartz LG, Braam B, Verhaar MC, Cramer MJ, Goldschmeding R, Gaillard CA, Doevendans PA, Joles JA (2010) Transient nitric oxide reduction induces permanent cardiac systolic dysfunction and worsens kidney damage in rats with chronic kidney disease. Am J Physiol Regul Integr Comp Physiol 298:R815–R823
68. Bongartz LG, Cramer MJ, Doevendans PA, Joles JA, Braam B (2005) The severe cardiorenal syndrome: 'Guyton revisited'. Eur Heart J 26:11–17
69. Siddesha JM, Valente AJ, Sakamuri SS, Yoshida T, Gardner JD, Somanna N, Takahashi C, Noda M, Chandrasekar B (2013) Angiotensin II stimulates cardiac fibroblast migration via the differential regulation of matrixins and reck. J Mol Cell Cardiol 65:9–18
70. Balakumar P, Jagadeesh G (2014) A century old renin-angiotensin system still grows with endless possibilities: At1 receptor signaling cascades in cardiovascular physiopathology. Cell Signal 26:2147–2160
71. Nishikimi T, Inaba-Iemura C, Ishimura K, Tadokoro K, Koshikawa S, Ishikawa K, Akimoto K, Hattori Y, Kasai K, Minamino N, Maeda N, Matsuoka H (2009) Natriuretic peptide/natriuretic peptide receptor-a (NPR-a) system has inhibitory effects in renal fibrosis in mice. Regul Pept 154:44–53
72. Hoang V, Alam M, Addison D, Macedo F, Virani S, Birnbaum Y (2016) Efficacy of angiotensin-converting enzyme inhibitors and angiotensin-receptor blockers in coronary artery disease without heart failure in the modern statin era: a meta-analysis of randomized-controlled trials. Cardiovasc Drugs Ther 30(2):189–198. https://doi.org/10.1007/s10557-016-6652-7
73. Yancy CW, Jessup M, Bozkurt B et al (2013) ACCF/AHA guideline for the management of heart failure. Circulation 128:e240–e327
74. Zhou X, Zhang P, Liang T, Chen Y, Liu D, Yu H (2019) Relationship between circulating levels of angiotensin-converting enzyme 2-angiotensin-(1–7)-MAS axis and coronary heart disease. Heart Vessels 35(2):153–161. https://doi.org/10.1007/s00380-019-01478-y
75. Zhang YH, Zhang YH, Dong XF, Hao QQ, Zhou XM, Yu QT, Li SY, Chen X, Tengbeh AF, Dong B, Zhang Y (2015) ACE2 and Ang-(1–7) protect endothelial cell function and prevent early atherosclerosis by inhibiting inflammatory response. Inflamm Res 64(3–4):253–260
76. Yang JM, Dong M, Meng X, Zhao YX, Yang XY, Liu XL, Hao PP, Li JJ, Wang XP, Zhang K, Gao F, Zhao XQ, Zhang MX, Zhang Y, Zhang C (2013) Angiotensin-(1–7) dose-dependently inhibits atherosclerotic lesion formation and enhances plaque stability by targeting vascular cells. Arterioscler Thromb Vasc Biol 33(8):1978–1985
77. Authors/Task Force members, Windecker S, Kolh P, Alfonso F, Collet JP, Cremer J, Falk V, Filippatos G, Hamm C, Head SJ, Juni P, Kappetein AP, Kastrati A, Knuuti J, Landmesser U, Laufer G, Neumann FJ, Richter DJ, Schauerte P, Sousa Uva M, Stefanini GG, Taggart DP, Torracca L, Valgimigli M, Wijns W, Witkowski A (2014) 2014 ESC/EACTS Guidelines on myocardial revascularization: the task force on myocardial revascularization of the european society of cardiology (ESC) and the European Association for Cardio-Thoracic

Surgery (EACTS) developed with the special contribution of the European Association of Percutaneous Cardiovascular Interventions (EAPCI). Eur Heart J 35(37):2541–2619
78. Amsterdam EA, Wenger NK, Brindis RG, Casey DE Jr, Ganiats TG, Holmes DR Jr, Jaffe AS, Jneid H, Kelly RF, Kontos MC, Levine GN, Liebson PR, Mukherjee D, Peterson ED, Sabatine MS, Smalling RW, Zieman SJ, Members AATF (2014) 2014 AHA/ACC guideline for the management of patients with non-ST-elevation acute coronary syndromes: a report of the American College of Cardiology/American Heart Association Task Force on Practice Guidelines. Circulation 130(25):e344–e426
79. Liu W, Zhou X, Yu F, Hu J, Hu W (2013) Arg^{972} Insulin receptor substrate-1 is associated with decreased serum angiotensin-converting enzyme 2 levels in acute myocardial infarction patients: in vivo and in vitro evidence. Cardiovasc Diabetol 12:151. https://doi.org/10.1186/1475-2840-12-151
80. Burchill LJ, Velkoska E, Dean RG, Griggs K, Patel SK, Burrell LM (2012) Combination renin-angiotensin system blockade and angiotensin-converting enzyme 2 in experimental myocardial infarction: implications for future therapeutic directions. Clin Sci (Lond) 123:649–658. https://doi.org/10.1042/CS20120162
81. Burrell LM, Risvanis J, Kubota E, Dean RG, MacDonald PS, Lu S, Tikellis C, Grant SL, Lew RA, Smith AI, Cooper ME, Johnston CI (2005) Myocardial infarction increases ACE2 expression in rat and humans. Eur Heart J 114:1–7
82. Perez JTO, Riera M, Genover XB, De Caralt TM, Perea RJ (2011) Serum ACE2 activity correlates with infarct size and left ventricular dysfunction during acute myocardial infarction. J Cardiovas Magn Res 13(Suppl 1):142. https://doi.org/10.1186/1532-429X-13-S1-P142
83. Porzio O, Federici M, Hribal ML, Lauro D, Accili D, Lauro R, Borboni P, Sesti G (1999) The Gly972–>Arg amino acid polymorphism in IRS-1 impairs insulin secretion in pancreatic beta cells. J Clin Invest 104:357–364. https://doi.org/10.1172/JCI5870
84. Ahn WJ, Rha S-W, Choi BG, Jeong MH (2023) The impact of angiotensin-converting-enzyme inhibitors versus angiotensin receptor blockers on 3-year clinical outcomes in elderly (≥65) patients with acute myocardial infarction without hypertension. Heart Vessels 38(7):898–908. https://doi.org/10.1007/s00380-023-02244-x
85. McAlister FA (2012) Angiotensin-converting enzyme inhibitors or angiotensin receptor blockers are beneficial in normotensive atherosclerotic patients: a collaborative meta-analysis of randomized trials. Eur Heart J 33:505–514
86. McMurray J, Solomon S, Pieper K, Reed S, Rouleau J, Velazquez E, White H, Howlett J, Swedberg K, Maggioni A, Køber L, Van de Werf F, Califf R, Pfeffer M (2006) The effect of valsartan, captopril, or both on atherosclerotic events after acute myocardial infarction: an analysis of the Valsartan in Acute Myocardial Infarction Trial (VALIANT). J Am Coll Cardiol 47:726–733
87. Borghi C, Bacchelli S, Esposti DD, Bignamini A, Magnani B, Ambrosioni E (1999) Effects of the administration of an angiotensin-converting enzyme inhibitor during the acute phase of myocardial infarction in patients with arterial hypertension. SMILE Study Investigators. Survival of myocardial infarction long-term evaluation. Am J Hypertens 12:665–672
88. Gustafsson F, Torp-Pedersen C, Køber L, Hildebrandt P (1997) Effect of angiotensin converting enzyme inhibition after acute myocardial infarction in patients with arterial hypertension. TRACE study group. Trandolapril Cardiac Event J Hypertens 15:793–798
89. Her AY, Choi BG, Rha SW, Kim YH, Choi CU, Jeong MH (2020) The impact of angiotensin-converting-enzyme inhibitors versus angiotensin receptor blockers on 3-year clinical outcomes in patients with acute myocardial infarction without hypertension. PLoS One 15:e0242314
90. Patarroyo Aponte MM, Francis GS (2012) Effect of angiotensin-converting enzyme inhibitors and angiotensin receptor antagonists in atherosclerosis prevention. Curr Cardiol Rep 14(4):433–442. https://doi.org/10.1007/s11886-012-0275-9
91. Lonn E (2002) Angiotensin-converting enzyme inhibitors and angiotensin receptor blockers in atherosclerosis. Curr Atheroscler Rep 4(5):363–372

92. Ferrario C (2009) Effect of angiotensin receptor blockade on endothelial function: focus on olmesartan medoxomil. Vasc Health Risk Manag 5(1):301–314. This is a complete review regarding effects of ARBs on atherosclerosis prevention. It also gives a great explanation of the pathophysiology of RAAS and atherosclerosis
93. Shahin Y, Khan JA, Samuel N, Chetter I (2011) Angiotensin converting enzyme inhibitors effect on endothelial dysfunction: a meta-analysis of randomized controlled trials. Atherosclerosis 216(1):7–16. This meta-analysis shows the effect of ACEIs on endothelial dysfunction, which is the first step for atherosclerosis
94. Fox KM, For The EURopean trial On reduction of cardiac events with Perindopril in stable coronary Artery disease Investigators (2003) Efficacy of perindopril in reduction of cardiovascular events among patients with stable coronary artery disease: randomised, double-blind, placebo-controlled, multicentre trial (the EUROPA study). Lancet 362:782–788
95. Nakamura M, Funakoshi T, Arakawa N et al (1994) Effect of angiotensin-converting enzyme inhibitors on endothelium-dependent peripheral vasodilation in patients with chronic heart failure. J Am Coll Cardiol 24(5):1321–1327
96. Millgård J, Hägg A, Sarabi M, Lind L (1998) Captopril, but not nifedipine, improves endothelium-dependent vasodilation in hypertensive patients. J Hum Hypertens 12(8):511–516
97. Mühlen BV, Millgård J, Lind L (2001) Effects of digoxin, furosemide, enalaprilat and metoprolol on endothelial function in young normotensive subjects. Clin Exp Pharmacol Physiol 28(5–6):381–385
98. Fliser D, Buchholz K, Haller H (2004) European trial on Olmesartan and Pravastatin in Inflammation and Atherosclerosis (EUTOPIA) Investigators. Antiinflammatory effects of angiotensin II subtype 1 receptor blockade in hypertensive patients with microinflammation. Circulation 110(9):1103–1107
99. Ellis KL, Palmer BR, Frampton CM, Troughton RW, Doughty RN, Whalley GA, Ellis CJ, Pilbrow AP, Skelton L, Yandle TG, Richards AM, Cameron VA (2012) Genetic variation in the renin–angiotensin–aldosterone system is associated with cardiovascular risk factors and early mortality in established coronary heart disease. J Hum Hypertens 27(4):237–244. https://doi.org/10.1038/jhh.2012.24
100. Kurdi M, De Mello WC, Booz GW (2005) Working outside the system: an update on the unconventional behavior of the renin-angiotensin system components. Int J Biochem Cell Biol 37:1357–1367
101. Pitt B, Zannad F, Remme WJ et al (1999) The effect of spironolactone on morbidity and mortality in patients with severe heart failure. Randomized Aldactone Evaluation Study Investigators. N Engl J Med 341:709–717. https://doi.org/10.1056/NEJM199909023411001
102. Jeunemaitre X (2008) Genetics of the human renin angiotensin system. J Mol Med 86:637–641
103. Zullo AR, Riester MR, Erqou S, Wu W-C, Rudolph JL, Steinman MA (2020) Comparative effectiveness of angiotensin II receptor blockers and angiotensin-converting enzyme inhibitors in older nursing home residents after myocardial infarction: a retrospective cohort study. Drugs Aging 37(10):755–766. https://doi.org/10.1007/s40266-020-00791-w
104. Swedberg K, Held P, Kjekshus J, Rasmussen K, Ryden L, Wedel H (1992) Effects of the early administration of enalapril on mortality in patients with acute myocardial infarction. Results of the Cooperative New Scandinavian Enalapril Survival Study II (CONSENSUS II). N Engl J Med 327(10):678–684
105. Gruppo Italiano per lo Studio Della Sopravvivenza Nell'Infarto Miocardico (1996) Six-month effects of early treatment with lisinopril and transdermal glyceryl trinitrate singly and together withdrawn six weeks after acute myocardial infarction: the GISSI-3 trial. Gruppo Italiano per lo Studio della Sopravvivenza nell'Infarto Miocardico. J Am Coll Cardiol 27(2):337–344
106. Fourth International Study of Infarct Survival Collaborative Group (1995) A randomized factorial trial assessing oral captopril, oral mononitrate, and intravenous magnesium sulphate in 58,050 patients with suspected acute myocardial infarction. ISIS-4. Lancet 345:669–685

107. Ambrosioni E, Borghi C, Magnani B, The Survival of Myocardial Infarction Long-Term Evaluation (SMILE) Study Investigators (1995) The effect of the angiotensin-converting enzyme inhibitor zofenopril on mortality and morbidity after anterior myocardial infarction. N Engl J Med 332:80–85
108. The Acute Infarction Ramipril Efficacy (AIRE) Study Investigators (1993) Effect of ramipril on mortality and morbidity of survivors of acute myocardial infarction with clinical evidence of heart failure. The Acute Infarction Ramipril Efficacy (AIRE) Study Investigators. Lancet 342(8875):821–828
109. Kober L, Torp-Pedersen C, Carlsen JE, Bagger H, Eliasen P, Lyngborg K et al (1995) A clinical trial of the angiotensin-converting-enzyme inhibitor trandolapril in patients with left ventricular dysfunction after myocardial infarction. Trandolapril Cardiac Evaluation (TRACE) Study Group. N Engl J Med 333:1670–1676
110. Winkelmayer WC, Fischer MA, Schneeweiss S et al (2006) Angiotensin inhibition after myocardial infarction: does drug class matter? J Gen Intern Med 21(12):1242–1247. https://doi.org/10.1111/j.1525-1497.2006.00590.x
111. Carpenter GI, Hastie CL, Morris JN et al (2006) Measuring change in activities of daily living in nursing home residents with moderate to severe cognitive impairment. BMC Geriatr 6:7. https://doi.org/10.1186/1471-2318-6-7
112. Zhuang S, Wang HF, Wang X et al (2016) The association of renin–angiotensin system blockade use with the risks of cognitive impairment of aging and Alzheimer's disease: a meta-analysis. J Clin Neurosci 33:32–38. https://doi.org/10.1016/j.jocn.2016.02.036
113. Zhuang S, Wang HF, Li J et al (2016) Renin–angiotensin system blockade use and risks of cognitive decline and dementia: a meta-analysis. Neurosci Lett 624:53–61. https://doi.org/10.1016/j.neulet.2016.05.003
114. Stuhec M, Keuschler J, Serra-Mestres J et al (2017) Effects of different antihypertensive medication groups on cognitive function in older patients: a systematic review. Eur Psychiatry 46:1–15. https://doi.org/10.1016/j.eurpsy.2017.07.015
115. Barthold D, Joyce G, Wharton W et al (2018) The association of multiple anti-hypertensive medication classes with Alzheimer' disease incidence across sex, race, and ethnicity. PLoS One 13(11):e0206705. https://doi.org/10.1371/journal.pone.0206705

Chapter 4
Role of ACE Inhibitors in Transforming Renin–Angiotensin System

Mukesh Nandave

Introduction by the Editor

All the available anti-hypertensive agents are known to reduce the risk of stroke, myocardial infarction, heart failure, and other cardiovascular disease. However, Blockade of Renin-Angiotensin-Aldosterone System (RAAS) with angiotensin receptor converting Enzyme (ACE) inhibitor is considered as one of the notable advances in therapeutic intervention in the treatment of hypertension, coronary heart disease, heart failure, diabetic nephropathy. ACE inhibitor and angiotensin receptor blockers (ARBs) are two important drug classes of RAAS inhibitors recommended by international guidelines for the treatment of hypertension. By targeting RAAS, 50% of patients are successfully treated in cardiovascular segment in addition to diabetes, cancer, and Alzheimer's. This transformation took place around five decades back by the unexpected discovery of bradykinin facilitating peptide from venom of snake which led to the discovery of ACE inhibitor, namely captopril. The discovery of ACE inhibitors is the major factor contributing to RAAS transformation [1]. Current guidelines for the arterial hypertension management suggested the administration of ACE inhibitor as first line therapy for starting and maintaining anti-hypertensive treatments ideally in combination with diuretic or calcium channel blockers. According to the reports, anti-hypertensive agents such as ACE inhibitor have some biological properties that reduce the diabetes risk and also improve the outcome of heart failure. In a study, it is reported that ACE inhibitors reduces the risk and mortality in patients of heart failure, diabetes and hypertension and the researchers suggested the use of ACE inhibitors as first line therapy in populations to reduce the cases of mortality and mortality [2]. ACE inhibitors are recommended

---

M. Nandave (✉)
Department of Pharmacology, Delhi Pharmaceutical Sciences and Research University, New Delhi, Delhi, India

M. Nandave (ed.), *Angiotensin-converting Enzyme Inhibitors vs. Angiotensin Receptor Blockers*, https://doi.org/10.1007/978-981-97-7380-0_4

in cardiovascular events like stroke, myocardial infarction, endothelial dysfunction, left ventricular hypertrophy or in metabolic syndrome and any stage of kidney disease. However, their use is contraindicated in some health conditions such as hyperkalemia, pregnancy, and bilateral renal stenosis.

Blood pressure control by ACE inhibitors is similar as other anti-hypertensive agents however in clinical practices it is observed that to have some efficacy differences among other anti-hypertensive agents. These differences can be attributed to the higher adherence and improved life quality associated with ACE inhibitors treatment in comparison to diuretics, beta blockers or calcium channel blockers [3]. The reduced adverse effects and perceived health advantages from treatment attributed to potential psychotropic effects reported in RAAS inhibitors. In a study, a secondary outcome associated with ACE inhibitors was observed, adults with hypertension treated with ACE inhibitors found to have improved mental health and quality of life [4]. ACE inhibitors found to reduce the risk of new onset-diabetes mellitus while calcium blockers and beta blockers may increase this risk. The association between anti-hypertensive agents and diabetes onset in underexplored. However, it may be attributed to RAAS blockade that results in the recruitment and differentiation of adipocytes leading to improved peripheral insulin effect and its secretion [5]. Clinical trials involving the comparison of ACE inhibitors or ARBs with other anti-hypertensive agents reported that RAAS inhibition significantly improves the insulin sensitivity in comparison to other anti-hypertensive agents. Therefore, it is proved that malfunction in RAAS may lead to insulin resistance. Moreover, other studies reported that long term treatment with ACE inhibitors failed to reduce the risk of diabetes in patients with impaired glucose tolerance. Thus, proving that the mechanism involved in hypertension associated insulin resistance is different from those contributing to insulin resistance in diabetes patients [6]. ACE inhibitors also have immunomodulator activity by inhibiting RAAS. They prevent the conversion of angiotensin I to angiotensin II leading to vasodilation and reduced blood pressure. ACE inhibitors alter the ACE mediated degradation of bradykinin and substance P that can influence immune cell function as these proteins play significant role in inflammation [7]. Additionally, these proteins promote mast cell degranulation and release of chemokine followed by recruitment of other immune cells [8]. This is the fundamental mechanism that explains the link between ACE inhibitors and immune system modulation [9].

This chapter explores the therapeutic role of ACE inhibitor by targeting or modulating RAAS. This chapter uncovers the efficacy and mechanism of ACE inhibitor in different diseases by facilitating alteration in RAAS. This chapter will analyze the practical examples of ACE inhibitor administration in cardiovascular diseases. This will include their fundamental role in hypertension along with their pivotal function in protecting the heart and kidney. Ultimately the goal of this chapter is to provide deeper knowledge on clinical applications of ACE inhibitors and mechanisms involved in transforming RAAS to clinicians, students, and researchers (Fig. 4.1).

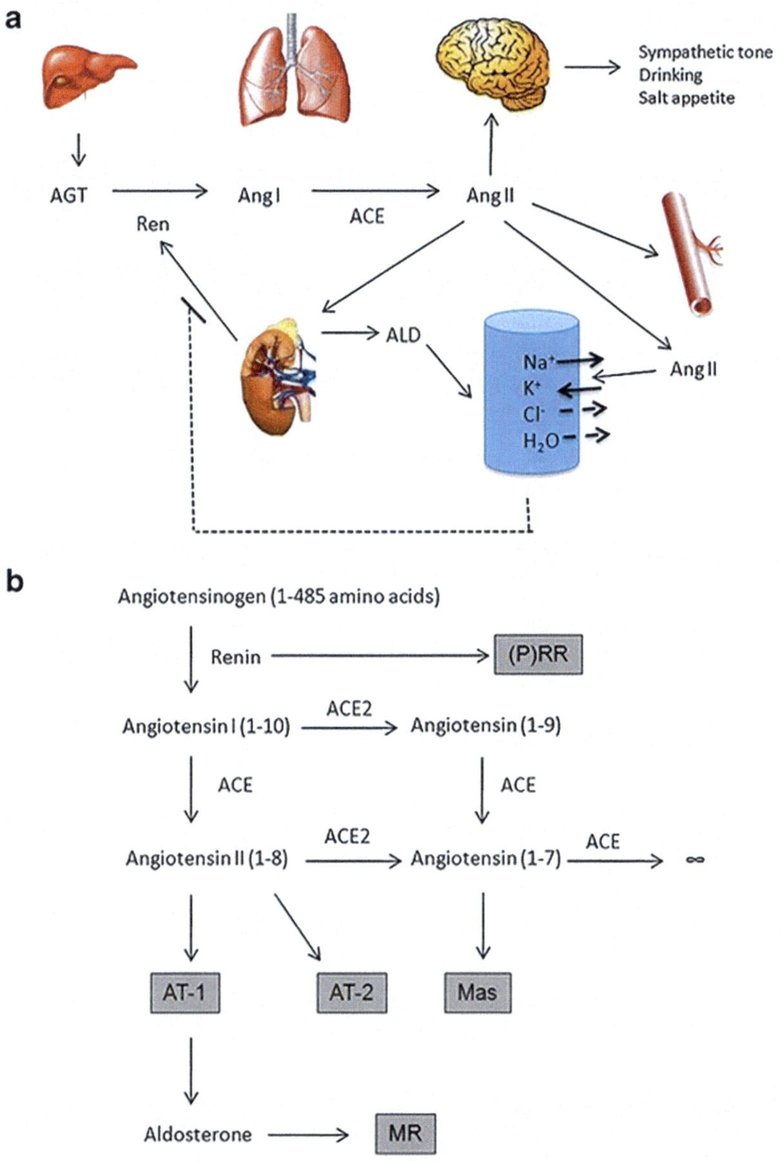

Fig. 4.1 Scheme of the components of the hormonal RAAS. a Liver-produced angiotensin (AGT) is cleaved by renin from the kidney to the decapeptide angiotensin I (Ang I), which in turn is converted to Ang II (largely in the lung). The effector Ang II directs the adrenal gland to release aldosterone (ALD), which directs the brain to increase sympathetic tone, drinking, and salt appetite and also increases vasomotor tone. ALD, sympathetic tone, and Ang II act independently to affect NaCl reabsorption in the kidney. A reverse feedback mechanism exists. b The components involve a series of proteins (substrates, enzymes, and products) that can be defined by genomic study and followed across evolution. *(P)RR* prorenin receptor, *ACE* and *ACE2* angiotensin converting enzymes 1 and 2, AT_1 and AT_2 angiotensin receptors 1 and 2, *Mas* Mas receptor, *MR* mineralocorticoid receptor. In addition to this hormonal RAAS, the system also acts locally at the tissue level, e.g., brain, adrenal gland, and heart. (Source: Fournier et al. [10])

Machine Generated Summaries

Disclaimer: The summaries in this chapter were generated from Springer Nature publications using extractive AI auto-summarization: An extraction-based summarizer aims to identify the most important sentences of a text using an algorithm and uses those original sentences to create the auto-summary (unlike generative AI). As the constituted sentences are machine selected, they may not fully reflect the body of the work, so we strongly advise that the original content is read and cited. The auto generated summaries were curated by the editor to meet Springer Nature publication standards. To cite this content, please refer to the original papers.

Machine generated keywords: bradykinin, perindopril, telmisartan, combination, ramipril, sbp, endothelial, mmhg, week, vascular, baseline, tolerability, captopril, enalapril, ace inhibitor.

ACE-Inhibitors in Hypertension: A Historical Perspective and Current Insights [11]

This is a machine-generated summary of:

Cutrell, Stacey; Alhomoud, Ibrahim S.; Mehta, Anurag; Talasaz, Azita H.; Van Tassell, Benjamin; Dixon, Dave L.: ACE-Inhibitors in Hypertension: A Historical Perspective and Current Insights [11].

Published in: Current Hypertension Reports (2023).

Link to original: https://doi.org/10.1007/s11906-023-01248-2

If you want to cite the papers, please refer to the original.

For technical reasons we could not place the page where the original quote is coming from.

Abstract-Summary "This review describes the discovery and development of ACE inhibitors as antihypertensive agents, compares their efficacy, tolerability, and safety to ARBs, and highlights the contemporary issues surrounding ACE inhibitor use for HTN."

"Angiotensin-converting enzyme (ACE) inhibitors are commonly prescribed medications for the management of hypertension (HTN) and other chronic conditions including heart failure and chronic kidney disease."

"ACE inhibitors are first-line therapy in HTN management along with thiazide diuretics, calcium channel blockers, and angiotensin receptor blockers (ARB)."

"Recent evidence has also suggested ARBs may have neuroprotective effects compared to other antihypertensives, including ACE inhibitors; however, this warrants further study."

"ACE inhibitors and ARBs have an equal class of recommendation for first-line treatment for the management of HTN."

"Recent evidence has shown ARBs to be just as effective as ACE inhibitors for HTN but with improved tolerability."

Introduction

"This is likely because ACE inhibitors are generically available, affordable, and recommended as a first-line option for the management of highly prevalent chronic conditions, such as hypertension (HTN), heart failure with reduced ejection fraction (HFrEF), and chronic kidney disease (CKD) [12–14]."

"ACE inhibitors are, however, associated with a modest, but significant, risk of bradykinin-mediated angioedema, acute kidney injury (AKI), hyperkalemia, and chronic cough."

"Although ARBs were initially more expensive than ACE inhibitors, both classes of medications are now generically available and similarly affordable."

"This has raised questions about whether ARBs should preferentially be used instead of ACE inhibitors for HTN given their more favorable safety profile and similar antihypertensive effectiveness."

Discovery and Development of ACE Inhibitors

"Discovery, researcher Maurio Rocha e Silva and his student, Sergio Ferreira, at the University of Sao Paulo, began to study the snake venom and identified a peptide in the venom, bradykinin potentiating factor (BPF), that caused the blood pressure (BP) lowering effects [15]."

"Finding, Vane proposed a research program in collaboration with Squibb Institute for Medical Research to develop the first orally active synthetic ACE inhibitor [16, 17]."

"After years of research and development, captopril, the first ACE inhibitor, was commercially released in 1981."

Antihypertensive Effects and Clinical Indications for ACE Inhibitors

"ACE inhibitors are considered first-line therapy in the management of HTN along with ARBs, thiazide diuretics, and calcium channel blockers (CCBs) [12]."

"A systematic review analyzed 92 randomized clinical trials that randomly assigned participants to an ACE inhibitor or placebo and evaluated the BP lowering effects of different ACE inhibitors in almost 13,000 participants [18]."

"Systematic reviews analyzing alternative first-line therapies have shown similar BP lowering effects with ACE inhibitors, thiazide diuretics (~9/4 mmHg), and ARBs (~8/5 mmHg) [19, 20]."

"Since thiazide diuretics, CCBs, ACE inhibitors, and ARBs share a similar class of recommendation for initial management in HTN, compelling indications should be a primary consideration when selecting first-line antihypertensive therapy."

Tolerability and Safety of ACE Inhibitors

"Chronic cough, hyperkalemia, acute kidney injury, and angioedema are expected potential adverse effects with ACE inhibitor use."

"Future use of ACE inhibitors is contraindicated in patients with a history of angioedema, but ARBs may be considered when RAS inhibition is necessary [7]."

"A related concern with ACE inhibitor (and ARB) use is the potential risk of lung cancer."

"Numerous observational studies and meta-analyses of ACE inhibitors, ARBs, and other antihypertensives and risk of cancer and/or lung cancer have shown conflicting results [21–26]."

"In studies showing an increased risk of lung cancer with ACE inhibitors, the absolute risk is quite small; however, this could be problematic given the millions of individuals around the world who use ACE inhibitors."

"ACE inhibitors along with other antihypertensives that affect the RAS can cause AKI and hyperkalemia [27]."

"To AKI, the incidence of hyperkalemia appears to be similar between ACE inhibitors and ARBs."

Contemporary Considerations

"Head-to-head trials comparing the antihypertensive effectiveness of ACE inhibitors and ARBs remain limited [28–31]."

"Most of the evidence comparing ACE inhibitors and ARBs has come from high-risk populations, which may limit application to the majority patients initiating antihypertensives [28–31]."

"A large-scale observational study of over 3 millions patients worldwide was designed to compare the effectiveness and safety of ACE inhibitors and ARBs when initiated as first-line treatment for HTN [32]."

"The study authors concluded that based on these results, ARBs should be selected over ACE inhibitors as first-line therapy for the management of HTN [32]."

"An observational study has shown a small reduction in dementia risk for ARBs compared with ACE inhibitors within the first 12 months of follow-up [33]."

"Other studies have demonstrated that ARBs cause slower cognitive decline compared to ACE inhibitors [34–36]."

Conclusion

"ACE inhibitors are effective antihypertensives for the management of HTN and provide important clinical benefits for patients with compelling chronic conditions (e.g., DM, HFrEF)."

"Chronic cough and angioedema occur at higher rates with ACE inhibitors than other antihypertensive agents, specifically ARBs."

"ACE inhibitors and ARBs are equally guideline-recommended first-line therapy in the management of HTN; however, recent evidence suggests ARBs to be just as effective as ACE inhibitors but with improved tolerability."

Reduced Hepatic Bradykinin Degradation Accounts for Cold-Induced BAT Thermogenesis and WAT Browning in Male Mice [37]

This is a machine-generated summary of:

Xiao, Fei; Jiang, Haizhou; Li, Zi; Jiang, Xiaoxue; Chen, Shanghai; Niu, Yuguo; Yin, Hanrui; Shu, Yousheng; Peng, Bo; Lu, Wei; Li, Xiaoying; Li, Zhigang; Lan, Shujue; Xu, Xiaoyan; Guo, Feifan: Reduced hepatic bradykinin degradation accounts for cold-induced BAT thermogenesis and WAT browning in male mice [37].

Published in: Nature Communications (2023).

Link to original: https://doi.org/10.1038/s41467-023-38141-0

If you want to cite the papers, please refer to the original.

For technical reasons we could not place the page where the original quote is coming from.

Abstract-Summary "We identify elevated serum bradykinin levels in response to acute cold exposure in male mice."

"A bolus of anti-bradykinin antibodies reduces body temperature during acute cold exposure, whereas bradykinin has the opposite effect."

"Acute cold exposure inhibits hepatic prolyl endopeptidase (PREP) activity, causing reduced liver bradykinin degradation and increased serum bradykinin levels."

"By blocking the breakdown of bradykinin, angiotensin-converting enzyme inhibitors (ACEIs) increase serum bradykinin levels and induce brown adipose tissue thermogenesis and white adipose tissue browning via B2R. Collectively, our data provide new insights into the mechanisms underlying organ crosstalk in whole-body physiology control during cold exposure and also suggest bradykinin as a possible anti-obesity target."

Introduction

"Adipose tissue plays an important role in protection against the cold through non-shivering thermogenesis (NST) [38]."

"Some brown fat-like cells may appear in the white adipose tissue (WAT) following external stimulation."

"Cold exposure enhances brown adipose tissue (BAT) activity and induces WAT browning to maintain body temperature."

"The crosstalk between liver and adipose tissue remains largely unknown, and more research is needed to identify additional mechanisms that drive thermogenesis during cold challenge."

"Considering these studies, the role of BK in adipose tissue thermogenesis and body temperature during cold exposure remains elusive."

"A bolus of anti-BK antibodies reduced body temperature during acute cold, whereas BK had the opposite effect."

"Further studies demonstrated that BK increased UCP1 expression, elevated BAT thermogenesis, and promoted WAT browning."

"By blocking BK breakdown, the angiotensin-converting enzyme inhibitors (ACEIs) could increase serum BK levels and had similar effects on adipose tissue as BK."

Results

"To elucidate the role of BK during acute cold exposure, mice were placed at room temperature (25 °C) or under cold conditions (4 °C) for different amounts of time, and the serum levels of BK as well as the other three kinins including des-Arg^{9}-BK, kallidin-like peptide (KLP, Arg-BK) and des-Arg^{10}-KLP were measured."

"Inducing WAT browning requires long-term treatment; therefore, we tested the effects of long-term BK treatment on UCP1 expression in WAT and BAT after injecting mice with 1 mg/kg BK once a day for 14 days at room temperature."

"To confirm the role of UCP1 in BK-mediated effects, we first performed time course experiments to elucidate changes in UCP1 expression and body temperature at room temperature."

"We first measured serum levels of the BK precursor HMWK in mice at room temperature or under conditions of acute cold exposure for different periods of time."

Discussion

"Our further study focused on BK and demonstrated a role for BK in regulating body temperature during acute cold exposure, as treatment with anti-BK antibodies reduced body temperature while BK had the opposite effect."

"PREP over-expression blocked cold-induced changes in hepatic and serum BK levels, BAT activity, WAT browning and body temperature."

"Our findings expand the physiological role of PREP in metabolism and demonstrate that the liver affects circulating levels of BK in response to acute cold exposure."

"Although BK can increase BAT thermogenesis and body temperature, we found that aged mice exhibited higher serum BK levels than young mice at room temperature."

"The effects of ACEIs on BAT activity and WAT browning were blocked in adipose tissue-specific B2R knockout mice, suggesting that BK mediates the effects of ACEIs in reducing fat mass."

"Our work identifies an important function of BK in regulating BAT thermogenesis and WAT browning during acute cold exposure."

Methods

"The adenoviruses expressing mouse PREP (Ad-PREP) were purchased from Hanbio Co.Ltd. Cells were infected with Ad-PREP or control adenoviruses at a dose of 10^{7} plaque-forming units/well in 12-well plates for 48 h. Rectal core temperature was measured by the digital thermometer (Physitemp Instruments, USA)."

"1 μM BK (Abcam, UK) was added to the fully differentiated cells for 48 h. For nitric oxide (NO) clearance experiments, 1 μM BK and 100 μM PTIO (Beyotime, China) were added simultaneously for 48 h on day 6."

"5 μL homogenates in PBS was used to determine the protein concentration by BCA Protein Assay Kit (Thermo, USA) for normalization."

"Before measurement, the cell plate was loaded with 5 μM Fluo-4 AM (Beyotime, China) and 2.5 mM probenecid (Aladdin, China) diluted in HBSS (Thermo, USA) for 1 h at 37 °C in the dark."

A Review of the Role of Bradykinin and Nitric Oxide in the Cardioprotective Action of Angiotensin-Converting Enzyme Inhibitors: Focus on Perindopril [39]

This is a machine-generated summary of:

Ancion, Arnaud; Tridetti, Julien; Nguyen Trung, Mai-Linh; Oury, Cécile; Lancellotti, Patrizio: A Review of the Role of Bradykinin and Nitric Oxide in the Cardioprotective Action of Angiotensin-Converting Enzyme Inhibitors: Focus on Perindopril [39].

Published in: Cardiology and Therapy (2019).

Link to original: https://doi.org/10.1007/s40119-019-00150-w

If you want to cite the papers, please refer to the original.

For technical reasons we could not place the page where the original quote is coming from.

Abstract-Summary "Chronic exposure to cardiovascular risk factors and oxidative stress results in an imbalance in these functions, creating an environment that favors reduced vasodilation and a proinflammatory and prothrombic state."

"The involvement of endothelial dysfunction in all stages of the cardiovascular continuum makes it an important target for treatment."

"One of the major endothelial-derived factors involved in the maintenance of endothelial function is nitric oxide (NO)."

"Among the ACE inhibitors, perindopril appears to have the greatest effects on bradykinin and has demonstrated efficacy in a number of markers of endothelial dysfunction including arterial stiffness and progression of atherosclerosis."

"There is also strong evidence supporting the use of perindopril-based therapy for the treatment of hypertension and for reducing the risk of cardiovascular morbidity and mortality in a wide range of patients across the cardiovascular continuum."

Introduction

"The earliest vascular abnormality in the continuum is endothelial dysfunction."

"Endothelial dysfunction is a reliable prognostic indicator of cardiovascular events, independently of traditional cardiovascular risk factors in patients with atherosclerotic coronary disease or at high cardiovascular risk [40]."

"To the correction of cardiovascular risk factors, re-establishing balanced endothelial function is therefore an important target for treatment."

"Two pathways that play a major role in endothelial homeostasis, and consequently endothelial dysfunction, are those of the renin–angiotensin and bradykinin–nitric oxide (NO) systems."

"This review will examine the role of angiotensin II and bradykinin in the pathophysiology of endothelial dysfunction, and the importance of endothelial dysfunction as a target for the prevention of cardiovascular disease."

Pathophysiology of Endothelial Dysfunction and Its Role in the Cardiovascular Continuum

"Angiotensin II also produces conditions favorable for atherogenesis by upregulating endothelial receptors for oxidized low-density lipoprotein (OxLDL), stimulating OxLDL uptake, and enhancing OxLDL-mediated ROS generation."

"When not sufficiently counterbalanced by the actions of bradykinin, these molecular effects of angiotensin II result in endothelial dysfunction."

"In endothelial cells, activation of B2R by bradykinin induces the release of NO, prostacyclin, endothelium-derived hyperpolarizing factor (EDHF), and tissue plasminogen activator, which exert diverse physiological actions on the cardiovascular system, including regulation of vascular tone and local blood flow to organs, coagulation, fibrinolysis, and water–electrolyte balance [41]."

"Experimental studies have demonstrated a protective role of B2R on cardiovascular function, as a result of its opposing effects on angiotensin II AT_1 receptor activation [42]."

"The anti-inflammatory effects and reduction in ROS induced by bradykinin have been shown to be mediated through the release of NO, a key regulator of endothelial function."

ACE Inhibition and Endothelial Function

"The possibility that ACE inhibitors could improve endothelial function was initially raised following reports from experimental studies that the renin–angiotensin system, and in particular angiotensin II, plays a major role in inhibiting NO production and activity, mainly by inducing ROS generation [43]."

"In the presence of these risk factors, chronic overexpression of tissue ACE disrupts the angiotensin II/bradykinin balance, increasing levels of angiotensin II and decreasing tissue levels of bradykinin, the net result being endothelial dysfunction."

"PERTINENT showed that perindopril improved endothelial dysfunction by increasing bradykinin and reducing angiotensin II levels, thereby restoring the angiotensin II/bradykinin balance."

"The combination of a lipophilic profile, high tissue affinity, and a high bradykinin/angiotensin I selectivity ratio provide perindopril with a complete and long-lasting inhibition of bradykinin degradation, and may offer a greater physiological impact compared with other ACE inhibitors [44]."

Cardioprotective Actions of Perindopril Translate into Improved Cardiovascular Outcomes

"In the blood pressure-lowering arm of the trial, patients (n = 19,257) at moderate cardiovascular risk were randomized to amlodipine 5–10 mg (with the addition of perindopril 4–8 mg as required) or the ß-blocker atenolol with the addition of diuretic as required [45]."

"Over a mean follow-up of 4.3 years, treatment with perindopril/indapamide fixed combination reduced the incidence of the composite primary endpoint of macrovascular (non-fatal stroke, non-fatal MI, and cardiovascular death) and microvascular (new or worsening nephropathy and retinopathy) events by 9% vs. placebo ($P < 0.05$)."

"After 1 year, the event rate was lower than expected and reduced the statistical power of the study, but perindopril still showed a strong tendency to reduce the primary endpoint (all-cause mortality, unplanned heart failure-related hospitalization with a minimum follow-up of 1 year) with a relative risk reduction of 31% ($P = 0.055$)."

Implications for Clinical Practice

"It is observed from the earliest stages of the cardiovascular disease continuum and its effects are cumulative, worsening endothelial dysfunction associated with progressive vascular damage."

"Certain cardiovascular drugs have pleiotropic effects that improve endothelial function independently of their primary indication."

"Among the antihypertensive agents, the ACE inhibitors appear to have the strongest effects on endothelial dysfunction."

"These properties may account, at least in part, for the documented superiority of this agent over other renin–angiotensin system inhibitors in the prevention and treatment of all stages of the cardiovascular continuum from hypertension to the most severe forms of cardiovascular disease."

"By attenuating the deleterious effects of endothelial dysfunction in addition to lowering blood pressure, the early initiation of agents such as ACE inhibitors and calcium channel blockers could interrupt and slow the development of endothelial dysfunction and progression to clinical disease at all stages of the cardiovascular continuum."

Conclusions

"The involvement of endothelial dysfunction in all stages of the cardiovascular continuum makes it an important target for treatment."

"NO is essential for endothelial function and its production is increased both directly and indirectly via inhibition of angiotensin II production and reduced degradation of bradykinin by the ACE inhibitors."

"Among the ACE inhibitors, perindopril appears to have the greatest effects on bradykinin and has demonstrated efficacy on a number of markers of endothelial dysfunction including arterial stiffness and progression of atherosclerosis."

"Evidence from a number of large, randomized controlled trials supports the use of perindopril-based therapy for the treatment of hypertension and for reducing the risk of cardiovascular morbidity and mortality in a wide range of patients across the cardiovascular continuum."

Polymorphisms in VEGFA Gene Affect the Antihypertensive Responses to Enalapril [46]

This is a machine-generated summary of:

Oliveira-Paula, G. H.; Lacchini, R.; Fontana, V.; Silva, P. S.; Biagi, C.; Tanus-Santos, Jose E.: Polymorphisms in VEGFA gene affect the antihypertensive responses to enalapril [46].

Published in: European Journal of Clinical Pharmacology (2015).

Link to original: https://doi.org/10.1007/s00228-015-1872-5

If you want to cite the papers, please refer to the original.

For technical reasons we could not place the page where the original quote is coming from.

Abstract-Summary "Angiotensin-converting enzyme inhibitors (ACEi) up-regulate the VEGF expression; thus, genetic polymorphisms in the VEGFA gene could affect the antihypertensive responses to these drugs."

"We compared the effect of VEGFA polymorphisms on changes in blood pressure after enalapril treatment."

"Individuals carrying the CA and AA genotypes for the g.-2578C>A polymorphism and the AGG haplotype showed more intense decrease in blood pressure in response to enalapril 20 mg/day."

"A multiple linear regression analysis showed that the AA genotype for the g.-2578C>A polymorphism and the AGG haplotype are associated with more intense decrease in blood pressure in response to enalapril 20 mg/day, while the CC genotype for the g.-2578C>A polymorphism and the CGG haplotype are associated with the opposite effect."

"These findings suggest that polymorphisms in VEGFA gene may affect the antihypertensive responses to enalapril."

Introduction

"It was shown that ACEi affect other relevant mediators, such as vascular endothelial growth factor (VEGF) [47, 48]."

"Considering the effect of VEGF on blood pressure, it is expected that it may be affected by antihypertensive drugs, including ACEi [49]."

"ACEi treatment increased VEGF expression in several experimental studies [47]."

"BR1 signaling, in turn, stimulates tissue VEGF expression [50], while BR2 stimulates endothelial NO production [51]."

"Li and others have suggested that ACEi may increase tissue VEGF levels through a possible interaction of BR2 with the angiotensin II type 2 receptor [50]."

"Since ACEi up-regulate VEGF expression, which promotes NO formation and vasodilation, it is possible that variations in the VEGFA gene could affect the antihypertensive response to ACEi."

"Studies demonstrated that these SNPs affect VEGF expression [52, 53]."

Methods

"The study participants included a total of 102 hypertensive patients with systolic blood pressure (SBP) $\geq$140 and $\leq$179 mmHg and diastolic blood pressure (DBP) $\geq$90 and $\leq$109 mmHg, recruited from Cardiology Division of the Araçatuba Health Center (Araçatuba, SP, Brazil)."

"Office SBP and DBP were recorded with a semiautomatic blood pressure monitor (OMRON® HEM-433 INT, Bannockburn, IL, USA) before and after the use of enalapril."

"Mean blood pressure (MBP) was calculated using the formula MBP = (SBP + 2 × DBP)/3."

"Changes in blood pressure were calculated as follows: (BP at baseline − BP after enalapril treatment) × (−1)."

"Age, gender, ethnicity, smoking status, VEGFA genotypes, and VEGFA haplotypes were included as independent variables in multiple linear regression models to explain changes in SBP, MBP, and DBP after enalapril treatment using JMP® software (SAS Institute, Cary, NC)."

Results

"The genotype distributions for VEGFA polymorphisms did not deviate from Hardy-Weinberg equilibrium ($P > 0.05$)."

"Baseline SBP, DBP, and MBP did not differ among the genotypes/alleles ($P > 0.05$; data not shown)."

"There were no differences in baseline SBP, DBP, and MBP stratified by genotypes/alleles between the group of patients treated with enalapril 10 mg/day and the group of patients treated with enalapril 20 mg/day ($P > 0.05$; data not shown)."

Discussion

"The main findings of this study were that (i) the variant genotypes for the g.-2578C>A polymorphism and the AGG haplotype in VEGFA gene were associated with better responses to enalapril 20 mg/day and (ii) the CC genotype for the g.-2578C>A polymorphism and the CGG haplotype were associated with worse responses to enalapril 20 mg/day."

"Although a previous study has showed that the eNOS and BDKRB2 genotypes affected the enalapril response independently of the doses used [54], our findings indicate that dose approach is important to evidence the effect of VEGFA polymorphisms on the antihypertensive response to enalapril, suggesting a gene-dose relationship."

"A higher dose of enalapril could effectively increase VEGF expression and this would be especially important in individuals carrying genetic polymorphisms that lead to lower VEGF expression, resulting in more intense decrease in blood pressure."

Nephroprotective Effects of Enalapril After [177Lu]-DOTATATE Therapy Using Serial Renal Scintigraphies in a Murine Model of Radiation-Induced Nephropathy [55]

This is a machine-generated summary of:

Ilhan, Harun; Wang, Hao; Gildehaus, Franz J.; Wängler, Carmen; Herrler, Tanja; Todica, Andrei; Schlichtiger, Julia; Cumming, Paul; Bartenstein, Peter; Hacker, Marcus; Haug, Alexander R.: Nephroprotective effects of enalapril after [177Lu]-DOTATATE therapy using serial renal scintigraphies in a murine model of radiation-induced nephropathy [55].

Published in: EJNMMI Research (2016).
Link to original: https://doi.org/10.1186/s13550-016-0219-2

If you want to cite the papers, please refer to the original.
For technical reasons we could not place the page where the original quote is coming from.

Abstract-Summary "We investigated the nephroprotective potential of the angiotensine converting enzyme inhibiting drug enalpril after [177Lu]-DOTATATE therapy in a murine model of radiation-induced nephropathy by renal scintigraphy."

"Baseline scintigraphy (n = 12) entailed 12-min dynamic acquisitions after injection of 25 MBq [99mTc]-MAG3, which was followed by radionuclide therapy at four escalating activities of [177Lu]-DOTATATE: group (Gp) 1: 10 MBq; Gp 2: 20 MBq; Gp 3: 40 MBq; Gp 4: 65 MBq."

"Daily administration by gavage of 10 mg/kg/d enalapril or water (control group) was initiated on the day of radionuclide therapy."

"At day 65 of follow-up, no significant change in the FUR relative to baseline (11.0 ± 0.3) was evident in radionuclide therapy groups 1 (11.2 ± 0.5) and 2 (10.1 ± 0.6), but FUR was significantly reduced in groups 3 (8.93 ± 0.6, $p < 0.05$) and 4 (6.0 ± 0.8, $p < 0.01$); we chose 40 MBq [177Lu]-DOTATATE (Gp 3) for the intervention study."

"At the last day of follow-up (day 86), FUR was unaltered in enalapril-treated mice (11.8 ± 0.5) relative to the baseline group (12.4 ± 0.3) and non-therapy group (11.9 ± 0.8), whereas FUR in the control group had undergone a significant decline (9.3 ± 0.5; $p < 0.01$)."

"Treatment with enalapril is effective for nephroprotection during radionuclide therapy with [177Lu]-DOTATATE in mice."

"Although these results are only limitedly transferable to human studies, enalapril might serve as a promising drug in the mitigation of nephropathy following treatment with [177Lu]-DOTATATE."

Background

"An important factor limiting benefits of this therapy is the occurrence of radiation-induced nephropathy, which arises due to renal clearance and megalin-receptor mediated tubular reabsorption of the chelated somatostatin analogues [56, 57]."

"Histopathological findings in kidneys after PRRT present a pattern of tubular and glomerular damage which seems similar to that evoked by external beam radiation [58]."

"The nephroprotective potential of angiotensin-converting-enzyme (ACE) inhibitors after external beam radiation of the kidneys in rats was first reported by Cohen and others in 1992 [59]."

"Given the similar pathologies and histopathological changes, we hypothesized that the pharmacological treatments effective in nephrotoxity induced by external beam radiation might also mitigate [177Lu]-DOTATATE induced nephrotoxicity."

Methods

"We investigated the activity-dependent impairment of renal function in mice treated with four activities of [177Lu]-DOTATATE: group 1 ($n = 6$), 10 MBq; group 2 ($n = 8$), 20 MBq; group 3 ($n = 7$), 40 MBq, and group 4 ($n = 7$), 65 MBq."

"Follow-up scintigraphies to assess renal function were carried out at days 9, 23, 44, and 65."

"Of the study, the nephroprotective properties of enalapril were evaluated in mice ($n = 7$) treated with 40 MBq [177Lu]-DOTATATE, as selected in part one."

"In this group, no PRRT was carried out and mice received MAG3 scintigraphy to identify therapy-independent changes in renal function over 3 months in healthy mice."

"MAG3 scintigraphy was obtained at baseline in order to determine the renal function prior to PRRT."

"Follow-up renal scintigraphies to assess renal function were carried out in all mice at days 9, 23, 44, 65, and 86."

Results

"During subsequent follow-up, FUR increased in group 1 (10 MBq), showing no significant difference at day 65 as compared to baseline values (11.2 ± 0.5 %IA/min vs. 11.0 ± 0.4 %IA/min)."

"At subsequent follow-up, FUR values tended to increase in the enalapril group, becoming non-significantly different from baseline (12.5 ± 0.3 %IA/min) at day 86 for enalapril treatment (11.8 ± 0.5 %IA/min), indicating rescue of renal function."

"Mean FUR values at the final day of follow-up revealed significant differences as compared to the water-treated control group, whereas no significant differences were measured in comparison to enalapril-treated mice underlining the nephroprotective effect of these treatment options (mean FUR after 3 months: 11.9 ± 0.8 %IA/min; $p < 0.05$ vs. water; p = n.s."

Discussion

"We investigated the nephroprotective characteristics of enalapril treatment in a mouse model of [177Lu]-DOTATATE therapy-induced nephropathy based upon encouraging results in studies based on external beam radiation [60–62]."

"Enalapril treatment likewise substantially rescued renal function, which was restored to baseline levels at day 86, as measured by FUR, and as also seen by renogram analysis."

"Renal histology was entirely normal in the enalapril-treatment group, providing further support for the potential clinical use of enalapril in reducing functional and histopathological changes in the kidney after PRRT with [177Lu]-DOTATATE."

"With the aid of renogram analysis and the calculation of the FUR, persistent impairment of renal function in mice after [177Lu]-DOTATATE therapy activity of at least 40 MBq is measurable by scintigraphy and was verified by histology."

Conclusions

"Treatment with enalapril for 3 months after radiotherapy with [177Lu]-DOTATATE mitigated renal damage in mice."

"Enalapril treatment could be an additional option for ameliorating the dose-limiting effects of radiation-induced kidney damage, thus allowing application of more effective therapy activities."

"Due to a moderate side effect profile and the applicability in patients with renal risk factors like hypertension and diabetes, which aggravate the nephrotoxicity of PRRT [63], enalapril treatment might be a promising therapy."

Unraveling the Pivotal Role of Bradykinin in ACE Inhibitor Activity [64]

This is a machine-generated summary of:

Taddei, Stefano; Bortolotto, L.: Unraveling the Pivotal Role of Bradykinin in ACE Inhibitor Activity [64].

Published in: American Journal of Cardiovascular Drugs (2016).

Link to original: https://doi.org/10.1007/s40256-016-0173-4

If you want to cite the papers, please refer to the original.

For technical reasons we could not place the page where the original quote is coming from.

Abstract-Summary "The first described effect of an angiotensin converting enzyme (ACE) inhibitor was an increased activity of bradykinin, one of the substrates of ACE."

"In the subsequent years, molecular models describing the mechanism of action of ACE inhibitors in decreasing blood pressure and cardiovascular risk have focused mostly on the renin-angiotensin system."

"The affinity of ACE appears to be higher for bradykinin than for angiotensin I, thereby suggesting that ACE inhibitors may be more effective inhibitors of bradykinin degradation than of angiotensin II production."

"Data describing the effect of ACE inhibition on bradykinin signaling support the hypothesis that the most cardioprotective benefits attributed to ACE inhibition may be due to increased bradykinin signaling rather than to decreased angiotensin II signaling, especially when high dosages of ACE inhibitors are considered."

Introduction

"The most recent evidence of the heterogeneity amongst RAS blockers was presented in a meta-analysis of data from 195,267 patients in whom the effect of ACE inhibitors and ARBs on major cardiovascular events was evaluated in comparison to placebo [65]."

"As ACE inhibitors do not bind selectively to one or the other catalytic domain, these data suggest that at a molecular level, ACE inhibitors may be more effective inhibitors of bradykinin degradation than of Ang II production."

"We will focus on data describing the cardiovascular effects of bradykinin and the effects of ACE inhibition on bradykinin signaling."

"We will explore the idea that current dosing regimens, which are largely based on the systemic effects of ACE inhibition on the Ang I pathway, could be considered in light of the data coming from the bradykinin system."

Bradykinin and Its Receptors

"In clinical studies, the role of bradykinin signaling in blood pressure regulation was underscored by a meta-analysis of 11 trials, which showed that the −58T/C (exon 1) polymorphism in the B2R gene, which reduces B2R transcription, was significantly associated with increased risk for essential hypertension [66]."

"Further evidence of the involvement of bradykinin signaling in renal health comes from studies that show significant associations between polymorphisms in the B1R and B2R genes and progression of renal dysfunction [67, 68]."

"Following ischemia/reperfusion injury in the kidney, DNA damage and apoptosis were significantly increased in $B2R^{-/-}/B1R^{-/-}$ mice compared with wild type mice [69]."

"When these mice were used in a model for renal ischemia/reperfusion injury, highest levels of oxidative DNA damage and apoptosis were found in the $B2R^{-/-}$ / $B1R^{-/-}$ mice, followed by the $B2R^{-/-}$ mice, and then wild type mice [69]."

"In rat aortic endothelial cells, bradykinin increased PAI-1 messenger RNA (mRNA) and protein expression, an effect that was inhibited by B2R antagonist HOE 140 [70]."

Bradykinin During Aging and Cardiovascular Disease

"This could be explained by the age-related decrease in the expression of the bradykinin B2R that has been observed in different rat models [71]."

"In the group of patients with coronary artery disease, its expression rapidly decreased between the ages of 50 and 65 [72]."

"Pathological situations such as hypertension seem to accelerate the bradykinin-related process of aging."

"In addition to the natural age-related decrease in expression and activity of B2R, hypertension and coronary artery disease further enhance the decline of bradykinin signaling by lowering levels of circulating kinins."

Angiotensin Converting Enzyme (ACE) Inhibitors and Bradykinin

"In studies of patients with heart failure, ACE inhibitor therapy caused a significant increase in forearm vasodilatation and blood flow in response to bradykinin infusion [73, 74]."

"The combination of a lipophilic profile, high tissue affinity, and a high bradykinin/Ang I selectivity ratio, however, suggests that perindopril could provide more complete, longer lasting inhibition of bradykinin metabolism, and therefore have an increased physiological impact compared with other ACE inhibitors."

"With respect to blood pressure reduction, the ACE inhibitor perindopril has demonstrated in several studies its ability to provide additional blood pressure reduction when the dose is increased from 5 mg to 10 mg."

"Even if cough were to be associated with the bradykinin pathway, it is important to note that ACE inhibitors tend to restore bradykinin to normal levels, as they are naturally low in hypertensive patients, rather than to increase them above physiological levels, as demonstrated with perindopril 10 mg in PERTINENT."

Conclusions

"These data suggest that our perspective, which has, to date, mostly been based on blood pressure effects and Ang I/Ang II plasma levels, could be expanded to include the data coming from the bradykinin system."

"Increases in bradykinin levels appear to be, not only a pleiotropic effect of ACE inhibitors, but also a fundamental element of their mode of action."

"The specific effect of ACE inhibitors on bradykinin rationally explains the differences in blood pressure reduction and cardiovascular protection noted between ACE inhibitors and ARBs."

Malaria Link of Hypertension: A Hidden Syndicate of Angiotensin II, Bradykinin and Sphingosine 1-Phosphate [75]

This is a machine-generated summary of:

Dhangadamajhi, Gunanidhi; Singh, Shailja: Malaria link of hypertension: a hidden syndicate of angiotensin II, bradykinin and sphingosine 1-phosphate [75].

Published in: Human Cell (2021).

Link to original: https://doi.org/10.1007/s13577-021-00513-3

If you want to cite the papers, please refer to the original.

For technical reasons we could not place the page where the original quote is coming from.

Abstract-Summary "Although malaria and hypertension seem to have no direct link, several studies in recent years support their possible link."

"In the present review, based on available literatures we highlight the present knowledge on the production and bioavailability of these molecules, the mechanism of their regulation of hypertension, and patho-physiological role in malaria."

"Further, a possible link between malaria and hypertension is hypothesized through various arguments based on experimental evidence."

"Understanding of their mechanisms of blood pressure regulation during malaria infection may open up avenues for drug therapeutics and management of malaria in co-morbidity with hypertension."

Introduction

"Increased incidence of hypertension in the most rural African region (of high malaria endemicity) [76] while refuting the western life-style attributed to the rise of BP [77], a prediction of about 3/4th of hypertensive patients of the World to be present by 2030 in economically developing countries where malaria is highly prevalent is alarming [78]."

"High proportions of known genetic variants for hypertension in the malaria-endemic population [79], and increased prevalence of their hypertension when they live in malaria-free regions [80, 81] suggest the operation of evolutionary force favoring the occurrence of hypertension in malaria-endemic regions."

"Three bioactive molecules such as Angiotensin II (Ang II), Bradykinin (BK) and S1P derived from these pathways play key role in vascular homeostasis, BP regulation, inflammation and malaria pathogenesis [82–84]."

"We have tried to highlight the present knowledge on production and bioavailability of these molecules, the mechanism of their regulation of hypertension, and patho-physiological role in malaria."

"Further, a possible link between malaria and hypertension through patho-physiological function of these molecules based on experimental evidences is hypothesized."

The RAAS Pathways and Regulation of BP

"The RAAS-mediated hypertension seems to be modulated by Ang II and Ang II-derived peptides signaling via different receptors (AT_1, AT_2, Mas, etc.)."

"The membrane-bound angiotensin-converting enzyme (ACE) on endothelial cells (EC) or selected tissues (such as heart, kidney, brain) extracellularly cleave Ang I into Ang II [85]."

"Although Ang II is also reported to be present within the cell, the intracellular receptor involved is largely unknown."

"Conversion of Ang II into either angiotensin (1–7) by ACE2 or its cleavage into angiotensin III, followed by Ang IV [86, 87] reduces the Ang II level which could have otherwise signaled through AT_1 receptor arm."

"Receptors activation by these Ang II derived peptides leads to the production of endothelium-derived hyperpolarizing factor (EDHF) and enhances cytosolic calcium ion concentration which is coupled to the production of nitric oxide (NO) and prostacyclin (PGI_2) in EC."

Angiotensin II and Malaria

"Ang II play a crucial role in malaria pathogenesis via two receptors, AT_1 and AT_2."

"While Ang II-AT_1 signaling has a detrimental role in malaria, Ang II-AT_2 axis of signaling has a direct protective role."

"While conversion of Ang II to Ang 1–7 seems to be beneficial, the role of other Ang II derived peptides (such as Ang III and Ang IV) and their signaling through corresponding receptors are not known."

"Ang II mediated protection appears to rely upon ACE/ACE2 ratio, their bioactivity, tissue-specific expression, and activation of receptors for Ang II and its derived peptides."

"We hypothesize that differential expression of receptors for Ang II and its derived peptides may likely to contribute inter-individual variation or age-related differences in the clinical manifestation of severe malaria."

Bradykinin Suppresses Hypertension

"Similar to Ang II derived active peptides, it induces the release of anti-hypertensive molecules such as NO, prostacyclin and EDHF from EC [88, 89]."

"The enhanced activity of ACE not only increases Ang II level, but also degrades the BK into inactive fragments [89]."

"ACE inhibition leading to reduced Ang II level and BK accumulation is suggested as alternative therapeutics to hypertension."

Bradykinin and Malaria

"Depending upon its systemic or local concentration, BK is thought to modulate parasite survival and host hemodynamics by signaling through its two receptors (B_1 and B_2)."

"In a recent in vitro study, impaired signaling of BK in P. chabaudi infected mice lacking B_1 receptor has led to its reduced survival and was suggested to be due to hepatic dysfunction [90]."

"Since there are multiple pathways of parasite invasion [91], successful establishment of infection through alternate pathways may lead to B_2 mediated BK deprivation in the surrounding medium."

"BK is proposed to contribute CM pathogenesis by favoring late-stage parasite (P. falciparum schizont) sequestration in microvessels and disrupting the integrity of IEJ through B_2 activation [92]."

S1P Signaling and Regulation of Hypertension

"Upon increased intracellular S1P, vasodilation in EC is suggested to be due to S1P export and subsequent autocrine signaling through the $S1PR_1$ receptor [93, 94]."

"Extracellular S1P has a BP-lowering effect mediated via $S1PR_1$ activation in EC [95, 96]."

"It is demonstrated that SPHK1-S1P signaling varies in EC and in VSMC of different developmental origin (such as pulmonary and systemic) due to differential expression of S1PRs in these cells and could be the underlying cause of SPHK1 induced pulmonary hypertension [97–99]."

"Collective evidences support, in addition to high plasma S1P level, sharp maintenance of S1P gradient between blood and tissues, distinct cell-specific activation of specific SPHK isoforms, differential expression of S1PRs on cells of the immune system and that of vascular bed of various tissue origin (pulmonary, brain and systemic) and subsequent S1P signaling modulate the onset of hypertension and its associated pathogenic condition."

S1P and Malaria

"Plasma S1P level is kept low in severe malaria because of the significant loss of two major S1P sources (RBC and platelets) [100–102], though thrombocytopenia in malaria could also be caused due to reduced plasma S1P [103]."

"The inverse relationship of plasma S1P with breakdown products of endothelial glycocalyx [104], endothelial dysfunction, and enhanced vascular permeability [105–107] facilitate iRBC sequestration [104, 108] and cause severe malaria when plasma S1P level is low."

"Deprivation of intracellular S1P in parasite-infected RBC, stimulation for augmented S1P release from cellular sources to circulation and/or exogenous supplementation of S1P could be the possible adjunctive therapeutics against severe malaria."

"Improved survival of experimental mice in late-stage infection upon FTY720 treatment in combination with low-dose artesunate (a potent antimalarial drug) is reported and suggested to be through FTY720 mediated breaching of BBB (by $S1PR_1$ antagonistic function) and effective drug delivery to the brain [109, 110]."

Malaria Link of Hypertension and Future Perspectives

"While increased level of Ang II and S1P are responsible for inducing hypertension, BK is arthero-protective and anti-hypertensive [111]."

"In endemic regions, repeated exposure to malaria infection may lead to perpetual protective inflammatory responses of enhanced Ang II and S1P, and/or reduced BK levels which in turn have the adverse sequel of encouraging hypertension."

"Parasite manipulation to host responses leading to reduced bioavailability of Ang II and S1P at their suitable site of action for malaria protection could be parasite's immune-escape mechanism of self-protection with a repercussion of hypertension."

"Since host responses to malaria infection (protective or parasite manipulated) seem to cause hypertension, adaptation to the duo of the diseases is reckoned among asymptomatic or healthy individuals from high endemicity regions for malaria."

"In agreement to this, despite high serum ACE activity (which indicates a high Ang II level) in endemic control, a positive correlation between ACE activity and hypertension is reported only among malaria patients in Nigeria [112]."

Future Perspectives

"Besides its direct effects through AT_1, Ang II induces hypertension by stimulating SPHK2-S1P production [113–115]."

"Hypoxia/Ang II induced SPHK1 derived S1P in lungs is documented for pulmonary hypertension/acute respiratory distress syndrome (ARDS) [98, 116]."

"Excessive production of Ang II and S1P, and their deregulated signaling play important role in the onset of hypertension."

"While prevention of Ang II production by ACE inhibition (e.g. with captopril) is demonstrated for early-stage malaria protection and BP regulation, it is shown un-effective in late-stage infection [90]."

"Whether Ang II-AT_1 blockade with losartan during malaria do favor Ang IV production or what role does Ang IV play in malaria pathogenesis is unknown."

"Validation of Ang II-AT_1 blockade and/or stimulation of Ang II-AT_2 axis or Ang1-7-Mas axis along with Ang IV/AT_4 cascade in malaria and hypertension co-morbidity would be a promising approach towards therapeutics development for malaria."

Conclusion

"The present review discussed the current knowledge on malaria pathophysiology with regards to hypertension and linked the two diseases through various arguments."

"While increased prevalence of hypertension in malaria-endemic region is proclaimed as an evolutionary adaptation against malaria, hypertension itself is a leading risk factor for death and the effect of pre-existing hypertension on malaria outcome is still unknown."

"Prevalence and pathogenesis of malaria in hypertensive individuals from varying malaria-endemic regions or assessment of Ang II and S1P signaling pathways together with BP monitoring in malaria eradicated population in cohort studies are warranted to uncover further insight."

"Although malaria link of hypertension is an emerging issue, several questions including those discussed above in this review are yet to be resolved for the strategic management of co-morbidity of malaria with hypertension."

Comparison of Endothelial Function Improvement Estimated with Reactive Hyperemia Index Between Ramipril and Telmisartan in Hypertensive Patients [117]

This is a machine-generated summary of:

Ki, You-Jeong; Seo, Jae-Bin; Kim, Hack-Lyoung; Lim, Woo-Hyun; Seo, Hye Yeon; Lee, Jin Yong; Chung, Woo-Young: Comparison of endothelial function improvement estimated with reactive hyperemia index between ramipril and telmisartan in hypertensive patients [117].

Published in: Clinical Hypertension (2017).

Link to original: https://doi.org/10.1186/s40885-016-0060-y

If you want to cite the papers, please refer to the original.

For technical reasons we could not place the page where the original quote is coming from.

Abstract-Summary "Twenty consecutive patients with hypertension (57.9 ± 11.3 years, 60% men) were assigned to receive treatment with ramipril or telmisartan for eight weeks (n = 10 per group)."

"Blood pressure (BP) and RHI were measured at baseline and after eight weeks treatment."

"Baseline systolic BP and pulse pressure (PP) were higher in telmisartan group than ramipril group (systolic BP, 159 ± 6.83 vs 150 ± 7.49, p = 0.028; PP, 75.0 ± 14.0 vs 60.3 ± 12.4, p = 0.034)."

"In both groups, systolic and diastolic BP decreased significantly after eight weeks treatment (p < 0.05 for each)."

"Although PP reduced in both group (ramipril group, 60.3 ± 12.4 mm Hg to 50.4 ± 7.60 mm Hg; telmisartan group, 75.0 ± 14.0 mm Hg to 57.4 ± 15.1 mm Hg), change was statistically remarkable only in telmisartan group."

"During eight weeks, there was no significant changes of RHI in both groups."

"There was a positive relationship between decrease of PP after 8 weeks and the improvement of endothelial function only in ramipril group, but not in telmisartan group (ramipril group, r = 0.671, p = 0.034; telmisartan group, r = −0.487, p = 0.153)."

"Despite PP reduction effect favoring endothelial function, it's not correlated with RHI improvement with telmisartan."

Background

"Both PAT and BAUS are validated method for evaluating peripheral endothelial function."

"Many studies have investigated the effect of AT II receptor blockers (ARBs) on endothelial function assessed by FMD."

"In a meta-analysis showed that ARBs improved the endothelial function compared with other antihypertensive agents and there was no difference between ARBs and angiotensin-converting enzyme inhibitors (ACEIs) [118]."

"In many studies, ACEIs and ARBs have beneficial effects on endothelium through inhibition of AT II [119, 120]."

"In one aspect where ARBs can block AT II action of, ARBs seems better in protecting endothelial function."

"Comparison of endothelial function improvement between ACEIs and ARBs has not been well studied."

"This study was performed to compare the effect of ACEIs or ARBs on peripheral endothelial function estimated with RHI in hypertensive patients."

Methods

"Subjects with following conditions were excluded: 1) patients of serum creatinine ≥1.5 mg/dL or during renal replacement therapy, 2) decompensated congestive heart failure, 3) systolic BP >180 mm Hg and diastolic BP >110 mm Hg, 4) acute coronary syndrome, 5) atrial fibrillation, 6) patients already receiving three-hypertensive therapy; high risk for the development of hypertensive catastrophe by cessation of medication 7) during pregnancy or planned for pregnancy subjects."

"The participants were randomly assigned in a 1:1 ratio to ramipril group or telmisartan group according to a random number, generated by a web based randomization program of Medical Research Collaboration Center (MRCC) web site (https://mrcc.snuh.org/) of our institute."

"All patients in each group underwent endothelial function test with PAT before the treatment and after 8 weeks treatment, respectively."

"The significance systolic BP, diastolic BP, PP and RHI changes were examined with Wilcoxon signed-rank tests for each group."

Results

"At 8 weeks follow up, BP was 130 ± 7/80 ± 5 mm Hg in ramipril group and 131 ± 14/73 ± 9 mm Hg in telmisartan group."

"BP reduction from baseline to the 8 weeks follow up was 21/11 mm Hg (systole/diastole) in the ramipril group and 28/11 mm Hg (systole/diastole) telmisartan group, respectively (p value, Wilcoxon signed-rank test: 0.005, 0.012, 0.005, 0.036, respectively)."

"The target BP (<140 mm Hg systolic and <90 mm Hg diastolic) was achieved in 9 (90%) patients in the ramipril group and 6 (60%) in the telmisartan group at 8 weeks follow up."

"At 8 weeks follow up, the RHI was 1.64 ± 0.33 in ramipril group and 1.59 ± 0.46 in telmisartan group (p = 0.256)."

Discussions

"The present study intended to investigate if ramipril and telmisartan affect endothelial function differently from each other after the treatment for eight weeks in hypertensive patients."

"Because any other factors associated with endothelial function such as lipid profile, smoking history, were not different between groups, the fact improvement of endothelial function is not correlated with decrease of PP in telmisartan group suggests telmisartan itself may negatively influence endothelium dependent vasodilatation."

"In his study, ACEIs, calcium antagonists, ARBs, and beta blockers similarly reduced BP, but only perindopril, one type of ACEI, improved endothelial function."

"It's notable the reduction of PP is well correlated with the improvement of endothelial function expressed as a RHI not in telmisartan group, but in ramipril group."

"PP reduction was not related with endothelial function improvement in telmisartan group."

"Other many studies show ARBs and ACEIs improved endothelial function without difference."

Conclusion

"In hypertensive patients, ramipril and telmisartan reduced systolic and diastolic BP after eight weeks treatment."

"PP lowering effect was shown statistically significant only in telmisartan group."

"Despite PP lowering effect, telmisartan didn't show endothelial function improvement proportional to reduced PP."

"These findings suggest telmisartan may negatively influence endothelium and emphasize the role of bradykinin mediated NO production pathway in the control of endothelial function, which is saved with ramipril treatment."

The Effects of a Perindopril-Based Regimen in Relation to Statin Use on the Outcomes of Patients with Vascular Disease: A Combined Analysis of the ADVANCE, EUROPA, and PROGRESS Trials [121]

This is a machine-generated summary of:

Radhoe, S. P.; Boersma, E.; Bertrand, M.; Remme, W.; Ferrari, R.; Fox, K.; MacMahon, S.; Chalmers, J.; Simoons, M. L.; Brugts, J. J.: The Effects of a

Perindopril-Based Regimen in Relation to Statin Use on the Outcomes of Patients with Vascular Disease: a Combined Analysis of the ADVANCE, EUROPA, and PROGRESS Trials [121].

Published in: Cardiovascular Drugs and Therapy (2022).
Link to original: https://doi.org/10.1007/s10557-022-07384-2

If you want to cite the papers, please refer to the original.

For technical reasons we could not place the page where the original quote is coming from.

Abstract-Summary "To study the effects of a perindopril-based regimen on cardiovascular (CV) outcomes in patients with vascular disease in relation to background statin therapy."

"A pooled analysis of the randomized ADVANCE, EUROPA, and PROGRESS trials was performed to evaluate CV outcomes in 29,463 patients with vascular disease treated with perindopril-based regimens versus placebo."

"Multivariable Cox regression analyses were performed to assess the effects of a perindopril-based regimen versus placebo in relation to statin use."

"In statin users (adjusted hazard ratio [aHR] 0.87, 95% confidence interval [CI] 0.77–0.98) and non-statin users (aHR 0.80, 95% CI 0.74–0.87), a perindopril-based regimen was associated with a significantly lower risk of the primary endpoint when compared to placebo."

"Our data suggest that the treatment benefits of a perindopril-based regimen in patients with vascular disease are independent of statin use."

Introduction

"Blood pressure-lowering drugs and cholesterol-lowering drugs such as angiotensin-converting enzyme (ACE) inhibitors and statins play an important role in the prevention and treatment of CVD, and they are often combined in clinical practice."

"ACE inhibitors are applied extensively in the management of patients with hypertension, (chronic) heart failure, and coronary disease, whereas statins are used for primary and secondary prevention of cardiovascular events by lowering LDL cholesterol levels."

"As CV diseases still constitute a major threat to global health, it is of great importance to elucidate the combined clinical effects of ACE inhibitors and statins in an attempt to further improve risk management in this large target population."

"The objective of this analysis was to study the effects of a perindopril-based regimen with or without background statin therapy in patients at increased cardiovascular risk."

Methods

"In the EUROPA trial, patients with stable coronary artery disease were randomized to 8 mg of perindopril or placebo [122]."

"Patients in the PROGRESS trial had a history of stroke or transient ischemic attack (TIA) and were randomized to receive perindopril 4 mg with or without 2.5 mg indapamide at the discretion of the physician or placebo [123]."

"Data were stratified according to statin use, and we preserved the randomization and treatment effect comparison between a perindopril-based regimen and placebo in all analyses."

"Effect estimates were adjusted for baseline age, sex, hypertension, diabetes mellitus, smoking, history of MI, history of percutaneous coronary intervention (PCI)/coronary artery bypass grafting (CABG), history of stroke/TIA, co-medication use (beta-blockers, antiplatelet agents, and calcium antagonists), indapamide use, and perindopril dosage (by trial)."

"Several subgroup analyses with regard to the primary composite endpoint and cardiovascular mortality were performed for patients with coronary artery disease (CAD), hypertension, diabetes, and previous stroke."

Results

"Among the 11,628 patients using a statin, 5770 (49.6%) were randomized to a perindopril-based regimen (statin/perindopril group) and 5858 (50.4%) to a placebo."

"Of the 17,835 patients not using a statin, 8960 (50.2%) were randomized to a perindopril-based regimen and 8875 (49.8%) to a placebo."

"In statin users, the primary endpoint occurred in 8.6% of patients randomized to a perindopril-based regimen versus 10.0% of patients in the placebo group (HR 0.87, 95% CI 0.77–0.98)."

"In the no-statin stratum, the primary outcome occurred in 11.1% of patients randomized to the perindopril group versus 13.5% of patients in the placebo group (HR 0.80, 95% CI 0.74–0.87)."

Discussion

"In this pooled analysis of three large placebo-controlled randomized clinical trials studying the effects of a perindopril-based regimen in patients with vascular disease, we have shown that a perindopril-based regimen significantly reduced the risk of a primary composite endpoint of cardiovascular mortality, nonfatal MI, and stroke independent of baseline statin use."

"Based on large clinical trials and meta-analyses, ACE inhibitors and statins are considered effective in reducing the risk of cardiovascular events in various groups of patients [124–136]."

"Our study is the first sufficiently powered study to directly compare the benefits of an ACE inhibitor versus placebo in the context of statin therapy in a randomized fashion and therefore adds importantly to the current literature by showing a positive additive effect of a perindopril-based regimen."

Limitations

"Of all, pooling data from the three large clinical trials resulted in a robust dataset with detailed information on the occurrence of cardiovascular adverse events, but heterogeneity between the trials may have occurred, for instance in definitions for endpoints, drug doses, and the primary diagnosis of the study patients."

"We assumed that the patients were similar in having vascular disease or being at high risk of CV events, which we believe justifies pooling, especially since all included trials studied a perindopril-based regimen in a randomized placebo-controlled setting."

"Stratification was based upon baseline statin use, whereas initiation or discontinuation of statins during trial conduct may have affected the results."

"A dose–response effect analysis and stratification of the perindopril treatment effect by baseline cholesterol levels were not possible because information on baseline cholesterol levels was unavailable in our pooled analysis nor in all individual trials."

Effects of Combination Therapy with Candesartan and Ramipril on Hypertension and Related Complications [137]

This is a machine-generated summary of:

Lee, Do-Hyung; Jo, Eun Ji; Ga, Eun-Ji; Han, Joo-Hui; Jung, Sang-Hyuk; Park, Hyun-Soo; Heo, Kyung-Sun; Myung, Chang-Seon: Effects of combination therapy with candesartan and ramipril on hypertension and related complications [137].

Published in: Journal of Pharmaceutical Investigation (2017).

Link to original: https://doi.org/10.1007/s40005-017-0339-3

If you want to cite the papers, please refer to the original.

For technical reasons we could not place the page where the original quote is coming from.

Abstract-Summary "The combination of candesartan and ramipril improved systolic blood pressure (SBP), mean arterial pressure (MAP), and heart rate (HR) significantly compared with monotherapy."

"Combined treatment with candesartan (3.06 mg/kg/day) and ramipril (0.96 mg/kg/day) significantly decreased cuff-induced neointima hyperplasia and media thickness in C57BL/6 mice."

"In oral glucose tolerance tests (OGTTs), the combination of candesartan and ramipril significantly controlled blood glucose levels within 2 h after glucose loading in low-dose (38 mg/kg, i.p.) streptozotocin-treated Wistar rats."

"The present study suggests that combination therapy with candesartan and ramipril may be a beneficial therapeutic strategy for the treatment of hypertensive patients with related complications, such as atherosclerosis and diabetes."

Introduction

"Renin is a glycoprotein enzyme synthesized by juxtaglomerular (JG) cells that cleaves angiotensinogen to angiotensin I. Under physiological conditions, angiotensin-converting enzyme (ACE) hydrolyzes angiotensin I to angiotensin II (the active form), the major effector of the RAS, which can bind to the angiotensin II type 1 (AT1) receptor and thus mediate nervous physiological actions including increased BP, cardiac vasoconstriction, insulin resistance, renal sodium retention, and aldosterone synthesis by the adrenal cortex (Atlas [138]; Carey and Siragy [139]; Ribeiro-Oliveira and others [140])."

"Many anti-hypertensive drugs have been developed, including thiazides, loop diuretics and potassium-sparing diuretics, angiotensin II receptor blockers (ARBs), ACE inhibitors (ACEIs), renin inhibitors, β-blockers, and calcium channel blockers (CCBs) (Nguyen and others [141])."

"European Society of Hypertension and European Society of Cardiology (ESH/ESC) guidelines also recommend using therapeutic drugs (including β-blockers) in treatment, and combination therapy is typically required for high-risk patients with cardiovascular disease (Mancia and others [142])."

"The combination of an ACE inhibitor and an ARB confers more pharmacological benefit than monotherapy on BP and heart weight (evaluated by hypertrophy) in spontaneously hypertensive rats (SHRs) (Menard and others [143])."

Materials and Methods

"Mouse anti-bromodeoxyuridine (BrdU) monoclonal antibody was purchased from Chemicon International, Inc. (Seongnam, Korea) and anti-mouse IgG from Vector (Burlingame, CA, USA)."

"Male SHRs (7–8 weeks of age; Charles River Laboratory, Wilmington, MA, USA), male C57BL/6 mice (10–12 weeks of age; Charles River Japan, Inc., Kanagawa, Japan), and Wistar rats (8–9 weeks of age; weight, 140–160 g) were purchased from Orient Bio, Inc. (Seongnam, Korea)."

"Measurements of systolic blood pressure (SBP), mean arterial pressure (MBP) and HR were made using a telemetry system (Data Sciences International, St. Paul, MN, USA) (Shin and others [144]; Lee and others [145]; Park and others [146])."

"Hemodynamic data of SHRs were measured at intervals of 5 min."

"The intima area (between the lumen and internal elastic lamina), medial area (between the internal and external elastic lamina), and intima/media ratio were assessed using Image J software (National Institutes of Health, Bethesda, MD, USA)."

Results and Discussion

"The combination of candesartan and ramipril produced a significant synergistic reduction of SBP in SHRs."

"These results also indicated that despite lowering BP, the combination of candesartan and ramipril did not result in side effects, such as reflex tachycardia or sympathetic activation (Loga-Zec and others [147])."

"We investigated the cardioprotective effects of candesartan and ramipril in SHRs."

"These results indicated that neither monotherapy nor combined therapy with candesartan and ramipril affected eNOS activation or NO formation."

"We next evaluated the effect of candesartan and ramipril in a cuff-induced vascular injury mouse model."

"Neither ramipril (0.96 mg/kg) alone nor in combination with candesartan showed any significant effect on the reduction of neointima formation."

"Combined treatment with candesartan and ramipril showed a greater inhibitory effect than monotherapy."

Conclusions

"Combination therapy with candesartan and ramipril showed a synergistic antihypertensive effect with no reflex tachycardia, suggesting that this combination may be appropriate for cases where there is a need for a large reduction in BP."

"This combination reduced cuff-induced DNA synthesis in the intima and media of blood vessels and controlled blood glucose levels against high-glucose input in diabetes."

"Combination therapy with candesartan and ramipril may be useful for treating hypertensive patients with complications, such as atherosclerosis and diabetes."

The Treatment Effect of an ACE-Inhibitor Based Regimen with Perindopril in Relation to Beta-Blocker Use in 29,463 Patients with Vascular Disease: A Combined Analysis of Individual Data of ADVANCE, EUROPA and PROGRESS Trials [148]

This is a machine-generated summary of:

Brugts, J. J.; Bertrand, M.; Remme, W.; Ferrari, R.; Fox, K.; MacMahon, S.; Chalmers, J.; Simoons, M. L.; Boersma, E.: The Treatment Effect of an ACE-Inhibitor Based Regimen with Perindopril in Relation to Beta-Blocker use in 29,463 Patients with Vascular Disease: a Combined Analysis of Individual Data of ADVANCE, EUROPA and PROGRESS Trials [148].

Published in: Cardiovascular Drugs and Therapy (2017).

Link to original: https://doi.org/10.1007/s10557-017-6747-9

If you want to cite the papers, please refer to the original.

For technical reasons we could not place the page where the original quote is coming from.

Abstract-Summary "In everyday practice, angiotensin converting enzyme inhibitors and beta-blockers are cornerstone treatments in patients with (cardio-)vascular disease."

"Multivariate Cox regression analyses were performed in patients randomized to a perindopril-based regimen or placebo (treatment effect), and data were stratified according to background beta-blocker treatment."

"The cumulative incidence of the primary endpoint over mean follow-up of 4.0 years (Sd 1.0) was significantly lower in the beta-blocker/perindopril group (9.6%; 545/5700 patients) as compared to beta-blocker/placebo (11.8%; 676/5718 patients) ($p < 0.01$)."

"Adding perindopril to existing beta-blocker treatment reduced the relative risk of the primary endpoint by 20% (hazard ratio (HR) 0.80; 95% confidence interval (CI) 0.71–0.90), non-fatal myocardial infarction by 23% (HR 0.77; 95% CI 0.65–0.91), and all-cause mortality by 22% (HR 0.78; 95% CI 0.68–0.88) as compared to placebo."

"The mortality benefit was only observed in patients with hypertension with background beta-blocker use."

"These data suggest that the beneficial cardioprotective effects of perindopril treatment are additive to the background beta-blockers use."

Introduction

"In order to reduce morbidity and mortality, guidelines for hypertension, coronary artery disease, and heart failure recommend treatment with beta-blockers and angiotensin-converting enzyme (ACE) inhibitors [142, 149, 150]."

"Consistent with these recommendations, a wide range of patients with cardiovascular diseases are treated daily with beta-blockers and ACE-inhibitors [151]."

"Large cross-sectional population studies have found, for instance, that beta-blockers and ACE-inhibitors are prescribed in 86 and 65% of patients with coronary disease and in 93 and 71% of patients with heart failure, respectively [152, 153]."

"As the ADVANCE and PROGRESS trials also included a large number of patients taking a beta-blocker as a background treatment [123, 154], a retrospective pooled analysis of the EUROPA, ADVANCE, and PROGRESS trials would offer outcome data for a large cohort of patients with a wide range of cardiovascular risk profiles."

Methods

"The rationale for combining these trials is based on the fact that all three trials studied the same agent, perindopril; we provided the opportunity to include individual data in this combined analysis, which made important subgroup analyses possible at the patient level with individual data access."

"Adjustments (full model) were made for baseline age, sex, hypertension, diabetes mellitus, smoking, history of MI, history of percutaneous coronary intervention/coronary artery bypass grafting, history of stroke/TIA, and co-medication use (antiplatelet agents, lipid-lowering agents, calcium antagonists, diuretics), indapamide use, and active treatment (perindopril) dosage (by trial)."

"As the definition of hypertension has changed since the EUROPA trial was performed, the primary endpoint was also assessed in additional post hoc subgroup analysis using a cut-off for hypertension of SBP/DBP $\geq$ 140/90 mmHg or the use of antihypertensive medication."

Results

"The primary endpoint (cardiovascular mortality/non-fatal MI/stroke) occurred in 1221 of the 11,418 patients in the beta-blocker stratum (10.7%; HR 0.80; 95% CI 0.71–0.90): 676 patients in the beta-blocker/placebo group (11.8%) and 545 patients in the beta-blocker/perindopril group (9.6%)."

"In the subgroup of hypertensive patients (n = 5838) using beta-blockers, perindopril treatment was associated with significant risk reduction compared to placebo for the endpoints of cardiovascular mortality/non-fatal MI/stroke (HR 0.77; 95% CI 0.66–0.89; p = 0.001), non-fatal MI (HR 0.74; 95% CI 0.58–0.94; p = 0.02), and all-cause mortality (HR 0.68; 95% CI 0.57–0.82; p = 0.001)."

"In the subgroup of non-hypertensive patients (n = 5580), perindopril significantly reduced cardiovascular mortality/non-fatal MI/stroke (HR 0.84; 95% CI 0.71–1.00; p = 0.04), and treatment benefit was consistent also without beta-blocker use."

Discussion

"In this retrospective pooled analysis of three large perindopril outcome trials in patients at high cardiovascular risk, we found that adding a perindopril-based regimen to existing beta-blocker treatment reduced the risk of the primary composite endpoint of cardiovascular mortality, non-fatal MI, and stroke by 20% and secondary endpoints such as non-fatal MI by 23%, all-cause mortality by 22%, and cardiovascular mortality by 27% compared to placebo."

"As the current analysis demonstrates a strong consistent treatment benefit of the ACE-inhibitor perindopril in patients with vascular disease on top of beta-blocker use and as this additive effect seems even more pronounced in patients with hypertension, the combination of perindopril and bisoprolol in a single-pill combination may offer treatment solutions to improve adherence."

"We did observe a mortality benefit of the combination perindopril on top of beta-blocker use overall and in hypertensive patients with a significant interaction effect between treatments used."

Conclusions

"In this meta-analysis, a consistent treatment benefit was observed with a perindopril-based regimen on a background of beta-blocker use."

"This treatment benefit was most pronounced relatively in patients with hypertension, which could suggest an additive effect of both treatments."

Randomized, Double-Blinded, Controlled Clinical Trial of the Effect of Captopril, Telmisartan and Their Combination on Systemic Inflammation of Patients on Hemodialysis [155]

This is a machine-generated summary of:

Ordaz-Medina, Susan M.; Cueto-Manzano, Alfonso M.; González-Plascencia, Juana; Montañez-Fernández, José L.; Ordaz-Medina, Elias J.; Martín-del-Campo, Fabiola; Cueto-Ramírez, Alfonso M.; Martínez-Martínez, Petra; Cortés-Sanabria, Laura; Rojas-Campos, Enrique; Trujillo-Hernández, Benjamín: Randomized, double-blinded, controlled clinical trial of the effect of captopril, telmisartan and their combination on systemic inflammation of patients on hemodialysis [155].

Published in: Scientific Reports (2022).

Link to original: https://doi.org/10.1038/s41598-022-22656-5

If you want to cite the papers, please refer to the original.

For technical reasons we could not place the page where the original quote is coming from.

Abstract-Summary "To evaluate individual and combined effect of captopril and telmisartan on systemic inflammation markers of hemodialysis (HD) patients."

"Patients on HD at least 2 months, with arteriovenous fistula, were randomly allocated to groups: (1) captopril/placebo (N 13); (2) telmisartan/placebo (N 13); (3) captopril + telmisartan (N 12); or (4) placebo/placebo (N 12)."

"During 3 months, patients received oral drugs as follows: captopril 50 mg/day, telmisartan 80 mg/day or placebo."

"Clinical and biochemical evaluations were performed monthly."

"Serum tumor necrosis factor alpha (TNFα), interleukin 6 (IL-6), and C-reactive protein (CRP) were measured at 0, 1 and 3 months."

"Baseline versus final inflammatory markers were: captopril/placebo TNFα, 2.47 (0.1–4.5) versus 1.73 (0.3–3.8) pg/ml; IL-6, 17.03 (7.2–23) versus 7.90 (0.7–19) pg/ml; CRP, 4.21 (1.6–18) versus 5.9 (3.0–28) mg/l; telmisartan/placebo

TNFα, 3.03 (2.3–4.6) versus 1.70 (1.2–2.0) pg/ml; IL-6, 14.10 (5.5–23) versus 9.85 (6.2–13) pg/ml; CRP, 5.74 (2.1–13) versus 10.60 (1.5–27) mg/l; captopril + telmisartan TNFα, 1.43 (0.7–5.4) versus 0.40 (0.1–2.1) pg/ml; IL-6, 10.05 (4.9–23) versus 4.00 (0.7–7.7) pg/ml ($p < 0.05$); CRP, 3.26 (0.7–12) versus 2.83 (0.6–6.5) mg/l; placebo/placebo TNFα, 3.13 (1.6–5.6) versus 1.64 (1.6–2.3) pg/ml; IL-6, 8.12 (5.4–16) versus 7.60 (2.4–15) pg/ml; CRP, 5.23 (1.9–16) versus 3.13 (1.5–18) mg/l. Monotherapy with captopril or telmisartan display a trend, but their combined treatment significantly decreased serum levels of IL-6."

Introduction

"Inflammation is highly prevalent in patients with end-stage kidney disease (ESKD) on dialysis, and has been associated with multiple factors such as malnutrition, overhydration, bioincompatibility of hemodialysis (HD) membranes and dialysate, uremia, dialysis vintage, dialysis dose, and vascular access, among others [156–161]."

"In an open crossover study with type 2 diabetes mellitus without kidney disease, ramipril, telmisartan, and particularly their combination, significantly decreased CRP compared to baseline [162]."

"Our group has previously shown in a double-blinded, controlled clinical trial in patients on HD [163], that enalapril did not significantly decrease serum levels of TNFα, IL-6 and CRP compared to placebo."

"Notwithstanding, current data are inconclusive and limited in this regard, particularly considering whether the chronic use of ACEIs, ARBs, or their combination, have a role in reducing inflammation in dialysis patients."

Methods

"We excluded patients with ESKD of inflammatory cause, infectious disease 2 months before the study or who were on treatment with antibiotics, pregnancy, cancer, liver disease, hypotension, AIDS, failed kidney graft, known hypersensitivity to captopril or telmisartan, and treatment with statins, immunosuppressive drugs, steroids, pentoxifylline, non-steroidal anti-inflammatory drugs, ACEIs or ARBs within four months previous to the study."

"During a period of three months, patients received the following oral drugs: captopril 50 mg/day, telmisartan 80 mg/day, or placebo (identical starch tablets)."

"Patients received the assigned treatment and had monthly clinical evaluations, for a 3-month period."

"At the 0, 1 and 3-month visits, a mid-week sample of blood was withdrawn at the beginning of HD session for the following measurements: glucose, urea, creatinine, albumin, electrolytes, lipids, complete blood count and inflammation markers (TNFα, IL-6 and CRP)."

Results

"One patient of group on Captopril + Placebo was eliminated because a clear non-adherence detected since the first month of follow-up; his results were similar to the other patients and were not eliminated from analysis."

"All these variables were within usual values for this kind of patients and were not different between groups."

"TNFα was significantly higher at baseline in patients with telmisartan compared to those with captopril or the combined treatment; it tended to decrease in all groups until the end of follow-up, but it reached statistical significance only at the 1-month evaluation in patients of telmisartan and placebo groups."

"Compared to baseline, CRP tended to increase at final evaluation in patients of telmisartan and captopril groups, whereas it remained roughly the same in those with combined drugs; in intergroup comparison, final CRP values were significantly lower in patients under treatment with both drugs than in patients on individual drugs."

Discussion

"This is the first randomized double-blinded, controlled clinical trial comparing the effect of the combination of captopril + telmisartan versus their individual treatment and placebo on systemic inflammation of HD patients."

"In the case of TNFα, the significant decrease in the groups with telmisartan and placebo were more probably due to the higher baseline values and a possible statistical effect of regression to the mean [164], whereas the lower CRP levels at final evaluation in the combined drug treatment were observed in relation to a trend to increase in captopril and telmisartan groups rather than to an intragroup decrease in the combined drugs group."

"Previous studies have shown that both ACEIs and ARBs may decrease some inflammation markers, including IL-6 and CRP [162, 163, 165], but this issue remains controversial [166]; moreover, there was no information whether these drugs may have an additive or synergistic effect in HD patients."

Conclusions

"Monotherapy with captopril or telmisartan display a trend, but the combined treatment significantly decreased serum levels of IL-6."

"No remarkable changes on TNFα and CRP were observed."

Development and Evaluation of Physiologically Based Pharmacokinetic Drug-Disease Models for Predicting Captopril Pharmacokinetics in Chronic Diseases [167]

This is a machine-generated summary of:

Rasool, Muhammad F.; Ali, Shazia; Khalid, Sundus; Khalid, Ramsha; Majeed, Abdul; Imran, Imran; Saeed, Hamid; Usman, Muhammad; Ali, Mohsin; Alali, Amer S.; AlAsmari, Abdullah F.; Ali, Nemat; Asiri, Ali Mohammed; Alasmari, Fawaz; Alqahtani, Faleh: Development and evaluation of physiologically based pharmacokinetic drug-disease models for predicting captopril pharmacokinetics in chronic diseases [167].

Published in: Scientific Reports (2021).

Link to original: https://doi.org/10.1038/s41598-021-88154-2

If you want to cite the papers, please refer to the original.

For technical reasons we could not place the page where the original quote is coming from.

Abstract-Summary "These PBPK models can incorporate disease-specific data and could be used to predict pharmacokinetics (PK) of administered drugs in different chronic conditions."

"The present study aimed to develop and evaluate PBPK drug-disease models for captopril after incorporating relevant pathophysiological changes occurring in adult chronic kidney disease (CKD) and chronic heart failure (CHF) populations."

"The developed disease models were successful in predicting captopril PK in all three stages of CKD (mild, moderate, and severe) and CHF, as the observed and predicted PK profiles and the $\text{ratio}_{(\text{obs/pred})}$ for the PK parameters were in close agreement."

"The developed captopril PBPK models can assist in tailoring captopril dosages in patients with different disease severity (CKD and CHF)."

Introduction

"Keeping in view the PK profile of captopril, if a PBPK model is developed that incorporates the pathophysiological changes occurring in CKD and CHF, it can be used to predict its ADME in patients with different degrees of renal and heart failure."

"After developing and evaluating the developed captopril PBPK disease model with the available clinical PK disease data, due to its mechanistic nature, it can be extended to other populations (geriatrics, liver cirrhosis, pregnant) with different disease severity and may be used to explore different what if clinical scenarios, such as CKD patients with CHF."

"The objectives of this study were, (1) to develop and evaluate PBPK drug-disease models for captopril after incorporating relevant pathophysiological changes occurring in CKD and CHF, (2) to predict and compare captopril PK in adult healthy, CKD, and CHF populations."

Materials and Methods

"Based on the presence of clear information on participants, PK data, and the PK profiles of captopril in literature, a total of 9 studies in a healthy population with 15 PK profiles (intravenous = 4 and oral = 11) were selected for model evaluation."

"After a successful evaluation of the developed model in healthy adults, the disease-specific pathophysiological changes are incorporated in the model to constitute the disease model, and then it is used to predict drug PK in disease populations."

"There are two renal failure populations within Simcyp which are based on pathophysiological information related to moderate and severe CKD (Sim-RenalGFR_30-60 and Sim-RenalGFR_less_30) that were used to predict captopril ADME in moderate and severe kidney disease."

"To account for the decrease in non-renal CL in CHF patients, a hepatic SF of 55% of the value used in healthy adults was used, which was based on a comparison of the observed and the predicted PK profiles of captopril."

Results

"It can be seen from the VPC that the model predictions were in agreement with the observed systemic captopril concentrations at all administered doses."

"The VPC shows that the predictions were in accordance with the observed data at all administered doses."

Discussion

"For the first time, a systematic model building approach was used to develop a PBPK model for predicting captopril ADME in healthy, CKD & CHF populations."

"There has been a previous report of a PBPK model for captopril that was used to predict its PK in healthy and severe CKD patients, and the predictions in moderate CKD were not evaluated against any clinical data [168]."

"The developed models were successfully evaluated after iv and oral captopril administration in healthy, CKD (mild, moderate, and severe) and CHF populations."

"The incorporation of organ blood flow reductions in the CHF population has resulted in a decrease in predicted CL/F, as it was 74.8 L/h in healthy adults [169], but was reduced to 66.54 L/h in CHF patients [170] after administering 25 mg oral captopril."

"This decrease in observed and predicted captopril CL/F in the CHF population was associated with the reductions in the organ/tissue blood flows, that were incorporated in the developed CHF model [171, 172]."

Limitations

"All the systemic captopril concentration vs. time data used for model evaluation was extracted carefully by scanning publication plots, although the extracted PK parameters were comparable to the reported PK parameters, but minor variations cannot be completely neglected."

"To decrease the predicted non-renal captopril CL in CKD and CHF populations, hepatic SF was used."

"The developed disease models may not reflect the complexity associated with the pathophysiologies of CKD and CHF, as a semi-mechanistic approach was used in the developed models by dividing the total CL into renal and non-renal parts."

Conclusion

"The developed PBPK models have successfully described captopril PK in healthy and disease (CKD and CHF) populations."

"The mechanistic nature of the developed captopril PBPK model in CKD can assist in tailoring captopril dosages in patients with impaired kidney functions according to the U.S. Food and Drug Administration (FDA) and European Medicines Agency (EMA) guidelines [173, 174]."

"By incorporating the reductions in organ blood flows, the captopril CHF model can be used to predict captopril exposure in patients with different disease severity."

Perindopril/Indapamide/Amlodipine in Hypertension: A Profile of Its Use [175]

This is a machine-generated summary of:

Syed, Yahiya Y.: Perindopril/Indapamide/Amlodipine in Hypertension: A Profile of Its Use [175].

Published in: American Journal of Cardiovascular Drugs (2022).

Link to original: https://doi.org/10.1007/s40256-022-00521-0

If you want to cite the papers, please refer to the original.

For technical reasons we could not place the page where the original quote is coming from.

Abstract-Summary "The single-pill combination (SPC) of perindopril (PER)/indapamide (IND)/amlodipine (AML) is a valuable and convenient treatment option for patients with hypertension controlled with two-drug SPC of PER/IND + AML given as two separate pills at the same dose level."

"Once-daily PER/IND/AML provided effective BP control, with good tolerability, in patients with uncontrolled hypertension in clinical trials and in large observational prospective studies."

"Switching from the two-pill PER/IND + AML regimen to single-pill PER/IND/AML reduces pill burden and simplifies drug administration, which may improve adherence to treatment, leading to better BP control and clinical outcomes."

What Is the Rationale for Using PER/IND/AML in Hypertension?

"Single-pill combinations (SPCs) of three drugs play a crucial role in the management of hypertension [176–179]."

"Angiotensin-converting enzyme inhibitors (ACEI) or angiotensin receptor blockers (ARB), diuretics and calcium channel blockers (CCB) form the core of drug treatment for hypertension, according to the current treatment guidelines [176–179]."

"Perindopril (PER), indapamide (IND) and amlodipine (AML) fulfil the criteria for the choice of core antihypertensive drugs [176–178]."

"PER, IND and AML as monotherapies and as two-drug SPCs (PER/IND, PER/AML, IND/AML) have long been available, and are routinely prescribed by health-care practitioners for the treatment of hypertension."

"In large observational studies, PER, IND and AML triple therapy administered as two separate pills (PER/IND + CCB or PER/AML + IND) effectively reduced BP in patients with hypertension uncontrolled on one or two drugs, including those with type 2 diabetes mellitus (T2DM), obesity and/or metabolic syndrome [180–183]."

How Do the Drugs in the Fixed-Dose Combination Work?

"There was no significant difference between AML, chlorthalidone and lisinopril in reducing fatal coronary heart disease (CHD) or nonfatal MI and all-cause mortality in patients aged ≥55 years with hypertension and at least one other CHD risk factor (ALLHAT) [184]."

"AML reduced adverse cardiovascular events in patients with CAD and normal BP (CAMELOT) [185]."

"Valsartan did not differ from AML in reducing cardiac morbidity and mortality in hypertensive patients with high cardiovascular risk (VALUE) [186]."

"PER/IND effectively reduced BP in several placebo-controlled and active comparator (losartan, atenolol, irbesartan) trials in patients with hypertension, including elderly patients and those with kidney function impairment [187]."

"In hypertensive patients with ≥3 other cardiovascular risk factors, AML ± PER was associated with reduced incidence of major cardiovascular events, all-cause mortality and new-onset diabetes, compared with atenolol ± bendroflumethiazide (ASCOT-BPLA) [188]."

What Is the Efficacy of PER/IND/AML in Clinical Studies?

"For central ambulatory BP, significant ($p \leq 0.05$) between-group differences in favour of PER/IND/AML was seen at 1 month for SBP (– 4.5, – 5.0 and −4.1 mmHg for 24-h, daytime and night-time, respectively) and DBP (−2.7 and −3.4 mmHg for 24-h and daytime) [189]."

"The BP control rate (target SBP/DBP 130/80 mmHg) was higher with the SPC than with the free-combination at 3 months (95.65% vs 80.49%; $p = 0.03$) but it did not differ significantly between the groups at 6 months (97.83% vs 92.68%), indicating BP control was achieved early with the SPC."

"The efficacy of PER/IND/AML was confirmed by central BP measurements in one study; the mean change from baseline in central SBP/DBP at 5 months was −24.7/−11.8 mmHg ($p \leq 0.001$ for both SBP and DBP), with 86.7% and 90% of patients achieving target central SBP and DBP, respectively [190]."

What Is the Effectiveness of PER/IND/AML in Clinical Practice?

"PER/IND/AML was effective in controlling BP in patients with uncontrolled hypertension in large observational prospective studies conducted in Hungary (PETRA [191]), Russia (TRIO [192], TRICOLOR [193]) and Greece (CONTROL-3 [194])."

"In these patients, the mean change from baseline in office SBP/DBP at 3 months on PER/IND/AML was −35.1/−16.0 mmHg, − 35.2/−15.6 mmHg and −37.7/−17.1 mmHg, respectively, and the corresponding BP control rates were 82.3%, 87% and 82.7% [192]."

"In CONTROL-3, 50.1% of 2285 patients were at high or very high risk for cardiovascular diseases; these patients showed a relatively greater degree of SBP reduction with PER/IND/AML [194]."

"In PETRA, 45.1%, 33.5% and 21.4% of patients were being treated with 5/1.25/5 mg, 10/2.5/5 mg and 10/2.5/10 mg strengths of PER/IND/AML, respectively, at the final visit (i.e. month 3), suggesting the lowest dose was adequate in nearly half of the target population [191]."

What Are the Other Benefits of PER/IND/AML?

"In PETRA, PER/IND/AML treatment was associated with significant ($p < 0.0001$) improvements in metabolic parameters, including total cholesterol (−8.6%), low-density lipoprotein cholesterol (−11.4%), triglyceride (−12.1%), fasting glucose (−6.6%), glycosylated hemoglobin (−6.5%) and serum urate (−6.1%) levels [191]."

"The therapeutic effect of PER/IND/AML was associated with improvements in health-related quality of life (HR-QOL) in hypertensive patients, as assessed by the 36-Item Short Form Survey [192] or the World Health Organization Quality-of-Life Scale (WHOQOL-BREF) [195]."

"In small clinical trials, after 3 months' PER/IND/AML treatment, investigators rated each patient's general condition or well being as 'excellent' or 'improved' in ≈ 89% of patients (the other rating categories were 'appropriate' or 'worse') [196, 197]."

"The use of triple-component SPC PER/IND/AML was associated with high adherence to treatment in the clinical practice setting [194, 198]."

"In clinical studies, compliance to PER/IND/AML treatment was high (87–98.5% of patients) [199–202] and was significantly ($p < 0.05$) higher than that seen with the free combination of PER + IND + AML (94% vs. 85% [200]; 87% vs. 61% [199])."

What Is the Tolerability of PER/IND/AML?

"PER/IND/AML was generally well tolerated in patients with hypertension, with no unexpected safety concerns [195–205]."

"None of the adverse reactions with PER, IND or AML were 'very common' (≥1/10 patients), with the exception of oedema related to AML [203]."

"In clinical studies, adverse events (AEs) with PER/IND/AML were of mild to moderate severity and the majority were not treatment-related [195–205]."

"The incidence of treatment-emergent AEs with PER/IND/AML 5/1.25/5 mg, 5/1.25/10 mg, 10/2.5/5 mg and 10/2.5/10 mg was 9.2%, 15.0% 14.8% and 12.9%, respectively, suggesting the SPC remained tolerable regardless of the dosage [202]."

"AEs leading to discontinuation of PER/IND/AML included oedema, cough, asthenia and dizziness, erectile dysfunction and hypertension [201, 202, 204]."

"AEs presumed to be related to study treatment by treating physicians occurred in 51 patients: the most common of these were leg oedema (0.07% of patients), unproductive cough (0.04%), tachycardia (0.03%), dizziness (0.03%) and hypotension (0.02%) [191]."

What Is the Current Clinical Position of PER/IND/AML?

"In Europe, it is indicated for patients who have already achieved BP control with the SPC of PER/IND + AML given as two separate pills at the same dose level."

"The antihypertensive efficacy of PER/IND/AML is similar to that of PER/IND + AML in patients with hypertension uncontrolled with one or two drugs."

"PER/IND/AML reduced BP, leading to a large proportion of patients achieving their target BP levels, in clinical trials and large prospective observational studies in a wide range of patient populations."

"PER/IND/AML reduces ambulatory, home and ambulatory central BP in patients with hypertension, providing additional support to its efficacy."

"PER/IND/AML provides rapid BP control in this population, while also reducing the risk of target organ damage and clinical worsening of their diseases."

"In patients receiving PER/IND + AML as two pills, switching to single-pill PER/IND/AML simplifies drug administration and may improve adherence, leading to better BP control and clinical outcomes."

Concomitant Treatment of Hypertensive Patients with Bisoprolol and Perindopril in Routine Clinical Practice: A Post Hoc Analysis of the CONFIDENCE II, PROTECT I, and PROTECT III Observational Studies [206]

This is a machine-generated summary of:

Abeel, Murielle; Gupta, Anil; Constance, Christian: Concomitant Treatment of Hypertensive Patients with Bisoprolol and Perindopril in Routine Clinical Practice:

A Post Hoc Analysis of the CONFIDENCE II, PROTECT I, and PROTECT III Observational Studies [206].

Published in: Advances in Therapy (2021).
Link to original: https://doi.org/10.1007/s12325-021-01958-6

If you want to cite the papers, please refer to the original.

For technical reasons we could not place the page where the original quote is coming from.

Abstract-Summary "This post hoc analysis of three observational studies provides effectiveness and safety data on treatment with perindopril on top of bisoprolol-based therapy, in routine clinical practice."

"Data were analyzed from three open-label, prospective, multicenter, observational studies of Canadian patients with mild-to-moderate hypertension, which shared the same inclusion and exclusion criteria, treatment duration, and primary outcome."

"This post hoc analysis focused on the subpopulation of patients treated with perindopril on top of bisoprolol-based therapy."

"Primary outcomes were mean changes in blood pressure (BP) and proportion of patients achieving BP control (<140/90 mmHg) in the full analysis set (FAS)."

"A total of 845 patients (mean age 68.3 ± 11.3 years, mean baseline BP 151.5/86.0 mmHg) were analyzed in the FAS."

"After 16 weeks, mean SBP/DBP decreased by − 20.4/−9.8 mmHg with statistically significant reductions observed at all visits in all three studies allowing 78% of patients to achieve the BP treatment goal."

"The addition of perindopril on top of bisoprolol-based therapy in patients with mild-to-moderate hypertension was associated with significant reductions in BP compared with baseline and with achievement of BP targets in the majority of patients."

Introduction

"In patients with hypertension and chronic coronary syndromes, angina, or chronic heart failure with reduced ejection fraction, beta-blockers, except if contraindicated, should be included in the therapeutic strategy."

"The combination of beta-blockers with ACE inhibitors plays a major therapeutic and preventive role in the management of coronary artery disease (CAD) and heart failure [153, 207], and many patients receive treatment with both agents in routine clinical practice [151]."

"Among beta-blockers, bisoprolol has shown a significant mortality benefit among patients with heart failure [208]."

"This post hoc analysis was performed in a subpopulation of patients selected from a large database from three observational studies that examined the efficacy and tolerability of perindopril in patients with hypertension receiving treatment with other antihypertensive agents, including beta-blockers, in a real-world setting."

Methods

"This post hoc analysis of the individual and combined studies focused on the subpopulation of patients treated with perindopril on top of bisoprolol-based therapy."

"Patients treated previously with an ACE inhibitor or an ARB and not controlled could be switched to perindopril at the time of study entry according to the judgement of the treating physician."

"The primary outcomes for these post hoc analyses were mean changes in BP from baseline following treatment with perindopril 4 and 8 mg/day on top of bisoprolol-based therapy as well as the proportion of patients achieving BP control (<140/90 mmHg, or <140/85 mmHg in patients with diabetes according to the thresholds recommended in European ESH/ESC guidelines [209]) in the intent-to-treat populations."

"Descriptive statistics, including the mean and standard deviation (SD) for continuous variables, and frequency distributions for categorical variables, were produced for patient demographics and baseline characteristics on the full analysis set (FAS), comprising all patients receiving concomitant perindopril and bisoprolol at baseline who had at least one follow-up BP measurement while on free combination treatment."

Results

"The merged population included 42,248 patients: 13,886 from the CONFIDENCE II study [210], 15,665 from the PROTECT I study [211], and 12,697 from the PROTECT III study [212]."

"In the subpopulation of patients receiving perindopril on top of bisoprolol-based therapy (merged data from three studies), a significant SBP decrease from baseline was observed at visit 2 (−14.7 ± 12.3 mmHg, $P < 0.001$); the decrease in DBP of −6.7 ± 8.2 mmHg did not reach statistical significance ($P = 0.059$)."

"The corresponding proportions with BP control in the individual studies were 60.4% of patients in CONFIDENCE II, 88.0% in PROTECT I, and 86.3% in PROTECT III."

"In the individual studies, at least one emergent adverse event was reported in 9%, 9%, and 4.7% of patients in CONFIDENCE II, PROTECT I, and PROTECT III, respectively."

Discussion

"This retrospective post hoc analysis in a merged patient population from three large observational studies showed that the addition of perindopril to background bisoprolol therapy was associated with statistically significant reductions in BP compared with baseline."

"Among the beta-blockers, bisoprolol was the first to demonstrate improved survival in a cardiovascular outcome trial, with a 34% relative risk reduction in all-cause mortality in patients with heart failure with reduced ejection fraction and NYHA class III–IV symptoms when added to standard therapy including ACE inhibitors and diuretics [208]."

"In a Canadian observational study in patients with hypertension and additional cardiovascular risk factors [213], the addition of perindopril to the subgroup of patients who were on beta-blocker therapy at baseline resulted in a reduction in mean SBP/DBP of −22.1/−9.7 mmHg after 10 weeks of treatment."

Conclusions

"The results of this retrospective post hoc analysis of three large observational studies show that addition of perindopril on top of bisoprolol-based therapy is commonly prescribed in routine clinical practice for patients with mild-to-moderate hypertension."

"Treatment effectiveness was confirmed by significant reductions in BP compared with baseline and achievement of BP targets by 78% of patients."

"The addition of perindopril to background bisoprolol was well tolerated, making it a safe and effective therapy option for patients in routine clinical practice."

Single-Pill Combination of Perindopril/Indapamide/Amlodipine in Patients with Uncontrolled Hypertension: A Randomized Controlled Trial [201]

This is a machine-generated summary of:

Nedogoda, Sergey V.; Stojanov, Vesna J.: Single-Pill Combination of Perindopril/Indapamide/Amlodipine in Patients with Uncontrolled Hypertension: A Randomized Controlled Trial [201].

Published in: Cardiology and Therapy (2017).

Link to original: https://doi.org/10.1007/s40119-017-0085-7

If you want to cite the papers, please refer to the original.

For technical reasons we could not place the page where the original quote is coming from.

Abstract-Summary "This international, multicenter, open-label, randomized controlled trial was conducted in men or women aged ≥18 years old with confirmed essential hypertension (SBP ≥140 and <160 mmHg and DBP ≥90 and <100 mmHg), uncontrolled on maximal dose antihypertensive monotherapy or with a single dose of dual therapy."

"The proportion of responders defined as those with normalized BP (SBP <140 mmHg and DBP <90 mmHg), and/or decrease of SBP ≥20 mmHg, and/or decrease of DBP ≥10 mmHg at week 12 (W12) compared with baseline was also assessed."

"Secondary efficacy endpoints included change in office supine SBP and DBP, response, and BP control at weeks 4 and 8."

"Mean supine SBP and DBP were 149.1 ± 4.7 and 94.1 ± 3.1 mmHg, respectively, with no relevant between-group difference."

"At week 12, both triple-therapy regimens were associated with clinically significant reductions in SBP compared with baseline (−21.5 ± 11.7 and −20.0 ± 12.9 mmHg, respectively)."

"The reduction in office supine SBP/DBP was already evident at week 4 and maintained for the duration of the study in both groups."

"The majority of patients were treatment responders at week 4 (89.2 and 82.9%, respectively) and had achieved BP control (87.8 vs. 78.6%, respectively), which was maintained until week 12 in both treatment groups."

"In adult patients with uncontrolled essential hypertension on treatment, single-pill triple-combination therapy with Per/Ind/Aml is as effective as the same dose dual-pill combination of Per/Ind + Aml."

Introduction

"The use of triple-combination therapy, targeting three different mechanisms of arterial hypertension pathogenesis, is becoming increasingly used to provide optimal BP control [214, 215] with fewer dose-related adverse effects."

"Each individual component is associated with a large evidence base of use in arterial hypertension, and single-pill combinations have also been extensively evaluated: perindopril/indapamide has shown efficacy in patients with recurrent stroke [123], diabetes mellitus [154], and in octogenarians with hypertension [216]; perindopril/amlodipine combination has been studied in detail in patients with hypertension at high cardiovascular risk [217]."

"Knowing that some physicians may be reluctant to prescribe fixed-dose triple-therapy combinations due to concerns over tolerability, the aim of the present study was to evaluate the clinical efficacy and safety of a triple combination of perindopril 5 mg/indapamide 1.25 mg/amlodipine 5 mg in a single-pill versus dual-pill combination perindopril 5 mg/indapamide 1.25 mg plus amlodipine 5 mg over 12 weeks, in treated patients with uncontrolled hypertension."

Methods

"Based on the intention-to-treat principle, the FAS corresponds to randomized patients having received at least one dose of study treatment and having a value at baseline and at least one post-baseline value for office supine SBP and DBP over the W0–W12 period."

"A number of secondary efficacy endpoints were also evaluated including: change from baseline to post-baseline value in office supine SBP and DBP over the W0–W4 and W0–W8 periods; response to antihypertensive treatment expressed as the rate of responders at each post-baseline visit over the W0–W4 and W0–W8 periods; and BP control expressed as the proportion of patients with BP control at post-baseline visit over W0–W12 period and at each post-baseline visit W4 and W8."

Results

"A response to antihypertensive treatment at the last post-baseline value was observed for the majority of patients in both treatment groups, and the frequency of responders was similar: 89.2% in the Per/Ind/Aml group versus 87.1% in the Per/Ind + Aml group; mean (SE) between-group difference 2.1% (5.4), 95% CI [−8.5; 12.6] in the FAS."

"Most patients were responders from the W4 visit (89.2 versus 82.9%, respectively; mean (SE) between-group difference 6.3% (5.8), 95% CI [−5.0; 17.7]."

"At W4, 87.8% of patients in the Per/Ind/Aml group versus 78.6% in the Per/Ind + Aml group achieved control of supine BP; mean (SE) between-group difference 9.3% (6.20), 95% CI [−2.89; 21.43]."

"Treatment-related EAEs were reported in only a few patients: (4.0%) in the Per/Ind/Aml group and (6.8%) in the Per/Ind + Aml group."

Discussion

"The study confirms previous observations from the PIANIST study [218] conducted in a high-risk population, in whom target BP levels were also achieved in more than 80% patients who had previously taken two antihypertensive drug combinations, albeit at higher doses of the three components than in the present study."

"The results suggest that the triple-therapy Per/Ind/Aml combination is suitable for a wide spectrum of patients with hypertension at both low and high cardiovascular risk."

"Parallel meta-analyses of ACE inhibitor and ARB trials vs. placebo or other active comparator, and meta-regression analyses that have adjusted for BP within the trials, have demonstrated that ACE inhibitors reduce the risk of myocardial infarction and mortality above and independently of BP lowering, whereas ARBs do not, reinforcing the need for an ACE inhibitor in a triple-therapy combination [219]."

"Control of hypertension was demonstrated from the week 4 visit in 88% of patients on the single-pill triple-drug combination compared with 79% on dual therapy + amlodipine."

Conclusions

"In patients with uncontrolled essential hypertension, single-pill triple therapy with perindopril 5 mg/indapamide 1.25 mg/amlodipine 5 mg was as effective as the same dose of a dual-pill combination of perindopril/indapamide plus separate amlodipine with earlier achievement of BP control."

"Patients already treated with an ACE inhibitor-based dual therapy who required three drugs in a single-pill were obliged to switch to other therapeutic classes."

"Perindopril/indapamide/amlodipine is currently the only triple-drug therapy incorporating an ACE inhibitor in a single pill, providing an evidence-based drug combination supported by international guidelines and recommendations for the treatment of hypertension."

The Combined Effects of Telmisartan and Ramipril on Hypertension and Cardiovascular Injury [220]

This is a machine-generated summary of:

Lee, Do-Hyung; Kim, Min-Tae; Lee, Hyung-Won; Han, Joo-Hui; Myung, Chang-Seon: The combined effects of telmisartan and ramipril on hypertension and cardiovascular injury [220].

Published in: Journal of Pharmaceutical Investigation (2022).

Link to original: https://doi.org/10.1007/s40005-022-00567-x

If you want to cite the papers, please refer to the original.

For technical reasons we could not place the page where the original quote is coming from.

Abstract-Summary "More than half of hypertensive patients receive combination therapy with two or more drugs."

"The effects of combination therapy with telmisartan (an angiotensin II receptor type 1 blocker) and ramipril (an angiotensin-converting enzyme inhibitor) on blood pressure control and cardiovascular protection were verified."

"The combination therapy with telmisartan and ramipril significantly decreased SBP and MAP."

"The results of this study suggest that combination therapy with telmisartan and ramipril is an effective strategy for the treatment of hypertension and complications of hypertensive disorders."

Introduction

"In hypertension management, nonpharmaceutical interventions such as salt intake limitation, weight loss, smoking cessation, exercise, and diet control can help reduce BP and risk factors for cardiovascular disease, as can reducing the dosage of medications for patients (Elmer and others [221])."

"The goal of drug therapy in hypertension is to significantly reduce the incidence of cardiovascular disease by lowering BP, and it is recommended to use angiotensin-converting enzyme inhibitors (ACEIs), angiotensin II receptor type 1 (AT_1) blockers (ARBs), calcium channel blockers (CCBs), thiazide diuretics, and β-blockers as first-line drugs for hypertension (Turnbull and others [222])."

"Only 30% of all hypertension cases can be controlled with monotherapy, and starting with a low-dose combination therapy improves the BP-lowering effect and minimizes the occurrence of adverse effects (Armario and Waeber [223])."

Materials and Methods

"Phosphate-buffered saline (PBS) was purchased from Gibco (Grand Island, NY, USA); polyethylene tubing-50 (PE-50) was purchased from Becton, Dickinson & Co. (Franklin Lakes, NJ, USA); and a mouse anti-bromodeoxyuridine (BrdU) monoclonal antibody was purchased from Chemicon International, Inc. (Seongnam, Korea)."

"The BP and heart rate (HR) of SHRs were measured using a telemetry system (Data Sciences International, St. Paul, MN, USA) as previously described (Shin and others [144]; Lee and others [145])."

"The SBP, mean arterial pressure (MAP), and HR were measured for 3 days prior to drug administration, and the average of these values was used as a baseline."

"To confirm the cardiovascular protective effect of the combination of telmisartan and ramipril, the expression of eNOS was measured using an ELISA kit (R&D Systems, MN, USA) as previously described (Park and others [224])."

"After placing a polyethylene tube (2-mm long PE-50 tube, 0.58 mm inner diameter) around the left femoral artery, each mouse was administered telmisartan and ramipril for 2 weeks."

Results

"Combination therapy with low-dose telmisartan and ramipril had the same BP-lowering effect as high-dose monotherapy of each drug without reflex tachycardia."

"These results suggested that the fixed-dose combination therapy with telmisartan and ramipril increased the expression of eNOS in the occluded tissue, thereby exhibiting a protective effect against heart damage induced by MI/R. To observe the effect of fixed-dose combination therapy with telmisartan and ramipril on cuff-induced neointimal hyperplasia, the thickness of the blood vessel intima and media after administration of both drugs alone or in combination for 14 days after cuff insertion and the degree of DNA synthesis were measured."

"These results indicated that a fixed-dose combination of telmisartan and ramipril protected against the blood vessel damage induced by cuff placement by inhibiting DNA synthesis in the intimal layer and significantly reducing the formation of the neointima."

Discussion

"Combination therapy with low doses (1/4 doses) of telmisartan and ramipril showed an antihypertensive effect similar to that of high-dose monotherapy with either drug."

"A fixed-dose combination of the two drugs did not result in a significant change in intimal thickness, but the increased eNOS expression induced vasodilation and appeared to have a protective effect against cardiac damage caused by myocardial ischemia."

"When losartan (ARB) and captopril (ACEI) were administered in combination at low doses to SHRs, BP-lowering effect was greater than monotherapy of each drug at high doses (Shin and others [144])."

"The combined treatment of valsartan (ARB) and ramipril at low doses effectively lowered BP, possibly inhibiting neointimal formation and DNA synthesis (Park and others [146])."

"The combination therapy of low-dose telmisartan and lercanidipine (CCB) is effective in lowering BP and also reduces adverse effects due to the maximal dose of each drug (Lee and others [145])."

Conclusion

"The findings indicate that when telmisartan and ramipril are administered in combination at low doses, BP can be effectively lowered to a similar extent as when the two drugs are administered alone at high doses."

"Use of the combination therapy can possibly reduce the degree and frequency of adverse effects caused by a high dose of each drug."

"The fixed-dose combination therapy showed a beneficial protective effect against the occurrence of myocardial infarction due to cardiac ischemia and the occurrence of vascular damage due to neointima formation."

"These results suggest that this combination of these drugs at appropriate doses is an excellent strategy for the prevention and treatment of diseases such as hypertension, myocardial infarction, and atherosclerosis."

Bibliography

1. Stotter BR, Ferguson MA (2019) Should ACE inhibitors and ARBs be used in combination in children? Pediatr Nephrol 34(9):1521–1532. https://doi.org/10.1007/s00467-018-4046-8
2. Tai C, Gan T, Zou L et al (2017) Effect of angiotensin-converting enzyme inhibitors and angiotensin II receptor blockers on cardiovascular events in patients with heart failure: a meta-analysis of randomized controlled trials. BMC Cardiovasc Disord 17:257. https://doi.org/10.1186/s12872-017-0686-z
3. Omboni S, Volpe M (2019) Angiotensin receptor blockers versus angiotensin converting enzyme inhibitors for the treatment of arterial hypertension and the role of olmesartan. Adv Ther 36(2):278–297
4. Brownstein DJ, Salagre E, Köhler C et al (2018) Blockade of the angiotensin system improves mental health domain of quality of life: a meta-analysis of randomized clinical trials. Aust N Z J Psychiatry 52:24–38
5. Li Z, Li Y, Liu Y, Xu W, Wang Q (2017) Comparative risk of new-onset diabetes mellitus for antihypertensive drugs: a network meta-analysis. J Clin Hypertens (Greenwich) 19:1348–1356

6. Underwood PC, Adler GK (2013) The renin angiotensin aldosterone system and insulin resistance in humans. Curr Hypertens Rep 15:59–70
7. Kostis WJ, Shetty M, Chowdhury YS, Kostis JB (2017) ACE inhibitor-induced angioedema: a review. Curr Hypertens Rep 20:1–7. https://doi.org/10.1007/s11906-018-0859-x
8. Hargreaves KM, Roszkowski MT, Swift JQ (1993) Bradykinin and inflammatory pain. Agents Actions 41:65–73
9. Byrd JB, Ram CVS, Lerma EV (2019) Pharmacologic treatment of hypertension, 4th edn. Elsevier Inc. https://doi.org/10.1016/B978-0-323-47871-7.00078-2
10. Fournier D, Luft FC, Bader M et al (2012) Emergence and evolution of the renin–angiotensin–aldosterone system. J Mol Med 90:495–508. https://doi.org/10.1007/s00109-012-0894-z
11. Cutrell S, Alhomoud IS, Mehta A, Talasaz AH, Tassell Benjamin V, Dixon DL (2023) ACE-inhibitors in hypertension: a historical perspective and current insights. Curr Hypertens Rep 25:243–250. https://doi.org/10.1007/s11906-023-01248-2
12. Whelton PK, Carey RM, Aronow WS et al (2018) 2017 ACC/AHA/AAPA/ABC/ACPM/AGS/APhA/ASH/ASPC/NMA/PCNA guideline for the prevention, detection, evaluation, and management of high blood pressure in adults: a report of the American College of Cardiology/American Heart Association task force on clinical practice guidelines [published correction appears in Hypertension. 2018 Jun;71(6):e140–e144]. Hypertension 71(6):e13–e115. https://doi.org/10.1161/HYP.0000000000000065
13. Kidney Disease: Improving Global Outcomes (KDIGO) Blood Pressure Work Group (2021) KDIGO 2021 clinical practice guideline for the management of blood pressure in chronic kidney disease. Kidney Int 99(3S):S1–S87. https://doi.org/10.1016/j.kint.2020.11.003
14. Heidenreich PA, Bozkurt B, Aguilar D et al (2022) 2022 AHA/ACC/HFSA guideline for the management of heart failure: a report of the American College of Cardiology/American Heart Association Joint Committee on clinical practice guidelines. J Am Coll Cardiol 79(17):e263–e421. https://doi.org/10.1016/j.jacc.2021.12.012
15. Ferreira SH (1965) Bradykinin-potentiating factor (BPF) present in the venom of bothrops jararca. Br J Pharmacol Chemother 24(1):163–169. https://doi.org/10.1111/j.1476-5381.1965.tb02091.x
16. Cushman DW, Ondetti MA (1991) History of the design of captopril and related inhibitors of angiotensin converting enzyme. Hypertension 17(4):589–592. https://doi.org/10.1161/01.hyp.17.4.589
17. Gavras H, Brunner HR, Turini GA et al (1978) Antihypertensive effect of the oral angiotensin converting-enzyme inhibitor SQ 14225 in man. N Engl J Med 298(18):991–995. https://doi.org/10.1056/NEJM197805042981803. First publication to report the potential of ACE inhibition for hypertension in humans
18. Heran BS, Wong MM, Heran IK, Wright JM (2008) Blood pressure lowering efficacy of angiotensin converting enzyme (ACE) inhibitors for primary hypertension. Cochrane Database Syst Rev. 2008(4):CD003823. https://doi.org/10.1002/14651858.CD003823.pub2. Published 2008
19. Heran BS, Wong MM, Heran IK, Wright JM (2008) Blood pressure lowering efficacy of angiotensin receptor blockers for primary hypertension. Cochrane Database Syst Rev. 2008(4):CD003822. https://doi.org/10.1002/14651858.CD003822.pub2. Published 2008
20. Musini VM, Nazer M, Bassett K, Wright JM (2014) Blood pressure-lowering efficacy of monotherapy with thiazide diuretics for primary hypertension. Cochrane Database Syst Rev (5):CD003824. https://doi.org/10.1002/14651858.CD003824.pub2. Published 2014
21. Hicks BM et al (2018) Angiotensin converting enzyme inhibitors and risk of lung cancer: population based cohort study. BMJ 363:k4209. https://doi.org/10.1136/bmj.k4209
22. Lin SY, Lin CL, Lin CC et al (2020) Association between angiotensin-converting enzyme inhibitors and lung cancer-a nationwide, population-based, propensity score-matched cohort study. Cancers (Basel). 12(3):747. https://doi.org/10.3390/cancers12030747. Published 2020
23. Kristensen KB, Hicks B, Azoulay L, Pottegård A (2021) Use of ACE (angiotensin-converting enzyme) inhibitors and risk of lung cancer: a nationwide nested case-

control study. Circ Cardiovasc Qual Outcomes 14(1):e006687. https://doi.org/10.1161/CIRCOUTCOMES.120.006687
24. Wang Z, Wei L, Yin C, Li W, Wan B (2023) Angiotensin receptor blocker associated with a decreased risk of lung cancer: an updated meta-analysis. J Pers Med. 13(2):243. https://doi.org/10.3390/jpm13020243. Published 2023
25. Batais M, Almigbal T, Alotaibi K et al (2021) Angiotensin converting enzyme inhibitors and risk of lung cancer: a systematic review and meta-analysis. Medicine (Baltimore) 100(17):e25714. https://doi.org/10.1097/MD.0000000000025714
26. Wu Z, Yao T, Wang Z et al (2023) Association between angiotensin-converting enzyme inhibitors and the risk of lung cancer: a systematic review and meta-analysis. Br J Cancer 128(2):168–176. https://doi.org/10.1038/s41416-022-02029-5
27. Momoniat T, Ilyas D, Bhandari S (2019) ACE inhibitors and ARBs: managing potassium and renal function. Cleve Clin J Med 86(9):601–607. https://doi.org/10.3949/ccjm.86a.18024
28. Investigators O, Yusuf S, Teo KK, Pogue J, Dyal L, Copland I et al (2008) Telmisartan, ramipril, or both in patients at high risk for vascular events. N Engl J Med 358(15):1547–1559
29. Bremner AD, Baur M, Oddou-Stock P, Bodin F (1997) Valsartan: long-term efficacy and tolerability compared to lisinopril in elderly patients with essential hypertension. Clin Exp Hypertens 19(8):1263–1285
30. Barnett AH, Bain SC, Bouter P, Karlberg B, Madsbad S, Jervell J et al (2004) Angiotensin-receptor blockade versus converting-enzyme inhibition in type 2 diabetes and nephropathy. N Engl J Med 351(19):1952–1961
31. Spinar J, Vítovec J, Souček M, Dušek L, Pavlík T, CORD investigators (2010) CORD: COmparison of Recommended Doses of ace inhibitors and angiotensin II receptor blockers. Int J Cardiol 144(2):293–294. https://doi.org/10.1016/j.ijcard.2009.02.022
32. ••Chen R, Suchard MA, Krumholz HM et al (2021) Comparative first-line effectiveness and safety of ACE (angiotensin-converting enzyme) inhibitors and angiotensin receptor blockers: a multinational cohort study. Hypertension 78(3):591–603. https://doi.org/10.1161/HYPERTENSIONAHA.120.166. ARBs have similar antihypertensive effectiveness as ACE inhibitors but with a better safety profile
33. Goh KL, Bhaskaran K, Minassian C, Evans SJ, Smeeth L, Douglas IJ (2015) Angiotensin receptor blockers and risk of dementia: cohort study in UK Clinical Practice Research Datalink. Br J Clin Pharmacol 79(2):337–350. https://doi.org/10.1111/bcp.12511
34. Ho JK, Nation DA (2017) Alzheimer's Disease Neuroimaging Initiative. Memory is preserved in older adults taking AT1 receptor blockers. Alzheimers Res Ther. 9(1):33. https://doi.org/10.1186/s13195-017-0255-9. Published 2017
35. Hajjar I, Okafor M, McDaniel D et al (2020) Effects of candesartan vs lisinopril on neurocognitive function in older adults with executive mild cognitive impairment: a randomized clinical trial. JAMA Netw Open 3(8):e2012252. https://doi.org/10.1001/jamanetworkopen.2020.12252. Published 2020. Randomized trial demonstrating potential neurocognitive benefits with candesartan compared to lisinopril
36. Deng Z, Jiang J, Wang J et al (2022) Angiotensin receptor blockers are associated with a lower risk of progression from mild cognitive impairment to dementia. Hypertension 79(10):2159–2169. https://doi.org/10.1161/HYPERTENSIONAHA.122.19378
37. Xiao F, Jiang H, Li Z, Jiang X, Chen S, Niu Y, Yin H, Shu Y, Peng B, Lu W, Li X, Li Z, Lan S, Xu X, Guo F (2023) Reduced hepatic bradykinin degradation accounts for cold-induced BAT thermogenesis and WAT browning in male mice. Nat Commun 14(1):2523. https://doi.org/10.1038/s41467-023-38141-0
38. Bartelt A, Heeren J (2014) Adipose tissue browning and metabolic health. Nat Rev Endocrinol 10:24–36
39. Ancion A, Tridetti J, Nguyen Trung M-L, Oury C, Lancellotti P (2019) A review of the role of bradykinin and nitric oxide in the cardioprotective action of angiotensin-converting enzyme inhibitors: focus on perindopril. Cardiol Ther 8:179–191. https://doi.org/10.1007/s40119-019-00150-w

40. Lerman A, Zeiher AM (2005) Endothelial function: cardiac events. Circulation 111:363–368
41. Su JB (2006) Kinins and cardiovascular diseases. Curr Pharm Des 12:3423–3435
42. Su JB (2014) Different cross-talk sites between the renin–angiotensin and the kallikrein–kinin systems. J Renin-Angiotensin-Aldosterone Syst 15:319–328
43. Virdis A, Neves MF, Amiri F, Touyz RM, Schiffrin EL (2004) Role of NAD(P)H oxidase on vascular alterations in angiotensin II-infused mice. J Hypertens 22:535–542
44. Ceconi C, Francolini G, Bastianon D et al (2007) Differences in the effect of angiotensin-converting enzyme inhibitors on the rate of endothelial cell apoptosis in vitro and in vivo studies. Cardiovasc Drugs Ther 21(6):423–429
45. Poulter NR, Wedel H, Dahlöf B, ASCOT Investigators et al (2005) Role of blood pressure and other variables in the differential cardiovascular event rates noted in the Anglo-Scandinavian Cardiac Outcomes Trial-Blood Pressure Lowering Arm (ASCOT-BPLA). Lancet 366:907–913
46. Oliveira-Paula GH, Lacchini R, Fontana V, Silva PS, Biagi C, Tanus-Santos JE (2015) Polymorphisms in VEGFA gene affect the antihypertensive responses to enalapril. Eur J Clin Pharmacol 71:949–957. https://doi.org/10.1007/s00228-015-1872-5
47. Ebrahimian TG, Tamarat R, Clergue M, Duriez M, Levy BI, Silvestre JS (2005) Dual effect of angiotensin-converting enzyme inhibition on angiogenesis in type 1 diabetic mice. Arterioscler Thromb Vasc Biol 25(1):65–70
48. Yazawa H, Miyachi M, Furukawa M, Takahashi K, Takatsu M, Tsuboi K, Ohtake M, Murase T, Hattori T, Kato Y, Murohara T, Nagata K (2011) Angiotensin-converting enzyme inhibition promotes coronary angiogenesis in the failing heart of Dahl salt-sensitive hypertensive rats. J Card Fail 17(12):1041–1050
49. Ferroni P, Della-Morte D, Palmirotta R, Rundek T, Guadagni F, Roselli M (2012) Angiogenesis and hypertension: the dual role of anti-hypertensive and anti-angiogenic therapies. Curr Vasc Pharmacol 10(4):479–493
50. Li P, Kondo T, Numaguchi Y, Kobayashi K, Aoki M, Inoue N, Okumura K, Murohara T (2008) Role of bradykinin, nitric oxide, and angiotensin II type 2 receptor in imidapril-induced angiogenesis. Hypertension 51(2):252–258
51. Thuringer D, Maulon L, Frelin C (2002) Rapid transactivation of the vascular endothelial growth factor receptor KDR/Flk-1 by the bradykinin B2 receptor contributes to endothelial nitric-oxide synthase activation in cardiac capillary endothelial cells. J Biol Chem 277(3):2028–2032
52. Lambrechts D, Storkebaum E, Morimoto M, Del-Favero J, Desmet F, Marklund SL, Wyns S, Thijs V, Andersson J, van Marion I, Al-Chalabi A, Bornes S, Musson R, Hansen V, Beckman L, Adolfsson R, Pall HS, Prats H, Vermeire S, Rutgeerts P, Katayama S, Awata T, Leigh N, Lang-Lazdunski L, Dewerchin M, Shaw C, Moons L, Vlietinck R, Morrison KE, Robberecht W, Van Broeckhoven C, Collen D, Andersen PM, Carmeliet P (2003) VEGF is a modifier of amyotrophic lateral sclerosis in mice and humans and protects motoneurons against ischemic death. Nat Genet 34(4):383–394
53. Shahbazi M, Fryer AA, Pravica V, Brogan IJ, Ramsay HM, Hutchinson IV, Harden PN (2002) Vascular endothelial growth factor gene polymorphisms are associated with acute renal allograft rejection. J Am Soc Nephrol 13(1):260–264
54. Silva PS, Fontana V, Luizon MR, Lacchini R, Silva WA Jr, Biagi C, Tanus-Santos JE (2013) eNOS and BDKRB2 genotypes affect the antihypertensive responses to enalapril. Eur J Clin Pharmacol 69(2):167–177
55. Ilhan H, Wang H, Gildehaus FJ, Wängler C, Herrler T, Todica A, Schlichtiger J, Cumming P, Bartenstein P, Hacker M, Haug AR (2016) Nephroprotective effects of enalapril after [177Lu]-DOTATATE therapy using serial renal scintigraphies in a murine model of radiation-induced nephropathy. EJNMMI Res 6:64. https://doi.org/10.1186/s13550-016-0219-2
56. Duncan JR, Stephenson MT, Wu HP, Anderson CJ (1997) Indium-111-diethylenetriaminepentaacetic acid-octreotide is delivered in vivo to pancreatic, tumor cell, renal, and hepatocyte lysosomes. Cancer Res 57:659–671

57. de Jong M, Barone R, Krenning E, Bernard B, Melis M, Visser T et al (2005) Megalin is essential for renal proximal tubule reabsorption of (111)In-DTPA-octreotide. J Nucl Med 46:1696–1700
58. Cohen EP, Robbins ME (2003) Radiation nephropathy. Semin Nephrol 23:486–499
59. Cohen EP, Fish BL, Moulder JE (1992) Treatment of radiation nephropathy with captopril. Radiat Res 132:346–350
60. Moll S, Nickeleit V, Mueller-Brand J, Brunner FP, Maecke HR, Mihatsch MJ (2001) A new cause of renal thrombotic microangiopathy: yttrium 90-DOTATOC internal radiotherapy. Am J Kidney Dis 37:847–851
61. Moulder JE, Fish BL, Cohen EP (1993) Treatment of radiation nephropathy with ACE inhibitors. Int J Radiat Oncol Biol Phys 27:93–99
62. Juncos LI, Carrasco Duenas S, Cornejo JC, Broglia CA, Cejas H (1993) Long-term enalapril and hydrochlorothiazide in radiation nephritis. Nephron 64:249–255
63. Bodei L, Cremonesi M, Ferrari M, Pacifici M, Grana CM, Bartolomei M et al (2008) Long-term evaluation of renal toxicity after peptide receptor radionuclide therapy with 90Y-DOTATOC and 177Lu-DOTATATE: the role of associated risk factors. Eur J Nucl Med Mol Imaging 35:1847–1856
64. Taddei S, Bortolotto L (2016) Unraveling the pivotal role of bradykinin in ACE inhibitor activity. Am J Cardiovas Drug 16:309–321. https://doi.org/10.1007/s40256-016-0173-4
65. Thomopoulos C, Parati G, Zanchetti A (2015) Effects of blood pressure lowering on outcome incidence in hypertension: 4. Effects of various classes of antihypertensive drugs–overview and meta-analyses. J Hypertens 33(2):195–211
66. Li YY, Zhang H, Xu J et al (2012) Bradykinin beta2 receptor -58T/C gene polymorphism and essential hypertension: a meta-analysis. PLoS One 7(8):e43068
67. Bachvarov DR, Landry M, Pelletier I et al (1998) Characterization of two polymorphic sites in the human kinin B1 receptor gene: altered frequency of an allele in patients with a history of end-stage renal failure. J Am Soc Nephrol 9(4):598–604
68. Jozwiak L, Drop A, Buraczynska K et al (2004) Association of the human bradykinin B2 receptor gene with chronic renal failure. Mol Diagn 8(3):157–161
69. Kakoki M, McGarrah RW, Kim HS et al (2007) Bradykinin B1 and B2 receptors both have protective roles in renal ischemia/reperfusion injury. Proc Natl Acad Sci 104(18):7576–7581
70. Kimura S, Tsuji H, Nishimura H et al (2002) Bradykinin enhances in vitro procoagulant and antifibrinolytic properties of rat vascular endothelial cells. Thromb Res 106(1):41–50
71. Kuoppala A, Shiota N, Lindstedt KA et al (2003) Expression of bradykinin receptors in the left ventricles of rats with pressure overload hypertrophy and heart failure. J Hypertens 21(9):1729–1736
72. Liesmaa I, Shiota N, Kokkonen JO et al (2012) Bradykinin type-2 receptor expression correlates with age and is subjected to transcriptional regulation. Int J Vasc Med 2012:159646
73. Witherow FN, Dawson P, Ludlam CA et al (2002) Marked bradykinin-induced tissue plasminogen activator release in patients with heart failure maintained on long-term angiotensin-converting enzyme inhibitor therapy. J Am Coll Cardiol 40(5):961–966
74. Lang NN, Cruden NL, Tse GH et al (2008) Vascular B1 kinin receptors in patients with congestive heart failure. J Cardiovasc Pharmacol 52(5):438–444
75. Dhangadamajhi G, Singh S (2021) Shailja Malaria link of hypertension: a hidden syndicate of angiotensin II, bradykinin and sphingosine 1-phosphate. Hum Cell 34:734–744. https://doi.org/10.1007/s13577-021-00513-3
76. Koopman JJ, van Bodegom D, Jukema JW, Westendorp RG (2012) Risk of cardiovascular disease in a traditional African population with a high infectious load: a population-based study. PLoS One 7(10):e46855
77. Volpe M, Battistoni A (2019) An evolutionary rebus: the complex link between malaria and hypertension. J Hypertens 37(7):1344–1346
78. Kearney PM, Whelton M, Reynolds K, Whelton PK, He J (2004) Worldwide prevalence of hypertension: a systematic review. J Hypertens 22(1):11–19

79. Dhangadamajhi G, Mohapatra BN, Kar SK, Ranjit M (2010) Gene polymorphisms in angiotensin I converting enzyme (ACE I/D) and angiotensin II converting enzyme (ACE2 C→ T) protect against cerebral malaria in Indian adults. Infect Genet Evol 10(2):337–341
80. Cappuccio FP (1997) Ethnicity and cardiovascular risk: variations in people of African ancestry and South Asian origin. J Hum Hypertens 11(9):571–576
81. Sampson UK, Edwards TL, Jahangir E, Munro H, Wariboko M, Wassef MG et al (2014) Factors associated with the prevalence of hypertension in the southeastern United States: insights from 69 211 blacks and whites in the southern community cohort study. Circ Cardiovasc Qual Outcomes 7(1):33–54
82. Ferrari R et al (2013) RAAS inhibition and mortality in hypertension: from pharmacology to clinical evidence. Glob Cardiol Sci Pract 2013(3):34–278
83. Intapad S (2019) Sphingosine-1-phosphate signaling in blood pressure regulation. Am J Physiol-Ren Physiol 317(3):F638–F640
84. Katsi V, Katsimichas T, Pittaras A, Grassos C, Katsimichas A, Tousoulis D et al (2012) Hypertension and bradykinin: a dangerous affair? Cardiovasc Endocrinol Metab 1(2):24–30
85. Foulquier S, Paulis L, Kaschina E, Namsolleck P, Unger T (2018) Hormonal systems. In: Disorders of blood pressure regulation. Springer, pp 81–106
86. Royea J, Hamel E (2020) Brain angiotensin II and angiotensin IV receptors as potential Alzheimer's disease therapeutic targets. GeroScience 42:1–20
87. Wright JW, Harding JW (2019) Contributions by the brain renin-angiotensin system to memory, cognition, and Alzheimer's disease. J Alzheimers Dis 67(2):469–480
88. Khalil RA (2013) Hypertension and vascular dysfunction. In: Interdisciplinary concepts in cardiovascular health. Springer, pp 1–37
89. Moreau ME, Garbacki N, Molinaro G, Brown NJ, Marceau F, Adam A (2005) The kallikrein-kinin system: current and future pharmacological targets. J Pharmacol Sci 99(1):6–38
90. Ventura PD, Carvalho CP, Barros NM, Martins-Silva L, Dantas EO, Martinez C et al (2019) Malaria infection promotes a selective expression of kinin receptors in murine liver. Malar J 18(1):213
91. Singh S, Chitnis CE (2017) Molecular signaling involved in entry and exit of malaria parasites from host erythrocytes. Cold Spring Harb Perspect Med 7(10):a026815
92. Silva LS, Pinheiro AS, Teixeira DE, Silva-Aguiar RP, Peruchetti DB, Scharfstein J et al (2019) Kinins released by erythrocytic stages of Plasmodium falciparum enhance adhesion of infected erythrocytes to endothelial cells and increase blood brain barrier permeability via activation of bradykinin receptors. Front Med 6:75
93. Cantalupo A, Zhang Y, Kothiya M, Galvani S, Obinata H, Bucci M et al (2015) Nogo-B regulates endothelial sphingolipid homeostasis to control vascular function and blood pressure. Nat Med 21(9):1028–1037
94. Cantalupo A, Gargiulo A, Dautaj E, Liu C, Zhang Y, Hla T et al (2017) S1PR1 (sphingosine-1-phosphate receptor 1) signaling regulates blood flow and pressure. Hypertension 70(2):426–434
95. Kurano M, Yatomi Y (2017) Sphingosine 1-phosphate and atherosclerosis. J Atheroscler Thromb 25:RV17010–RV17026
96. Tölle M, Levkau B, Keul P, Brinkmann V, Giebing G, Schönfelder G et al (2005) Immunomodulator FTY720 induces eNOS-dependent arterial vasodilatation via the lysophospholipid receptor S1P3. Circ Res 96(8):913–920
97. MacRitchie N, Volpert G, Al Washih M, Watson DG, Futerman AH, Kennedy S et al (2016) Effect of the sphingosine kinase 1 selective inhibitor, PF-543 on arterial and cardiac remodelling in a hypoxic model of pulmonary arterial hypertension. Cell Signal 28(8):946–955
98. Siedlinski M, Nosalski R, Szczepaniak P, Ludwig-Gałęzowska AH, Mikołajczyk T, Filip M et al (2017) Vascular transcriptome profiling identifies Sphingosine kinase 1 as a modulator of angiotensin II-induced vascular dysfunction. Sci Rep 7:44131
99. Pyne NJ, Pyne S (2017) Sphingosine kinase 1: a potential therapeutic target in pulmonary arterial hypertension? Trends Mol Med 23(9):786–798

100. Punsawad C, Viriyavejakul P (2019) Expression of sphingosine kinase 1 and sphingosine 1-phosphate receptor 3 in malaria-associated acute lung injury/acute respiratory distress syndrome in a mouse model. PLoS One 14(9):e0222098
101. Birhanu M, Asres Y, Adissu W, Yemane T, Zemene E, Gedefaw L (2017) Hematological parameters and hemozoin-containing leukocytes and their association with disease severity among malaria infected children: a cross-sectional study at Pawe General Hospital, Northwest Ethiopia. Interdiscip Perspect Infect Dis 2017:1–7
102. Dhangadamajhi G, Panigrahi S, Roy S, Tripathy S (2019) Effect of Plasmodium falciparum infection on blood parameters and their association with clinical severity in adults of Odisha. India Acta Trop 190:1–8
103. Zhang L, Orban M, Lorenz M, Barocke V, Braun D, Urtz N et al (2012) A novel role of sphingosine 1-phosphate receptor S1pr1 in mouse thrombopoiesis. J Exp Med 209(12):2165–2181
104. Yeo TW, Weinberg JB, Lampah DA, Kenangalem E, Bush P, Chen Y et al (2019) Glycocalyx breakdown is associated with severe disease and fatal outcome in Plasmodium falciparum malaria. Clin Infect Dis 69(10):1712–1720
105. Cannon RE, Peart JC, Hawkins BT, Campos CR, Miller DS (2012) Targeting blood-brain barrier sphingolipid signaling reduces basal P-glycoprotein activity and improves drug delivery to the brain. Proc Natl Acad Sci U S A 109(39):15930–15935
106. Oggungwan K, Glaharn S, Ampawong S, Krudsood S, Viriyavejakul P (2018) FTY720 restores endothelial cell permeability induced by malaria sera. Sci Rep 8(1):1–6
107. Yanagida K, Liu CH, Faraco G, Galvani S, Smith HK, Burg N et al (2017) Size-selective opening of the blood–brain barrier by targeting endothelial sphingosine 1–phosphate receptor 1. Proc Natl Acad Sci 114(17):4531–4536
108. Hempel C, Sporring J, Kurtzhals JAL (2019) Experimental cerebral malaria is associated with profound loss of both glycan and protein components of the endothelial glycocalyx. FASEB J 33(2):2058–2071
109. Dhangadamajhi G, Singh S (2020) Sphingosine 1-Phosphate in malaria pathogenesis and its implication in therapeutic opportunities. Front Cell Infect Microbiol 10:10
110. Finney CA, Hawkes CA, Kain DC, Dhabangi A, Musoke C, Cserti-Gazdewich C et al (2011) S1P is associated with protection in human and experimental cerebral malaria. Mol Med 17(7):717–725
111. Li P, Kondo T, Numaguchi Y, Kobayashi K, Aoki M, Inoue N et al (2008) Role of bradykinin, nitric oxide, and angiotensin II type 2 receptor in imidapril-induced angiogenesis. Hypertension 51(2):252–258
112. Abdulazeez A, Ya'u M, Kurfi B et al (2017) Association of hypertension and activity of angiotensin converting enzyme in malaria patients attending Sheik Muhammad Jidda General Hospital, Kano State, Nigeria. Niger J Basic Clin Sci 14(2):121
113. Meissner A, Miro F, Jimenez-Altayo F, Jurado A, Vila E, Planas AM (2017) Sphingosine-1-phosphate signalling—a key player in the pathogenesis of Angiotensin II-induced hypertension. Cardiovasc Res 113(2):123–133
114. Guzik TJ, Hoch NE, Brown KA, McCann LA, Rahman A, Dikalov S et al (2007) Role of the T cell in the genesis of angiotensin II–induced hypertension and vascular dysfunction. J Exp Med 204(10):2449–2460
115. Itani HA, McMaster WG Jr, Saleh MA, Nazarewicz RR, Mikolajczyk TP, Kaszuba AM et al (2016) Activation of human T cells in hypertension: studies of humanized mice and hypertensive humans. Hypertension 68(1):123–132
116. Yang K, Jiang K, Xu Z, Song Y, Wang J (2019) Targeting sphingosine kinase 1 for the treatment of pulmonary arterial hypertension. Future Med Chem 11(22):2939–2953
117. Ki Y-J, Seo J-B, Kim H-L, Lim W-H, Seo HY, Lee JY, Chung W-Y (2017) Comparison of endothelial function improvement estimated with reactive hyperemia index between ramipril and telmisartan in hypertensive patients. Clin Hyperten 23:4. https://doi.org/10.1186/s40885-016-0060-y

118. Li S, Wu Y, Yu G, Xia Q, Yawei X (2014) Angiotensin II receptor blockers improve peripheral endothelial function: a meta-analysis of randomized controlled trials. PLoS One 9(3):e90217
119. Anderson TJ (1999) Assessment and treatment of endothelial dysfunction in humans. J Am Coll Cardiol 34(3):631–638
120. Watanabe T, Barker TA, Berk BC (2005) Angiotensin II and the endothelium: diverse signals and effects. Hypertension 45(2):163–169
121. Radhoe SP, Boersma E, Bertrand M, Remme W, Ferrari R, Fox K, MacMahon S, Chalmers J, Simoons ML, Brugts JJ (2022) The effects of a perindopril-based regimen in relation to statin use on the outcomes of patients with vascular disease: a combined analysis of the ADVANCE, EUROPA, and PROGRESS trials. Cardiovasc Drugs Ther 38:131–139. https://doi.org/10.1007/s10557-022-07384-2
122. Fox KM, For The EURopean trial On reduction of cardiac events with Perindopril in stable coronary Artery disease Investigators (2003) Efficacy of perindopril in reduction of cardiovascular events among patients with stable coronary artery disease: randomised, double-blind, placebo-controlled, multicentre trial (the EUROPA study). Lancet 362:782–788
123. PROGRESS Collaborative Group (2001) Randomized trial of a perindopril-based blood-pressure-lowering regimen among 6105 individuals with previous stroke or transient ischemic attack. Lancet 358(9287):1033–1041
124. Baigent C, Keech A, Kearney PM, Blackwell L, Buck G, Pollicino C et al (2005) Efficacy and safety of cholesterol-lowering treatment: prospective meta-analysis of data from 90,056 participants in 14 randomised trials of statins. Lancet 366(9493):1267–1278
125. Cholesterol Treatment Trialists C, Kearney PM, Blackwell L, Collins R, Keech A, Simes J et al (2008) Efficacy of cholesterol-lowering therapy in 18,686 people with diabetes in 14 randomised trials of statins: a meta-analysis. Lancet 371(9607):117–125
126. Cholesterol Treatment Trialists C, Baigent C, Blackwell L, Emberson J, Holland LE, Reith C et al (2010) Efficacy and safety of more intensive lowering of LDL cholesterol: a meta-analysis of data from 170,000 participants in 26 randomised trials. Lancet 376(9753):1670–1681
127. Cholesterol Treatment Trialists C, Mihaylova B, Emberson J, Blackwell L, Keech A, Simes J et al (2012) The effects of lowering LDL cholesterol with statin therapy in people at low risk of vascular disease: meta-analysis of individual data from 27 randomised trials. Lancet 380(9841):581–590
128. Cholesterol Treatment Trialists C, Fulcher J, O'Connell R, Voysey M, Emberson J, Blackwell L et al (2015) Efficacy and safety of LDL-lowering therapy among men and women: meta-analysis of individual data from 174,000 participants in 27 randomised trials. Lancet 385(9976):1397–1405
129. Yusuf S, Pitt B, Davis CE, Hood WB, Cohn JN (1991) Effect of enalapril on survival in patients with reduced left ventricular ejection fractions and congestive heart failure. N Engl J Med 325(5):293–302. https://doi.org/10.1056/NEJM199108013250501
130. Konstam MA, Rousseau MF, Kronenberg MW, Udelson JE, Melin J, Stewart D, Dolan N, Edens TR, Ahn S, Kinan D (1992) Effects of the angiotensin converting enzyme inhibitor enalapril on the long-term progression of left ventricular dysfunction in patients with heart failure. SOLVD Investigators. Circulation 86:431–438. https://doi.org/10.1161/01.CIR.86.2.431
131. Pfeffer MA, Braunwald E, Moyé LA et al (1992) Effect of captopril on mortality and morbidity in patients with left ventricular dysfunction after myocardial infarction: results of the survival and ventricular enlargement trial. N Engl J Med 327(10):669–677. https://doi.org/10.1056/NEJM199209033271001
132. The Acute Infarction Ramipril Efficacy (AIRE) Study Investigators (1993) Effect of ramipril on mortality and morbidity of survivors of acute myocardial infarction with clinical evidence of heart failure. Lancet 342(8875):821–828
133. Kober L, Torp-Pedersen C, Carlsen JE, Bagger H, Eliasen P, Lyngborg K et al (1995) A clinical trial of the angiotensin-converting-enzyme inhibitor trandolapril in patients with left ventricular dysfunction after myocardial infarction. Trandolapril Cardiac Evaluation (TRACE) Study Group. N Engl J Med 333:1670–1676

134. Dahlöf B, Sever PS, Poulter NR et al (2005) Prevention of cardiovascular events with an antihypertensive regimen of amlodipine adding perindopril as required versus atenolol adding bendroflumethiazide as required, in the Anglo-Scandinavian Cardiac Outcomes Trial-Blood Pressure Lowering Arm (ASCOT-BPLA): a multicentre randomised controlled trial. Lancet 366:895–906. https://doi.org/10.1016/S0140-6736(05)67185-1
135. Yusuf S, Sleight P, Pogue J et al (2000) Effects of an angiotensin-converting enzyme inhibitor, ramipril, on cardiovascular events in high-risk patients. The Heart Outcomes Prevention Evaluation Study Investigators. N Engl J Med 342:145–153
136. van Vark LC, Bertrand M, Akkerhuis KM, Brugts JJ, Fox K, Mourad JJ, Boersma E (2012) Angiotensin-converting enzyme inhibitors reduce mortality in hypertension: a meta-analysis of randomized clinical trials of renin-angiotensin-aldosterone system inhibitors involving 158,998 patients. Eur Heart J 33:2088–2097
137. Lee D-H, Jo EJ, Ga E-J, Han J-H, Jung S-H, Park H-S, Heo K-S, Myung C-S (2017) Effects of combination therapy with candesartan and ramipril on hypertension and related complications. J Pharm Investig 47:365–371. https://doi.org/10.1007/s40005-017-0339-3
138. Atlas SA (2007) The renin-angiotensin aldosterone system: pathophysiological role and pharmacologic inhibition. J Manag Care Pharm 13:S9–S20
139. Carey RM, Siragy HM (2003) Newly recognized components of the renin-angiotensin system: potential roles in cardiovascular and renal regulation. Endocr Rev 24:261–271
140. Ribeiro-Oliveira A, Nogueira AI, Pereira RM, Boas WW, Dos Santos RA, Simoes e Silva AC. (2008) The renin-angiotensin system and diabetes: an update. Vasc Health Risk Manag 4:787–803
141. Nguyen Q, Dominguez J, Nguyen L, Gullapalli N (2010) Hypertension management: an UPDATE. Am Health Drug Benefits 3:47–56
142. Mancia G, Fagard R, Narkiewicz K, Redon J, Zanchetti A, Bohm M, Christiaens T, Cifkova R, De Backer G, Dominiczak A, Galderisi M, Grobbee DE, Jaarsma T, Kirchhof P, Kjeldsen SE, Laurent S, Manolis AJ, Nilsson PM, Ruilope LM, Schmieder RE, Sirnes PA, Sleight P, Viigimaa M, Waeber B, Zannad F (2014) 2013 ESH/ESC guidelines for the management of arterial hypertension. The task force for the management of arterial hypertension of the European Society of Hypertension (ESH) and of the European Society of Cardiology (EGC). J Hypertens 31:1281–1357
143. Ménard J, Campbell DJ, Azizi M, Gonzales MF (1997) Synergistic effects of ACE inhibition and Ang II antagonism on blood pressure, cardiac weight, and renin in spontaneously hypertensive rats. Circulation 96(9):3072–3080. https://doi.org/10.1161/01.CIR.96.9.3072
144. Shin CY, Choi WS, Yi I, Nan MH, Myung CS (2009) Synergistic decrease in blood pressure by captopril combined with losartan in spontaneous hypertensive rats. Arch Pharm Res 32:955–962
145. Lee JJ, Shin CY, Park HJ, Zhang WY, Kim Y, Kim IS, Lee KH, Myung CS (2010) Drug synergism of antihypertensive action in combination of telmisartan with lercanidipine in spontaneous hypertensive rats. Arch Pharm Res 33:1411–1418
146. Park HS, Han JH, Jung SH, Jo EJ, Myung CS (2016) The combination of valsartan and ramipril protects against blood vessel injury and lowers blood pressure. J Pharm Investig 46:265–272
147. Loga-Zec S, Asceric M, Loga-Andrijic N, Kapetanovic B, Zerem E (2014) The incidence of antihypertensive drug-induced side effects in patients with diabetes mellitus type 2 and hypertension. Med Arch 68:372–375
148. Brugts JJ, Bertrand M, Remme W, Ferrari R, Fox K, MacMahon S, Chalmers J, Simoons ML, Boersma E (2017) The treatment effect of an ACE-inhibitor based regimen with perindopril in relation to beta-blocker use in 29,463 patients with vascular disease: a combined analysis of individual data of ADVANCE, EUROPA and PROGRESS trials. Cardiovasc Drugs Ther 31:391–400. https://doi.org/10.1007/s10557-017-6747-9
149. Rosendorff C, Lackland DT, Allison M, Aronow WS, Black HR, Blumenthal RS et al (2015) Treatment of hypertension in patients with coronary artery disease: a scientific statement

from the American Heart Association, American College of Cardiology, and American Society of Hypertension. J Am Coll Cardiol 65(18):1998–2038
150. Ponikowski P, Voors AA, Anker SD, Bueno H, Cleland JGF, Coats AJS, Falk V, González-Juanatey JR, Harjola VP, Jankowska EA, Jessup M, Linde C, Nihoyannopoulos P, Parissis JT, Pieske B, Riley JP, Rosano GMC, Ruilope LM, Ruschitzka F, Rutten FH, van der Meer P (2016) 2016 ESC guidelines for the diagnosis and treatment of acute and chronic heart failure. Eur Heart J 37:2129–2200. https://doi.org/10.1093/eurheartj/ehw128
151. Thoenes M, Neuberger HR, Volpe M, Khan BV, Kirch W, Bohm M (2010) Antihypertensive drug therapy and blood pressure control in men and women: an international perspective. J Hum Hypertens 24(5):336–344
152. Kotseva K, Wood D, De Bacquer D, De Backer G, Ryden L, Jennings C et al (2016) EUROASPIRE IV: a European Society of Cardiology survey on the lifestyle, risk factor and therapeutic management of coronary patients from 24 European countries. Eur J Prev Cardiol 23(6):636–648
153. Maggioni AP, Anker SD, Dahlström U, Heart Failure Association of the ESC et al (2013) Are hospitalized or ambulatory patients with heart failure treated in accordance with European Society of Cardiology guidelines? Evidence from 12,440 patients of the ESC Heart Failure Long-Term Registry. Eur J Heart Fail 15:1173–1184
154. Patel A, Group AC, MacMahon S, Chalmers J, Neal B, Woodward M et al (2007) Effects of a fixed combination of perindopril and indapamide on macrovascular and microvascular outcomes in patients with type 2 diabetes mellitus (the ADVANCE trial): a randomised controlled trial. Lancet 370(9590):829–840
155. Ordaz-Medina SM, Cueto-Manzano AM, González-Plascencia J, Montañez-Fernández JL, Ordaz-Medina EJ, Martín-del-Campo F, Cueto-Ramírez AM, Martínez-Martínez P, Cortés-Sanabria L, Rojas-Campos E, Trujillo-Hernández B (2022) Randomized, double-blinded, controlled clinical trial of the effect of captopril, telmisartan and their combination on systemic inflammation of patients on hemodialysis. Sci Rep 12:17568. https://doi.org/10.1038/s41598-022-22656-5
156. Pecoits-Filho R, Lindholm B, Stenvinkel P (2002) The malnutrition, inflammation, and atherosclerosis (MIA) syndrome—the heart of the matter. Nephrol Dial Transpl 17(Suppl 11):28–31
157. Jacobs LH et al (2010) Inflammation, overhydration and cardiac biomarkers in haemodialysis patients: a longitudinal study. Nephrol Dial Transpl 25:243–248
158. Dai L, Golembiewska E, Lindholm B, Stenvinkel P (2017) End-stage renal disease, inflammation and cardiovascular outcomes. Contrib Nephrol 191:32–43
159. Schindler R (2004) Causes and therapy of microinflammation in renal failure. Nephrol Dial Transpl 19(Suppl 5):V34–V40
160. Cobo G, Lindholm B, Stenvinkel P (2018) Chronic inflammation in end-stage renal disease and dialysis. Nephrol Dial Transpl 33(Suppl 3):iii35–iii40
161. Movilli E et al (2006) The kind of vascular access influences the baseline inflammatory status and epoetin response in chronic hemodialysis patients. Blood Purif 24:387–393
162. Koulouris S et al (2005) Comparison of the effects of ramipril versus telmisartan in reducing serum levels of high-sensitivity C-reactive protein and oxidized low-density lipoprotein cholesterol in patients with type 2 diabetes mellitus. Am J Cardiol 95:1386–1388
163. Ordaz-Medina S et al (2010) Is systemic inflammation of hemodialysis patients improved with the use of enalapril? Results of a randomized, double-blinded, placebo-controlled clinical trial. ASAIO J 56:37–41
164. Daly LE, Bourke GJ (eds) (2000) Interpretation and uses of medical statistics, 5th edn. Blackwell Science Ltd, Oxford, pp 335–337
165. Gamboa JL et al (2012) Comparative effects of angiotensin-converting enzyme inhibition and angiotensin-receptor blockade on inflammation during hemodialysis. J Am Soc Nephrol 23:334–342

166. Peters CD et al (2017) Long-term effects of angiotensin II blockade with irbesartan on inflammatory markers in hemodialysis patients: a randomized double blind placebo controlled trial (SAFIR study). Hemodial Int 21:47–62
167. Rasool MF, Ali S, Khalid S, Khalid R, Majeed A, Imran I, Saeed H, Usman M, Ali M, Alali AS, AlAsmari AF, Ali N, Asiri AM, Alasmari F, Alqahtani F (2021) Development and evaluation of physiologically based pharmacokinetic drug-disease models for predicting captopril pharmacokinetics in chronic diseases. Sci Rep 11:8589. https://doi.org/10.1038/s41598-021-88154-2
168. Takubo H, Taniguchi T, Iwanaga K, Nomura Y (2020) Evaluation of the changes in exposure to thiol compounds in chronic kidney disease patients using the PBPK model. Xenobiotica 51:31–39
169. Chik Z et al (2014) A bioequivalence comparison of two captopril formulations (25 mg tablets): an open-label, randomized, two-treatment, two-way crossover study in healthy volunteers. J Bioequivalence Bioavailab 6:80
170. Shaw T et al (1985) Plasma free captopril concentrations during short and long term treatment with oral captopril for heart failure. Heart 54:160–165
171. Leithe ME, Margorien RD, Hermiller JB, Unverferth DV, Leier CV (1984) Relationship between central hemodynamics and regional blood flow in normal subjects and in patients with congestive heart failure. Circulation 69:57–64
172. Lee RE, Beard JD, Aldoori MI (1993) Cardiac output and regional flow in health and disease. Springer, pp 505–522
173. Food and Drug Administration, Center for Drug Evaluation and Research (CDER) (2010) Guidance for industry: pharmacokinetics in patients with impaired renal function—study design, data analysis, and impact on dosing and labeling. http://www.fda.gov/downloads/Drugs/GuidanceComplianceRegulatoryInformation/Guidances/UCM204959.pdf. Accessed 10 Aug 2020
174. European Medicines Agency, Committee for Medicinal Products for Human Use (CHMP) (2016) Guideline on the evaluation of the pharmacokinetics of medicinal products in patients with decreased renal function. http://www.ema.europa.eu/docs/en_GB/document_library/Scientific_guideline/2016/02/WC500200841.pdf. Accessed 20 Jul 2020
175. Syed YY (2022) Perindopril/indapamide/amlodipine in hypertension: a profile of its use. Am J Cardiovas Drug 22:219–230. https://doi.org/10.1007/s40256-022-00521-0
176. Williams B, Mancia G, Spiering W et al (2018) 2018 ESC/ESH Guidelines for the management of arterial hypertension. Eur Heart J 39(33):3021–3104
177. National Institute for Health and Care Excellence (2019) Hypertension in adults: diagnosis and management. NICE guideline [NG136]. https://www.nice.org.uk/guidance/ng136. Accessed 14 Sep 2021
178. Unger T, Borghi C, Charchar F et al (2020) 2020 International Society of Hypertension global hypertension practice guidelines. Hypertension 75(6):1334–1357
179. World Health Organization (2021) Guideline for the pharmacological treatment of hypertension in adults. Web Annex A. Summary of evidence. World Health Organization, Geneva. Licence: CC BY-NC-SA 3.0 IGO
180. Pall D, Szanto I, Szabo Z (2014) Triple combination therapy in hypertension: the antihypertensive efficacy of treatment with perindopril, amlodipine, and indapamide SR. Clin Drug Investig 34(10):701–708
181. Tóth K (2014) Antihypertensive efficacy of triple combination perindopril/indapamide plus amlodipine in high-risk hypertensives: results of the PIANIST study (Perindopril-Indapamide plus AmlodipiNe in high rISk hyperTensive patients). Am J Cardiovasc Drugs 14(2):137–145
182. Dezsi CA, Glezer M, Karpov Y et al (2021) Effectiveness of perindopril/indapamide single-pill combination in uncontrolled patients with hypertension: a pooled analysis of the FORTISSIMO, FORSAGE, ACES and PICASSO observational studies. Adv Ther 38(1):479–494

183. Farsang C, Dezsi CA, Brzozowska-Villatte R et al (2021) Beneficial effects of a perindopril/indapamide single-pill combination in hypertensive patients with diabetes and/or obesity or metabolic syndrome: a post hoc pooled analysis of four observational studies. Adv Ther 38(4):1776–1790
184. ALLHAT Officers Coordinators for the ALLHAT Collaborative Research Group (2002) Major outcomes in high-risk hypertensive patients randomized to angiotensin-converting enzyme inhibitor or calcium channel blocker vs diuretic: the Antihypertensive and Lipid-Lowering Treatment to Prevent Heart Attack Trial (ALLHAT). JAMA 288(23):2981–2997
185. Nissen SE, Tuzcu EM, Libby P et al (2004) Effect of antihypertensive agents on cardiovascular events in patients with coronary disease and normal blood pressure: the CAMELOT study: a randomized controlled trial. JAMA 292(18):2217–2225
186. Julius S, Kjeldsen SE, Weber M et al (2004) Outcomes in hypertensive patients at high cardiovascular risk treated with regimens based on valsartan or amlodipine: the VALUE randomised trial. Lancet 363(9426):2022–2031
187. Matheson AJ, Cheer SM, Goa KL (2001) Perindopril/indapamide 2/0.625 mg/day: a review of its place in the management of hypertension. Drugs 61(8):1211–1229
188. Dahlof B, Sever PS, Poulter NR et al (2005) Prevention of cardiovascular events with an antihypertensive regimen of amlodipine adding perindopril as required versus atenolol adding bendroflumethiazide as required, in the Anglo-Scandinavian Cardiac Outcomes Trial-Blood Pressure Lowering Arm (ASCOT-BPLA): a multicentre randomised controlled trial. Lancet 366(9489):895–906
189. Topouchian J, Mourad JJ, De Champvallins M et al (2019) Feasibility of 24-h central blood pressure monitoring: experience from multinational clinical trial assessing the efficacy of perindopril/indapamide/amlodipine. J Hypertens 37(12):2442–2451
190. Netchessova TA, Charnyak SV, Yakubova LV (2018) Effect of perindopril/indapamide/amlodipine fixed-dose combination on peripheral and central hemodynamics and vascular wall stiffness parameters in patients with uncontrolled hypertension. Eur Heart J 39(Suppl 1):397
191. Abraham G, Dezsi CA (2017) The antihypertensive efficacy of the triple fixed combination of perindopril, indapamide, and amlodipine: the results of the PETRA Study. Adv Ther 34(7):1753–1763
192. Mareev VY, Minina YV, Begrambekova YL et al (2020) Therapeutic approaches to the rational use of triple combination therapy with a fixed combination of amlodipine, indapamide and perindopril arginine (TRIPLE COMBINATION) in patients with hypertension who do not control blood pressure on conventional treatment: description and main results of the TRIO program. Kardiologiia 60(5):62–73
193. Logunova N, Khomitskaya Y, Karpov Y et al (2021) Antihypertensive effectiveness and tolerability of perindopril/indapamide/amlodipine triple single-pill combination in the treatment of patients with arterial hypertension (TRICOLOR). J Hypertens 39(Suppl 1):e373
194. Tsioufis K, Douma S, Kallistratos MS et al (2019) Effectiveness and adherence to treatment with perindopril/indapamide/amlodipine single-pill combination in a Greek population with hypertension. Clin Drug Investig 39(4):385–393
195. Thacker H, Konda Reddy KM, Murthy LS et al (2020) Blood-pressure lowering efficacy and safety of perindopril/indapamide/amlodipine single-pill combination in hypertensive patients: phase III trial in India. J Assoc Physicians India 68(10):39–43
196. Popescu L, Balan H (2019) Fixed full-dose combination perindopril/indapamide/amlodipine in severe diabetic hypertensives. J Hypertens 37(Suppl 1):e174
197. Popescu L, Balan H (2018) Low fixed-doses combination perindopril/indapamide/amlodipine-effects in grade 2 hypertensives not adequately controlled. J Hypertens 36(Suppl 1):e152–e153
198. Kobalava ZD, Troitskaya EA, Tolkacheva VV (2018) Combined therapy of arterial hypertension with triple fixed-dose combination of amlodipine/indapamide/perindopril arginine in real clinical practice: the organization and the main results of the DOKAZATEL'STVO (Proof) Study. Kardiologiia 58(9):21–30

199. Koval SM, Snihurska IO, Starchenko TG et al (2019) Efficacy of fixed dose of triple combination of perindopril-indapamide-amlodipine in obese patients with moderate-to-severe arterial hypertension: an open-label 6-month study. Biomed Res Ther 6(11):3501–3512
200. Marazzi G, Pelliccia F, Campolongo G et al (2016) Greater cardiovascular risk reduction with once-daily fixed combination of three antihypertensive agents and statin versus free-drug combination: the ALL-IN-ONE trial. Int J Cardiol 222:885–887
201. Nedogoda SV, Stojanov VJ (2017) Single-pill combination of perindopril/indapamide/amlodipine in patients with uncontrolled hypertension: a randomized controlled trial. Cardiol Ther 6(1):91–104
202. Mourad JJ, Amodeo C, de Champvallins M et al (2017) Blood pressure-lowering efficacy and safety of perindopril/indapamide/amlodipine single-pill combination in patients with uncontrolled essential hypertension: a multicenter, randomized, double-blind, controlled trial. J Hypertens 35(7):1481–1495
203. European Medicines Agency (2019) Triplixam (perindopril arginine/indapamide/amlodipine): summary of product characteristics. http://mri.cts-mrp.eu/download/NL_H_2636_001_FinalSPC.pdf. Accessed 14 Sep 2021
204. Mazza A, Lenti S, Schiavon L et al (2017) Fixed-dose triple combination of antihypertensive drugs improves blood pressure control: from clinical trials to clinical practice. Adv Ther 34(4):975–985
205. Brguljan J, Chazova IE, Gaciong Z et al (2021) PRECIOUS trial confirms safety and efficacy of guideline's single-pill combination strategy. J Hypertens 39(Suppl. 1):e415
206. Abeel M, Gupta A, Constance C (2021) Concomitant treatment of hypertensive patients with bisoprolol and perindopril in routine clinical practice: a post hoc analysis of the CONFIDENCE II, PROTECT I, and PROTECT III observational studies. Adv Ther 39(1):391–404. https://doi.org/10.1007/s12325-021-01958-6
207. Kotseva K, De Backer G, De Bacquer D et al (2019) Lifestyle and impact on cardiovascular risk factor control in coronary patients across 27 countries: results from the European Society of Cardiology ESC-EORP EUROASPIRE V registry. Eur J Prev Cardiol 26(8):824–835
208. CIBIS-II Investigators and Committees (1999) The cardiac insufficiency Bisoprolol Study II (CIBIS-II): a randomised trial. Lancet 353(9146):9–13
209. Montalescot G, Sechtem U, Achenbach S et al (2013) ESC guidelines on the management of stable coronary artery disease: the task force on the management of stable coronary artery disease of the European Society of Cardiology. Eur Heart J 34:2949–3003
210. Tsoukas G, Anand S, Yang K et al (2011) Dose-dependent antihypertensive efficacy and tolerability of perindopril in a large, observational, 12-week, general practice-based study. Am J Cardiovasc Drugs 11(1):45–55
211. Jain S, Boucher D, Chen JSL (2014) Effectiveness of perindopril in the management of hypertension: identification of patient and physician determinants of response to treatment. J Hypertens 32(e-suppl.1):e342
212. Jain S, Birbrager DR, Kumar N, Sampalis J (2014) Effectiveness of a support program designed to sensitize and assist hypertensive patients to decrease their salt consumption. J Hypertens 32(suppl1):e61–e62
213. Ogilvie RI, Anand S, Roy P, De Souza S (2008) Perindopril for control of blood pressure in patients with hypertension and other cardiovascular risk factors: an open-label, observational, multicentre, general practice-based study. Clin Drug Investig 28(11):673–686
214. Wald DS, Law M, Morris JK, Bestwick JP, Wald NJ (2009) Combination therapy vs. monotherapy in reducing blood pressure: meta-analysis on 11,000 participants from 42 trials. Am J Med 122:290–300
215. Neutel JM, Smith DH (2013) Hypertension management: rationale for triple therapy based on mechanisms of action. Cardiovasc Ther 31:251–258
216. Beckett N, Peters R, Fletcher AE, For thc HYVET Study Group et al (2008) Treatment of hypertension in patients 80 years of age or older. N Engl J Med 358:1887–1898

217. Dahlof B, Sever P, Poulter N, For the ASCOT investigators et al (2005) Prevention of cardiovascular events with an antihypertensive regimen of amlodipine adding perindopril as required versus atenolol adding bendroflumethiazide as required, in the Anglo-Scandinavian Cardiac Outcomes Trial-Blood Pressure Lowering Arm (ASCOT-BPLA): a multicentre randomised controlled trial. Lancet 366:895–890
218. Tóth K, Investigators PIANIST (2014) Antihypertensive efficacy of triple combination perindopril/indapamide plus amlodipine in high-risk hypertensives: results of the PIANIST study (Perindopril-Indapamide plus AmlodipiNe in high rISk hyperTensive patients). Am J Cardiovasc Drugs 14:137–145
219. Strauss MH, Hallb AS (2016) The divergent cardiovascular effects of angiotensin converting enzyme inhibitors and angiotensin receptor blockers on myocardial infarction and death. Prog Cardiovasc Dis 58:473–482
220. Lee D-H, Kim M-T, Lee H-W, Han J-H, Myung C-S (2022) The combined effects of telmisartan and ramipril on hypertension and cardiovascular injury. J Pharm Investig 52:443–451. https://doi.org/10.1007/s40005-022-00567-x
221. Elmer PJ, Obarzanek E, Vollmer WM, Simons-Morton D, Stevens VJ, Young DR, Lin PH, Champagne C, Harsha DW, Svetkey LP, Ard J, Brantley PJ, Proschan MA, Erlinger TP, Appel LJ, Group PCR (2006) Effects of comprehensive lifestyle modification on diet, weight, physical fitness, and blood pressure control: 18-month results of a randomized trial. Ann Intern Med 144:485–495
222. Turnbull F, Neal B, Algert C, Chalmers J, Chapman N, Cutler J, Woodward M, Macmahon S. Blood Pressure Lowering Treatment Trialists' Collaboration(2005) Effects of different blood pressure-lowering regimens on major cardiovascular events in individuals with and without diabetes mellitus: results of prospectively designed overviews of randomized trials. Arch Intern Med 165:1410–1419
223. Armario P, Waeber B (2013) Therapeutic strategies to improve control of hypertension. J Hypertens 31(Suppl 1):S9–S12
224. Park HS, Lee DH, Han JH, Jung SH, Lee M, Jang KW, Myung CS (2020) The effects of combined treatment of losartan and ramipril on hypertension and related complications. J Pharm Investig 50:573–581
225. von Lueder TG, Krum H (2013) RAAS inhibitors and cardiovascular protection in large scale trials. Cardiovasc Drugs Ther 27(2):171–179
226. Etyang AO, Kapesa S, Odipo E, Bauni E, Kyobutungi C, Abdalla M et al (2019) Effect of previous exposure to malaria on blood pressure in Kilifi, Kenya: a Mendelian randomization study. J Am Heart Assoc 8(6):e011771
227. Etyang AO, Smeeth L, Cruickshank JK, Scott JAG (2016) The malaria-high blood pressure hypothesis. Circ Res 119(1):36–40
228. Eze IC, Bassa FK, Essé C, Koné S, Acka F, Laubhouet-Koffi V et al (2019) Epidemiological links between malaria parasitaemia and hypertension: findings from a population-based survey in rural Côte d'Ivoire. J Hypertens 37(7):1384–1392
229. Gallego-Delgado J, Walther T, Rodriguez A (2016) The high blood pressure-malaria protection hypothesis. Circ Res 119(10):1071–1075
230. Don-Doncow N, Zhang Y, Matuskova H, Meissner A (2019) The emerging alliance of sphingosine-1-phosphate signalling and immune cells: from basic mechanisms to implications in hypertension. Br J Pharmacol 176(12):1989–2001
231. Nwokocha CR, Bafor EE, Ajayi OI, Ebeigbe AB (2020) The malaria-high blood pressure hypothesis: revisited. Am J Hypertens 33:695–702
232. Raposeiras-Roubin S, Abu-Assi E, Redondo-Dieguez A, Gonzalez-Ferreiro R, Lopez-Lopez A, Bouzas-Cruz N et al (2015) Prognostic benefit of beta-blockers after acute coronary syndrome with preserved systolic function. Still relevant today? Rev Esp Cardiol 68(7):585–591. https://doi.org/10.1016/j.rec.2014.07.028
233. Law MR, Morris JK, Wald NJ (2009) Use of blood pressure lowering drugs in the prevention of cardiovascular disease: meta-analysis of 147 randomised trials in the context of expectations from prospective epidemiological studies. BMJ 338:b1665

234. Zhang H, Yuan X, Zhang H, Chen S, Zhao Y, Hua K et al (2015) Efficacy of long-term beta-blocker therapy for secondary prevention of long-term outcomes after coronary artery bypass grafting surgery. Circulation 131(25):2194–2201
235. Choo EH, Chang K, Ahn Y, Jeon DS, Lee JM, Kim DB et al (2014) Benefit of beta-blocker treatment for patients with acute myocardial infarction and preserved systolic function after percutaneous coronary intervention. Heart 100(6):492–499
236. Brugts JJ, den Uil CA, Danser AHJ et al (2009) The renin-angiotensin-aldosterone system: approaches to guide angiotensin-converting enzyme inhibition in patients with coronary artery disease. Cardiology 112:303–312
237. Brugts JJ, van Vark L, Akkerhuis M et al (2015) Impact of renin-angiotensin system inhibitors on mortality and major cardiovascular endpoints in hypertension: a number-needed-to-treat analysis. Int J Cardiol 181:425–429

Chapter 5
The Effect of ACE Inhibitors Vs. Angiotensin Receptor Blockers on Insulin Resistance in Hypertensive Patients

Mukesh Nandave

Introduction by the Editor

According to the reports and evidence it is concluded that insulin resistance is more than just a metabolic disorder, it is complex multifaceted syndrome that can affect regulation of blood pressure. The dysfunction of neuro-immune and neuro humoral systems plays a significant role in pathophysiology of insulin resistance and hypertension. Insulin resistance is a major contributor for type 2 diabetes, therefore responsible for high number of morbidity and mortality. Insulin resistance prevalence is increasing day by day especially in hypertensive and obese individuals. According to studies, a high number of diabetes mellitus cases are observed in hypertensive patients. To design a more personalized and effective treatment of insulin resistance in hypertensive patients, it is necessary to study the specific mechanism involved in insulin resistance. Alteration in Renin-Angiotensin-Aldosterone System (RAAS) initiates pathophysiology associated with insulin resistance in humans. However, different individuals respond differently to RAAS inhibition in case of insulin resistance. Therefore, understanding differences among individuals in the association between RAAS and insulin resistance could provide valuable information to improve personalized treatment and achieve better outcomes. The mechanism involving the effect of RAAS on glucose metabolism and blood pressure regulation is extensively studied however current advancements in understanding the effect of tissue specific RAAS within adipocytes, skeletal muscle, pancreas, vasculature and heart led to the comprehension how activated tissue RAAS contributes to the insulin resistance and eventually diabetes. Angiotensin II in RAAS is the major component responsible for insulin resistance [1]. However, renin, ACE2 and aldosterone also contribute to the insulin resistance. Clinical trials involving the

M. Nandave (✉)
Department of Pharmacology, Delhi Pharmaceutical Sciences and Research University, New Delhi, Delhi, India

M. Nandave (ed.), *Angiotensin-converting Enzyme Inhibitors vs. Angiotensin Receptor Blockers*, https://doi.org/10.1007/978-981-97-7380-0_5

comparison of ACE inhibitors or ARBs with other anti-hypertensive agents reported that RAAS inhibition significantly improves the insulin sensitivity in comparison to other anti-hypertensive agents [1]. Therefore, it is proved that malfunction in RAAS may lead to insulin resistance. Moreover, other studies reported that long term treatment with ACE inhibitors does not decrease the risk of diabetes in patients with impaired glucose tolerance. Thus, proving that the mechanism involved in hypertension associated insulin resistance is different from those contributing to insulin resistance in diabetes patients.

Angiotensin II acting via angiotensin type 1 receptor (AT1) impaired the insulin action by the production reactive oxygen species (ROS) through NADPH oxidase. ROS is an important intracellular messenger, and their production is associated with angiotensin II linked insulin resistance. These mechanisms may lead to inflammation that interferes with insulin signaling pathways. Molecular abnormalities that lead to insulin resistance include alternations in insulin receptor structure, number, binding or affinity. For example, hyperglycemia associated insulin resistance is also result of ROS generation that inhibits insulin receptor autophosphorylation. Other mechanism that results into insulin signaling pathways inhibition includes kinase induced serine/threonine phosphorylation of insulin receptor and substrate, proteosome facilitated degradation of insulin receptor substrate. Insulin resistance also increased the incidence of hypertension associated complications such as atherosclerosis, left ventricular hypertrophy and chronic kidney disease (CKD). In a study involving experiment on smooth muscle cells from rat thoracic aorta, reported that angiotensin II induces ROS mediated insulin receptor substrate 1 (IRS-1) phosphorylation on Ser307 eventually resulting in proteosome dependent degradation thus reducing the IRS-1 level [2]. Angiotensin associated insulin resistance is also proved by in-vivo study, continuous administration of angiotensin II in rats results into hypertension and decreases the insulin mediated glucose uptake during hyper insulinemic-euglycemic clamp tests and plasma cholesteryl ester hydroperoxide levels was found to be increasing indication increased oxidative stress. However, treatment with tempol, compound mimicking superoxide dismutase restored the levels of cholesteryl ester hydroperoxide and enhanced the insulin sensitivity. This experiment suggested that angiotensin II induced insulin resistance can reversed by reducing the oxidative stress [3, 4].

Clinical trial shows that treatment with Angiotensin Receptor Converting Enzyme (ACE) inhibitor and Angiotensin Receptor blockers (ARBs) improves insulin sensitivity in comparison to other anti-hypertensive agents [1]. It is believed that ACE inhibitors and ARBs provide benefits in hypertensive diabetic patients however it is observed in prior research that these therapies are not consistently prescribed for these patients [5–7].

This chapter explains the comparative efficacy of ACE inhibitors and ARBs on insulin resistance in hypertensive patients. These two classes of drugs targets RAAS but by different mechanism to improve insulin sensitivity (Fig. 5.1).

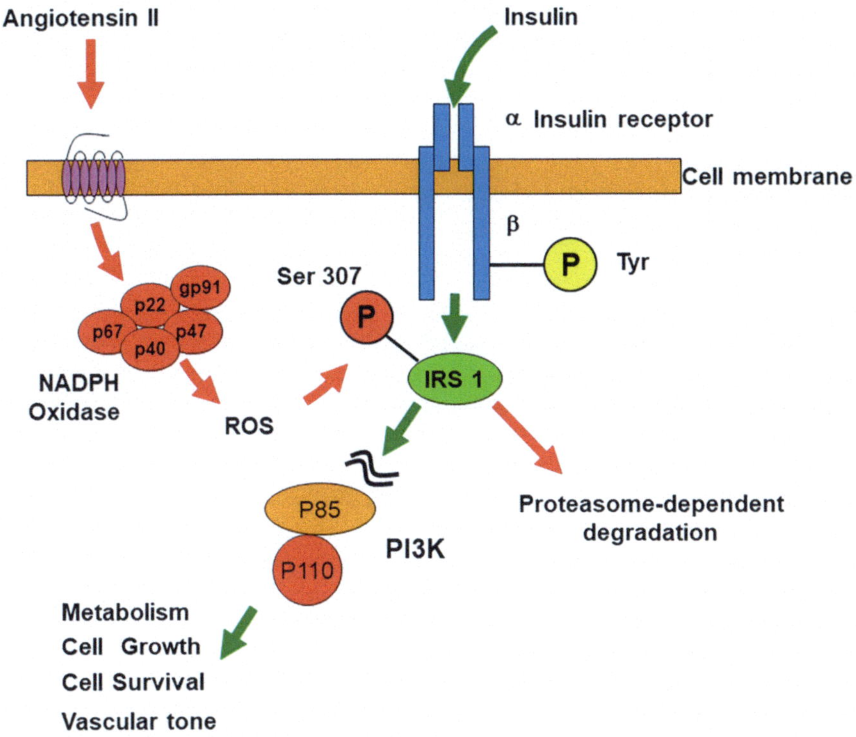

Fig. 5.1 Molecular mechanisms that account for angiotensin II-induced insulin resistance. The binding of insulin to its own receptor evokes the tyrosine autophosphorylation of the β subunit, which, in turn activates, in sequence, the insulin receptor substrate-1 and phosphatidylinositol 3-kinase (green arrows). This cascade, accounts for the biological effects of insulin. Angiotensin II stimulation, through the activation of NADPH oxidase, stimulates the generation of reactive oxygen species, which, in turn promote the threonine phosphorylation of insulin receptor substrate-1 (red arrows). This induces the proteasome-dependent degradation of insulin receptor substrate-1, interrupting the insulin signalling cascade. *Ser* serine, *P* phospho, *Tyr* tyrosine, *ROS* reactive oxygen species, *PI3K* phosphatidylinositol 3-kinase, *IRS-1* insulin receptor substrate-1. (Source: Mancusi et al. [4])

Machine Generated Summaries

Disclaimer: The summaries in this chapter were generated from Springer Nature publications using extractive AI auto-summarization: An extraction-based summarizer aims to identify the most important sentences of a text using an algorithm and uses those original sentences to create the auto-summary (unlike generative AI). As the constituted sentences are machine selected, they may not fully reflect the body of the work, so we strongly advise that the original content is read and cited. The auto generated summaries were curated by the editor to meet Springer Nature publication standards. To cite this content, please refer to the original papers.

Machine generated keywords: insulin, metabolic, insulin resistance, glucose, resistance, type diabete, obesity, combination, diabetic, ccb, substrate, sensitivity, diabetes, beta, dual.

The Renin Angiotensin Aldosterone System and Insulin Resistance in Humans [1]

This is a machine-generated summary of:

Underwood, Patricia C.; Adler, Gail K.: The Renin Angiotensin Aldosterone System and Insulin Resistance in Humans [1].

Published in: Current Hypertension Reports (2012).

Link to original: https://doi.org/10.1007/s11906-012-0323-2

If you want to cite the papers, please refer to the original.

For technical reasons we could not place the page where the original quote is coming from.

Abstract-Summary "Alterations in the renin angiotensin aldosterone system (RAAS) contribute to the underlying pathophysiology of insulin resistance in humans; however, individual differences in the treatment response of insulin resistance to RAAS blockade persist."

"Angiotensin II (ANGII) is the predominant RAAS component contributing to insulin resistance; however, other players such as aldosterone, renin, and ACE2 are also involved."

"This review examines the role of local ANGII activity on insulin resistance development in skeletal muscle, adipocytes, and pancreas, followed by a discussion of the other RAAS components implicated in insulin resistance, including ACE2, Ang1-7, renin, and aldosterone."

Introduction

"The prevalence of insulin resistance is increasing; this is particularly relevant in hypertensive and obese individuals who are at high cardiovascular risk [8, 9]."

"Understanding the specific mechanisms contributing to development of insulin resistance on an individual level is essential for designing more effective and personalized prevention and treatment strategies."

"The renin angiotensin aldosterone system (RAAS) contributes to the underlying pathophysiology of insulin resistance; however, the optimum approaches to target the RAAS for personalized prevention and treatment of insulin resistance are still under debate."

"Blockade of the RAAS has been shown to prevent insulin resistance and type 2 diabetes in some [10–12], but not all, studies [13, 14], suggesting that inter-individual differences contribute to the effects of the RAAS on the development of insulin resistance."

"This review will discuss the pertinent studies linking the RAAS to insulin resistance in humans, and will highlight possible mechanisms for inter-individual differences in the relationship between RAAS and insulin resistance."

Overview of the Renin Angiotensin Aldosterone System

"ANGII exerts physiologic effects through both the angiotensin type 1 receptor (AT_1R) and angiotensin type 2 receptor (AT_2R) in the vasculature, kidney, skeletal muscle, heart, adipocytes, pancreas, and adrenal tissues [15, 16]."

"AT_1R mediated ANGII effects include: 1) vasoconstriction of the vascular smooth muscle cells of the arteriole, 2) sodium retention in the renal proximal tubules, and 3) aldosterone release from the adrenal zonaglomerulosa [17]."

"The effects of the systemic RAAS on blood pressure regulation, glucose metabolism and inflammation have been studied extensively; however, recent discoveries on the influence of local tissue RAAS in the skeletal muscle, heart, vasculature, adipocytes, and pancreas have led to an improved understanding of how activated tissue RAAS influences the development of insulin resistance and diabetes in humans [18]."

"This review examines the role of local ANGII activity on insulin resistance development in skeletal muscle, adipocytes, and pancreas, followed by a discussion of the other RAAS components implicated in insulin resistance, including ACE2, Ang1-7, renin, and aldosterone."

RAAS "Blockade" Insulin Sensitivity and Type 2 Diabetes Mellitus: Large-Scale Human Trials

"Trials comparing the effects of angiotensin-converting-enzyme inhibitor (ACEI) or angiotensin II receptor blocker (ARB) treatment versus other anti-hypertensive medications (hydrochlorothiazide, β-blockers, calcium channel blockers) consistently demonstrate that RAAS blockade results in significant improvements in insulin sensitivity compared to other anti-hypertensive agents [19, 20], raising the possibility that RAAS is involved in the pathophysiology of insulin resistance, and thus the development of type 2 diabetes."

"The lack of consistency between these two large trials is consistent with prior studies evaluating the effects of ACEI or ARB on the development of diabetes in clinical trials where diabetes risk was not the primary endpoint."

"These large-scale human trials demonstrate heterogeneity in the relationship between the RAAS and development of DM, with some studies demonstrating significant benefit of ACEI or ARB therapy."

ANGII Action in Skeletal Muscle

"The effects of ANGII on skeletal muscle glucose uptake is related to 1) alterations in skeletal muscle blood flow, as well as 2) non-hemodynamic effects of ANGII on insulin signaling and insulin stimulated glut-4 glucose uptake [21–23]."

"Animal studies demonstrate that ANGII reduces (and ARB improves) the effects of insulin on both microvascular blood volume and glucose extraction [24]."

"Several human studies confirmed this relationship, demonstrating that ANGII decreases microvascular blood flow to the skeletal muscle and these effects are reversed with ARB administration [25•, 26]."

"Studies demonstrated that the influence of ANGII on insulin signaling and glucose uptake in skeletal muscle cell is independent of the effects of ANGII on blood flow to the muscle [21, 27]."

"Our understanding of the relationship between RAAS and glucose homeostasis is further complicated by early studies examining the effects of an acute ANGII infusion on insulin stimulated glucose uptake, assessed by the euglycemic insulin clamp technique."

Adipose Tissue

"The possibility that a local RAS directly affects adipogenesis, obesity, and insulin resistance in humans was introduced after Karlsson and others [28] demonstrated that angiotensinogen and ACE were present in adipose tissue of obese humans, raising the possibility that ANGII was made locally and could exert local effects on insulin resistance."

"Many human studies have shown that both the local and systemic renin-angiotensin system (RAS) are activated in obese individuals [29, 30] and are associated with insulin resistance."

"One of the effects of the local adipose RAS on insulin resistance is believed to be through increased adipocyte differentiation leading to obesity and insulin resistance [31–36]."

"Goossens and others [32] demonstrated that 26 weeks of valsartan treatment reduced subcutaneous adipose tissue size, decreased markers of adipogenesis (PPARγ) and inflammatory markers (CD68, CD163), and improved adipocyte function in obese humans."

Pancreas

"Below, mechanisms contributing to this association have been clarified, and include direct RAS effects on 1) pancreatic blood flow, 2) insulin secretion, and 3) inflammation and pancreatic fibrosis [18, 37]."

"Direct ANGII infusion to the pancreas led to reduced whole pancreatic and islet blood flow in rats; effects that were reversed with ARB administration [38]."

"Recent studies in both animal models and humans provide strong support for a direct role of ANGII on insulin secretion."

"ANGII administration decreased insulin secretion in isolated mouse pancreatic beta cells in a dose dependent manner [39]."

"In animal models, ANGII infusion decreased insulin secretion [40] and ARB administration improved insulin secretion in response to western diet and glucose supplementation [34, 41]."

"26 weeks of treatment with the ARB valsartan led to improvements in both phase 1 and phase 2 insulin secretion when compared with placebo controls [11]."

Non-ANGII Factors

"Heretofore, we have discussed the negative relationship between the ACE/ANGII/AT_1R axis and insulin resistance demonstrating that increases in ANGII activity lead to alterations in: 1) insulin signaling and glucose uptake, 2) insulin secretion, and 3) inflammation which portend the development of insulin resistance."

"Understanding the interplay between ANGII and ACE2 in the development of insulin resistance has led to an investigation of the effects of treatment of either the ACE/ANGII/AT1R or ACE2/Ang1-7/MAS receptor axis abnormalities."

"Blockade of the mineralocorticoid receptor (spironolactone), but not AT1R blockade (irbesartan), improved chlorthalidone-induced insulin resistance in hypertensive individuals, suggesting a causative relationship between activated mineralocorticoid receptor, increased aldosterone, and greater levels of insulin resistance [42]."

"Closer examination of the mechanism underlying the relationship between renin inhibition and improved insulin sensitivity found that aliskiren treatment led to improvements in systemic insulin resistance and improved insulin signaling and glucose uptake in skeletal muscle in a rat model of RAAS activation (TG(mRen2)27) [43]."

Genetics

"Human genetic studies examining the relationship between RAAS candidate gene variants and insulin resistance provides some insight into the observed inter-individual differences between altered RAAS physiology and insulin resistance discussed thus far."

"Variants within two RAAS candidate genes, ACE and AGT, consistently demonstrate a relationship with insulin resistance [44, 45•], suggesting that a subgroup of individuals are at increased risk for insulin resistance secondary to alterations in the RAAS."

"Analyzing variants of genes in a more homogeneous subset of individuals (i.e., an intermediate phenotype), pooling the results of these studies using meta-analysis, or evaluating the effects of other genes that regulate the expression of the AGT gene, ACE gene, or the RAAS may provide clarification on the role of genes and the RAAS on the development of insulin resistance."

Conclusion

"The studies described in this review clearly delineate a relationship between the RAAS and insulin resistance in humans."

"Since the randomized control trials that evaluated the outcomes of RAAS blockade on insulin resistance and type 2 diabetes often have conflicting results, it is important for us to understand the basic pathophysiologic mechanisms underlying the relationship between the RAAS and insulin resistance."

"Further, genetic studies demonstrate that some individuals are predisposed to an increased risk for altered RAAS activity and insulin resistance."

"Identifying those individuals at greatest risk for altered RAAS and insulin resistance and targeting them with personalized treatment with RAAS blockade would likely result in more consistent results in evaluating the relationship between RAAS blockade and altered glucose metabolism."

"Understanding this relationship is important when prescribing anti-hypertensive medications in those at risk for insulin resistance."

Insulin Resistance: An Additional Risk Factor in the Pathogenesis of Cardiovascular Disease in Type 2 Diabetes [46]

This is a machine-generated summary of:

Patel, Tushar P.; Rawal, Komal; Bagchi, Ashim K.; Akolkar, Gauri; Bernardes, Nathalia; Dias, Danielle da Silva; Gupta, Sarita; Singal, Pawan K.: Insulin resistance: an additional risk factor in the pathogenesis of cardiovascular disease in type 2 diabetes [46].

Published in: Heart Failure Reviews (2015).

Link to original: https://doi.org/10.1007/s10741-015-9515-6

If you want to cite the papers, please refer to the original.

For technical reasons we could not place the page where the original quote is coming from.

Abstract-Summary "Obesity plays a central role in occurrence of various diseases like hyperinsulinemia, hyperglycemia and hyperlipidemia, which lead to insulin resistance and metabolic derangements like cardiovascular diseases (CVDs) mediated by oxidative stress."

"Insulin resistance (IR) leads to micro or macro angiopathy, peripheral arterial dysfunction, hampered blood flow, hypertension, as well as the cardiomyocyte and the endothelial cell dysfunctions, thus increasing risk factors for coronary artery blockage, stroke and heart failure suggesting that there is a strong association between IR and CVDs."

"The plausible linkages between these two pathophysiological conditions are altered levels of insulin signaling proteins such as IR-β, IRS-1, PI3K, Akt, Glut4 and PGC-1α that hamper insulin-mediated glucose uptake as well as other functions of insulin in the cardiomyocytes and the endothelial cells of the heart."

"It evidently becomes important to unravel the mechanisms of the association between IR and CVDs in order to formulate novel efficient drugs to treat patients suffering from insulin resistance-mediated cardiovascular diseases."

"The possible associations between insulin resistance and cardiovascular diseases are reviewed here."

Introduction

"In diabetic patients, 65% of the deaths are listed due to CVD [47]."

"Several hypothesis such as hyperglycemia, oxidative stress, inflammation, obesity, sedentary life style, genetic predisposition etc have emerged to connect the dots between diabetes and CVD."

"In aggressive conventional therapy for diabetes the risk of CVD is reduced by about 42%."

"A high-quality management of diabetes alone does not explain the high incidence of CVD in these patients."

"One of the overlooked links that is common in type 2 diabetic patients is the occurrence of insulin resistance (IR)."

Pathophysiology of Cardiovascular Diseases in Diabetes

"Persistent hyperglycemia causes microvascular and macrovascular complications in both type 1 and type 2 diabetes."

"Some of the main etiological factors for CVD are as follows: Much of the enduring pathology of diabetes occurs as a consequence of persistent hyperglycemia leading to increased reactive oxygen species (ROS) production by mitochondria, which is the main source of oxidative stress involving complications of diabetic pathologies including CVD [47–49]."

"In type 1 diabetes, endothelial dysfunction is an essential determinant of inflammatory activities and considered as an early CVD marker."

"It is reported that approximately 10–30% type 1 diabetic and 60% type 2 diabetics suffer from hypertension and thus high risk of CVD."

"EURODIAB study reported that poor glycemic control is strong risk factor for CAN which is the predictor of CVD morbidity and mortality in type 1 diabetes [50]."

"All the above factors play an important role in diabetes related CVD risk."

Molecular Mechanism of Insulin Resistance

"Muscle, adipose and liver are the most affected organs due to overload of lipid accumulation and thus, lead to peripheral insulin resistance [51]."

"Free fatty acids (FFA) circulate and deposit into the skeletal muscle myocytes and intramuscular lipid accumulation occurs, which further aggravates the insulin resistance condition by downregulating the expression as well as reducing total insulin receptor number [52]."

"The later, activates NFκB-mediated cellular toxicity by activating various PKCs and downregulating tyrosine phosphorylation of insulin receptors."

"Insulin resistance can also be due to an increase in the activity as well as amount of the enzymes that normally reverse insulin action, including the phosphotyrosine phosphatases, e.g., PTP1b, and the PIP phosphatases, e.g., PTEN and SHIP."

"All these events lead to a concomitant reduction in insulin stimulated glycogen synthesis and glucose uptake which leads to activation of the phosphoenolpyruvate carboxykinase, the rate limiting enzyme of gluconeogenesis."

Mechanism of Oxidative Stress in Diabetes and Insulin Resistance

"These include the activation of polyol pathway, glucose auto oxidation, formation of advanced glycation end (AGEs) products, increased FFA, leptin levels and increased mitochondrial ROS generation [49, 53]."

"Ketoaldehyde, protein reactive dicarbonyl sugar, is a product of glucose autoxidation and a member of AGE, which not only yields H_2O_2 but also the other highly reactive oxidants that become an important source of diabetes mellitus (DM)-induced oxidative stress [49]."

"Oxidative stress increases with age as well as severity of DM, which stimulates Maillard reaction where these dicarbonyl intermediates attach non-enzymatically to protein amino-structures generating ROS which can promote oxidation of glycation products leading to AGE formation, AGEs precursors can further bind to AGE receptors on the surface of endothelial cells and macrophages resulting in receptor-mediated production of oxygen free radicals and dysregulating their functions [54, 55]."

Association of IR and CVD

"It has been observed that the hypertensive patients have higher fasting and post-prandial insulin levels than normal subjects [56]."

"Hyperfibrinogenemia is a powerful independent risk factor for CVD caused by elevated levels of fibrinogen, which have also been observed in the insulin-resistant state [57, 58]."

"Further, abatement of insulin-mediated glucose uptake and decrease in insulin stimulated blood flow has been observed in insulin-resistant obese patients."

"In more specific vascular studies, it was observed that in insulin-resistant obese patients the ability of insulin to decrease aortic wave reflection was severely blunted, as determined from augmentation index."

"This defect was a consequence of impaired insulin action, as it was not observed in the basal state suggesting that IR extends to large conduit vessels as well as to vessels regulating peripheral blood flow thereby increasing the risk toward cardiovascular diseases [59–61]."

Inflammatory Responses in Obesity, IR and CVD

"IR in hyperinsulinemia, hypertension, hyperlipidemia leads to type 2 DM, and an increased risk of atherosclerotic CVDs are the adverse effects of central obesity [62]."

"Various bioactive compounds released by adipose tissue provoke IR, alterations in lipids, coagulation, fibrinolysis, inflammation that leads to endothelial dysfunction and atherosclerosis [63]."

"Excess of adipose tissue expansion and hypoxic conditions activate inflammatory responses that secrete various pro-inflammatory cytokines."

"Netrin-1 is responsible for retention of macrophages into adipose tissue via Unc5b receptor and hence leads to increased IR in obesity [64]."

"Infiltration of macrophages into adipose tissue leads to expansion of the tissue causing chronic low-grade inflammation."

"Elevated central obesity is associated with worsened cardiovascular risk profiles, IR, hyperlipidemia, increasing the influx of FFA into cardiomyocytes."

"Various NADPH oxidases (NOXs) present in macrophages are responsible for generation of ROS in adipose tissue which aids in cardiovascular diseases [65]."

Interplay of Fat Cells Macrophages, Endothelial Cells in IR and CVD

"As explained in the earlier section, adipose tissue harbors two types of macrophages of which M1-macrophages is predominant in obesity, secreting TNF-α and IL-6 thereby enhancing inflammation [66]."

"Macrophage-derived TNF-α activates adipocytes, thereby further inducing lipolysis and enhancing the expression of various genes [intracellular adhesion molecule-1 (ICAM-1), IL-6, macrophage chemo attractant protein-1 (MCP-1)]."

"Endothelial cells are crucial target during diabetes and whole body IR because of obesity and adipocyte inflammation which leads to a reduction in NO synthesis."

"The fat cell macrophages that are hyperactivated during obesity in addition to inflammation initiate the whole body IR."

Cross-Talk of Signaling Pathways in Development of IR in the Heart

"Insulin signaling is a complex cascade wherein, the effector signaling proteins like IRS-(1/2)/PI3K/Akt have various downstream substrates, potentially activated by insulin thus, depicting varied biological roles of insulin."

"LCFA uptake in cardiomyocytes occurs through insulin stimulated activation of PI3K and then translocation of the LCFA transporter FAT/CD36 to the plasma membrane [67]."

"Insulin functions as an important vasodilator by stimulating increased production of the potent vasodilator NO from vascular endothelium through the activation of eNOS by PI3K/PKB/Akt pathway [68]."

"Angiotensin II, a component of renin-angiotensin system (RAS) via stimulation of the angiotensin II, type I receptor (AT1R) activates JNK and MAP-kinase pathways, leading to increased serine phosphorylation of IRS-1 and 2 proteins ultimately inhibiting PI3K signaling and further causing deleterious effects [69]."

"Impaired mitochondrial oxidative phosphorylation (OXPHO) and mitochondrial biogenesis contributes to an inhibition of insulin metabolic signaling [70]."

IR Related to CVDs and Potential Therapeutic Approaches

"Mitochondrial function and insulin sensitivity can be improved by increased expression of UCP2/3 or decrease in ROS production by antioxidants [71]."

"Adjustment of insulin signaling can also be done by using thiazolidinediones and metformin–insulin sensitizers, which are reported to reduce ROS production, increase expression of PGC-1α, and stimulate AMPK, thus improving mitochondrial function by reducing oxidative stress and stimulating mitochondrial biogenesis [71]."

"Adiponectin directly stimulates the production of NO from vascular endothelium using a PI3-kinase-dependent signaling mechanism similar to that of insulin, thus opposing atherogenesis and improve endothelial function [72]."

"Pharmacological inhibitors such as angiotensin-converting enzyme (ACE) inhibitors reduce circulating angiotensin II levels, and angiotensin receptor blockers (ARBs) block the actions of angiotensin II ultimately helping in lowering of blood pressure, improving endothelial function and reduce circulating markers of inflammation, augmentation of insulin stimulated glucose uptake."

Conclusions

"The complex interplay of IR and CVD has been studied extensively to elucidate the mechanistic pathway underlying the pathogenesis of the disease."

"The major causes of IR are hyperglycemia, oxidative stress and dyslipidemia which present as risk factors for CVD."

"Drugs regulating type 2 DM and hyperlipidemia have side effects associated with CVD and associated complications suggesting potential dual links between IR, type 2 DM and CVD at the molecular level."

"Given the serious consequences of the global CVD epidemic, understanding of the mechanisms that link IR with the development of CVD and comorbidities should be considered as a high priority in further research."

Insulin Resistance the Hinge Between Hypertension and Type 2 Diabetes [73]

This is a machine-generated summary of:

Mancusi, Costantino; Izzo, Raffaele; di Gioia, Giuseppe; Losi, Maria Angela; Barbato, Emanuele; Morisco, Carmine: Insulin Resistance the Hinge Between Hypertension and Type 2 Diabetes [73].

Published in: High Blood Pressure & Cardiovascular Prevention (2020).

Link to original: https://doi.org/10.1007/s40292-020-00408-8

If you want to cite the papers, please refer to the original.

For technical reasons we could not place the page where the original quote is coming from.

Abstract-Summary "Insulin resistance is defined as a less than expected biologic response to a given concentration of the hormone and plays a pivotal role in the pathogenesis of diabetes."

"The dysregulation of neuro-humoral and neuro-immune systems is involved in the pathophysiology of both insulin resistance and hypertension."

"These mechanisms induce a chronic low grade of inflammation that interferes with insulin signalling transduction."

"Molecular abnormalities associated with insulin resistance include the defects of insulin receptor structure, number, binding affinity, and/or signalling capacity."

"Hyperglycaemia impairs insulin signalling through the generation of reactive oxygen species, which abrogate insulin-induced tyrosine autophosphorylation of the insulin receptor."

"Insulin resistance plays a key role also in the pathogenesis and progression of hypertension-induced target organ damage, like left ventricular hypertrophy, atherosclerosis and chronic kidney disease."

Essential Hypertension and Type 2 Diabetes the Link

"In women only established hypertension significantly increased the risk of T2D. Although these studies clearly demonstrated the link between hypertension and T2D, they lacked of rigorous criteria to diagnosis T2D, since in many cases the diagnosis was based on self-reported incident diabetes."

"We extended these epidemiological data demonstrating that in a cohort of hypertensives, those with an uncontrolled hypertension had a higher risk of developing T2D. In particular, in nondiabetic hypertensive subjects, uncontrolled BP was associated with twofold increased risk of incident T2D independently of age, body mass index (BMI), baseline BP, or fasting glucose [74]."

"The strong association between hypertension and diabetes has been further documented by the evidence that patients with essential hypertension and concomitant hypertension-related target organ damage (TOD), such as left ventricular hypertrophy (LVH)end/or carotid atherosclerosis (CA), are at higher risk of incident T2D, compared to those without TOD."

Insulin Resistance and Hypertension

"Molecular and pathophysiological mechanisms underlying the reciprocal relationship between insulin resistance and hypertension result in a vicious cycle which reinforces the link between metabolic and hemodynamic disorders."

"Insulin resistance affects negatively myocardial energetic efficiency in hypertensive patients [75] and in unselected population [76]."

"The association between hypertension, insulin resistance, and resultant hyperinsulinemia is well documented [77]."

"The association of insulin resistance and essential hypertension does not occur in secondary hypertension [78]."

"These data suggest the existence of a common genetic pathway for essential hypertension and insulin resistance, a concept that is also supported by the finding of altered glucose metabolism in normotensive offspring of hypertensive patients [79]."

"Insulin resistance state is characterized by lower expression levels and impaired translocation of GLUT 4."

"Mitochondrial dysfunction, which also plays a key role in the genesis of insulin resistance, is affected by epigenetic modifications."

Insulin Resistance Directly Affects Blood Pressure Control

"In healthy subjects, insulin evokes a net reflex in sympathetic outflow and at the same time it blunts the vasoconstrictive effect resulting from this sympathetic activation."

"In hypertensive patients insulin evokes a sympathetic activation that is three times greater than in normal subjects, and moreover its vaso-relaxant action is impaired [80]."

"Insulin resistance and the resultant hyperinsulinemia are involved in the development of hypertension-related TOD, through the abnormalities of the counter-regulatory effects of insulin."

Molecular Mechanisms of Insulin Resistance

"The binding of insulin to the α subunit of its receptor activates the tyrosine kinase of the β subunit of the receptor, leading to autophosphorylation, as well as tyrosine phosphorylation of several IR substrates (IRS), including IRS-1 and IRS-2 [81]."

"Abnormalities of the IR function that may contribute to insulin resistance include the defects of receptor structure, number, binding affinity, and/or its signalling capacity."

"Phosphorylation of IRS-1 on Ser307 results in its dissociation from the IR and triggers proteasome-dependent degradation, also impairing insulin signalling."

"The mechanistic role of abnormalities of IR or IRS-1 signalling in the pathogenesis of insulin resistance and hypertension is supported by several pioneering studies performed in genetically engineered mice."

"The results of these studies demonstrate that the abnormalities of IR or IRS signalling play a mechanistic role in the development of hypertension, independently form glucose homeostasis and plasma insulin levels, and indicate that insulin resistance by itself is involved the pathogenesis of hypertension."

Insulin Resistance and Neuro-hormonal Activities in Hypertension

"The key role of ROS in the pathogenesis of Ang II-induced insulin resistance has been also confirmed by in vivo studies."

"In rats chronic infusion of Ang II induced hypertension and reduced insulin-evoked glucose uptake during hyperinsulinemic-euglycemic clamp, and increased plasma cholesterylester hydroperoxide levels, indicating an increased oxidative stress."

"In the endothelial cells, Ang II induces insulin resistance through the phosphorylation of IRS-1 at Ser312 and Ser616 via JNK- and ERK1/2-dependent mechanisms, respectively."

"It has been documented that increased sympathetic tone resulting in an abnormal stimulation of β-ARs, is able to induce insulin resistance through the activation of different serine/threonine kinases that blunt insulin signal by phosphorylating IR or IRS-1."

"β-ARs stimulation results in an impairment of insulin signalling and insulin-induced glucose uptake, which profoundly differs between the two cell types regarding the kinetic and molecular mechanisms involved."

Insulin Resistance and Hypertension Related Target Organ Damage

"LVH, CA, and renal dysfunction are expression of hypertension-evoked TOD, and are independent risk factors for both fatal and nonfatal cardio- and cerebro-vascular events [82–86].Several studies have shown that insulin resistance promotes the development of left ventricular hypertrophy, carotid atherosclerosis and chronic kidney disease (CKD)."

"The production of NO by endothelial cells, stimulated by insulin or insulin-like growth factor, leads to a host of anti-inflammatory and antithrombotic effects, which are antiatherogenic."

"The TNF-α gene locus seems to be involved in insulin resistance-associated hypertension [87]."

"TNF-α also determines endothelial dysfunction linked to insulin resistance [88]."

"Insulin resistance is associated with activation of both renin-angiotensin system and sympathetic nervous system activities, contributing to increased renal sodium reabsorption, associated fluid retention and hypertension [89]."

"These changes in combination with the raise in BP levels associated with the insulin-resistant state increase the tubular reabsorption and maintain sodium balance."

Conclusions

"These data encourage the adoption of a holistic strategy to prevent the development of insulin resistance."

"It is noteworthy that consistent body of evidence supports the notion that exercise training is able to modify the epigenetics changes that are involved in the development of insulin resistance [90]."

"The dysregulation of renin-angiotensin system plays a pivotal role in the development of insulin resistance; thus, the prevention of incident T2D in patients with hypertension requires the inhibition of RAS with AT1 antagonist or ACE inhibitors [91]."

"The prevention of the insulin resistance-induced continuum of CV disease requires an integrated approach which involves non pharmacologic and pharmacologic therapies."

Interactions Between Diabetic and Hypertensive Drugs: A Pharmacogenetics Approach [92]

This is a machine-generated summary of:

Ansari, Asma Imran; Rizvi, Aliya Abbas; Verma, Shrikant; Abbas, Mohammad; Siddiqi, Zeba; Mishra, Divakar; Verma, Sushma; Raza, Syed Tasleem; Mahdi, Farzana: Interactions between diabetic and hypertensive drugs: a pharmacogenetics approach [92].

Published in: Molecular Genetics and Genomics (2023).

Link to original: https://doi.org/10.1007/s00438-023-02011-7

If you want to cite the papers, please refer to the original.

For technical reasons we could not place the page where the original quote is coming from.

Abstract-Summary "The polytherapy might lead to several drug–drug interactions (DDIs), which cause certain life-threatening complications such as diabetic nephropathy and hypoglycaemia."

"In this review we focused on drug–drug interactions and impact of genetic factors on drug responses for better disease management."

"Drug–drug interactions (DDIs) may act either synergistically or antagonistically."

"A combination of metformin with angiotensin II receptor antagonist or angiotensin-converting enzyme inhibitors (ACEIs) synergistically improves glucose absorption, whereas the same hypertensive drug combination with sulphonylurea might cause severe hypoglycaemia sometimes."

"All of these findings established a connection between drug–drug interaction and genetics, which might be used for effective disease management."

Introduction

"According to the American Diabetes Association (ADA), different classes of medications reduce blood glucose levels in various ways and are thus used as antidiabetic drugs."

"Moving forward, the American Diabetes Association (ADA) has recommended that both angiotensin-converting enzyme inhibitors (ACEIs) and angiotensin receptor blockers (ARBs) be used as a first-line therapy for hypertension in diabetic patients."

"A high blood glucose level activates RAAS and increases angiotensin II levels."

"Other people metabolize drugs so quickly that after they take a usual dose, the drug levels in the blood never become high enough for the drug to be effective."

"This review aims to illuminate the role of genetic factors involved in the drug metabolism of both antihypertensive and antidiabetic drugs and their interaction (DDI) to form a qualitative as well as a quantitative framework for well-suited combination therapy and dosing regimen."

Pharmaceutical Interactions in Polytherapy

"These include diverse pharmacokinetic (PK) and pharmacodynamic (PD) interactions."

"PK describes a drug's absorption, distribution, metabolism, and excretion properties (known as ADME), whereas PD describes how biological processes in the body respond to or are impacted by a drug (Palleria and others [93])."

"In the simplest terms, pharmacokinetics is what the body does to the drug and pharmacodynamics is what the drug does to the body."

[Section 3]

"Histamine receptor H_2 blocker, which reduces the amount of acid produced by the body, when given together with the hypoglycaemic drug tolbutamide and antihypertensive drug class beta-blockers, facilitates its absorption (Palleria and others [93])."

"Metoclopramide, for example, can help to speed up the emptying of the stomach and also limit the amount of time that a drug is in contact with the mucosal area where it is absorbed, causing less drug absorption (Custodio and others [94])."

"Emergence of complexes: In this instance, tetracyclines (such as doxycycline or minocycline) in the digestive tract may interact with metal ions (such as calcium, magnesium, aluminium, or iron) to produce complexes that are ineffectively absorbed."

"A number of medications, including antacids, magnesium salt preparations, aluminium, and calcium preparations containing iron can significantly reduce the absorption of tetracyclines (Palleria and others [93])."

[Section 4]

"Additivity is the term used when the overall effect of a drug is the sum of the pharmacological effects."

"Synergy exists when the combined effects of the drugs are more than additive."

"Antagonism occurs when the combined effects of the drugs are less than additive."

"An example of an antagonist effect is when ACE inhibitors combined with thiazide diuretics can cause hypotension and over-the-top diuresis."

Antidiabetic and Antihypertensive Drug–Drug Interactions

"Hypertension in diabetic patients increases the risk of cardiovascular problems significantly, and these two disorders together predispose to coronary artery diseases (Lago and others [95])."

"In an effort to achieve the desired blood pressure and normal blood glucose level in good time, more than one therapy is needed."

"Since diabetes is associated with severe comorbidities, some DDIs between antihypertensive and antidiabetic drugs are perhaps the reason behind it."

"By comprehending the mechanics of medications and the elements that contribute to them, we can forecast and probably halt these harmful interactions."

[Section 6]

"Metformin targets the AMP-activated protein kinase (AMPK) pathway to carry out its whole activity."

"Active AMPK acts on glucose uptake pathway by inhibiting a protein TBC1 domain family member 1 (TBC1D1)."

"This protein prevents glucose uptake by inhibiting glucose transporter 4 (GLUT4) translocation in insulin-sensitive cells, i.e., adipose tissues, heart, and muscle cells."

"Metformin inhibits TBC1D1, thereby activating GLUT4 induced glucose transport (Hernandez and others [96])."

"This action stimulates GLUT4, in response, to an enhancement in glucose uptake in insulin-sensitive tissues (Berger and others [97])."

[Section 7]

"Uehara and others found that ACE inhibitors causes a significant increase in plasma bradykinin concentrations in T2DM patient (Uehara and others [98])."

"Since metformin also stimulates glucose uptake through GLUT4, ACE inhibitor treatment may affect T2DM individuals in positive ways as mentioned in certain studies (Custodio and others [94])."

"Zou and others [99] studied two genes, ACE I/D [insertion/deletion (I/D) genotypes of a 287-bp Alu repeat] and bradikinin type 2 receptor gene (BDKRB2) + 9/−9 bp [insertion or deletion of 9 base pairs from the BDKRB2 gene] in the Chinese population."

"They found genotypic combination (ACE I/D and BDKRB2 genes i.e., ACE II -B2R+ 9 bp, ACE DD -B2R + 9 bp, or ACE DD-B2R -9 bp), were associated with worsening of diabetic nephropathy, including oxidative damage, mitochondrial dysfunction, inflammatory responses, glomerular lesions, and collagen buildup in the renal tissues (Zou and others [99])."

[Section 8]

"Sulphonylureas are the insulin secretagogues which increase insulin sensitivity, leading to regulation of glucose level."

"Sulphonylurea acts by binding to its receptor called sulphonylurea receptor SUR-1."

"This levels up calcium in the cell and results in subsequent insulin release."

"Inhibition of angiotensinogen II downstream the effects of the angiotensin II type 1(AT1) receptor and the angiotensin II type 2 (AT2) receptor results in salt and water retention, cell proliferation, and vasoconstriction (Schinner and others [100])."

"ACE inhibitors cause a significant increase in plasma bradykinin concentrations (Uehara and others [98])."

"Another Brazilian study by de Oliveira Alvim and others [101], showed that reduced transcriptional activity of B2 receptor of bradykinin receptor gene BDKRB2 was conferred by + 9 allele carrier individuals compared to those who were −9 allele carriers and it was associated with lower bradykinin activity as well as reduced glucose uptake."

[Section 9]

"Rosiglitazone (TZD class of antidiabetic drug) is an agonist of the PPAR-γ, which is found in insulin-dependent glucose-requiring tissues and causes insulin sensitization (Young and others [102])."

"A study discovered that telmisartan, when administered orally, decreased glucose, insulin, and lipid levels in their study on rats fed a high-fat and high-carbohydrate diet (Schoonjans and others [103])."

"When a telmisartan dose of approximately 80 mg/day was administered to that patient, hypertension was relieved, insulin resistance was decreased, and blood glucose levels were normalized."

"Plasma triglyceride levels decreased, suggesting that telmisartan may have impacts on insulin sensitivity and triglyceride levels because of its capacity to activate PPARγ (Pershadsingh and Kurtz and others [104])."

"The PPARγ agonists, rosiglitazone and pioglitazone, which are extensively used antidiabetic drugs, are limited by their proclivity for causing fluid retention, peripheral oedema, and heart failure, especially in patients on insulin (Sunder and others [105]; White and others [106])."

[Section 10]

"Segment 1 of proximal convoluted tubule of the kidneys expresses sodium–glucose co-transporter-2 (SGLT2) proteins."

"Sodium–glucose co-transporter-2 inhibitors (SGLT2Is) reduce plasma glucose levels in an insulin-independent manner and lower the risk of hypoglycaemia by preventing significant reabsorption of glucose and increasing urine glucose and sodium excretion (Abdul and others [107]) ."

"SGLT2 also significantly affects osmotic diuresis and natriuresis, causing a decrease in blood pressure."

"Inhibition of Sodium-Potassium-Chloride Cotransporters (NKCC2) causes low reabsorption of sodium chloride renal proximal tubule."

"A study by Karg and others [108], in Germany, stated that 6 weeks of SGLT2 inhibitor treatment in type 2 diabetic individuals reduces tissue sodium and water concentration."

[Section 11]

"In diabetic individuals, the use of beta-adrenergic blocking medications may have adverse effects (Prudente and others [109])."

"During concurrent treatment of glipizide (sulphonylurea) with propranolol (beta-blocker) on albino diabetic rats reveals that repeated injection of propranolol considerably boosted the hypoglycaemic activity of glipizide (Parameshappa and others [110]) ."

"In both healthy and diabetic animals, non-selective beta-blockers can postpone the restoration of insulin-induced low blood sugar levels."

"A study in individuals with essential hypertension found that cilnidipine (CCB) increased the glucose infusion rate (GIR) (Yagi and others [111])."

"Another finding stated that high-fat diet-fed mice with a defective N-type calcium channel had higher glucose tolerance and lower insulin levels than wild-type mice (Takahashi and others [112])."

"These investigations led us to the conclusion that CCBs and beta-blockers may occasionally induce severe hypoglycaemia and other harmful effects."

Conclusion and Future Prospects

"Use of angiotensin II receptor antagonists (ACEIs) in diabetic patients taking metformin led to enhanced glucose absorption resulting in better hyperglycaemia control."

"Angiotensin II receptor blockers sometimes show side effects in patients prescribed second-line antidiabetic drugs such as sulfonylureas and TDZs."

"In case of TZDs, angiotensin II receptor antagonist neutralizes these side effects."

"Diabetic patients with any type of cardiovascular disease should be prescribed a combination of SGLT2 inhibitors and ACEIs."

"We uncovered the favourable and adverse effect of polytherphy and provide manageable drug combination, which might be able to raise the living standards for diseased individuals."

Combined Angiotensin Receptor Modulation in the Management of Cardio-Metabolic Disorders [113]

This is a machine-generated summary of:

Paulis, Ludovit; Foulquier, Sébastien; Namsolleck, Pawel; Recarti, Chiara; Steckelings, Ulrike Muscha; Unger, Thomas: Combined Angiotensin Receptor Modulation in the Management of Cardio-Metabolic Disorders [113].

Published in: Drugs (2015).

Link to original: https://doi.org/10.1007/s40265-015-0509-4

If you want to cite the papers, please refer to the original.

For technical reasons we could not place the page where the original quote is coming from.

Abstract-Summary "Cardiovascular and metabolic disorders, such as hypertension, insulin resistance, dyslipidemia or obesity are linked with chronic low-grade inflammation and dysregulation of the renin–angiotensin system (RAS)."

"RAS inhibition by ACE inhibitors or angiotensin AT1 receptor (AT1R) blockers is the evidence-based standard for cardiovascular risk reduction in high-risk patients, including diabetics with albuminuria."

"A concept of dual AT1R/AT2R modulation emerges as a putative means for risk reduction in cardio-metabolic diseases."

"The approach employing simultaneous RAS blockade (AT1R) and RAS stimulation (AT2R) is distinct from previous attempts of double intervention in the RAS by dual blockade."

"Dual blockade abolishes the AT1R-linked RAS almost completely with subsequent risk of hypotension and hypotension-related events, i.e. syncope or renal dysfunction."

"To dual RAS blockade, the add-on of AT2R stimulation does not exert significant blood pressure effects, but it may complement and enhance the anti-inflammatory and antifibrotic/de-stiffening effects of the AT1R blockade and improve the metabolic profile."

Introduction

"Cardiovascular mortality remains high world-wide."

"Cardiovascular morbidity and mortality are strongly determined by the presence of metabolic alterations such as different pro-thrombotic states, dyslipidemia, obesity and insulin resistance (with or without its overt clinical manifestation), which are clinically grouped in the metabolic syndrome."

"The cardio-metabolic syndrome, depending on the definition, usually features at least three of the following dysregulations: obesity (or central obesity), dyslipidemia [hypertriglyceridemia or low high-density lipoprotein (HDL) levels], hypertension or impaired glucose metabolism (impaired fasting glucose, insulin resistance, hyperinsulinemia or diabetes mellitus), while the World Health Organization adds microalbuminuria as a criterion as well [114]."

"Insulin resistance blunts the vasodilator effects of insulin, and chronic hyperinsulinemia increases sympathetic nervous activity, reduces natriuresis, promotes vascular smooth muscle growth, endothelial dysfunction and hypertriglyceridemia with subsequent atherosclerosis, hypertension and vascular events such as myocardial infarction, stroke or peripheral arterial occlusion disease [115]."

Behind the Scenes: Pathophysiological Considerations

"In the adipose tissue of healthy, lean subjects, $CD4^+$ T_{reg} cells prevail, producing type 2 T-helper cell (T_h2) anti-inflammatory cytokines such as the IL-4 and IL-13 and thereby stimulating the differentiation of the residing macrophages towards the alternatively activated M2 (F4/80$^+$, CD11b$^+$) CD11c$^-$ phenotype [116]."

"Adiponectin inhibits the nuclear factor (NF)-κB pathway as well as tumor necrosis factor (TNF)-α signaling and promotes the expression of the peroxisome proliferator-activated receptor (PPAR)-γ co-activator in macrophages, further promoting their M2 phenotype [117]."

"In macrophages and adipocytes, these pathways lead to the transactivation of overlapping sets of pro-inflammatory molecules [118, 119] and promote cellular insulin resistance as well as leptin secretion in adipocytes."

"In both macrophages and adipocytes, the loss of nuclear receptor corepressor activity can be prevented by PPAR-γ activation (e.g. by thiazolidinediones) resulting in reduced inflammation and improved insulin sensitivity."

"The pro-inflammatory activity of Ang II via its AT1R is well recognized [120]."

RAS Modulation in Cardio-Metabolic Disease

"The cardio-protective effects of AT2R stimulation were not associated with a reduction in blood pressure in these or other experiments when compound 21 was administered peripherally."

"In type 2 diabetic KKAy mice, compound 21 improved insulin sensitivity, increased adiponectin and reduced TNF-α levels, while protecting the pancreatic β-cells."

"The beneficial effects of AT2R activation were blocked by PPAR-γ inhibition [121]."

"The effects of AT2R stimulation were broader compared to the effects of the ARB (valsartan in this study), which improved glucose tolerance only."

"Although the effects in Zucker rats were not associated with blood pressure-lowering effect by AT2R stimulation, compound 21 prevented salt-sensitive hypertension in these rats."

"We need to be cautious when attributing the effects of ACE2/Ang (1–7) stimulation to the activation of a particular receptor (AT2R or the Mas)."

Combined Angiotensin Receptor Modulation

"Because these considerations represent a translational approach with a very specific aim, only few experimental studies have investigated the effects of the combination of AT1R blockade with AT2R stimulation."

"A clinical rationale for combined angiotensin receptor modulation includes the AT1R blockade aimed at achieving target blood pressure values and the AT2R stimulation aimed to reduce arterial stiffness in the long term."

"The mechanisms responsible for these beneficial effects of the combined angiotensin receptor blockade were largely attributed to the anti-inflammatory effects of compound 21."

"There is only one study which has investigated the effects of combined AT2R stimulation + AT1R blockade specifically in the setting of a metabolic disorder."

"Due to these additional beneficial effects of the add-on AT2R stimulation to AT1R blockade, such combination represents an interesting perspective for future clinical investigation."

Conclusion

"The combined modulation of angiotensin receptors by AT1R blockade and simultaneous AT2R stimulation provides an intriguing novel therapeutic concept."

"Patients with chronic low-grade inflammation and/or isolated systolic hypertension might benefit from the anti-inflammatory and de-stiffening effects of the AT2R stimulation additive to the AT1R blockade."

"Future studies on the combined angiotensin receptor modulation in the field of cardio-metabolic diseases represent an attractive and highly sought endeavor."

Anti-hypertensive Drug Treatment of Patients with and the Metabolic Syndrome and Obesity: A Review of Evidence, Meta-Analysis, Post Hoc and Guidelines Publications [122]

This is a machine-generated summary of:

Owen, Jonathan G.; Reisin, Efrain: Anti-hypertensive Drug Treatment of Patients with and the Metabolic Syndrome and Obesity: a Review of Evidence, Meta-Analysis, Post hoc and Guidelines Publications [122].

Published in: Current Hypertension Reports (2015).

Link to original: https://doi.org/10.1007/s11906-015-0558-9

If you want to cite the papers, please refer to the original.

For technical reasons we could not place the page where the original quote is coming from.

Abstract-Summary "Epidemiological studies have shown an increasing prevalence of obesity and the metabolic syndrome worldwide."

"The ideal pharmacological antihypertensive regimen should target the underlying mechanisms involved in this syndrome, including sympathetic activation, increased renal tubular sodium reabsorption, and overexpression of the renin-angiotensin-aldosterone system by the adipocyte."

"Few prospective trials have been conducted in the search of the ideal antihypertensive regimen in patients with obesity and the metabolic syndrome."

"We summarize previously published ad hoc studies, prospective studies, and guideline publications regarding the treatment of hypertension in patients with obesity and the metabolic syndrome."

"Caution exists regarding the use of thiazide diuretics due to potential metabolic derangements, there is insufficient data to show worsened cardiovascular or renal outcomes in patients treated with these drugs."

"Renin-angiotensin-aldosterone system (RAAS) inhibition with an ACE or an ARB and treatment with calcium channel blockers appears safe and well tolerated in obesity-related hypertension and in patients with metabolic syndrome."

Introduction

"The metabolic syndrome (MS) is a disorder most typically characterized by insulin resistance (IR), visceral fat accumulation, atherogenic plasma lipid derangements, and elevated blood pressure."

"In response to IR, the pancreas secretes progressively increasing quantities of insulin to meet metabolic demand and maintain normal plasma glucose."

"Epidemiological studies show a rapidly increasing prevalence of obesity and the metabolic syndrome worldwide and especially in developed countries like the USA [123, 124]."

"Drug therapies to help achieve weight loss goals and improve insulin sensitivity may play an increasingly important role in this condition [125–127]."

"The ideal antihypertensive regimen should target the underlying mechanisms involved in this syndrome."

"Many antihypertensive medications have significant positive and negative effects on glucose intolerance and other features common in the metabolic syndrome."

Pathophysiology of Hypertension in Obesity and Metabolic Syndrome

"It appears additionally likely that adipose tissue itself, and importantly inflamed adipose tissue as seen in visceral fat deposits, plays a crucial role in the development of hypertension in the metabolic syndrome via upregulation of RAAS and due to the increased secretion of adipokines which lead to, among other effects, sympathetic over-activation and decreased vascular smooth muscle expression of nitric oxide [128–132]."

"Further supporting the contribution of this mechanism in obesity-related hypertension is the observation that angiotensinogen knockout mice appear immune to the development of obesity, metabolic syndrome, and hypertension [133, 134]."

"Further, there is increased recognition that aldosterone may promote inflammation and fibrosis within the kidney, heart and vascular system, and recent studies showing favorable effects on insulin resistance, adipokine production, fat differentiation, and vascular tone with aldosterone antagonism make this a promising target for obesity-related hypertension [135, 136]."

"The likely contribution of the sympathetic nervous system in obesity-related hypertension is underscored by the frequent observation of increased sympathetic tone in obese patients [128, 130, 137, 138]."

Therapeutic Drug Classes and Evidence on Their Effect in Metabolic Syndrome

"This study showed a significantly increased rate of the development of diabetes in the chlorthalidone group compared to lisinopril, but not amlodipine in the patients with preexisting metabolic syndrome (17.1 vs. 12.6 vs. 16%, respectively)."

"In the patients without preexisting metabolic syndrome, there was an increased risk in development of overt diabetes with chlorthalidone as compared to either lisinopril or amlodipine (7.7 vs 4.7 vs 4.2%, respectively) at 4 years of follow-up."

"Given the suggestion that absolute blood pressure reduction was the primary predictor of risk rather than metabolic effect, a post hoc analysis of ALLHAT conducted by Reisin et al sought to determine if there were differences in blood pressure lowering effects between chlorthalidone vs. lisinopril or amlodipine when patients were stratified into groups of normal weight (BMI < 25, overweight (BMI = 25–29.9) or obese (BMI > 30)."

Review of Current Guideline Publications

"To recommending lifestyle modification with emphasis on weight loss in these patients, the guidelines recommended that the initial antihypertensives used in this population be either calcium channel blockers or RAAS inhibitors as metabolic syndrome is a prediabetic state, and thiazide diuretics and traditional beta-blockers have been shown to worsen insulin sensitivity and accelerate progression to diabetes."

"The JNC 8 guidelines made no specific recommendations on hypertension management in the subset of patients with obesity and metabolic syndrome."

"This guideline is notable, however in that it did specifically recommend ACE/ARB as the first-line therapy for patients with hypertension and age younger than 55, whereas those older than 55 or of African descent should receive a calcium channel blocker."

"These guidelines do recommend a calcium channel blocker over a thiazide diuretic in patients with overt diabetes."

Conclusion

"The optimal antihypertensive drug therapy for patients with obesity and/or the metabolic syndrome has not been defined."

"A drug therapy will target the underlying mechanisms of hypertension in this population, has minimal metabolic side effects, and has proven outcomes data in long-term clinical trials."

"Given the apparent favorable metabolic effects, vasodilating beta-blockers should be used in preference to traditional beta-blockers when these medications are required for therapy in this population."

"More investigation on this population is needed to define the ideal antihypertensive drug therapy, and future investigations into aldosterone antagonism and novel antihypertensives targeting the underlying physiology are anxiously awaited."

Comparison Between Calcium Channel Blocker with Angiotensin Converting Enzyme Inhibitor or Angiotensin II Type 1 Receptor Blocker Combination on the Development of New-Onset Diabetes in Hypertensive Korean Patients [139]

This is a machine-generated summary of:

Kim, Yong Hoon; Her, Ae-Young; Rha, Seung-Woon; Choi, Byoung Geol; Choi, Se Yeon; Byun, Jae Kyeong; Kang, Dong Oh; Jang, Won Young; Kim, Woohyeun; Baek, Ju Yeol; Choi, Woong Gil; Kang, Tae Soo; Ahn, Jihun; Park, Sang-Ho; Park, Sung Hun; Hong, Ji Yeon; Park, Ji Young; Lee, Min-Ho; Choi, Cheol Ung; Park, Chang Gyu; Seo, Hong Seog: Comparison between calcium channel blocker with angiotensin converting enzyme inhibitor or angiotensin II type 1 receptor blocker combination on the development of new-onset diabetes in hypertensive Korean patients [139].

Published in: Journal of Diabetes & Metabolic Disorders (2020).

Link to original: https://doi.org/10.1007/s40200-020-00521-4

If you want to cite the papers, please refer to the original.

For technical reasons we could not place the page where the original quote is coming from.

Abstract-Summary "The aim of this study was to evaluate which combination therapy, calcium channel blocker (CCB) with angiotensin converting enzyme inhibitor (ACEI) or CCB with angiotensin II type 1 receptor blocker (ARB), is best in reducing/preventing the development of NODM during 4-year follow-up periods in non-diabetic hypertensive Korean patients."

"A total of 1221 consecutive hypertensive patients without a history of diabetes mellitus who had been prescribed CCB were retrospectively enrolled and divided into the two groups, an ACEI group (combination CCB with ACEI, n = 251) and an ARB group (combination CCB with ARB, n = 970)."

"During 4-year follow-up periods, there were similar incidence of NODM (Hazard ratio [HR]; 1.198, 95% confidence interval [CI]; 0.591–2.431, P = 0.616), MACE (HR; 1.324, 95% CI; 0.714–2.453, P = 0.373), total death, MI and PCI between the two groups after PSM analysis."

"CCB with ACE or CCB with ARB combination strategies are equally acceptable in hypertensive Korean patients regarding the occurrence of NODM."

Introduction

"Previous prospective studies reported the positive relationship between antihypertensive drugs and NODM [140–143]."

"These effects of these antihypertensive drugs on blood glucose level are different according to the class of antihypertensive drugs [144, 145]."

"Because, most of the previous studies investigated the cause-effect relationship only between a single class of antihypertensive agent and NODM [146–148], the results between combination therapy of antihypertensive drugs and the incidence of NODM is scarce [149]."

"The aims of this study was to investigate which combination therapy, CCB with ACEI or CCB with ARB, is best to prevent the development of NODM in Korean population during 4-year follow-up periods in non-diabetic hypertensive Korean patients."

Materials and Methods

"The mean prescription duration of the ACEI group was 1651 ± 1088 days and the ARB group was 1802 ± 1008 days in all patients."

"We tested all available variables that could be of potential relevance: gender, age, body mass index (BMI), systolic blood pressure (SBP), diastolic blood pressure (DBP), heart rate, dyslipidemia, previous MI, previous PCI, previous cerebrovascular accident (CVA), previous heart failure (HF), coronary artery spasm, atrial fibrillation and arrhythmia, current smokers, current alcoholics, laboratory findings (fasting blood glucose, HbA1c, total cholesterol, triglyceride, high-density lipoprotein [HDL]-cholesterol, low-density lipoprotein [LDL]-cholesterol, high-sensitivity C-reactive protein [hs-CRP], Hb, serum creatinine), medications (BBs, diuretics, nitrate, lipid lowering agents, aspirin, clopidogrel, cilostazole)."

"The following factors were co-analyzed in multivariate Cox-regression analysis: ACEI group vs. ARB group, age (≥65 years), gender (men), BMI (≥24 kg/m^2), SBP, DBP, dyslipidemia, previous MI, previous PCI, previous CVA, previous HF, current smokers, current alcoholics, BBs, diuretics, nitrates, lipid lowering agent, and clopidogrel."

Results

"In the total study population, men, previous MI, previous PCI and the use of BBs, nitrates and clopidogrel variables were significantly higher in the ACEI group compared to the ARB group."

"In the total study population, the cumulative incidence of NODM (7.0% vs. 9.2%, Log rank P = 0.471) was not statistically different between the two groups."

"The incidence of MACE (10.9% vs. 5.9%, Log rank P = 0.003) and PCI (9.2% vs. 3.4%, Log rank P < 0.001) were significantly higher in the ACEI group."

"After PSM, the incidences of NODM (7.3% vs. 9.0%, Log rank P = 0.615, hazard ratio [HR]; 1.198, 95% confidence interval [CI]; 0.591–2.431, P = 0.616) and MACE (11.3% vs. 10.0%, Log rank P = 0.371, HR; 1.324, 95% CI; 0.714–2.453, P = 0.373) were similar between the two groups."

Discussion

"Those patients who were treated with CCB were considered as the baseline study population and the two combination groups (ACEI group vs. ARB group) were compared in aspects with the comparative superiority of beneficial effects on the incidence of NODM."

"Another study demonstrated ACEI and ARB had comparable effects on the development of NODM [150]."

"Their report said that in patients at high-risk without heart failure, ARB was similar to ACEI in preventing incident risk of all-cause death, MI, NODM."

"Although in our study CCB with ACEI combination therapy did not show significant differences on the development of NODM compared to CCB with ARB combination therapy up to 4-year follow-up periods, our results are meaningful because our study appears to be the first study comparing the effect of antihypertensive drug combinations on the incidence of NODM in hypertensive Korean patients."

Conclusion

"CCB with ACEI combination therapy did not show significant differences on the development of NODM and individual and composite MACE compared with CCB with ARB combination therapy up to 4-year follow-up periods in Korean patients."

"These two treatment strategies are considered to be equally acceptable in hypertensive Korean patients in the aspect of the occurrence of NODM."

The Benefits of Angiotensin-Converting Enzyme Inhibitors/ Angiotensin II Receptor Blockers Combined with Calcium Channel Blockers on Metabolic, Renal, and Cardiovascular Outcomes in Hypertensive Patients: A Meta-Analysis [151]

This is a machine-generated summary of:

Pongpanich, Punnaka; Pitakpaiboonkul, Pasvich; Takkavatakarn, Kullaya; Praditpornsilpa, Kearkiat; Eiam-Ong, Somchai; Susantitaphong, Paweena: The benefits of angiotensin-converting enzyme inhibitors/angiotensin II receptor blockers combined with calcium channel blockers on metabolic, renal, and cardiovascular outcomes in hypertensive patients: a meta-analysis [151].

Published in: International Urology and Nephrology (2018).

Link to original: https://doi.org/10.1007/s11255-018-1991-x

If you want to cite the papers, please refer to the original.

For technical reasons we could not place the page where the original quote is coming from.

Abstract-Summary "Most patients need more than one drug to achieve blood pressure (BP) target."

"We conducted a meta-analysis to explore the benefits of angiotensin-converting enzyme inhibitors (ACEIs)/angiotensin II receptor blockers (ARBs) combined with calcium channel blockers (CCBs) on metabolic, renal, and cardiovascular outcomes in hypertensive patients."

"A systematic literature search was conducted in MEDLINE, Scopus, Cochrane Central Register of Controlled Trials, and Clinical Trials.gov (until April 7, 2016) to identify randomized controlled trials (RCTs) comparing the benefits of ACEIs/ARBs combined with CCBs versus other dual or triple combinations on clinical outcomes in hypertensive patients."

"When compared with other combinations, the combination of ACEIs/ARBs and CCBs had comparable WMD of systolic as well as diastolic BP (73 study arms) but provided better benefits on metabolic parameters, such as HDL, FBS, HbA1C, and serum uric acid; renal functions, including serum creatinine and estimated glomerular filtration rate; and cardiovascular diseases, including reduction of all cardiovascular events, myocardial infarction, and syncope/hypotension."

"The combination of ACEIs/ARBs with CCBs has superior benefits on metabolic, renal, and cardiovascular outcomes in hypertensive patients."

"This combination should be considered whenever monotherapy does not achieve the guideline target."

Introduction

"Due to excellent BP lowering efficacy and less adverse metabolic side effects, the combination of ACEIs/ARBs with CCBs has been widely used in several recent RCTs and appears to provide satisfactory outcomes [152–157]."

"The first meta-analysis in eight RCTs containing 20,451 patients by Chi and others [156] showed that ACEIs/ARBs with CCB combination was superior to other dual antihypertensive combinations by lowering incidence of cardiovascular events and adverse events while preserving renal function."

"The second meta-analysis [157] in 14 RCTs with 18,125 patients by Cheng and others [157] demonstrated that ACEIs/ARBs with CCB combination had a stronger effect on the maintenance of renal function than ACEIs/ARBs plus diuretic."

"The present meta-analysis was conducted to compare the effects of the combination of ACEIs/ARBs and CCBs in general hypertensive patients with all other combinations, dual or triple antihypertensive agents, regarding metabolic, renal, and cardiovascular outcomes, and adverse side effects."

Method

"We investigated sources of heterogeneity for the outcomes of interest by performing random effects model meta-regression analyses based on a priori selected study characteristics, including country (Africa, Asia, Europe, Multinational, North America, South America), trial design (crossover vs. parallel-arm), population setting (diabetic, non-diabetic vs. mixed populations), age (<60 vs. ≥60 years), method of BP measurement (ambulatory vs. office), duration of follow-up (<6 vs. >6 months), type of combination therapies (ACEI vs. ARB), type of control therapies (ACEI + CCB + BB, ACEI + CCB + TD, ACEI + TD, ARB + CCB + BB, ARB + CCB + TD, ARB + TD, CCB + BB, CCB + TD, BB + TD), and study quality (fair vs. good)."

Results

"By subgroup analysis, studies that compared the combination therapy of ACEIs/ARBs and CCBs with triple therapy showed a significant increase in BP parameters including SBP for ARBs or ACEIs, CCB and TD combination, and DBP for ARBs or ACEIs, CCB and TD or BB combination."

"The significant effect of combination of ACEIs/ARBs with CCB therapy on augmented HDL levels were demonstrated in studies of parallel design, fair study quality, age <60 years, both DM and non-DM, duration of follow-up over 6 months, using ARB + TD, and CCB + BB as control group."

"The significant increase of serum potassium was observed in all subgroups except studies in Asia, fair quality, mean age >60 years, mixed population, follow-up above 6 months, studies that using ACEIs + CCBs + BB, ACEIs + TD, CCBs + BB as control group."

Discussion

"The results in the present meta-analysis, which included nearly 50,000 participants, demonstrated that the combination of ACEIs/ARBs with CCBs in general hypertensive patients, when compared with other dual/triple antihypertensive combinations, yielded comparable BP control and could provide superior benefits on (1) metabolic parameters including FBS, HbA1C, serum uric acid, and HDL, (2) renal functions comprising serum creatinine and estimated GFR, and (3) cardiovascular outcomes including reductions of all cardiovascular events, myocardial infarction, and syncope/hypotension."

"In the present meta-analysis, the combination of ACEIs/ARBs with CCBs significantly reduced FBS, HbA1C, and serum uric acid when compared with other combinations."

"The present meta-analysis demonstrated that the combination of ACEIs/ARBs with CCBs, when compared with other dual or triple antihypertensive combination, could preserve renal function, reduced the incidences of all cardiovascular events and myocardial infarction, but had comparable incidences of all-cause mortality cardiovascular mortality and stroke."

The Different Therapeutic Choices with ARBs. Which One to Give? When? Why? [158]

This is a machine-generated summary of:

Dézsi, Csaba András: The Different Therapeutic Choices with ARBs. Which One to Give? When? Why? [158].

Published in: American Journal of Cardiovascular Drugs (2016).

Link to original: https://doi.org/10.1007/s40256-016-0165-4

If you want to cite the papers, please refer to the original.

For technical reasons we could not place the page where the original quote is coming from.

Abstract-Summary "Each angiotensin receptor blocker (ARB) is important in the treatment of hypertension, according to the results of recent years."

Introduction

"The appearance of angiotensin receptor blockers (ARBs) amongst the therapeutic options in the treatment of cardiovascular diseases (CVDs) was a new milestone in the history of hypertension treatment."

"ARBs have shown excellent efficacy, they have no negative metabolic effects and they cause no accumulation of bradykinin."

"According to the latest international guidelines, ACEIs or ARBs should be preferred in patients with co-morbid microalbuminuria, renal dysfunction and chronic kidney disease (CKD), metabolic syndrome and diabetes mellitus (DM), atherosclerosis, chronic stable angina and previous myocardial infarction (MI), atrial fibrillation (AF) as well as heart failure (HF) [159, 160]."

"As to which particular ARB should be preferred in case of different co-morbid conditions, no guidance is available."

"Several studies are available where certain ARBs have shown additional beneficial effect; the present review of the available evidence should provide help in treatment selection for individual patients."

Prevention of Cardiovascular Events and Mortality

"Losartan has also shown benefits in reducing the relative risk of the composite endpoint of death, MI or stroke by 13% compared with atenolol in the LIFE study, with more benefit amongst diabetic patients, where mortality was reduced by 39% [161]."

"In HF patients not receiving ACEIs, valsartan reduced all-cause mortality by 33% and composite mortality and morbidity risk by 44% compared with placebo in the Val-HeFT trial."

"The consequent CHARM trial showed that candesartan also caused a significant reduction in the risk of CV deaths and hospital admissions for HF compared with placebo [162]."

"The MOSES trial, investigating high-risk hypertensive stroke patients, showed that compared to nitrendipine, eprosartan therapy resulted in significantly fewer cerebrovascular events during the 2.5 years of follow-up [163]."

Prevention of Diabetes Mellitus and Associated Risk Factors

"ARB therapy can reduce the incidence of new onset diabetes compared with placebo in patients with high CV risk and/or hypertension [150, 164]."

"The meta-analysis of LIFE, SCOPE and VALUE trials has shown that losartan, candesartan as well as valsartan can cause a clinically significant decrease in the incidence of new onset diabetes, with a combined estimated relative risk (RR) of 0.80 for all the three agents [165]."

"The meta-analysis of the TRANSCEND and PRoFESS trials has shown that treatment with telmisartan is associated with a 16% reduction in the risk of new onset DM compared with placebo [166]."

"In a population-based cohort study among older diabetic patients, telmisartan and valsartan (with an adjusted hazard ratio of 0.85 and 0.86, respectively) were both associated with a lower risk of admission to hospital for acute MI, stroke or HF, compared with irbesartan."

Renal End-Organ Protection

"Compared with placebo, losartan given in addition to conventional antihypertensive treatment reduced the risk of ESRD by 28% and decreased the level of urinary protein excretion by 35% in patients with coexistent diabetic nephropathy in the RENAAL study [167]."

"In the IDNT trial, irbesartan reduced the risk of doubling serum creatinine levels by 33% and the onset of ESRD by 23% compared with placebo in hypertensive patients with nephropathy due to DM."

"The addition of valsartan to conventional therapy significantly slowed the rate of renal function decline, reduced the doubling of serum creatinine levels and delayed the appearance of ESRD in hypertensive patients with advanced CKD compared with placebo [168]."

"In patients with type II diabetes and microalbuminuria with or without hypertension, valsartan significantly reduced elevated urine albumin excretion compared with baseline in the MARVAL trial."

Obesity and Metabolic Syndrome

"The PPAR-γ agonist telmisartan improves both hemodynamic and metabolic abnormalities found in hypertensive patients with obesity."

"The results of a recent meta-analysis showed that telmisartan therapy significantly improves metabolic parameters such as fasting glucose, insulin, hemoglobin A1c: glycosylated hemoglobin (HbA1c) levels and HOMA index in patients with metabolic syndrome."

"The ATHLETE study also showed that in obese patients with hypertension and IR, telmisartan significantly improved the hyperinsulin response to glucose loading [169]."

"In obese but otherwise healthy subjects, valsartan did decrease fasting plasma insulin levels, and in patients with impaired glucose metabolism, valsartan treatment reduced abdominal subcutaneous adipocyte size as well as adipose tissue macrophage infiltration markers, and increased fasting and postprandial adipose tissue blood flow compared with placebo [32, 170]."

"The results of the K-MetS study [171], which are expected to be released in 2016, aside from providing information on the antihypertensive efficacy of fimasartan-based treatment, are going to provide valuable information concerning other potential effects detected in patients with metabolic syndrome in case of such treatments."

Hyperuricemia

"The renal uric acid transporter (URAT1) was shown to be involved in the effect of ARBs on SUA level."

"Such trans-stimulatory effects may lead to an increase of SUA level [172]."

"Losartan increased the excretion of uric acid and decreased the SUA level in both healthy and hypertensive subjects."

"Eprosartan had no effect on SUA concentrations or urine uric acid excretion in patients with mild-to-moderate essential hypertension [173]."

Erectile Dysfunction

"In large prospective studies, the use of valsartan increased the rate of sexual intercourses per week and caused a reduction in ED, with improved orgasmic function, intercourse and overall sexual satisfaction in hypertensive men [174, 175]."

"In comparative studies, long-term use of valsartan was also shown to significantly improve sexual activity in comparison with the β-blockers carvedilol and atenolol, with the latter also reducing serum testosterone levels [176, 177]."

"Treatment with losartan improved erectile function, sexual satisfaction and frequency of sexual activity in hypertensive patients."

"In hypertensive patients with the metabolic syndrome, treatment with irbesartan alone or in combination with hydrochlorothiazide was associated with an improvement of sexual desire, frequency of sexual contacts and erectile function."

"Irbesartan also improved erectile function recovery in prostatectomized patients [178, 179]."

The Future of Angiotensin Receptor Blockers: Protection of Cognitive Function

"In hypertensive rats, olmesartan treatment restored the cognitive decline and ameliorated leakage from brain microvessels."

"Telmisartan seems to protect against hypertension-associated cognitive decline not only by its AT_1 receptor blockade, but also partly because of its PPAR-γ activation in the hippocampus."

"Co-administration of a PPAR-γ antagonist with telmisartan partially attenuated the protective effect of telmisartan on cognitive decline [180]."

"Telmisartan was also shown to significantly restore cognitive functions impaired by chronic stress and decrease forgetfulness [181]."

"The OSCAR study, evaluating the effect of 6 months of eprosartan therapy on cognitive function resulted in significant improvement on the overall mean Mini-Mental State Examination (MMSE) in patients with essential hypertension [182]."

"Lack of significant cognitive decline was observed with telmisartan in patients with probable AD after 6 months of treatment, while patients treated with amlodipine showed a worsening on the AD Assessment Scale-Cognitive Subscale score."

Conclusions

"For hypertensive patients at a higher risk of stroke, losartan should be the first therapeutic option; telmisartan, eprosartan and candesartan have also shown risk reduction in this subpopulation."

"In the case of patients with a history of AF, the use of telmisartan can be recommended; losartan, candesartan and valsartan have shown a reduced incidence of new-onset AF; therefore their use may also be beneficial in patients at risk of AF."

"In patients at risk of developing DM, many ARBs (such as losartan, telmisartan, irbesartan, candesartan and valsartan) have shown protective properties."

"In terms of cardioprotection in patients with DM, both telmisartan and valsartan have shown lower risk of admission to hospital due to MI, stroke or HF."

"The most investigated ARBs in patients with ED are valsartan, irbesartan and losartan; the latter two have also been studied in coexisting metabolic syndrome and DM."

Neprilysin Inhibition: A New Therapeutic Option for Type 2 Diabetes? [183]

This is a machine-generated summary of:

Esser, Nathalie; Zraika, Sakeneh: Neprilysin inhibition: a new therapeutic option for type 2 diabetes? [183].

Published in: Diabetologia (2019).
Link to original: https://doi.org/10.1007/s00125-019-4889-y

If you want to cite the papers, please refer to the original.
For technical reasons we could not place the page where the original quote is coming from.

Abstract-Summary "Preclinical studies have also reported that neprilysin inhibition, alone or in combination with renin–angiotensin system blockers, elicits beneficial effects on glucose homeostasis."

"We evaluate existing evidence from preclinical and clinical studies in which neprilysin is deleted/inhibited, we highlight potential mechanisms underlying the beneficial glycaemic effects of neprilysin inhibition, and discuss possible deleterious effects that may limit the efficacy and safety of neprilysin inhibitors in the clinic."

"We also review the favourable impact neprilysin inhibition can have on diabetic complications, in addition to glucose control."

"We conclude that neprilysin inhibitors may be a useful therapeutic option for treating type 2 diabetes; however, their combination with angiotensin II receptor blockers is needed to circumvent deleterious consequences of neprilysin inhibition alone."

Introduction

"Neprilysin activity is increased in plasma and metabolic tissues of mice with diet-induced obesity, and its levels correlate with decreased insulin sensitivity and reduced beta cell function [184, 185]."

"While there is some evidence that plasma neprilysin levels positively correlate with BMI and other features of the metabolic syndrome in humans [184, 186], this needs to be confirmed by additional studies."

"In both humans [187–189] and animals [190–193], they have also been shown to improve insulin sensitivity, beta cell function and glucose tolerance in diabetic and obese states."

"Neprilysin inhibitors are now approved for use in humans with heart failure, a population in which approximately 35% also have type 2 diabetes [194], it is both timely and important to better understand the molecular mechanisms underpinning their glucoregulatory effects."

"We also discuss considerations for the clinical use of neprilysin inhibitors in the prevention and treatment of type 2 diabetes."

Evidence for a Beneficial Effect of Neprilysin Inhibition on Glucose Homeostasis

"In the third study, among 73 individuals with heart failure, including 16 with diabetes, a change of treatment from either an ACE inhibitor or ARB to ARNi for 3 months resulted in a decrease of plasma neprilysin activity that was associated with reduced fructosamine levels, a marker of protein glycation [189]."

"These data demonstrate improvements in determinants of glucose tolerance and support the use of neprilysin inhibition to improve the metabolic derangements of type 2 diabetes."

"Some studies support a glucose-lowering effect of neprilysin inhibition via increased plasma levels of these substrates, including GLP-1 [185, 189, 190, 195], bradykinin [191, 196] and natriuretic peptides, atrial natriuretic peptide (ANP) and B-type natriuretic peptide (BNP) [197]."

"One potential mechanism by which neprilysin inhibition improves glucose homeostasis may be by increasing levels, and thereby the insulinotropic effects, of GLP-1 [190, 198]."

"We demonstrated in vivo in high-fat fed, neprilysin-deficient mice that elevated active GLP-1 levels in plasma were associated with improved glucose tolerance as a result of enhanced beta cell function and insulin sensitivity [185]."

Arguments Against a Beneficial Effect of Neprilysin Inhibition on Glucose Homeostasis

"To the above-mentioned positive effects of reduced neprilysin activity on glucose homeostasis, some studies on deficiency/pharmacological inhibition of neprilysin have raised some uncertainty with respect to the potential glycaemic effects of neprilysin inhibitors [184, 199–204]."

"Regarding pharmacological studies in animals, while subcutaneous or intravenous administration of a neprilysin inhibitor for an acute period (up to 2 h) [190–193] had a positive impact on glucose homeostasis, its oral administration for a 3 month period (12–14 weeks) failed to improve oral [202] or intraperitoneal [201, 203, 204] glucose tolerance in high-fat-fed or diabetic rodents, suggesting that either the bioavailability of inhibitor is lower when given orally or compensatory mechanisms are activated over time that result in loss of inhibitor efficacy."

"Studies that employed an intraperitoneal [201, 203, 204] rather than oral route of glucose administration during the tolerance test would have excluded any effect of neprilysin inhibition to enhance the incretin effect."

"An important consideration with neprilysin inhibition is that it also increases levels of substrates capable of impairing insulin sensitivity and secretion (see text box), which might be a possible explanation for the negative findings in the studies above."

Considerations for Clinical Use of Neprilysin Inhibitors in Type 2 Diabetes

"A study in pigs demonstrated that dual neprilysin and DPP-4 inhibition may have additive effects and therapeutic potential for type 2 diabetes, as combined neprilysin and DPP-4 inhibition was more effective at maintaining active GLP-1 levels and enhancing insulin secretion than inhibition of either alone [190]."

"Results from another study suggest that any residual neprilysin activity may negate the beneficial effects of combined neprilysin plus DPP-4 inhibition [202]."

"Dual ACE–neprilysin inhibition in rodents is more effective than inhibition of either ACE [191, 196, 205, 206] or neprilysin [191, 201, 203] alone at improving insulin sensitivity and glucose tolerance, suggesting there is a synergistic or additive effect of combining ACE and neprilysin inhibitors."

"We showed that in amyloid-prone mouse islets, neprilysin inhibition increased amyloid formation and beta cell apoptosis, whereas upregulation of neprilysin had the opposite effect [207]."

"It is also possible that the increase in GLP-1 with neprilysin inhibition may limit islet amyloid-induced beta cell apoptosis [208]."

Areas for Future Work

"To resolve some of the uncertainties in the field with respect to the role of neprilysin in modulating glucose homeostasis, we suggest future work that encompasses the following areas."

"More research is needed to elucidate whether substrates that are hydrolysed by neprilysin in vitro (see text box) have clinical relevance with respect to glucose homeostasis in vivo."

"It is also unclear how neprilysin action in metabolic tissues aside from the pancreas, such as liver, adipose tissue, kidney and intestine, contributes to regulation of glucose homeostasis."

"Tissue-specific deletion of neprilysin in rodent models will help delineate the relative importance of the different neprilysin substrates in modulating glucose levels, and aid the development of targeted therapies that avoid undesirable off-target effects."

Conclusion

"The increase in angiotensin II levels associated with neprilysin inhibition limits its use as monotherapy in type 2 diabetic patients and a neprilysin inhibitor should necessarily be prescribed together with an ARB, which is preferred to an ACE inhibitor to avoid angioedema."

"The beneficial glycaemic effects of neprilysin inhibition can be exploited, while limiting harmful side effects of increased angiotensin II levels at the metabolic, cardiovascular and renal levels."

"Carefully designed and controlled preclinical studies are necessary for understanding the molecular mechanisms by which neprilysin inhibitors work."

Bibliography

1. Underwood PC, Adler GK (2013) The renin angiotensin aldosterone system and insulin resistance in humans. Curr Hypertens Rep 15(1):59–70. https://doi.org/10.1007/s11906-012-0323-2
2. Taniyama Y, Hitomi H, Shah A, Alexander RW, Griendling KK (2005) Mechanisms of reactive oxygen species-dependent downregulation of insulin receptor substrate-1 by angiotensin II. Arterioscler Thromb Vasc Biol 25:1142–1147
3. Ogihara T, Asano T, Ando K, Chiba Y, Sakoda H, Anai M, Shojima N, Ono H, Onishi Y, Fujishiro M, Katagiri H, Fukushima Y, Kikuchi M, Noguchi N, Aburatani H, Komuro I, Fujita T (2002) Angiotensin II-induced insulin resistance is associated with enhanced insulin signaling. Hypertension 40:872–879
4. Mancusi C, Izzo R, di Gioia G, Losi MA, Barbato E, Morisco C (2020) Insulin resistance the hinge between hypertension and type 2 diabetes. High Blood Press Cardiovasc Prev. 27(6):515–526
5. Yang Y, Thumula V, Pace PF, Banahan BF, Wilkin NE, Lobb WB (2010) Nonadher-ence to angiotensin-converting enzyme inhibitors and/or angiotensin II receptor blockers among high-risk patients with diabetes in Medicare part D programs. J Am Pharm Assoc 50(4):527–531
6. Aparasu RR, Aparasu A (2008) Hypertension management in outpatient visits by diabetic patients. Res Social Adm Pharm 4(3):284–291
7. Johnson ML, Singh H (2005) Patterns of antihypertensive therapy among patients with diabetes. J Gen Intern Med 20(9):842–846
8. Davila EP, Florez LE, Fleming LE et al (2010) Prevalence of the metabolic syndrome among U.S. workers. Diabetes Care 33(11):2390–2395
9. Ford ES, Li C, Sattar N (2008) Metabolic syndrome and incident diabetes: current state of the evidence. Diabetes Care 31:1898–1904
10. McMurray JJ, Holman RR, Haffner SM et al (2010) Effect of valsartan on the incidence of diabetes and cardiovascular events. N Engl J Med 362:1477–1490. The NAVIGATOR study, one of the first prospective randomized control trials powered to evaluate the effect of RAAS blockade (valsartan) on incidence of diabetes as a primary endpoint. Individuals receiving valsartan had a 14 % reduction in the incidence of diabetes compared to the placebo control group
11. van der Zijl NJ, Moors CC, Goossens GH, Hermans MM, Blaak EE, Diamant M (2011) Valsartan improves {beta}-cell function and insulin sensitivity in subjects with impaired glucose metabolism: a randomized controlled trial. Diabetes Care 34:845–851. This is the first randomized control trial in humans that evaluated the effect of an ARB versus placebo on beta cell function. Chronic valsartan treatment, compared with placebo control, improved glucose stimulated insulin secretion during an oral glucose tolerance test as well as insulin sensitivity assessed by euglycemic clamp, suggesting that ARB blockade has an effect not only on glucose uptake, but also pancreatic insulin secretion
12. Abuissa H, Jones PG, Marso SP, O'Keefe JH (2005) Angiotensin-converting enzyme inhibitors or angiotensin receptor blockers for prevention of type 2 diabetes: a meta-analysis of randomized clinical trials. J Am Coll Cardiol 46:821–826
13. Perlstein TS, Henry RR, Mather KJ et al (2012) Effect of angiotensin receptor blockade on insulin sensitivity and endothelial function in abdominally obese hypertensive patients with impaired fasting glucose. Clin Sci (Lond) 122:193–202

14. Lteif AA, Chisholm RL, Gilbert K, Considine RV, Mather KJ (2012) Effects of losartan on whole body, skeletal muscle and vascular insulin responses in obesity/insulin resistance without hypertension. Diabetes Obes Metab 14:254–261
15. Muniyappa R, Yavuz S (2012) Metabolic actions of angiotensin II and insulin: a microvascular endothelial balancing act. Mol Cell Endocrinol 378:59–69. https://doi.org/10.1016/j.mce.2012.05.017
16. Yatabe J, Yoneda M, Yatabe MS et al (2011) Angiotensin III stimulates aldosterone secretion from adrenal gland partially via angiotensin II type 2 receptor but not angiotensin II type 1 receptor. Endocrinology 152:1582–1588
17. Marcus Y, Shefer G, Stern N (2012) Adipose tissue renin-angiotensin-aldosterone system (RAAS) and progression of insulin resistance. Mol Cell Endocrinol 378:1–14. https://doi.org/10.1016/j.mce.2012.06.021
18. Leung PS (2007) Mechanisms of protective effects induced by blockade of the renin-angiotensin system: novel role of the pancreatic islet angiotensin-generating system in type 2 diabetes. Diabet Med 24:110–116
19. Grassi G, Seravalle G, Dell'Oro R et al (2003) Comparative effects of candesartan and hydrochlorothiazide on blood pressure, insulin sensitivity, and sympathetic drive in obese hypertensive individuals: results of the CROSS study. J Hypertens 21:1761–1769
20. Jin HM, Pan Y (2007) Angiotensin type-1 receptor blockade with losartan increases insulin sensitivity and improves glucose homeostasis in subjects with type 2 diabetes and nephropathy. Nephrol Dial Transplant 22:1943–1949
21. Henriksen EJ, Prasannarong M (2012) The role of the renin angiotensin system in the development of insulin resistance in skeletal muscle. Mol Cell Endocrinol 378:15–22. https://doi.org/10.1016/j.mce.2012.04.011
22. Velloso LA, Folli F, Sun XJ, White MF, Saad MJ, Kahn CR (1996) Cross-talk between the insulin and angiotensin signaling systems. Proc Natl Acad Sci U S A 93:12490–12495
23. Manrique C, Lastra G, Gardner M, Sowers JR (2009) The renin angiotensin aldosterone system in hypertension: roles of insulin resistance and oxidative stress. Med Clin North Am 93:569–582
24. Chai W, Wang W, Liu J et al (2010) Angiotensin II type 1 and type 2 receptors regulate basal skeletal muscle microvascular volume and glucose use. Hypertension 55:523–530
25. Goossens GH, Blaak EE, Saris WH, van Baak MA (2004) Angiotensin II-induced effects on adipose and skeletal muscle tissue blood flow and lipolysis in normal-weight and obese subjects. J Clin Endocrinol Metab 89:2690–2696. A physiologic human study that evaluated the effects of ANGII infusion on lipolysis in skeletal muscle and adipose tissue, demonstrating that ANGII inhibits lipolysis (which may increase insulin resistance) in these tissues in both obese and healthy individuals. A limitation of this study is that measurements of insulin resistance were not measured to determine whether they correlated with decreases in lipolysis
26. Sauder MA, Liu J, Jahn LA, Fowler DE, Chai W, Liu Z (2012) Candesartan acutely recruits skeletal and cardiac muscle microvasculature in healthy humans. J Clin Endocrinol Metab 97:E1208–E1212
27. Diamond-Stanic MK, Henriksen EJ (2010) Direct inhibition by angiotensin II of insulin-dependent glucose transport activity in mammalian skeletal muscle involves a ROS-dependent mechanism. Arch Physiol Biochem 116:88–95
28. Karlsson C, Lindell K, Ottosson M, Sjöström L, Carlsson B, Carlsson LM (1998) Human adipose tissue expresses angiotensinogen and enzymes required for its conversion to angiotensin II. J Clin Endocrinol Metab 83:3925–3929
29. Bentley-Lewis R, Adler GK, Perlstein T et al (2007) Body mass index predicts aldosterone production in normotensive adults on a high-salt diet. J Clin Endocrinol Metab 92:4472–4475
30. Goossens GH, Blaak EE, Arner P, Saris WH, van Baak MA (2007) Angiotensin II: a hormone that affects lipid metabolism in adipose tissue. Int J Obes 31:382–384
31. Lee MH, Song HK, Ko GJ et al (2008) Angiotensin receptor blockers improve insulin resistance in type 2 diabetic rats by modulating adipose tissue. Kidney Int 74:890–900

32. Goossens GH, Moors CC, van der Zijl NJ et al (2012) Valsartan improves adipose tissue function in humans with impaired glucose metabolism: a randomized placebo-controlled double-blind trial. PLoS One 7:e39930
33. Chu KY, Lau T, Carlsson PO, Leung PS (2006) Angiotensin II type 1 receptor blockade improves beta-cell function and glucose tolerance in a mouse model of type 2 diabetes. Diabetes 55:367–374
34. Cole BK, Keller SR, Wu R, Carter JD, Nadler JL, Nunemaker CS (2010) Valsartan protects pancreatic islets and adipose tissue from the inflammatory and metabolic consequences of a high-fat diet in mice. Hypertension 55:715–721. An elegant study demonstrating that valsartan blocks western diet induced increases in inflammation, insulin levels, and glucose stimulated insulin secretion in a mouse model of the metabolic syndrome. Results of this study demonstrate that the RAAS influences the relationship between high fat diet and a worsening metabolic profile and suggests that blocking the RAAS in individuals eating a high fat diet, a common problem in today's society, may be beneficial
35. Muñoz C, Giani JF, Dominici FP, Turyn D, Toblli JE (2009) Long-term treatment with an angiotensin II receptor blocker decreases adipocyte size and improves insulin signaling in obese Zucker rats. J Hypertens 27:2409–2420
36. Fujisaka S, Usui I, Kanatani Y et al (2011) Telmisartan improves insulin resistance and modulates adipose tissue macrophage polarization in high-fat-fed mice. Endocrinology 152:1789–1799
37. Yuan L, Li X, Xu GL, Qi CJ (2010) Effects of renin-angiotensin system blockade on islet function in diabetic rats. J Endocrinol Investig 33:13–19
38. Carlsson PO, Berne C, Jansson L (1998) Angiotensin II and the endocrine pancreas: effects on islet blood flow and insulin secretion in rats. Diabetologia 41:127–133
39. Lau T, Carlsson PO, Leung PS (2004) Evidence for a local angiotensin-generating system and dose-dependent inhibition of glucose-stimulated insulin release by angiotensin II in isolated pancreatic islets. Diabetologia 47:240–248
40. Juan CC, Chien Y, Wu LY et al (2005) Angiotensin II enhances insulin sensitivity in vitro and in vivo. Endocrinology 146:2246–2254
41. Rodriguez R, Viscarra JA, Minas JN, Nakano D, Nishiyama A, Ortiz RM (2012) Angiotensin receptor blockade increases pancreatic insulin secretion and decreases glucose intolerance during glucose supplementation in a model of metabolic syndrome. Endocrinology 153:1684–1695. A novel study demonstrating the effects of ARB treatment (olmesartan) on pancreatic insulin secreation and GLP-1 signalling in a rat model of the metabolic syndrome-OLETF rats. Interestingly, olmesartan resulted in improvements in glucose stimulated pancreatic insulin secretion, decreases in pancreatic AT1R activation, and increases in GLP-1 signaling without changes in insulin signaling in the skeletal muscle. This is the first study to suggest that the relationship between RAAS blockade and improvements in insulin resistance may be mediated by changes in GLP-1 signaling
42. Raheja P, Price A, Wang Z et al (2012) Spironolactone prevents chlorthalidone-induced sympathetic activation and insulin resistance in hypertensive patients. Hypertension 60:319–325
43. Lastra G, Habibi J, Whaley-Connell AT et al (2009) Direct renin inhibition improves systemic insulin resistance and skeletal muscle glucose transport in a transgenic rodent model of tissue renin overexpression. Endocrinology 150:2561–2568
44. Guo X, Cheng S, Taylor KD et al (2005) Hypertension genes are genetic markers for insulin sensitivity and resistance. Hypertension 45:799–803
45. Bonnet F, Patel S, Laville M et al (2008) Influence of the ACE gene insertion/deletion polymorphism on insulin sensitivity and impaired glucose tolerance in healthy subjects. Diabetes Care 31:789–794. The largest human genetics study (N = 1,286) that demonstrates a strong positive association between ACE gene insertion/deletion polymorphism and increased insulin resistance in humans

46. Patel TP, Rawal K, Bagchi AK, Akolkar G, Bernardes N, Dias D d S, Gupta S, Singal PK (2015) Insulin resistance: an additional risk factor in the pathogenesis of cardiovascular disease in type 2 diabetes. Heart Fail Rev 21:11–23. https://doi.org/10.1007/s10741-015-9515-6
47. Ceriello A (2005) Postprandial hyperglycemia and diabetes complications is it time to treat? Diabetes 54(1):1–7
48. Ceriello A (2003) New insights on oxidative stress and diabetic complications may lead to a "causal" antioxidant therapy. Diabetes Care 26(5):1589–1596
49. Farahmand F, Lou H, Singal PK (2003) Oxidative stress in cardiovascular complications of diabetes. In: Pierce GN, Nagano M, Zahradka P, Dhalla NS (eds) Atherosclerosis, hypertension and diabetes. Kluwer Academic Publications, Boston, pp 427–437
50. Astrup AS, Tarnow L, Rossing P, Hansen BV, Hilsted J, Parving H-H (2006) Cardiac autonomic neuropathy predicts cardiovascular morbidity and mortality in type 1 diabetic patients with diabetic nephropathy. Diabetes Care 29(2):334–339
51. Morino K, Petersen KF, Shulman GI (2006) Molecular mechanisms of insulin resistance in humans and their potential links with mitochondrial dysfunction. Diabetes 55(Supplement 2):S9–S15
52. DeFronzo RA, Tripathy D (2009) Skeletal muscle insulin resistance is the primary defect in type 2 diabetes. Diabetes Care 32(suppl 2):S157–S163
53. Brownlee M (2001) Biochemistry and molecular cell biology of diabetic complications. Nature 414(6865):813–820
54. Wolff SP, Dean R (1987) Glucose autoxidation and protein modification. The potential role of 'autoxidative glycosylation' in diabetes. Biochem J 245:243–250
55. Yan S, Stern D, Schmidt A (1997) What's the RAGE? The receptor for advanced glycation end products (RAGE) and the dark side of glucose. Eur J Clin Investig 27(3):179–181
56. Shen D-C, Shieh S-M, Fuh M-T, Wu D-A, Chen Y-D, Reaven G (1988) Resistance to insulin-stimulated-glucose uptake in patients with hypertension*. J Clin Endocrinol Metab 66(3):580–583
57. Sowers JR, Sowers PS, Peuler JD (1994) Role of insulin resistance and hyperinsulinemia in development of hypertension and atherosclerosis. J Lab Clin Med 123(5):647–652
58. Chen Y-Q, Su M, Walia RR, Hao Q, Covington JW, Vaughan DE (1998) Sp1 sites mediate activation of the plasminogen activator inhibitor-1 promoter by glucose in vascular smooth muscle cells. J Biol Chem 273(14):8225–8231
59. Laine H, Yki-Jarvinen H, Kirvela O, Tolvanen T, Raitakari M, Solin O, Haaparanta M, Knuuti J, Nuutila P (1998) Insulin resistance of glucose uptake in skeletal muscle cannot be ameliorated by enhancing endothelium-dependent blood flow in obesity. J Clin Invest 101(5):1156
60. Westerbacka J, Vehkavaara S, Bergholm R, Wilkinson I, Cockcroft J, Yki-Järvinen H (1999) Marked resistance of the ability of insulin to decrease arterial stiffness characterizes human obesity. Diabetes 48(4):821–827
61. Steinberg HO, Chaker H, Leaming R, Johnson A, Brechtel G, Baron AD (1996) Obesity/insulin resistance is associated with endothelial dysfunction. Implications for the syndrome of insulin resistance. J Clin Invest 97(11):2601
62. Després J-P (2006) Abdominal obesity: the most prevalent cause of the metabolic syndrome and related cardiometabolic risk. Eur Heart J Suppl 8(suppl B):B4–B12
63. Van Gaal LF, Mertens IL, Christophe E (2006) Mechanisms linking obesity with cardiovascular disease. Nature 444(7121):875–880
64. Ramkhelawon B, Hennessy EJ, Ménager M, Ray TD, Sheedy FJ, Hutchison S, Wanschel A, Oldebeken S, Geoffrion M, Spiro W (2014) Netrin-1 promotes adipose tissue macrophage retention and insulin resistance in obesity. Nat Med 20(4):377–384
65. De Marchi E, Faldassari B, Bononi A, Wieckowski M, Pinton P (2013) Oxidative stress in cardiovascular diseases and obesity: role of p66Shc and protein kinase C. Oxidative Med Cell Longev 2013:564961. https://doi.org/10.1155/2013/564961
66. Lumeng CN, Bodzin JL, Saltiel AR (2007) Obesity induces a phenotypic switch in adipose tissue macrophage polarization. J Clin Invest 117(1):175

67. Bertrand L, Horman S, Beauloye C, Vanoverschelde J-L (2008) Insulin signalling in the heart. Cardiovasc Res 79(2):238–248
68. Dimmeler S, Fleming I, Fisslthaler B, Hermann C, Busse R, Zeiher AM (1999) Activation of nitric oxide synthase in endothelial cells by Akt-dependent phosphorylation. Nature 399(6736):601–605
69. Mehta PK, Griendling KK (2007) Angiotensin II cell signaling: physiological and pathological effects in the cardiovascular system. Am J Phys Cell Physiol 292:C82–C97
70. Petersen KF, Dufour S, Befroy D, Garcia R, Shulman GI (2004) Impaired mitochondrial activity in the insulin-resistant offspring of patients with type 2 diabetes. N Engl J Med 350(7):664–671
71. Kim J-a, Wei Y, Sowers JR (2008) Role of mitochondrial dysfunction in insulin resistance. Circ Res 102(4):401–414
72. Chen H, Montagnani M, Funahashi T, Shimomura I, Quon MJ (2003) Adiponectin stimulates production of nitric oxide in vascular endothelial cells. J Biol Chem 278(45):45021–45026
73. Mancusi C, Izzo R, di Gioia G, Losi MA, Barbato E, Morisco C (2020) Insulin resistance the hinge between hypertension and type 2 diabetes. High Blood Press Cardiovas Prev 27:515–526. https://doi.org/10.1007/s40292-020-00408-8
74. Izzo R, de Simone G, Chinali M, Iaccarino G, Trimarco V, Rozza F et al (2009) Insufficient control of blood pressure and incident diabetes. Diabetes Care 32:845–850
75. Mancusi C, Losi MA, Izzo R, Canciello G, Manzi MV, Sforza A, De Luca N, Trimarco B, de Simone G (2017) Effect of diabetes and metabolic syndrome on myocardial mechano-energetic efficiency in hypertensive patients. The Campania Salute Network. J Hum Hypertens 31:395–399
76. Mancusi C, de Simone G, Best LG, Wang W, Zhang Y, Roman MJ, Lee ET, Howard BV, Devereux RB (2019) Myocardial mechano-energetic efficiency and insulin resistance in non-diabetic members of the Strong Heart Study cohort. Cardiovasc Diabetol 18:56
77. Ferrannini E, Buzzigoli G, Bonadonna R, Giorico MA, Oleggini M, Graziadei L, Pedrinelli R, Brandi L, Bevilacqua S (1987) Insulinresistance in essentialhypertension. N Engl J Med 317:350–357
78. Reaven GM, Lithell H, Landsberg L (1996) Hypertension and associated metabolic abnormalities–the role of insulin resistance and the sympathoadrenal system. N Engl J Med 334:374–381
79. Grunfeld B, Balzareti M, Romo M, Gimenez M, Gutman R (1994) Hyperinsulinemia in normotensive offspring of hypertensive parents. Hypertension 23:12–15
80. Lembo G, Napoli R, Capaldo B, Rendina V, Iaccarino G, Volpe M, Trimarco B, Sacca L (1992) Abnormal sympathetic overactivity evoked by insulin in the skeletal muscle of patients with essential hypertension. J Clin Invest 90:24–29
81. Lee J, Pilch PF (1994) The insulin receptor: structure, function, and signaling. Am J Phys 266:C319–C334
82. Levy D, Garrison RJ, Savage DD, Kannel WB, Castelli WP (1990) Prognostic implications of echocardiographically determined left ventricular mass in the Framingham heart study. N Engl J Med 322:1561–1566
83. Bots ML, Hoes AW, Koudstaal PJ, Hofman A, Grobbee DE (1997) Common carotid intima-media thickness and risk of stroke and myocardial infarction: the Rotterdam study. Circulation 96:1432–1437
84. Schiffrin EL, Lipman ML, Mann JF (2007) Chronic kidney disease: effects on the cardiovascular system. Circulation 116:85–97
85. Carpinella G, Pagano G, Buono F, Petitto M, Guarino G, Orefice G, Rengo G, Trimarco B, Morisco C (2015) Prognostic value of combined target-organ damage in patients with essential hypertension. Am J Hypertens 28:127–134
86. Meccariello A, Buono F, Verrengia E, Orefice G, Grieco F, Romeo F, Trimarco B, Morisco C (2016) Microalbuminuria predicts the recurrence of cardiovascular events in patients with essential hypertension. J Hypertens 34:646–653

87. Pausova Z, Deslauriers B, Gaudet D, Tremblay J, Kotchen TA, Larochelle P, Cowley AW, Hamet P (2000) Role of tumor necrosis factor-alpha gene locus in obesity and obesity-associated hypertension in frenchcanadians. Hypertension 36:14–19
88. Winkler G, Lakatos P, Salamon F, Nagy Z, Speer G, Kovacs M, Harmos G, Dworak O, Cseh K (1999) Elevated serum tnf-alpha level as a link between endothelial dysfunction and insulin resistance in normotensive obese patients. Diabet Med 16:207–211
89. Zhang R, Reisin E (2000) Obesity-hypertension: the effects on cardiovascular and renal systems. Am J Hypertens 13:1308–1314
90. Dos Santos JM, Moreli ML, Tewari S, Benite-Ribeiro SA (2015) The effect of exercise on skeletal muscle glucose uptake in type 2 diabetes: an epigenetic perspective. Metabolism 64:1619–1628
91. Borghi C, Task Force SIIA, Rossi F, Task SIF, Force. (2015) Role of the renin-angiotensin-aldosterone system and its pharmacological inhibitors in cardiovascular diseases: complex and critical issues. High Blood Press Cardiovasc Prev 22:429–444
92. Ansari AI, Rizvi AA, Verma S, Abbas M, Siddiqi Z, Mishra D, Verma S, Raza ST, Mahdi F (2023) Interactions between diabetic and hypertensive drugs: a pharmacogenetics approach. Mol Gen Genomics 298(4):803–812. https://doi.org/10.1007/s00438-023-02011-7
93. Palleria C, Di Paolo A, Giofrè C, Caglioti C, Leuzzi G, Siniscalchi A, De Sarro G, Gallelli L (2013) Pharmacokinetic drug-drug interaction and their implication in clinical management. J Res Med Sci 18(7):601–610. PMID: 24516494
94. Custodio JM, Wu CY, Benet LZ (2008) Predicting drug disposition, absorption/elimination/transporter interplay and the role of food on drug absorption. Adv Drug Deliv Rev 60(6):717–733. https://doi.org/10.1016/j.addr.2007.08.043. Epub 2007 Nov 28 PMID: 18199522
95. Lago RM, Singh PP, Nesto RW (2007) Diabetes and hypertension. Nat Clin Pract Endocrinol Metab 3(10):667. https://doi.org/10.1038/ncpendmet0638. PMID: 17893686
96. Hernandez R, Teruel T, Lorenzo M (2003) Rosiglitazone produces insulin sensitisation by increasing expression of the insulin receptor and its tyrosine kinase activity in brown adipocytes. Diabetologia 46(12):1618–1628. https://doi.org/10.1007/s00125-003-1236-z. Epub 2003 Nov 1 PMID: 14595539
97. Berger J, Bailey P, Biswas C, Cullinan CA, Doebber TW, Hayes NS, Saperstein R, Smith RG, Leibowitz MD (1996) Thiazolidinediones produce a conformational change in peroxisomal proliferator-activated receptor-gamma: binding and activation correlate with antidiabetic actions in db/db mice. Endocrinology 137(10):4189–4195. https://doi.org/10.1210/endo.137.10.8828476. PMID: 8828476
98. Uehara M, Kishikawa H, Isami S, Kisanuki K, Ohkubo Y, Miyamura N, Miyata T, Yano T, Shichiri M (1994) Effect on insulin sensitivity of angiotensin converting enzyme inhibitors with or without a sulphydryl group: bradykinin may improve insulin resistance in dogs and humans. Diabetologia 37(3):300–307. https://doi.org/10.1007/BF00398058. PMID: 8174845
99. Zou H, Wu G, Lv J, Xu G (2017) Relationship of angiotensin I-converting enzyme (ACE) and bradykinin B2 receptor (BDKRB2) polymorphism with diabetic nephropathy. Biochim Biophys Acta Mol basis Dis 1863(6):1264–1272. https://doi.org/10.1016/j.bbadis.2017.04.002. Epub 2017 Apr 5. Erratum in: BiochimBiophysActa. 2017 Dec 26;: PMID: 28390948
100. Schinner S, Dellas C, Schroder M, Heinlein CA, Chang C, Fischer J, Knepel W (2002) Repression of glucagon gene transcription by peroxisome proliferator-activated receptor gamma through inhibition of Pax6 transcriptional activity. J Biol Chem 277(3):1941–1948. https://doi.org/10.1074/jbc.M109718200. Epub 2001 Nov 13 PMID: 11707457
101. de Oliveira AR, Santos PC, Nascimento RM, Coelho GL, Mill JG, Krieger JE, Pereira AC (2012) BDKRB2 +9/−9 polymorphism is associated with higher risk for diabetes mellitus in the Brazilian general population. Exp Diabetes Res 2012:480251. https://doi.org/10.1155/2012/480251. Epub 2012 Nov 29. PMID: 23243416

102. Young PW, Buckle DR, Cantello BC, Chapman H, Clapham JC, Coyle PJ, Haigh D, Hindley RM, Holder JC, Kallender H, Latter AJ, Lawrie KW, Mossakowska D, Murphy GJ, Roxbee Cox L, Smith SA (1998) Identification of high-affinity binding sites for the insulin sensitizer rosiglitazone (BRL-49653) in rodent and human adipocytes using a radioiodinated ligand for peroxisomal proliferator-activated receptor gamma. J Pharmacol Exp Ther 284(2):751–759. PMID: 9454824
103. Schoonjans K, Martin G, Staels B, Auwerx J (1997) Peroxisome proliferator-activated receptors, orphans with ligands and functions. Curr Opin Lipidol 8(3):159–166. https://doi.org/10.1097/00041433-199706000-00006. PMID: 9211064
104. Pershadsingh HA, Kurtz TW (2004) Insulin-sensitizing effects of telmisartan: implications for treating insulin-resistant hypertension and cardiovascular disease. Diabetes Care 27(4):1015. https://doi.org/10.2337/diacare.27.4.1015. PMID: 15047668
105. Sunder M, Chang AR, Henry RR (2003) Thiazolidinediones, peripheral edema, and type 2 diabetes: incidence, pathophysiology, and clinical implications. Endocr Pract 9(5):406–416
106. White M, Racine N, Ducharme A, de Champlain J (2001) Therapeutic potential of angiotensin II receptor antagonists. Expert Opin Investig Drugs 10(9):1687–1701. https://doi.org/10.1517/13543784.10.9.1687. PMID: 11772278
107. Abdul-Ghani MA, Norton L, Defronzo RA (2011) Role of sodium–glucose cotransporter 2 (SGLT 2) inhibitors in the treatment of type 2 diabetes. Endocr Rev 32(4):515–531. https://doi.org/10.1210/er.2010-0029. Epub 2011 May 23 PMID: 21606218
108. Karg MV, Bosch A, Kannenkeril D, Striepe K, Ott C, Schneider MP, Boemke-Zelch F, Linz P, Nagel AM, Titze J, Uder M, Schmieder RE (2018) SGLT-2-inhibition with dapagliflozin reduces tissue sodium content: a randomised controlled trial. Cardiovasc Diabetol 17(1):5. https://doi.org/10.1186/s12933-017-0654-z. PMID: 29301520
109. Prudente S, Di Paola R, Pezzilli S, Garofolo M, Lamacchia O, Filardi T, Mannino GC, Mercuri L, Alberico F, Scarale MG, Sesti G, Morano S, Penno G, Cignarelli M, Copetti M, Trischitta V (2018) Pharmacogenetics of oral antidiabetes drugs: evidence for diverse signals at the IRS1 locus. Pharmacogenomics J 18(3):431–435. https://doi.org/10.1038/tpj.2017.32. Epub 2017 Jul 11 PMID: 28696414
110. Parameshappa B, Rao NV, Gouda TS, Sen S, Chakraborty R, Basha MA, Reddy AS, Kumar SS (2010) A study on drug-drug interaction between anti-hypertensive drug (propranolol) and anti-diabetic drug (glipizide). Ann Biol Res 1(3):35–40
111. Yagi S, Goto S, Yamamoto T, Kurihara S, Katayama S (2003) Effect of cilnidipine on insulin sensitivity in patients with essential hypertension. Hypertens Res 26(5):383–387. https://doi.org/10.1291/hypres.26.383. PMID: 12887129
112. Takahashi E, Ito M, Miyamoto N, Nagasu T, Ino M, Tanaka I (2005) Increased glucose tolerance in N-type Ca^{2+} channel alpha(1B)-subunit gene-deficient mice. Int J Mol Med 15(6):937–944. PMID: 15870896
113. Paulis L, Foulquier S, Namsolleck P, Recarti C, Steckelings UM, Unger T (2015) Combined angiotensin receptor modulation in the management of cardio-metabolic disorders. Drugs 76:1–12. https://doi.org/10.1007/s40265-015-0509-4
114. Magliano DJ, Shaw JE, Zimmet PZ (2006) How to best define the metabolic syndrome. Ann Med 38:34–41
115. Katovich MJ, Pachori A (2000) Effects of inhibition of the renin–angiotensin system on the cardiovascular actions of insulin. Diabetes Obes Metab 2(1):3–14
116. Feuerer M, Herrero L, Cipolletta D, Naaz A, Wong J, Nayer A, Lee J, Goldfine AB, Benoist C, Shoelson S, Mathis D (2009) Lean, but not obese, fat is enriched for a unique population of regulatory T cells that affect metabolic parameters. Nat Med 15(8):930–939
117. Odegaard JI, Ricardo-Gonzalez RR, Red Eagle A, Vats D, Morel CR, Goforth MH, Subramanian V, Mukundan L, Ferrante AW, Chawla A (2008) Alternative M2 activation of Kupffer cells by PPARdelta ameliorates obesity-induced insulin resistance. Cell Metab 7(6):496–507

118. Ogawa S, Lozach J, Jepsen K, Sawka-Verhelle D, Perissi V, Sasik R, Rose DW, Johnson RS, Rosenfeld MG, Glass CK (2004) A nuclear receptor corepressor transcriptional checkpoint controlling activator protein 1-dependent gene networks required for macrophage activation. Proc Natl Acad Sci USA 101(40):14461–14466
119. Huang W, Ghisletti S, Perissi V, Rosenfeld MG, Glass CK (2009) Transcriptional integration of TLR2 and TLR4 signaling at the NCoR depression checkpoint. Mol Cell 35:48–57
120. Dagenais NJ, Jamali F (2005) Protective effects of angiotensin II interruption: evidence for antiinflammatory actions. Pharmacotherapy 25:1213–1229
121. Oshima K, Mogi M, Jing F, Iwanami J, Tsukuda K, Min LJ, Ogimoto A, Dahlöf B, Steckelings UM, Unger T, Higaki J, Horiuchi M (2012) Direct angiotensin II type 2 receptor stimulation ameliorates insulin resistance in type 2 diabetes mice with PPARγ activation. PLoS One 7(11):e48387
122. Owen JG, Reisin E (2015) Anti-hypertensive drug treatment of patients with and the metabolic syndrome and obesity: a review of evidence, meta-analysis, post hoc and guidelines publications. Curr Hypertens Rep 17:558. https://doi.org/10.1007/s11906-015-0558-9
123. Ogden CL, Carroll MD (2010) Prevalence of overweight, obesity, and extreme obesity among adults: United States, trends 1960–1962 through 2007–2008. National Center for Health Statistics
124. Chan JC, Malik V, Jia W, Kadowaki T, Yajnik CS, Yoon KH et al (2009) Diabetes in Asia: epidemiology, risk factors, and pathophysiology. JAMA 301(20):2129
125. Orchard TJ, Temprosa M, Goldberg R, Haffner S, Ratner R, Marcovina S et al (2005) The effect of metformin and intensive lifestyle intervention on the metabolic syndrome: the diabetes prevention program randomized trial. Ann Intern Med 142:611–619
126. Knowler WC, Barrett-Connor E, Fowler SE, Hamman RF, Lachin JM, Walker EA et al (2002) Diabetes prevention program research group. Reduction in the incidence of type 2 diabetes with lifestyle intervention or metformin. N Engl J Med 346(6):393–403
127. Apovian CM, Aronne L, Rubino D, Still C, Wyatt H, Burns C et al (2013) A randomized, phase 3 trial of naltrexone SR/bupropion SR on weight and obesity-related risk factors (COR-II). Obesity 21(5):935–943
128. Landsberg L, Aronne LJ, Beilin LJ, Burke V, Igel LI, Loyd-Jones D et al (2013) Obesity related hypertension: pathogenesis, cardiovascular risk, and treatment—a position paper of the obesity society and the American society of hypertension. Obesity 21(1):8–24. A position paper on obesity-related hypertension
129. de Faria AP, Modolo R, Fontana V, Moreno H (2014) Adipokines: novel players in resistant hypertension. J Clin Hypertens 16(10):754–759
130. Rahmouni K (2014) Obesity associated hypertension: recent progress in deciphering the pathogenesis. Hypertension 64:215–221. An excellent review that examine the pathogenesis of obesity hypertension
131. Yvan-Charvet L, Quignard-Boulange A (2011) Role of adipose tissue renin-angiotensin system in metabolic and inflammatory diseases associated with obesity. Kidney Int 79:162–168
132. Frigolet ME, Torres N, Tovar AR (2013) The renin-angiotensin system in adipose tissue and its metabolic consequences during obesity. J Nutr Biochem 24:2003–2015
133. Massiera F, Seydoux J, Geloen A et al (2001) Angiotensinogen-deficient mice exhibit impairment of diet-induced weight gain with alteration in adipose tissue development and increased locomotor activity. Endocrinology 142:5220–5225
134. Kouyama R, Suganami T, Nishida J et al (2005) Attenuation of diet-induced weight gain and adiposity through increased energy expenditure in mice lacking angiotensin II type 1a receptor. Endocrinology 146:3481–3489
135. De Souza F, Muxfeldt E, Fiszman R, Salles G (2010) Efficacy of spironolactone therapy in patients with true resistant hypertension. Hypertension 55:147–152
136. Nagase M, Fujita T (2009) Mineralocorticoid receptor activation in obesity hypertension. Hypertens Res 32(8):649–657

137. Troisi RJ, Weiss ST, Parker DR, Sparrow D, Young JB, Landsberg L (1991) Relation of obesity and diet to sympathetic nervous system activity. Hypertension 17:669–677
138. Raumouni K, Correla MI, Haynes WG, Mark AL (2005) Obesity associated hypertension: new insights into mechanisms. Hypertension 25:9–14
139. Kim YH, Her A-Y, Rha S-W, Choi BG, Choi SY, Byun JK, Kang DO, Jang WY, Kim W, Baek JY, Choi WG, Kang TS, Ahn J, Park S-H, Park SH, Hong JY, Park JY, Lee M-H, Choi CU, Park CG, Seo HS (2020) Comparison between calcium channel blocker with angiotensin converting enzyme inhibitor or angiotensin II type 1 receptor blocker combination on the development of new-onset diabetes in hypertensive Korean patients. J Diabetes Metab Disord. 19(1):405–413. https://doi.org/10.1007/s40200-020-00521-4
140. Rajala U, Qiao Q, Laakso M, Keinänen-Kiukaanniemi S (2000) Antihypertensive drugs as predictors of type 2 diabetes among subjects with impaired glucose tolerance. Diabetes Res Clin Pract 50(3):231–239
141. ALLHAT Officers and Coordinators for the ALLHAT Collaborative Research Group. The Antihypertensive and Lipid-Lowering Treatment to Prevent Heart Attack Trial (2002) Major outcomes in high-risk hypertensive patients randomized to angiotensin-converting enzyme inhibitor or calcium channel blocker vs diuretic: the Antihypertensive and Lipid-Lowering Treatment to Prevent Heart Attack Trial (ALLHAT). JAMA 288:2981–2997
142. Pepine CJ, Handberg EM, Cooper-DeHoff RM, Marks RG, Kowey P, Messerli FH, Mancia G, Cangiano JL, Garcia-Barreto D, Keltai M, Erdine S, Bristol HA, Kolb HR, Bakris GL, Cohen JD, Parmley WW, Investigators I (2003) A calcium antagonist vs a non-calcium antagonist hypertension treatment strategy for patients with coronary artery disease. The International Verapamil-Trandolapril Study (INVEST): a randomized controlled trial. JAMA 290:2805–2816
143. Vardeny O, Uno H, Braunwald E, Rouleau JL, Gersh B, Maggioni AP et al (2011) Opposing effects of beta blockers and angiotensin-converting enzyme inhibitors on development of new-onset diabetes mellitus in patients with stable coronary artery disease. Am J Cardiol 107(12):1705–1709
144. Houston MC (1988) The effects of antihypertensive drugs on glucose intolerance in hypertensive nondiabetics and diabetics. Am Heart J 115(3):640–656
145. Lithell HO (1991) Effect of antihypertensive drugs on insulin, glucose, and lipid metabolism. Diabetes Care 14(3):203–209
146. Kuti EL, Baker WL, White CM (2007) The development of new-onset type 2 diabetes associated with choosing a calcium channel blocker compared to a diuretic or beta-blocker. Curr Med Res Opin 23(6):1239–1244
147. Ogihara T, Ueshima K, Nakao K, Fukiyama K, Oba K, Yasuno S et al (2011) Long-term effects of candesartan and amlodipine on cardiovascular morbidity and mortality in Japanese high-risk hypertensive patients: the Candesartan Antihypertensive Survival Evaluation in Japan Extension Study (CASE-J Ex). Hypertens Res 34(12):1295–1301
148. Fonseca V, Sharma PP, Shah M, Deedwania P (2011) Risk of new-onset diabetes mellitus associated with beta-blocker treatment for hypertension. Curr Med Res Opin 27(4):799–807
149. Burke TA, Sturkenboom MC, Ohman-Strickland PA, Wentworth CE, Rhoads GG (2007) The effect of antihypertensive drugs and drug combinations on the incidence of new-onset type-2 diabetes mellitus. Pharmacoepidemiol Drug Saf 16(9):979–987
150. Andraws R, Brown DL (2007) Effect of inhibition of the renin-angiotensin system on development of type 2 diabetes mellitus (meta-analysis of randomized trials). Am J Cardiol 99(7):1006–1012
151. Pongpanich P, Pitakpaiboonkul P, Takkavatakarn K, Praditpornsilpa K, Eiam-Ong S, Susantitaphong P (2018) The benefits of angiotensin-converting enzyme inhibitors/angiotensin II receptor blockers combined with calcium channel blockers on metabolic, renal, and cardiovascular outcomes in hypertensive patients: a meta-analysis. Int Urol Nephrol. 50(12):2261–2278. https://doi.org/10.1007/s11255-018-1991-x

152. Wu L, Deng SB, She Q (2014) Calcium channel blocker compared with angiotensin receptor blocker for patients with hypertension: a meta-analysis of randomized controlled trials. J Clin Hypertens (Greenwich) 16:838–845
153. Cicero AFG, Gerocarni B, Rosticci M, Borghi C (2012) Blood pressure and metabolic effect of a combination of lercanidipine with different antihypertensive drugs in clinical practice. Clin Exp Hypertens 34(2):113–117
154. Huang RS, Cheng YM, Zeng XX, Kim S, Fu P (2016) Renoprotective effect of the combination of renin-angiotensin system inhibitor and calcium channel blocker in patients with hypertension and chronic kidney disease. Chin Med J (England) 129:562–569
155. Jamerson K, Weber MA, Bakris GL, Dahlöf B, Pitt B, Shi V, Hester A, Gupte J, Gatlin M, Velazquez EJ, ACCOMPLISH Trial Investigators (2008) Benazepril plus amlodipine or hydrochlorothiazide for hypertension in high-risk patients. N Engl J Med 359:2417–2428
156. Chi C, Tai C, Bai B, Yu S, Karamanou M, Wang J, Protogerou A, Blacher J, Safar ME, Zhang Y, Xu Y (2016) Angiotensin system blockade combined with calcium channel blockers is superior to other combinations in cardiovascular protection with similar blood pressure reduction: a meta-analysis in 20,451 hypertensive patients. J Clin Hypertens (Greenwich) 18:801–808
157. Cheng Y, Huang R, Kim S, Zhao Y, Li Y, Fu P (2016) Renoprotective effects of renin-angiotensin system inhibitor combined with calcium channel blocker or diuretic in hypertensive patients: a PRISMA-compliant meta-analysis. Medicine (Baltimore) 95(28):e4167. https://doi.org/10.1097/MD.0000000000004167
158. Dézsi CA (2016) The different therapeutic choices with ARBs. Which one to give? When? Why? Am J Cardiovas Drugs 16:255–266. https://doi.org/10.1007/s40256-016-0165-4
159. James PA, Oparil S, Carter BL et al (2014) 2014 evidence-based guideline for the management of high blood pressure in adults: report from the panel members appointed to the Eighth Joint National Committee (JNC 8). JAMA 311(5):507–520
160. Rosendorff C et al (2015) Treatment of hypertension in patients with coronary artery disease: a scientific statement from the American Heart Association, American College of Cardiology, and American Society of Hypertension. J Am Soc Hypertens 9(6):453–498
161. Scheen AJ (2002) Clinical study of the month. The LIFE study: cardiovascular protection of hypertensive patients by losartan. Rev Med Liege 57(4):240–244
162. Pfeffer MA, Swedberg K, Granger CB, Held P, McMurray JJ, Michelson EL et al (2003) Effects of candesartan on mortality and morbidity in patients with chronic heart failure: the CHARM-Overall programme. Lancet 362(9386):759–766
163. Schrader J, Luders S, Kulschewski A, Hammersen F, Plate K, Berger J et al (2005) Morbidity and mortality after stroke, eprosartan compared with nitrendipine for secondary prevention: principal results of a prospective randomized controlled study (MOSES). Stroke 36(6):1218–1226
164. Tocci G (2011) Angiotensin-converting enzyme inhibitors, angiotensin II receptor blockers and diabetes: a meta-analysis of placebo-controlled clinical trials. Am J Hypertens 24(5):582–590
165. Cheung BMY et al (2006) Meta-analysis of large outcome trials of angiotensin receptor blockers in hypertension. J Hum Hypertens 20:37–43
166. Kurtz TW, Klein U (2009) Next generation multifunctional angiotensin receptor blockers. Hypertens Res 32(10):826–834
167. Brenner BM, Cooper ME, de Zeeuw D et al (2001) Effects of losartan on renal and cardiovascular outcomes in patients with type 2 diabetes and nephropathy. N Engl J Med 345:861–869
168. Yasuda T et al (2013) Effects of valsartan on progression of kidney disease in Japanese hypertensive patients with advanced, predialysis, chronic kidney disease: Kanagawa Valsartan Trial (KVT). Hypertens Res 36(3):240–246
169. Mori Y et al (2011) Influence of telmisartan on insulin response after glucose loading in obese patients with hypertension: ARB Trial of Hypertension in Obese Patients with

Hyperinsulinemia Assessed by Oral Glucose Tolerance Test (ATHLETE). Adv Ther 28(8):698–706
170. Brook RD et al (2007) Valsartan improves insulin sensitivity without altering vascular function in healthy overweight adults without the metabolic syndrome. Metab Syndr Relat Disord 5(3):255–261
171. Kim C, Kim MY, Kang DR et al (2013) The efficacy of fimasartan for cardiovascular events and metabolic syndrome (K-MetS Study): rationale, design and participant characteristics. Pulse 1(3–4):177–185
172. Iwanaga T et al (2007) Concentration-dependent mode of interaction of angiotensin II receptor blockers with uric acid transporters. JPET 320:211–217
173. Ilson BE et al (1998) The effects of eprosartan, an angiotensin II AT1 receptor antagonist, on uric acid excretion in patients with mild to moderate essential hypertension. J Clin Pharmacol 38(5):437–441
174. Della Chiesa A et al (2003) Sexual activity in hypertensive men. J Hum Hypertens 17(8):515–521
175. Dusing R (2003) Effect of the angiotensin II antagonist valsartan on sexual function in hypertensive men. Blood Press Suppl 2:29–34
176. Fogari R, Zoppi A, Poletti L et al (2001) Sexual activity in hypertensive men treated with valsartan or carvedilol: a crossover study. Am J Hypertens 14(1):27–31
177. Fogari R et al (2002) Effect of antihypertensive treatment with valsartan or atenolol on sexual activity and plasma testosterone in hypertensive men. Eur J Clin Pharmacol 58(3):177–180
178. Baumhäkel M et al (2008) Effect of irbesartan on erectile function in patients with hypertension and metabolic syndrome. Int J Impot Res 20(5):493–500
179. Segal RL et al (2012) Irbesartan promotes erection recovery after nerve-sparing radical retropubic prostatectomy: a retrospective long-term analysis. BJU Int 110(11):1782–1786
180. Kishi T et al (2012) Telmisartan protects against cognitive decline via up-regulation of brain-derived neurotrophic factor/tropomyosin-related kinase B in hippocampus of hypertensive rats. J Cardiol 60:489–494
181. Wincewicz D, Braszko JJ (2014) Telmisartan attenuates cognitive impairment caused by chronic stress in rats. Pharmacol Rep 66:436–441
182. Hanon O et al (2008) Effects of hypertension therapy based on eprosartan on systolic arterial blood pressure and cognitive function: primary results of the Observational Study on Cognitive function And Systolic Blood Pressure Reduction open-label study. J Hypertens 26(8):1642–1650
183. Esser N, Zraika S (2019) Neprilysin inhibition: a new therapeutic option for type 2 diabetes? Diabetologia 62:1113–1122. https://doi.org/10.1007/s00125-019-4889-y
184. Standeven KF, Hess K, Carter AM et al (2011) Neprilysin, obesity and the metabolic syndrome. Int J Obes 35(8):1031–1040. https://doi.org/10.1038/ijo.2010.227
185. Willard JR, Barrow BM, Zraika S (2017) Improved glycaemia in high-fat-fed neprilysin-deficient mice is associated with reduced DPP-4 activity and increased active GLP-1 levels. Diabetologia 60(4):701–708. https://doi.org/10.1007/s00125-016-4172-4
186. Rice GI, Jones AL, Grant PJ et al (2006) Circulating activities of angiotensin-converting enzyme, its homolog, angiotensin-converting enzyme 2, and neprilysin in a family study. Hypertension 48(5):914–920. https://doi.org/10.1161/01.HYP.0000244543.91937.79
187. Jordan J, Stinkens R, Jax T et al (2017) Improved insulin sensitivity with angiotensin receptor neprilysin inhibition in individuals with obesity and hypertension. Clin Pharmacol Ther 101(2):254–263. https://doi.org/10.1002/cpt.455
188. Seferovic JP, Claggett B, Seidelmann SB et al (2017) Effect of sacubitril/valsartan versus enalapril on glycaemic control in patients with heart failure and diabetes: a post-hoc analysis from the PARADIGM-HF trial. Lancet Diabetes Endocrinol 5(5):333–340. https://doi.org/10.1016/S2213-8587(17)30087-6

189. Nougué H, Pezel T, Picard F et al (2018) Effects of sacubitril/valsartan on neprilysin targets and the metabolism of natriuretic peptides in chronic heart failure: a mechanistic clinical study. Eur J Heart Fail 21:598–605. https://doi.org/10.1002/ejhf.1342
190. Plamboeck A, Holst JJ, Carr RD, Deacon CF (2005) Neutral endopeptidase 24.11 and dipeptidyl peptidase IV are both mediators of the degradation of glucagon-like peptide 1 in the anaesthetised pig. Diabetologia 48(9):1882–1890. https://doi.org/10.1007/s00125-005-1847-7
191. Arbin V, Claperon N, Fournié-Zaluski MC et al (2001) Acute effect of the dual angiotensin-converting enzyme and neutral endopeptidase 24-11 inhibitor mixanpril on insulin sensitivity in obese Zucker rat. Br J Pharmacol 133(4):495–502. https://doi.org/10.1038/sj.bjp.0704098
192. Chipkin RE, Kreutner W, Billard W (1984) Potentiation of the hypoglycemic effect of insulin by thiorphan, an enkephalinase inhibitor. Eur J Pharmacol 102(1):151–154. https://doi.org/10.1016/0014-2999(84)90349-2
193. Wu HT, Chang CK, Cheng KC et al (2010) Increase of plasma insulin by racecadotril, an inhibitor of enkephalinase, in Wistar rats. Horm Metab Res 42(04):261–267. https://doi.org/10.1055/s-0029-1246190
194. Kristensen SL, Preiss D, Jhund PS et al (2016) Risk related to pre-diabetes mellitus and diabetes mellitus in heart failure with reduced ejection fraction. Circ Heart Fail 9:e002560
195. Vodovar N, Nougué H, Launay JM et al (2017) Sacubitril/valsartan in PARADIGM-HF. Lancet Diab Endocrinol 5(7):495–496. https://doi.org/10.1016/S2213-8587(17)30177-8
196. Wang CH, Leung N, Lapointe N et al (2003) Vasopeptidase inhibitor omapatrilat induces profound insulin sensitization and increases myocardial glucose uptake in Zucker fatty rats. Circulation 107(14):1923–1929. https://doi.org/10.1161/01.CIR.0000062646.09566.CC
197. Northridge D, Alabaster C, Connell JC et al (1989) Effects of UK 69 578: a novel atriopeptidase inhibitor. Lancet 334(8663):591–593. https://doi.org/10.1016/S0140-6736(89)90714-9
198. Hupe-Sodmann K, McGregor GP, Bridenbaugh R et al (1995) Characterisation of the processing by human neutral endopeptidase 24.11 of GLP-1(7–36) amide and comparison of the substrate specificity of the enzyme for other glucagon-like peptides. Regul Pept 58(3):149–156. https://doi.org/10.1016/0167-0115(95)00063-H
199. Becker M, Siems W-E, Kluge R et al (2010) New function for an old enzyme: NEP deficient mice develop late-onset obesity. PLoS One 5(9):e12793. https://doi.org/10.1371/journal.pone.0012793
200. Davidson E, Coppey L, Lu B et al (2009) The roles of streptozotocin neurotoxicity and neutral endopeptidase in murine experimental diabetic neuropathy. Exp Diabetes Res 2009:431980
201. Coppey L, Lu B, Gerard C, Yorek MA (2012) Effect of inhibition of angiotensin-converting enzyme and/or neutral endopeptidase on neuropathy in high-fat-fed C57Bl/6J mice. J Obes 2012:326806
202. Simonsen L, Pilgaard S, Carr RD et al (2009) Inhibition of neutral endopeptidase 24.11 does not potentiate the improvement in glycemic control obtained with dipeptidyl peptidase-4 inhibition in diabetic Goto–Kakizaki rats. Horm Metab Res 41(11):851–853. https://doi.org/10.1055/s-0029-1225609
203. Davidson EP, Coppey LJ, Holmes A, Yorek MA (2012) Effect of inhibition of angiotensin converting enzyme and/or neutral endopeptidase on vascular and neural complications in high fat fed/low dose streptozotocin-diabetic rats. Eur J Pharmacol 677(1–3):180–187. https://doi.org/10.1016/j.ejphar.2011.12.003
204. Davidson EP, Coppey LJ, Dake B, Yorek MA (2011) Effect of treatment of Sprague Dawley rats with AVE7688, enalapril, or candoxatril on diet-induced obesity. J Obes 2011:686952
205. Aguilar-Salinas CA, Arellano SA, Villanueva-Sanchez O et al (2001) Effects of omapatrilat on blood pressure and insulin sensitivity in an animal model of insulin resistance. Blood Press 10(3):164–169. https://doi.org/10.1080/080370501753182389
206. Arbin V, Claperon N, Fournié-Zaluski MC et al (2003) Effects of dual angiotensin-converting enzyme and neutral endopeptidase 24-11 chronic inhibition by mixanpril on insulin sensitivity in lean and obese Zucker rats. J Cardiovasc Pharmacol 41(2):254–264. https://doi.org/10.1097/00005344-200302000-00015

207. Zraika S, Aston-Mourney K, Marek P et al (2010) Neprilysin impedes islet amyloid formation by inhibition of fibril formation rather than peptide degradation. J Biol Chem 285(24):18177–18183. https://doi.org/10.1074/jbc.M109.082032
208. Aston-Mourney K, Hull RL, Zraika S et al (2011) Exendin-4 increases islet amyloid deposition but offsets the resultant beta cell toxicity in human islet amyloid polypeptide transgenic mouse islets. Diabetologia 54(7):1756–1765. https://doi.org/10.1007/s00125-011-2143-3

Chapter 6
Role of ACE Inhibitors and Angiotensin Receptor Blockers in Acute Heart Failure

Mukesh Nandave

Introduction by the Editor

Acute heart failure is a life-threatening medical condition requiring immediate development of novel therapeutic intervention. Acute heart failure is characterized by sudden onset and worsening of the symptoms requiring immediate treatment. Treatment of acute heart failure is a complex process due to some reasons such as diverse patient population, lack of pathogenesis knowledge, inadequate evidence-based guidelines. The primary goal of the treatment is to alleviate the congestion and improve the symptoms. Improved understanding of underlying pathophysiology of heart failure can promote development of novel therapy for the treatment [1]. Renin–angiotensin–aldosterone system (RAAS) plays a significant role in the pathophysiology of heart failure. In acute heart failure, dysregulation of RAAS leads to sodium retention, vasoconstriction, and adverse remodeling processes thus worsening the condition. RAAS inhibition has a significant role in reducing morbidity and mortality in heart failure patients especially with reduced ejection fraction (HFrEF). Effectiveness of RAAS inhibition has been proved in several significant clinical trials that lead to their inclusion as essential element of guideline-directed medical therapies (GDMT) for HFrEF. However, it is uncertain whether RAAS inhibition is effective in reducing mortality and morbidity in heart failure patients with preserved ejection fraction (HFpEF) but it could have potential role in reducing hospitalization and mortality rate in careful selected patients [2].

Angiotensin converting enzyme (ACE) inhibitors and angiotensin receptor blockers (ARB) are not only found to be effective in management of hypertension but also found to be effective in heart failure. ACE inhibitors alleviate ventricular

M. Nandave (✉)
Department of Pharmacology, Delhi Pharmaceutical Sciences and Research University, New Delhi, Delhi, India

M. Nandave (ed.), *Angiotensin-converting Enzyme Inhibitors vs. Angiotensin Receptor Blockers*, https://doi.org/10.1007/978-981-97-7380-0_6

remodeling by working on cellular level including on fibrosis, hypertrophy, and apoptosis therefore ameliorate ventricular function in heart failure patients [1]. ACE inhibitors reduces death rate in patients with heart failure and vascular dysfunction as well as in high-risk patients of myocardial infarction and stroke [3]. According to the reports ARBs also found to reduce the rate of hospitalization and death in heart failure patients who cannot tolerate ACE inhibitors.

Although ACE inhibitors and ARBs are prescribed in heart failure, their clinical and prognostic impact in acute phase of acute heart failure is still unclear due to limited data on their safety and efficacy. Limited quality research data is available on initiation, continuation and withdraw of ACE inhibitors and ARBs in acute heart failure which is characterized by increased and dysfunction RAAS activation irrespective of underlying ejection fraction [4]. Continuation of RAAS inhibition therapy after hospital discharge is found to be associated with reduced rate of mortality and readmission of patients with HFrEF [5].

Successful development of angiotensin converting enzyme ACE inhibitors and ARB that block RAAS shows importance and success of this treatment strategy. However, there are some complications related with ACE inhibitors and ARBs in acute heart failure patients such as hypotension, angioedema, hyperkalemia and worsening kidney function [4].

In post hoc analysis of the REALITY-AHF trial, it was observed that ACE inhibitors and ARBs has significantly improved the 1-year outcomes after hospitalization. This improvement is attributed to the early initiation of these medications. It was reported that patients who were administered with ACE inhibitors and ARBs within 48 h of admission have better outcomes than patients who received these medications later. These results indicate that administration timings of ACE inhibitors and ARBs in acute heart failure patients may affect their prognosis. It is noteworthy, the positive impact of early administration of ACE inhibitors and ARBs was consistent regardless of whether patient had HFpEF or HFrEF, despite prior trials suggesting that these therapies have better impact on HFrEF. The underlying mechanism for beneficial effect of ACE inhibitors and ARBs may vary between acute heart failure and chronic heart failure [6].

This chapter explores the significant role played by ACE inhibitors, ARBs in acute heart failure, focusing on their underlying mechanism of action, safety considerations, clinical efficacy, current guidelines and controversies over their prescription in heart failure. This chapter explores the various research data available on management of acute heart failure and ACE inhibitors/ARBs improving patient outcomes (Fig. 6.1).

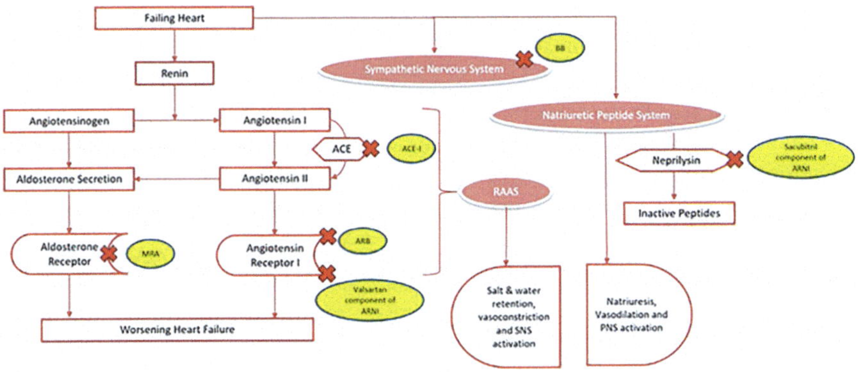

Fig. 6.1 Neurohormonal activation in heart failure and its therapeutic antagonism. (Source: Dalal et al. [7])

Machine Generated Summaries

Disclaimer: The summaries in this chapter were generated from Springer Nature publications using extractive AI auto-summarization: An extraction-based summarizer aims to identify the most important sentences of a text using an algorithm and uses those original sentences to create the auto-summary (unlike generative AI). As the constituted sentences are machine selected, they may not fully reflect the body of the work, so we strongly advise that the original content is read and cited. The auto generated summaries were curated by the editor to meet Springer Nature publication standards. To cite this content, please refer to the original papers.

Machine generated keywords: ang, plasma, aceisarb, aceiarb, aceang, ras, play key, key role, axis, hfpef, allcause, admission, hospitalization, peptide, acei.

The Predictability of Renin–Angiotensin–Aldosterone System Factors for Clinical Outcome in Patients with Acute Decompensated Heart Failure [8]

This is a machine-generated summary of:

Nakada, Yasuki; Takahama, Hiroyuki; Kanzaki, Hideaki; Sugano, Yasuo; Hasegawa, Takuya; Ohara, Takahiro; Amaki, Makoto; Funada, Akira; Yoshida, Akemi; Yasuda, Satoshi; Ogawa, Hisao; Anzai, Toshihisa: The predictability of renin–angiotensin–aldosterone system factors for clinical outcome in patients with acute decompensated heart failure [8].

Published in: Heart and Vessels (2015).

Link to original: https://doi.org/10.1007/s00380-015-0688-7

If you want to cite the papers, please refer to the original.
For technical reasons we could not place the page where the original quote is coming from.

Abstract-Summary "Although counter-regulation between B-type natriuretic peptide (BNP) levels and renin–angiotensin–aldosterone system (RAAS) activation in heart failure (HF) has been suggested, whether the regulation is preserved in acute decompensated heart failure (ADHF) patients remains unclear."

"This study aimed to determine: (1) the relationship between RAAS activation and clinical outcomes in ADHF patients, and (2) the relationships between plasma BNP levels and degrees of activation in RAAS factors."

"This study included ADHF patients (n = 103, NYHA3-4, plasma BNP > 200 pg/ml)."

"We studied the predictability of RAAS factors for cardiovascular events and the relationships between plasma BNP levels and the degrees of activation in RAAS factors, which were evaluated by plasma renin activity (PRA) and aldosterone concentration (PAC)."

"PRA was a strong predictor of cardiovascular (CV) events over 1 year, even after accounting for plasma BNP levels (hazard ratio (HR): 1.04, CI [1.02–1.06], $p < 0.01$) and medication such as RAAS blockers (HR: 1.03, CI [1.01–1.05], $p < 0.01$), whereas PAC was borderline-significant (univariate analysis, $p = 0.06$)."

"Elevated RAAS factors were found in a substantial number of ADHF patients with high plasma BNP levels in the association with hemodynamic state, which predicts poor clinical outcomes."

Introduction

"A counter-regulatory relationship between BNP levels and an activation of RAAS has been suggested in patients with HF [9, 10]."

"Although several studies have focused on the plasma levels of neurohormones in patients with compensated HF [11, 12] and RAAS activity in community based population [13], the assessment of RAAS activation in ADHF patients has not been established for clinical risk stratification."

"Since the pathophysiology of ADHF may include hemodynamic disorders, this hemodynamic interaction underlying the balances between plasma BNP levels and RAAS activation should be considered in ADHF patients."

"The aims of the present study were (1) to evaluate the predictability of RAAS factors for clinical outcomes in ADHF patients; (2) to investigate whether the counter-regulation between plasma BNP levels and the degree of activation of RAAS factors is preserved in ADHF patients."

Methods

"The present study aimed to investigate neurohormonal activities in ADHF patients with the elevation of plasma BNP levels."

"We set the entry criteria as (1) HF symptoms (NYHA3–4), (2) plasma BNP levels at admission ≥200 pg/ml, and (3) underwent blood testing (PRA, PAC and plasma BNP level) within the first 6 days after admission."

"Of these patients, 103 ADHF patients who fulfilled the criteria were identified via medical records."

"We set the cut-off criteria of plasma BNP levels as 200 pg/ml."

"We collected the data of plasma BNP levels which are measured on the day closest to PRA and PAC measurements."

"Body weight (BW) was measured on admission day and the day before hospital discharge. %".

"In ADHF patients, LV ejection fraction (EF) was measured using the Teichholz method [14]."

"Associations between plasma BNP levels and PRA were examined using linear regression."

Results

"Even after the adjustment for diuretics, PRA was strongly associated with clinical events (HR: 1.03, 95% CI 1.01–1.05, $p < 0.01$). In contrast, the predictive value of PAC was borderline-significant (HR: 1.01, CI 1.00–1.02, $p = 0.06$, univariate model), even after adjusting for age, gender and systolic blood pressure, BUN, log BNP ($p = 0.01$–0.10 [models 1–6])."

"The high PRA group had significantly lower mean age, systolic/diastolic blood pressure, LVEF, larger left ventricle dimensions and lower levels of eGFR compared with the low PRA group."

"By adjusting for age, gender, blood pressure, renal function and medication such as diuretics, ACEi, ARB and AA (a lower row), a significant relationship was found between log BNP and log PRA ($p = 0.01$)."

Discussion

"These findings significantly imply that the counter regulation between circulating BNP levels and RAAS activation was disrupted in a substantial number of patients with ADHF, which indicates poor clinical outcomes in ADHF patients."

"The adjustments for blood pressure and eGFR had the critical influence on the relationship between BNP and PRA, suggesting important roles for the hemodynamics state on neurohormonal balances in ADHF patients."

"We suggest that the acute changes of systemic hemodynamics in ADHF patients might influence PRA before changing entire RAAS activation."

"We focused on ADHF in this study and our findings suggest that there is an important role of RAAS factors relating to systemic hemodynamics and renal perfusion, which might shed a light on the different aspects of systemic hemodynamics from the HF pathophysiology which was proposed by plasma BNP levels in ADHF patients."

Limitations

"Despite the small sample of ADHF patients, the present study confirms the importance of PRA in the prediction of the clinical outcomes even in patients with high plasma BNP levels."

"All blood tests in this study were routine clinical examinations and RAAS factors measurements were not done for all patients, based on the physicians' decision."

"We could not exclude the possibility that the lower burden of diuretics might be associated with the lower PRA in the HFpEF patients."

"There might be insufficient evidence to determine the influence of diuretics use on PRA in HFpEF patients in this study due to a small number of patients with HFpEF (n = 9)."

Conclusion

"The activation of RAAS factors was observed in a substantial number of ADHF patients even those with high plasma BNP levels, and was strongly associated with poor clinical outcomes."

"This suggests the counter-regulation between BNP level and RAAS activation was disrupted in the association with hemodynamic state and medication effects."

"The measurements of RAAS factors help to stratify ADHF patients at risk for further cardiovascular events."

Role of ACE2 in Diastolic and Systolic Heart Failure [15]

This is a machine-generated summary of:

Wang, Wang; Bodiga, Sreedhar; Das, Subhash K.; Lo, Jennifer; Patel, Vaibhav; Oudit, Gavin Y.: Role of ACE2 in diastolic and systolic heart failure [15].

Published in: Heart Failure Reviews (2011).

Link to original: https://doi.org/10.1007/s10741-011-9259-x

If you want to cite the papers, please refer to the original.

For technical reasons we could not place the page where the original quote is coming from.

Abstract-Summary "A novel angiotensin-converting enzyme (ACE) homolog, named ACE2, is a monocarboxypeptidase which metabolizes several peptides."

"ACE2 degrades Angiotensin (Ang) II, a peptide with vasoconstrictive/proliferative effects, to generate Ang-(1–7), which acting through its receptor Mas exerts vasodilatory/anti-proliferative actions."

"The first one is formed by the classical pathway involving the ACE-Ang II-AT_1 receptor axis and the second arm is constituted by the ACE2-Ang 1–7/Mas receptor axis."

"ACE2 is also a negative regulator of Ang II-induced myocardial hypertrophy, fibrosis, and diastolic dysfunction."

"The ACE2-Ang 1–7/Mas axis may represent new possibilities for developing novel therapeutic strategies for the treatment of hypertension and cardiovascular diseases."

Background

"The RAS consist of a series of enzymatic reactions culminating in the generation of angiotensin II (Ang II) in plasma as well as in various tissues including the heart and kidneys."

"Angiotensin-converting enzyme 2 (ACE2) was discovered in 2000 [16, 17] and the functional importance of this enzyme has become unequivocal."

"Blockade of angiotensin (Ang) II synthesis by angiotensin-converting enzyme (ACE) inhibitors or its actions by Ang II receptor blockers (ARBs) increases ACE2 expression in the heart [18, 19]."

"Ang-(1–7) is a biologically active metabolite of the renin-angiotensin system (RAS) whose actions are often opposite to those attributed to Ang II, the major component of the RAS [20, 21]."

"While the ACE-Ang II-AT_1 receptor is a well-established axis of the RAS leading to vasoconstrictive/proliferative effects, the ACE2/Ang 1–7/Mas axis provides a vasoprotective/antiproliferative mechanism resulting in the counter-regulation of the RAS."

Biochemical Aspects of ACE2

"Both ACE and ACE2 are endothelium-bound carboxypeptidases which are both widely expressed including the heart, kidney, brain, and vasculature."

"ACE2 can directly metabolize Ang II to generate Ang-(1–7) but is also able to cleave Ang I to generate the inactive Ang-(1–9) peptide [17, 22]."

"Analysis of angiotensin peptide processing in the intact heart showed that ACE2 is mainly responsible for Ang II to Ang-(1–7) metabolism while carboxypeptidase A generates Ang-(1–9) from Ang I [23]."

"In the absence of ACE2, increased plasma and myocardial Ang II levels are likely a direct result of reduced metabolism of plasma Ang II."

"ACE2 is predicted to antagonize the pressor, hypertrophic, and pro-oxidative effects of Ang II by decreasing the levels of Ang II due to increased degradation while directly promoting the formation of Ang-(1–7) [24, 25, 26]."

"ACE2 hydrolyzes both apelin-13 and apelin-36 peptides with high catalytic efficiency [22]."

ACE2 as a Cardioprotective Enzyme: Role in Systolic Dysfunction

"Oudit GY and others [27] reported that the ACE2 protein and activity are significantly augmented in failing human heart ventricles resulting in an increased Ang-(1–7)-forming activity using Ang II as the substrate."

"Burrell and others observed an increase in ACE2 expression in infarcted rat hearts after 28 days and in failing human hearts independently of AT_1 receptor blockade [28]."

"ACE2-deficient mice also present increased plasma and heart Ang II levels in the heart leading to cardiac dysfunction, a phenotype which is critically dependent on the genetic background [27, 29]."

"In response to pressure-overload induced biomechanical stress from pressure, loss of ACE2 worsened the pathological remodeling and results in a rapid progression to systolic dysfunction and heart failure [25, 30]."

"In human heart failure, plasma ACE2 activity is increased and correlates with adverse clinical outcomes [31, 32]."

ACE2 as a Negative Regulator of Ang II-Induced Diastolic Dysfunction

"ACE2 negatively regulates the pathophysiological effects of a pressor and subpressor dose of Ang II on myocardial structure and function [24]."

"Ang II-induced myocardial fibrosis, pathological hypertrophy, and diastolic dysfunction were prevented by recombinant ACE2 [24]."

"In response to exogenous Ang II and pressure-overload, ACE2 levels were decreased thereby perpetuating the pathological effects of Ang II."

"The direct effect of Ang II on adult ventricular cardiomyocytes and cardiac fibroblasts was suppressed by recombinant human ACE2 in an Ang-(1–7)-dependent manner [24]."

"Overexpression of ACE2 protects the heart against myocardial injuries induced by Ang II infusion in rats [33]."

"We proposed that ACE2 functions as negative regulator of the RAS predominantly in the setting of increased Ang II such as in heart disease."

ACE2 in Vascular Diseases

"The in vitro biochemical activity of ACE2 supports its role as a potential regulator of blood pressure homeostasis, via its modulation of the RAS as well as other regulatory peptide pathways [16, 17, 22, 34]."

"In these models of hypertension, ACE2 mRNA and protein levels were greatly reduced in association with increased blood pressure [35]."

"These genetic data argue for a pathophysiological role of ACE2 in hypertension in diet-induced and spontaneous hypertensive rat models."

"Western blot analysis revealed a 40% decrease in ACE2 in the RVLM of spontaneously hypertensive rat compared with Wistar–Kyoto rats while overexpression of ACE2 overcomes its intrinsic decrease in the RVLM and decreases high blood pressure in the spontaneously hypertensive rat [36]."

"Overexpression of ACE2 in the central nervous system modulates local Ang II/ Ang-(1–7) levels, modulates autonomic function and attenuates neurogenic hypertension [37]."

"Overexpression of ACE2 in the vasculature reduces blood pressure and improves endothelial function in hypertensive rats [38]."

Ang 1–7-Mas Axis

"In the intact and failing human hearts, there is a clear dependence of Ang II as substrate for Ang-(1–7) generation [39, 40]."

"Ang-(1–7) functions as a possible antagonist of Ang II actions and potentiates bradykinin activity on the B_2 receptor resulting in nitric-oxide-dependent vasodilation [41, 42]."

"Ang-(1–7) can suppress Ang II-mediated myocardial hypertrophy and fibrosis independent of blood pressure [21, 43]."

"Ang-(1–7) has beneficial effects on the failing heart by activating the sodium pump, hyperpolarising the cell membrane, increasing conduction velocity, and shortening action potential duration [44]."

Pharmacological Approaches to Enhance Ang-(1–7) Effects and ACE2 Action

"There are alternate pathways for converting Ang I to Ang II which do not require ACE [45]."

"ACE-independent Ang II formation in the heart is due to a serine proteinase belonging to the chymase family [45, 46] and the major cellular source of this chymase is the mast cell [47, 48]."

"A clinical consequence of these pathways is seen in patients who take ACE inhibitors chronically, where incomplete suppression of Ang II levels in plasma is often observed [49, 50]."

"The generation of tissue Ang II by non-ACE-related enzymes such as chymase suggests that enhancing ACE2 action may indeed have a unique therapeutic role [24, 47]."

"We need to better define the subpopulations of patients with heart failure in order to selectively target the appropriate subgroup where the ratio of Ang II/Ang-(1–7) remains elevated."

Conclusions

"Pharmacological therapies based on the RAS blockade are used extensively for the treatment of hypertension and cardiovascular diseases including heart failure."

"In spite of their success in pharmacological blockade of the RAS, the prevalence of heart failure has risen steadily in the last several decades."

"These observations indicate that novel and innovative approaches must be discovered in an attempt to promote a more effective treatment for heart failure."

"Due to its unique characteristics, the ACE2/Ang 1–7/Mas axis represents a promising endogenous target for the development of novel drugs targeting diastolic and systolic heart failure."

Future Perspective

"The novel role of ACE2 in hydrolyzing several other peptides such as the apelin peptides, opioids, and kinin metabolites raises the possibility that peptide systems other than angiotensin and its derivatives may also have an important role in regulating cardiovascular and renal function."

"Apelin is a powerful inotrope, peripheral vasodilator and may be involved in fluid homeostasis, making it an attractive target for heart failure therapy."

"Drugs targeting ACE2 represent potential candidates to prevent and treat diastolic and systolic heart failure."

"As we move forward, any novel therapy aimed at enhancing ACE2 action will have to be tested against ACE inhibition, angiotensin receptor blocker, and beta-blockers all of which have been shown to reduce the morbidity and mortality in patients with heart failure."

Angiotensin-Converting Enzyme 2 as a Therapeutic Target for Heart Failure [51]

This is a machine-generated summary of:

Chamsi-Pasha, Mohammed A. R.; Shao, Zhili; Tang, W. H. Wilson: Angiotensin-Converting Enzyme 2 as a Therapeutic Target for Heart Failure [51].

Published in: Current Heart Failure Reports (2013).

Link to original: https://doi.org/10.1007/s11897-013-0178-0

If you want to cite the papers, please refer to the original.

For technical reasons we could not place the page where the original quote is coming from.

Abstract-Summary "The renin-angiotensin system (RAS) plays a major role in the pathophysiology of cardiovascular disorders."

"Angiotensin-converting enzyme 2 (ACE2), a newly discovered homolog of ACE, plays a key role as the central negative regulator of the RAS."

"We aim to focus on the conceptual facts of the ACE2-Ang(1–7) axis with regards to clinical implications and therapeutic targets in cardiovascular disorders, with emphasis on the potential therapeutic role in cardiovascular diseases."

Introduction

"Angiotensin II (Ang-II), the main active substrate of RAS pathway, binds to type-1 receptors (AT1R), thereby promoting vasoconstriction, fibrosis, and salt retention."

"While the ACE/Ang-II/AT1R is a well-established axis of the RAS leading to vasoconstrictive and proliferative effects, the ACE2 linking to angiotensin (1–7) [Ang(1–7)] and its G-protein coupled protein receptor (Mas), provides a vasoprotective and anti-proliferative mechanism, resulting in counter regulation of RAS [52]."

"We attempt to emphasize the role of the ACE2/Ang-(1–7) pathway as a central regulator of the RAS, and as a potential target for therapy in patients across the spectrum of cardiovascular diseases particularly in the setting of heart failure (HF)."

Biochemical Aspects of ACE2 and Ang(1–7) Production

"ACE2 catalyzes the conversion of Ang I to angiotensin-(1–9) which, in turn, can be converted to Ang(1–7) by ACE."

"ACE2 also directly hydrolyzes Ang-II to Ang(1–7) with high catalytic affinity [22]."

"Ang(1–7) is a biologically active metabolite that counterbalances the cardiovascular effects of Ang-II."

"Increased cardiovascular expression of ACE2 and plasma Ang(1–7) levels have been demonstrated with treatment of angiotensin receptor blockers (ARB) as well as mineralocorticoid receptor antagonists (MRA) in animals and humans [19–50, 52, 53]."

"In the absence of ACE2, increased plasma and myocardial Ang-II levels have been attributed to reduced metabolism of plasma Ang-II [24, 26]."

"Production of Ang-II is decreased with increased levels in Ang-I with ACE inhibitors."

"Ang(1–7) is increased primarily due to decreased degradation of Ang-I. In contrast, increased circulating levels of Ang-II by ARB drives the catabolism to the unopposed AT2 receptors, and, hence, to increased levels of Ang(1–7)."

Cardioprotective Role of ACE2 Against Angiontensin II in Animal Studies

"Several observations and experimental evidence from animal models have suggested a beneficial role of the ACE2-Ang(1–7) axis on cardiovascular function."

"Loss of ACE2 enhances the susceptibility to myocardial dysfunction, while enhancing ACE2 action prevents adverse pathological remodeling and slows the progression to HF [27, 54]."

"A deficiency of ACE2 can lead to increased tissue and circulating levels of Ang-II and reduced levels of Ang(1–7) as demonstrated in animal models, which result in early cardiac hypertrophy and fibrosis that is reversible with double knockout mice of ACE and ACE2 genes or following treatment with ACE inhibitors or angiotensin receptor blockers (ARB) [27, 54]."

"Loss of ACE2 worsens the pathological remodeling and results in a rapid progression to reduced systolic function and HF in a pressure-overload mouse model [30]."

Role of ACE2 in Cardiac Remodeling and Systolic Dysfunction in Humans

"In patients with HF, elevated levels of Ang-II and myocardial ACE mRNA level activity have been reported [55]."

"The clinical relevance of ACE2 in the setting of systolic dysfunction was further demonstrated by the detection of soluble ACE2 (sACE2) activity in patients with systolic HF [56]."

"Increasing sACE2 plasma activity strongly correlated with a clinical diagnosis of HF regardless of etiology and tracked with worsening functional class and higher natriuretic peptide levels, while independent of other disease states and medication use [56]."

"Perspective, ARBs would appear to have an advantage since they tend to increase Ang-II levels, an effect that along with its promotion of ACE2 activity, would raise the levels of the protective peptide Ang(1–7)."

"Studies demonstrating incremental benefit of MRAs in patients with systolic HF have supported its broad adoption, yet to our knowledge, no studies on long term effects of MRA on ACE2 or Ang(1–7) metabolism and effects in humans have been conducted."

Role of ACE2 in Diastolic Dysfunction and Hypertension

"ACE2 negatively regulates the pathophysiological effects of a pressor and suppressor dose of Ang-II on myocardial structure and function [24]."

"ACE2 is also a negative regulator of Ang-II-induced myocardial hypertrophy, fibrosis, and diastolic dysfunction [52]."

"With the paucity of effective drug therapies, strategies to enhance ACE2 effects in patients with HFpEF are promising, although studies showing reversal and recovery of myocardial stiffness after its development are lacking."

"Based on in vitro biochemical data and in vivo findings, a reduction in ACE2 levels could lead to elevated Ang-II levels, thus promoting increased blood pressure [24, 57]. Overexpression of ACE2 in the vasculature reduces blood pressure and improves endothelial function in hypertensive rats [58]."

"Ang(1–7) levels are elevated with treatment of ACE inhibitors and ARB, which might suggest the contribution of this peptide in their antihypertensive effects [59]."

"Localized ACE2/Ang(1–7) axis in the brain may also modulate centrally-mediated hypertension."

Utilization of ACE2 Activators in Cardiovascular Diseases: Future Prospects

"ACE and ACE2 have distinct effects on the metabolism of RAS effector peptides that regulate cardiovascular structure and function, drugs which can modify the homeostatic balance of expressions and activities of these enzymes can be viewed as potential therapeutic tools to treat a variety of cardiovascular diseases [60]."

"RhACE2 suppresses the direct effect of Ang-II on cardiomyocytes and fibroblasts in a pressure-overloaded model of HF [24]."

"Ang(1–7) peptide was shown to rescue systolic dysfunction in ACE2-null mice in a pressure-overloaded induced HF model [61]."

"The effects of these newly-developed reagents directly targeting ACE2 or Mas receptor must be compared with the drugs currently used to treat HF patients (i.e., ARBs and MRAs) to determine if targeting the ACE2/Ang(1–7) pathway alone or targeting multiple components of the RAS offers any advantages beyond those of existing therapies [62]."

Conclusion

"The discovery of ACE2 and its role in counteracting the effect of Ang-II through Ang(1–7) formation represents a new avenue for our understanding of the role of the RAS on cardiac pathology."

"The emerging concept is that an imbalance in ACE2/Ang-(1–7) and ACE/Ang-II axes is critical in the development of cardiovascular diseases."

"The central role of ACE2, therefore, appears to counter ACE activity by reducing Ang-II bioavailability and increasing Ang(1–7) formation."

Effect of Angiotensin-Converting Enzyme Inhibitors and Angiotensin II Receptor Blockers on Cardiovascular Events in Patients with Heart Failure: A Meta-Analysis of Randomized Controlled Trials [63]

This is a machine-generated summary of:

Tai, Chenhui; Gan, Tianyi; Zou, Liling; Sun, Yuxi; Zhang, Yi; Chen, Wei; Li, Jue; Zhang, Jian; Xu, Yawei; Lu, Huihe; Xu, Dachun: Effect of angiotensin-converting enzyme inhibitors and angiotensin II receptor blockers on cardiovascular events in patients with heart failure: a meta-analysis of randomized controlled trials [63].

Published in: BMC Cardiovascular Disorders (2017).

Link to original: https://doi.org/10.1186/s12872-017-0686-z

If you want to cite the papers, please refer to the original.

For technical reasons we could not place the page where the original quote is coming from.

Abstract-Summary "Heart failure (HF) remains a significant cause of morbidity and mortality."

"Multiple trials over the past several years have examined the effects of both angiotensin-converting enzyme inhibitors (ACEIs) and angiotensin II receptor blockers (ARBs) in the treatment of left ventricular dysfunction, both acutely after myocardial infarction and in chronic heart failure."

"Our study was conducted to assess efficacy of ACEIs and ARBs in reducing all-cause and cardiovascular mortality in heart failure patients."

"We included randomized clinical trials compared ACEIs and ARBs treatment (any dose or type) with placebo treatment, no treatment, or other anti-HF drugs treatment, reporting cardiovascular or total mortality with an observation period of at least 12 months."

"Of all 38 studies, 32 compared ACEIs with control therapy (included 13 arms that compared ACEIs with placebo, 10 arms in which the comparator was active treatment and 9 arms that compared ACEIs with ARBs), and six studies compared ARBs with placebo."

"ACEIs treatment in patients with HF reduced all-cause mortality to 11% (risk ratio (RR): 0.89, 95% confidence interval (CI): 0.83–0.96, $p = 0.001$) and the corresponding value for cardiovascular mortality was 14% (RR: 0.86, 95% CI: 0.78–0.94, $p = 0.001$)."

"ARBs had no beneficial effect on reducing all-cause and cardiovascular mortality."

"In head-to-head analysis, ACEIs was not superior to ARBs for all-cause mortality and cardiovascular deaths."

"In HF patients, ACEIs, but not ARBs reduced all-cause mortality and cardiovascular deaths."

Background

"A lot of clinical trials have confirmed that suppression of RAAS (angiotensin-converting enzyme inhibitors (ACEIs) and angiotensin II receptor blockers (ARBs)) reduces cardiovascular (CV) events in patients with heart failure [64–96]."

"Recent meta-analysis reported that in HF patients with hypertension [97] and diabetes [98], treatment with ACEIs resulted in a significant further reduction in all-cause and CV mortality, whereas ARBs had no benefit on these outcomes."

"These studies indicate that there are different clinical outcomes between ACEIs and ARBs among patients with heart failure."

"In light of these conflicting reports, the present meta-analysis was conducted to assess the efficacy of ACEIs and ARBs on all-cause and CV mortality in patients with heart failure."

Methods

"Studies were deemed eligible if they: 1) were RCTs, targeting HF patients with reduced ejection fraction (HFrEF, left ventricular ejection fraction ≤45%), with a median or mean follow-up of more than 12 months; 2) compared ACEIs and ARBs treatment (any dose or type) with placebo treatment, no treatment, or other anti-HF drugs treatment; 3) reported cardiovascular or total mortality."

"After excluding the unrelated studies, the following data were extracted: study characteristics (author, publication year, sample size, follow-up period), population baseline characteristics (age, sex, cause of heart failure, risk factors) and end-points."

"Studies were considered statistically heterogeneous if $I^2 > 50\%$ and $p \leq 0.05$."

"If heterogeneity between studies were identified, a random-effects model was applied."

"Meta-regression was conducted to explore the potential heterogeneity related to the participants (age, cause of HF, left ventricular ejection fraction, and follow-up weeks), the agent used (different types)."

Results

"Thirty-two studies [70–96, 99–103] reported the effect of ACEIs on all-cause mortality in a total of 39,254 HF patients with moderate heterogeneity in overall analysis ($I^2 = 44\%$, $p = 0.005$)."

"15 studies [64–96, 99–103] reported the effect of ARBs on all-cause mortality in a total of 28,814 HF patients with no significant heterogeneity in overall analysis ($I^2 = 26\%$, $p = 0.17$)."

"Seventeen studies [71–74, 76, 84, 86, 89, 90, 92–95, 99, 101–103] reported the effectiveness of ACEIs for CV mortality in a total of 28,302 HF patients with moderate heterogeneity in overall analysis ($I^2 = 51\%$, $p = 0.009$)."

"11 studies [64, 67–69, 93–95, 99, 101–103] reported the effectiveness of ARBs for CV mortality in a total of 27,991 HF patients with no significant heterogeneity in overall analysis ($I^2 = 40\%$, $p = 0.08$)."

"Meta-regression was conducted in different ages ($p = 0.97$), causes of HF ($p = 0.90$), left ventricular ejection fractions ($p = 0.09$), follow-up weeks ($p = 0.41$) to observe effects of ACEIs treatment on all-cause mortality."

Discussion

"ARBs have no significant effect on all-cause and CV mortality in HF patients."

"In head-to-head analysis, ACEIs are not superior to ARBs on all-cause and CV mortality."

"This meta-analysis provides compelling evidence that ACEIs are the most effective first-line treatment for preventing all-cause and CV mortality in HF patients."

"Several studies demonstrated that ACEIs reduced all-cause and CV mortality in HF patients, particularly after myocardial infarction [72, 74]."

"Besides, in some recent meta-analysis, Vark and others [97] and Cheng and others [98] presented that in patients with hypertension and diabetes, treatment with an ACEI resulted in a significant further reduction in all-cause and CV mortality, whereas ARBs had no benefit on these outcomes."

"Different types of ACEIs may influence the effect on all-cause mortality, which means that captopril may be superior to enalapril in reducing all-cause mortality in HF patients."

Conclusions

"In 47,662 subjects, our meta-analysis shows that ACEIs, but not ARBs reduce all-cause mortality and cardiovascular deaths in HF patients."

"ACEIs should be considered as first-line therapy to limit excess mortality and morbidity in this population."

Treatment with Optimal Dose Angiotensin-Converting Enzyme Inhibitors/Angiotensin Receptor Blockers Has a Positive Effect on Long-Term Survival in Older Individuals (Aged >70 Years) and Octogenarians with Systolic Heart Failure [104]

This is a machine-generated summary of:

Sargento, Luis; Simões, Andre Vicente; Longo, Susana; Lousada, Nuno; dos Reis, Roberto Palma: Treatment with Optimal Dose Angiotensin-Converting Enzyme Inhibitors/Angiotensin Receptor Blockers Has a Positive Effect on Long-Term Survival in Older Individuals (Aged >70 Years) and Octogenarians with Systolic Heart Failure [104].

Published in: Drugs & Aging (2016).

Link to original: https://doi.org/10.1007/s40266-016-0393-y

If you want to cite the papers, please refer to the original.

For technical reasons we could not place the page where the original quote is coming from.

Abstract-Summary "To evaluate the association of ACEI/ARB dose level with long-term survival in stable older patients (aged >70 years) and octogenarian outpatients with HFrEF."

"ACEIs/ARBs were prescribed to 91.3% of patients, and 52.9% received the high dose."

"Survival improved with increasing ACEI/ARB dose level in the total population (Hazard Ratio [HR] = 0.67; 95% confidence interval [CI] 0.55–0.82; $p < 0.001$), older patients aged >70 years (HR = 0.65; 95% CI 0.51–0.83; $p < 0.001$), and octogenarians (HR = 0.71; 95% CI 0.51–0.99; $p = 0.045$)."

"The low (HR = 0.35; 95% CI 0.16–0.76; $p = 0.008$) and high doses (HR = 0.13; 95% CI 0.06–0.32; $p < 0.001$) improved survival compared with not receiving ACEIs/ARBs."

"In octogenarians, all dose levels were associated with improved survival compared with not receiving ACEIs/ARBs, but there was no difference between ACEI/ARB doses."

"The achieved optimal dose of ACEIs/ARBs in ambulatory older people with HFrEF is associated with long-term survival."

Introduction

"In daily practice, achieving target doses is often challenging because of side effects or co-morbidity [105, 106], especially in older people with polypharmacy and multiple co-morbidities."

"Even in dedicated HF clinics, only half of the octogenarians were reported to achieve the ACEI/ARB target dose, and 21% achieved the BB target dose [105]."

"The target dose of ACEIs/ARBs was associated with reduced all-cause, 5-year mortality [105]."

"In the same cohort, only 36% of the patients received ≥50% of the target dose of ACEIs/ARBs and BBs."

"Whether the target dose of ACEIs/ARBs and BBs outperforms other doses is unknown."

"This study aimed to evaluate the association of ACEI/ARB therapy and the achieved dose with long-term survival in stable, ambulatory, older people (aged >70 years) and octogenarians with HFrEF."

Materials and Methods

"Patients were assessed at scheduled clinical visits in the HF unit with a 3-year follow-up."

"The secondary objectives were as follows. (1) The effect of ACEI/ARB prescription and the achieved doses on 3-year survival in octogenarians was examined. (2) The effect of ACEI/ARB prescription on 3-year survival in a propensity score-matched (PSM) population according to the ACEI/ARB dose level (low vs. high) was determined. (3) The effect of BB therapy on long-term survival was evaluated. (4) The relationships between baseline clinical and laboratory characteristics and outcome in older patients and older subgroups of patients were examined."

"Prospective recruited population of 138 older patients (aged ≥70 years), we retrospectively selected PSM cohorts according to ACEI/ARB low/high doses (1:1 ratio; n = 66; 52.3% of the total population receiving ACEIs/ARBs)."

Results

"Twelve (8.7%) patients did not receive ACEIs/ARBs and 52.9% received the high dose."

"Medical therapy was similar between the two age subgroups, but octogenarians received the high dose of ACEIs/ARBs, BBs, or a combination of both less frequently than patients aged 70–80 years."

"shows the clinical and demographic characteristics of the population according to the ACEI/ARB dose level (low vs. high)."

"The matched population was well balanced for all variables used in the general model, including renal dysfunction in the low and high doses (57.6 vs. 48.5%; p = 0.622)."

Discussion

"The present study shows the need to prescribe and up-titrate ACEIs/ARBs in older people, including octogenarians, with HFrEF, because there is a strong association between the dose level and long-term survival."

"Our findings indicate that the achieved dose level of ACEI/ARB therapy is associated with long-term survival in older patients with HFrEF."

"The beneficial effect of the ACEI/ARB dose level on survival was different according to the age subgroups."

"Our study suggests the clinical importance of prescribing ACEIs/ARBs to older patients and to up-titrate the dose because of its positive effect on survival."

"Non-octogenarian older patients should have the ACEI/ARB dose up-titrated to a high dose (≥50% TD) to improve survival."

"The low rate of older patients who achieved the TD also limited analysis at this dose level, but everything was done by the HC clinic team to achieve the TD."

Conclusions

"ACEI/ARB prescription and dose level optimization in older patients with HFrEF has a significant and positive effect on long-term survival."

"It is never too late to optimize HF therapy in older patients with HFrEF."

"Supplementary data mentioned in the text is available from the Drugs & Aging home page."

Effect of Prescribing Patterns of Renin–Angiotensin System Blockers and Beta-Blockers on Prognosis of Heart Failure [107]

This is a machine-generated summary of:

Kim, Hyun-Jin; Jo, Sang-Ho; Lee, Min-Ho; Seo, Won-Woo; Choi, Jin-Oh; Ryu, Kyu-Hyung: Effect of Prescribing Patterns of Renin–Angiotensin System Blockers and Beta-Blockers on Prognosis of Heart Failure [107].

Published in: Advances in Therapy (2020).

Link to original: https://doi.org/10.1007/s12325-020-01443-6

If you want to cite the papers, please refer to the original.

For technical reasons we could not place the page where the original quote is coming from.

Abstract-Summary "Use of angiotensin-converting enzyme inhibitors (ACEi)/ angiotensin receptor blockers (ARB) only, beta-blockers (BB) only, or both has been rarely compared in patients with heart failure (HF)."

"We evaluated the prescribing patterns of ACEi/ARB and BB on prognosis in HF according to left ventricular function."

"Patients were classified into four groups according to the prescription pattern at discharge: all ACEi/ARB and BB treatment group, only ACEi or ARB treatment group, only BB treatment group, and neither ACEi/ARB nor BB group."

"Use of both ACEi/ARB and BB had significantly lowest all-cause death rates among the four groups in all types of HF."

"Cox regression analysis showed that use of both drugs was independently associated with 51% reduced risk of all-cause death in patients with HF with preserved ejection fraction (HFpEF) and HF with mid-range ejection fraction (HFmrEF)."

"In patients with HF with reduced ejection fraction, use of ACEi/ARB and/or BB revealed an independent association with a reduced risk of all-cause death regardless of prescribing patterns."

Introduction

"Because the effectiveness of treatment with angiotensin-converting enzyme inhibitors (ACEi), angiotensin receptor blockers (ARB)—both renin–angiotensin system (RAS) blockers—and beta-blockers (BB) has been proven in patients with heart failure reduced ejection fraction (HFrEF), current guidelines recommend these medications [108, 109]."

"Compared to patients with HFrEF, no definitely proven treatments have been introduced for improved clinical outcomes in patients with heart failure with preserved ejection fraction (HFpEF) and heart failure with mid-range ejection fraction (HFmrEF) [108, 110]."

"The effects of ACEi, ARB, and BB on long-term clinical outcomes according to prescribing patterns such as combination therapy of ACEi/ARB and BB or monotherapy of ACEi, ARB, or BB alone have rarely been investigated in the HF field."

"We evaluated the actual prescribing patterns and prescribing status of ACEi/ ARB and BB in patients with HF at discharge, and their effect on long-term prognosis according to left ventricular ejection fraction (LVEF), especially in patients with HFpEF and HFmrEF."

Methods

"A minimum of 1 year of follow-up was strongly recommended to all patients and the outcome data were recorded prospectively in medical records and telephone correspondence, including death and rehospitalization due to HF."

"Among patients with an identified LVEF, 2825 patients suffering from acute HF who were able to determine whether they had received ACEi, ARB, and BB were finally analyzed."

"The patients were classified into two groups based on their LVEF as follows: HFrEF group whose LVEF was less than 40% versus HF with mid-range EF (HFmrEF) and HF with preserved EF (HFpEF) group whose LVEF was at least 40% [108]."

"The linear-by-linear test was also used to compare the prescribing patterns of ACEi/ARB and BB between the HFrEF group and HFmrEF and HFpEF group, and also used to extract the trend of study outcomes according to prescribing patterns of ACEi/ARB and BB."

Results

"There was no significant difference in prescription pattern for ACEi/ARB and BB at discharge between the two groups: 32.6% of patients with HFpEF and HFmrEF and 24.9% of patients with HFrEF did not receive ACEi/ARB and BB at discharge."

"Patients in the all ACEi/ARB and BB treatment groups had a significantly higher cumulative death-free survival rate in both the HFpEF and HFmrEF group and the HFrEF group."

"The four groups according to prescribing pattern of ACEi/ARB and BB had significantly different probabilities of all-cause death (long-rank test p for trend < 0.001) in patients with HFpEF and HFmrEF and also in patients with HFrEF."

"After adjusting for confounding factors, Cox regression analysis showed that use of all ACEi/ARB and BB at discharge was independently associated with 51% reduced risk of all-cause death in patients with HFpEF and HFmrEF."

Discussion

"Our results of the national registry of patients admitted with acute HF reflect real practice and reveal the beneficial effects of monotherapy of ACEi or ARB in patients with HFpEF and HFmrEF on the long-term prognosis differently from previous studies."

"Key trials for the effects of ACEi/ARB on clinical outcomes in patients with HFpEF have already shown negative results, and in recent years there have been few studies on the association between RAS inhibitors and HFpEF and HFmrEF."

"To RAS inhibitors, the role of BB in HFpEF and HFmrEF lowered the risk of all-cause death significantly when combined with ACEi or ARB, but monotherapy of BB showed no beneficial effect in this study."

"Despite the disappointing results of BB in patients with HFpEF and HFmrEF, which are not specifically recommended in the guidelines, a recent study using a systemic review and meta-analysis reported a 21% risk reduction in all-cause death at short-term follow-up of 3–12 months [111]."

Conclusions

"Prescribing patterns of ACEi, ARB, and BB were diverse in patients with HF and there was a difference in the degree of risk reduction in all-cause death."

"ACEi, ARB, and BB were still inadequately prescribed to patients and should be actively given to patients with HF to improve their clinical outcomes."

"Clinicians should consider prescribing ACEi/ARB first to patients with HFpEF and HFmrEF prior to BB."

Renin–Angiotensin–Aldosterone System Optimization for Acute Decompensated Heart Failure Patients (ROAD-HF): Rationale and Design [112]

This is a machine-generated summary of:

Dass, Bhagwan; Dimza, Michelle; Singhania, Girish; Schwartz, Cody; George, Jerin; Bhatt, Avni; Radhakrishnan, Nila; Bansari, Asha; Bozorgmehri, Shahab; Mohandas, Rajesh: Renin–Angiotensin–Aldosterone System Optimization for Acute Decompensated Heart Failure Patients (ROAD-HF): Rationale and Design [112].

Published in: American Journal of Cardiovascular Drugs (2019).

Link to original: https://doi.org/10.1007/s40256-019-00389-7

If you want to cite the papers, please refer to the original.

For technical reasons we could not place the page where the original quote is coming from.

Abstract-Summary "The administration of ACEIs/ARBs in acute decompensated heart failure (ADHF) can increase the risk of morbidity and mortality secondary to worsening renal function (WRF)."

"The aim of our study is to determine whether withholding ACEIs/ARBs during the initial 72 h of admission in patients with ADHF will prevent WRF and allow more effective diuresis."

"Four hundred and thirty patients will be randomized to the intervention (withholding ACEIs/ARBs) or control (continue/start ACEIs/ARBs) arms for 72 h. Primary outcomes include rates of acute kidney injury (AKI), patient global assessment, and change in kinetic eGFR over 72 h, while secondary outcomes include change in weight, fluid balance, change in signs and symptoms of congestion, change in renal function, change in urinary biomarkers (tissue inhibitor of metalloproteinases 2 [TIMP-2] × insulin-like growth factor-binding protein 7 [IGFBP7]), patients experiencing treatment failure, hospital length of stay (LOS), cost analysis, mortality within 30 days, and hospital readmissions over 30 days and 1 year."

"Holding ACEIs/ARBs might help preserve renal function, and decrease hospital LOS, readmission rates, and cost of care in ADHF."

Introduction

"While the benefits of using angiotensin-converting enzyme inhibitors (ACEIs) and angiotensin receptor blockers (ARBs) in chronic heart failure are well-documented, their role in acute decompensated heart failure (ADHF) is less clear."

"The introduction of ACEIs can be associated with worsening of renal function in some patients."

"Recent studies have found worsening renal function (WRF) during index hospitalization is strongly associated with increased mortality, hospital length of stay (LOS), readmission rates, and cost of care [113, 114]."

"The Renin Angiotensin Aldosterone Optimization in Acute Decompensated Heart Failure (ROAD-HF) study is a randomized controlled trial (RCT) aimed at investigating the hypothesis that withholding ACEI/ARBs for the initial 72 h of ADHF hospitalization will reduce the rates of WRF, while allowing for more aggressive diuresis and clinical improvement."

Materials and Methods

"Secondary outcomes for ROAD-HF will include (a) change in weight; (b) net fluid balance; (c) freedom from signs and symptoms of congestion; (d) [TIMP-2] × [IGFBP7] biomarker (baseline level for all patients and reassessment at 48 h for the first 100 patients); (e) persistent or worsening heart failure; (f) treatment failure; (g) hospital LOS; (h) cost analysis of hospital stay; (i) death at 30 days; (j) readmission, or ED visit within 30 days; and (k) readmission rates at 1 year. [TIMP-2] × [IGFBP7] is a biomarker that predicts the risk of moderate or severe AKI within 12 h, in patients hospitalized to intensive care units [115]."

"A Data Safety Monitoring Board (DSMB), comprised of members outside of the study staff, will specifically focus on ensuring that all patients enrolled in the trial are restarted on their home ACEIs/ARBs after 72 h and prior to discharge from the hospital."

Discussion

"According to epidemiological studies, the lifetime risk for developing heart failure in Americans ≥40 years of age is about 20% [116]."

"The incidence of heart failure increases with age, from approximately 20 per 1000 individuals between 65 and 69 years of age, to >80 per 1000 individuals among those ≥85 years of age [117]."

"Although several therapies have been developed for heart failure, the overall mortality and adverse cardiovascular outcomes has not significantly improved over time."

"The long-term treatment of heart failure involves the use of ACEIs/ARBs as well as β-blockers to inhibit the maladaptive upregulation of the renin–angiotensin–aldosterone system (RAAS) and sympathetic nervous system that accompanies chronic heart failure."

"The use of ACEIs/ARBs during aggressive diuresis and hemodynamic instability blunts RAAS autoregulation and may result in WRF."

Conclusion

"The ROAD-HF study is an RCT aimed at assessing the impact of holding ACEI/ARB medication early in the treatment of ADHF."

"The study will compare two treatment strategies during aggressive diuresis—one group with continued ACEIs/ARBs and the other group without this therapy for the initial 72 h. Holding ACEIs/ARBs should mitigate the significant hemodynamic consequences on the RAAS during the aggressive diuresis phase of therapy."

"These data can be used to help standardize therapy for a diagnosis associated with such high morbidity and mortality."

Ace Inhibitor Therapy for Heart Failure in Patients with Impaired Renal Function: A Review of the Literature [118]

This is a machine-generated summary of:

Valika, Ali A.; Gheorghiade, Mihai: Ace inhibitor therapy for heart failure in patients with impaired renal function: a review of the literature [118].

Published in: Heart Failure Reviews (2012).

Link to original: https://doi.org/10.1007/s10741-011-9295-6

If you want to cite the papers, please refer to the original.

For technical reasons we could not place the page where the original quote is coming from.

Abstract-Summary "Neuro-hormonal antagonism plays a key role in the management of this syndrome, and angiotensin-converting enzyme inhibitors and angiotensin receptor blockers are one of the cornerstones of therapy."

"Cardiorenal physiology is becoming more recognized in these patients with advanced heart failure, and the role of neuro-hormonal blockade in this setting is vaguely defined in the literature."

"The purpose of this article is to review the role and pathophysiology of ace inhibition and angiotensin receptor blockade in patients with acute and chronic heart failure syndromes and concomitant cardiorenal physiology."

Pathophysiology

"These pressure differentials are in part mediated by a cascade of neuro-hormonal agents, allowing for auto-regulation of renal blood flow and GFR to be precisely controlled."

"A perceived reduction in renal perfusion, either from lower cardiac output or diminished arteriolar volume, would stimulate increased renin and angiotensin II production."

"Angiotensin II subsequently stimulates a preferential increase in effective efferent arteriolar resistance relative to the afferent system, thereby allowing for an increased pressure gradient to be further transmitted to the glomerus."

"In decompensated heart failure syndromes, a chronic reduction in renal perfusion pressure can lead to maximal activation of angiotensin II, whereby both afferent and efferent renal arteriolar constriction occurs."

Ace Inhibition Effect on GFR

"ACEi also act via the kallikrein-kinin pathway, whereby inhibition of kininase leads to accumulation of bradykinin levels and potentiates the therapeutic antihypertensive effects of ACEi via an increase in local endothelial nitric oxide production, further enhancing its long-term benefit [119]."

"In regard to its primary mechanism of action, the reduction in Angiotensin II levels also has the potential to mitigate the preferential increase in efferent arteriolar tone that occurs in the kidneys, potentially leading to a decline in the intraglomerular pressure gradient and subsequent decrease in GFR."

"In actuality, ACEi have been shown clinically to have a wide range of effects on the GFR."

"To the above, literature review would suggest that up to 24% of patients actually note a decrease in creatinine and hence improvement in GFR after starting ACEi therapy [120]."

ACE Inhibition in Worsening Renal Function

"In the CONSENSUS trial, in patients with initial worsening of renal function after starting ACEi, creatinine was noted to stabilize over a 6-month time period with continued enalapril therapy [120]."

"These patients, despite worsening renal function, may from the onset require continuation of ACEi therapy, with appropriate dose adjustments and close monitoring of mean arterial pressure, as counteracting the maladaptive responses to angiotensin II may help to actually stabilize GFR in the short term, and at the same time provide long-term cardiac benefit as previously described [121]."

"These studies would suggest that an impulsive reaction to discontinue ACEi in the setting of initial decline in renal function may not necessarily be beneficial, and an assessment of short-term risk of therapy versus long-term survival benefit needs to be addressed in clinical practice as well as in future trials."

Efficacy in Chronic Kidney Disease

"This was looked at in a randomized control study of benazepril versus placebo in 422 patients with non-diabetic chronic kidney disease, with a subgroup population noted to have serum creatinine ranging from 3.1 to 5.0 mg/dL. At a mean follow-up of 3.4 years, as compared with placebo, benazepril was associated with a 43% reduction in the risk of worsening renal function, end-stage renal disease, and death ($P = 0.005$) [122]."

"Not only is the progression of chronic kidney disease improved by ACEi and ARBs, but also the development of incident heart failure in patients with baseline CKD."

"Advanced kidney disease patients requiring renal replacement therapy also have limited data on the utility of ACEi, and few studies are known to have addressed this question in heart failure patients."

Timing of Therapy in Acute Heart Failure

"There are limited data on the utility of ACEi in the acute decompensated heart failure patient, where the goals of therapy are initially that of early decongestion."

"Prior, concomitant aggressive diuretic therapy and ACEi can lead to an initial decline in GFR."

"Further studies are needed to determine early versus late administration of ACEi therapy in the acute heart failure syndromes, as well as in patients with documented worsening renal function with initial diuretic therapy."

Conclusion

"ACEi have had a proven role as neuro-hormonal antagonists in improving survival in heart failure, and yet these protective strategies are often withheld in patients with concomitant acute or chronic kidney disease."

"A small rise in creatinine should not prohibit therapy, and even further worsening renal function can often be managed by decreasing or withholding diuretic therapy at the time of initiation of ACEi."

"This paradigm might be comparable to the role of beta-blocker therapy in heart failure, whereby there is often seen an initial decline in cardiac output with initiation of beta blockade, but overall improvement in long-term ejection fraction and survival."

"Timing of initiation of therapy remains to be studied, though general recommendations are to optimize fluid status first with diuretic therapy, with subsequent initiation of ACEi in patients with concomitant heart failure and renal dysfunction."

[Section 7]

"Heart failure encompasses a variety of clinical syndromes that are often difficult to manage and are associated with high morbidity and mortality."

"Neuro-hormonal antagonism plays a key role in the management of this syndrome, and angiotensin-converting enzyme inhibitors (ACEi) and angiotensin receptor blockers (ARB) are one of the cornerstones of therapy."

"Cardiorenal physiology is becoming more recognized in these patients with advanced heart failure, and the role of neuro-hormonal blockade in this setting is vaguely defined in the literature."

"The purpose of this article is to review the role and pathophysiology of ace inhibition and angiotensin receptor blockade in patients with acute and chronic heart failure syndromes and concomitant cardiorenal physiology."

Effects of Renin-Angiotensin System Blockade on Mortality and Hospitalization in Heart Failure with Preserved Ejection Fraction [123]

This is a machine-generated summary of:

Agarwal, Vikram; Briasoulis, Alexandros; Messerli, Franz H.: Effects of renin-angiotensin system blockade on mortality and hospitalization in heart failure with preserved ejection fraction [123].

Published in: Heart Failure Reviews (2012).

Link to original: https://doi.org/10.1007/s10741-012-9329-8

If you want to cite the papers, please refer to the original.

For technical reasons we could not place the page where the original quote is coming from.

Abstract-Summary "MEDLINE, EMBASE, and COCHRANE databases were searched from 1966 to 2011 for longitudinal studies examining HF-PEF patients receiving treatment with RAS inhibitors, either ACE inhibitors (ACE-I) or angiotensin receptor blockers (ARB) in addition to their standard treatment compared to those receiving standard treatment alone."

"We examined the all-cause mortality, cardiovascular mortality, and hospitalizations for heart failure."

"Among the randomized clinical trials, with the use of RAS inhibitors over standard treatment, there was no improvement in all-cause mortality (RR: 0.99; 95% CI: 0.88–1.12; p = 0.88), while there was a trend toward lowered rates of hospitalization (RR: 0.93; 95% CI: 0.86–1.01; p = 0.08)."

"Among the observational studies with the use of RAS inhibitors, there was a significant benefit in all-cause mortality (RR: 0.76; 95% CI: 0.62–0.93; p = 0.009), with no significant impact on the hospitalization rates."

"RAS inhibition in HF-PEF was not associated with significant reduction in all-cause or cardiovascular mortality, but randomized control trials appear to demonstrate a trend toward reduction in the risk for subsequent hospitalization."

"Further prospective randomized trials are warranted to confirm the effects of RAS inhibition on mortality and hospitalization."

Introduction

"Heart failure with preserved ejection fraction (HF-PEF) is the most common and fastest growing form of heart failure in the United States [124]."

"Renin-angiotensin system (RAS) inhibitors, including angiotensin-converting enzyme inhibitors (ACE-I) and angiotensin receptor blockade (ARB), constitute first-line treatment for patients with heart failure with reduced ejection fraction (HF-REF) with proven efficacy in reducing mortality and morbidity."

"The aim of this meta-analysis was to assess efficacy of RAS inhibition on mortality and hospitalizations due to heart failure in HF-PEF patients."

Materials and Methods

"Eligible studies were (1) prospective (randomized or non-randomized) or retrospective study designs assessing the effectiveness of RAS inhibitors (ACE-I or ARB) for HF-PEF (defined as signs or symptoms of heart failure and EF ≥40%); (2) studies reporting outcomes of interest, including mortality (all-cause and/or cardiac) and hospitalizations due to heart failure; and (3) studies with at least a 6-month follow-up in each study arm."

"An intention-to-treat traditional meta-analysis was performed in accordance with the recommendations from the Cochrane Collaboration and the preferred reporting items for systematic reviews and meta-analyses (PRISMA) statement (for randomized controlled trials) and meta-analysis of observational studies in epidemiology (MOOSE) statement for others."

"We separately examined if there were any differences in the outcomes between randomized and non-randomized studies, and various groups of RAS inhibitors, including ACE-I, ARB, and ACE-I/ARB combination."

"Since there was significant heterogeneity between the observational and randomized studies, the cumulative results of the two subgroups are reported separately."

Results

"There was no significant reduction in cardiovascular mortality with the use of RAS inhibitors compared to controls in both the randomized control trials (RR: 0.97; 95% CI: 0.86–1.1; p = 0.63) and the observational studies (RR: 052; 95% CI: 0.25–1.06; p = 0.07)."

"With the use of RAS inhibitors, the randomized control trials showed a trend toward lower rates of hospitalization (RR: 0.93; 95% CI: 0.86–1.01; p = 0.08), while the observational studies did not show any significant reduction in hospitalization rates (RR: 0.97; 95% CI: 0.77–1.21; p = 0.76)."

"On examining the individual subgroups among the randomized control trials, while the ARB subgroup showed a trend toward lower rates of hospitalization (RR: 0.94; 95% CI: 0.86–1.0; p = 0.14), there was no significant change in hospitalization rates with the use of ACE-I (RR: 0.85; 95% CI: 0.63–1.13; p = 0.26)."

Discussion

"While we found that regardless of the study design, there was little evidence of reduced all-cause or cardiovascular mortality, there was a trend toward lower rates of hospitalization among patients on RAS inhibitors, especially among the high-quality randomized clinical trials."

"Tighter control of blood pressure by various agents, including RAS inhibitors, potentially forms an important part of the armamentarium of management of HF-PEF."

"Conceivably, therefore, HF-PEF patients with higher systolic blood pressures may exhibit greater benefit, and consequently better outcomes, with the use of RAS inhibitors."

"The Treatment of Preserved Cardiac function heart failure with an Aldosterone Antagonist (TOPCAT) will focus on the effects of spironolactone in HF-PEF patients, with the primary end point examining a composite of cardiovascular mortality, aborted cardiac arrest, or hospitalization for the management of heart failure, and secondary end points including quality of life, non-fatal cardiovascular events, and new-onset atrial fibrillation [125]."

Conclusion

"In spite of the small reduction in hospitalization rates, especially with the use of ACE-Is and a trend toward decreased mortality, the inconsistency of the results between the studies along with the negative results of the larger trials allow no firm conclusions on therapy in patients with HF-PEF."

"For now, treatment of these patients should empirically focus on strict blood pressure control and paying attention to the other comorbidities often found in this patient population."

"Whether or not RAS inhibitors should be used as first-line drugs remains to be determined."

Safety and Prognostic Impact of Early Treatment with Angiotensin-Converting Enzyme Inhibitors or Angiotensin Receptor Blockers in Patients with Acute Heart Failure [126]

This is a machine-generated summary of:

Yoshioka, Kenji; Matsue, Yuya; Yamaguchi, Tetsuo; Kitai, Takeshi; Kagiyama, Nobuyuki; Okumura, Takahiro; Kida, Keisuke; Oishi, Shogo; Akiyama, Eiichi; Suzuki, Satoshi; Yamamoto, Masayoshi; Kuroda, Shunsuke; Matsumura, Akihiko; Hirao, Kenzo: Safety and Prognostic Impact of Early Treatment with Angiotensin-Converting Enzyme Inhibitors or Angiotensin Receptor Blockers in Patients with Acute Heart Failure [126].

Published in: American Journal of Cardiovascular Drugs (2019).

Link to original: https://doi.org/10.1007/s40256-019-00355-3

If you want to cite the papers, please refer to the original.

For technical reasons we could not place the page where the original quote is coming from.

Abstract-Summary "Although angiotensin-converting enzyme inhibitors (ACEIs) and angiotensin II receptor blockers (ARBs) have been recommended for patients with heart failure, their clinical and prognostic impact in the very acute phase of acute heart failure (AHF) is unclear, mainly because data on their safety and efficacy are lacking."

"Patients with AHF who did not take an ACEI or ARB at admission were enrolled."

"Patients who received these medications within 48 h of admission were categorized as the ACEI/ARB group, and all other patients were categorized as the no ACEI/ARB group."

"Of the 1682 patients in the REALITY-AHF cohort, 900 were enrolled in this study, and 288 (32%) were included in the ACEI/ARB group."

"Early initiation of ACEIs/ARBs within 48 h of admission for hospitalized patients with AHF was not associated with adverse events and correlated with improved outcomes at 1 year from admission."

Introduction

"Most of the studies that have shown beneficial effects tested the drugs in chronic heart failure; very little is known about the effect on outcomes of starting ACEIs/ARBs in the very acute phase of acute heart failure (AHF) in patients not receiving these medications at admission."

"It could be that early treatment with ACEIs/ARBs can be beneficial in terms of possibly improving hemodynamic status given that activation of the renin–angiotensin–aldosterone system is one of the key mechanisms of AHF, and some small studies in severe heart failure have shown hemodynamically beneficial effects from early administration of intravenous captopril [127, 128]."

"We investigated the safety and clinical implications of starting ACEIs/ARBs in the very acute phase of AHF."

Methods

"The present analysis focused on the clinical and prognostic impact of the very early introduction of ACEIs/ARBs within 48 h of hospital presentation in patients with AHF who were not receiving ACEIs/ARBs before admission."

"To evaluate the difference in the longitudinal trajectory of blood pressure over time between groups with and without ACEI/ARB treatment within 48 h while accounting for the within-individual correlation of repeated blood pressure measurement, we used a linear mixed-effect model."

"The propensity score was estimated based on a logistic model constructed with the following variables: age; sex; systolic blood pressure; history of hypertension, diabetes mellitus and coronary artery disease; left ventricular ejection fraction (LVEF); prescription of diuretics and β-blocker at admission; sinus rhythm on electrocardiogram at admission; white blood cell counts; hemoglobin; glucose levels; blood urea nitrogen; eGFR; and B-type natriuretic peptide (BNP), which were measured at admission."

Results

"Fewer patients in the early ACEI/ARB group were receiving heart failure medications at the time of admission and had preserved renal function than those in the late ACEI/ARB group."

"In univariate Cox regression analysis using the early ACEI/ARB group as a reference, only the no ACEI/ARB group (HR 3.11; 95% CI 2.21–4.37; $p < 0.001$) but not the late ACEI/ARB group (HR 1.31; 95% CI 0.84–2.03; $p = 0.233$) was associated with significantly worse prognosis."

"Both the no ACEI/ARB group (HR 2.54; 95% CI 1.50–4.31; $p < 0.001$) and the late ACEI/ARB group (HR 1.99; 95% CI 1.11–3.56; $p = 0.020$) were associated with a worse prognosis than was the early ACEI/ARB group after adjustment for covariates in the multivariable Cox regression analysis."

Discussion

"This is the first study to show the clinical and prognostic implications of ACEI/ARB treatment in the very acute phase of AHF in patients naïve to these drugs."

"ACEIs/ARBs have been one of the cornerstones of heart failure treatment; however, the optimal timing of starting ACEI/ARB in hospitalized patients with AHF not receiving ACEI/ARB treatment at the time of admission is unclear [71–73, 129]."

"Sanam and others [130] conducted a similar retrospective study using propensity score matching analysis and showed lower 30-day and 1-year mortality after discharge in hospitalized patients with AHF receiving ACEIs/ARBs at the time of discharge."

"Although these studies clarified the importance of starting ACEI/ARB treatment before discharge in patients hospitalized with AHF, especially those with reduced LVEF, when ACEI/ARB treatment should be started after admission remained unclear."

Antihypertrophic Effects of Combined Inhibition of the Renin–Angiotensin System (RAS) and Neutral Endopeptidase (NEP) in Progressive, Tachycardia-Induced Experimental Heart Failure [131]

This is a machine-generated summary of:

Birner, Christoph; Ulucan, Coskun; Bratfisch, Mona; Götz, Tobias; Dietl, Alexander; Schweda, Frank; Riegger, Günter A.; Luchner, Andreas: Antihypertrophic effects of combined inhibition of the renin–angiotensin system (RAS) and neutral endopeptidase (NEP) in progressive, tachycardia-induced experimental heart failure [131].

Published in: Naunyn-Schmiedeberg's Archives of Pharmacology (2012).
Link to original: https://doi.org/10.1007/s00210-012-0791-6

If you want to cite the papers, please refer to the original.
For technical reasons we could not place the page where the original quote is coming from.

Abstract-Summary "Vasopeptidase inhibition (VPI), a therapeutic strategy by dual inhibition of both ACE and neutral endopeptidase 24.11, has not shown a prognostic benefit over ACE inhibition in chronic severe heart failure (CHF)."

"The effects of early treatment by VPI on cardiac remodelling have not been well assessed."

"We analysed the effects of early chronic VPI (50 mg/kg/day Omapatrilat) on cardiac remodelling and neurohumoral function during the progression of rapid ventricular pacing-induced heart failure in rabbits (early left ventricular dysfunction [ELVD]: 10 days at 330 bpm, CHF: further 10 days at 360 bpm)."

"This increase was markedly attenuated by VPI (both $p < 0.05$ vs. placebo)."

"CHF was associated with a further increase in atrial mass and an increase in LV mass (both $p < 0.05$), which was again attenuated by VPI (atrial mass, $p < 0.05$ vs. untreated)."

"LV BNP mRNA was significantly increased in CHF ($p < 0.05$ vs. control), and chronic VPI completely abolished this increase in ELVD and significantly attenuated it in CHF ($p < 0.05$ vs. CHF-placebo)."

"Beyond that, the increase of cGMP was augmented by chronic VPI ($p < 0.05$ vs. placebo in CHF) in heart failure and that of Aldosterone was attenuated ($p < 0.05$ vs. placebo in ELVD), whereas PRA was temporarily increased ($p < 0.05$ vs. placebo in ELVD)."

"Combined inhibition of ACE and NEP by VPI significantly inhibits early cardiac remodelling and LV BNP gene expression."

Introduction

"With respect to chronic experimental heart failure, NEP inhibition has recently shown to delay the onset of sodium retention during the transition from early to severe heart failure and improve the natriuretic response to volume expansion while enhancing the natriuretic peptides and depressing aldosterone activation in tachycardia-induced heart failure (Martin and others [132])."

"It was our objective to assess the effects of combined inhibition of the RAS and NEP upon cardiac remodelling and neurohumoral function."

"Given the recently demonstrated effects of chronic inhibition of NEP as demonstrated in the canine model (Martin and others [132]), we hypothesized that dual inhibition of ACE and NEP might as well attenuate cardiac remodelling in the progressive rabbit model."

"In order to address our hypothesis, we assessed the effects of chronic RAS and NEP inhibition by the vasopeptidase inhibitor Omapatrilat in rabbits with chronic progressive tachycardia-induced heart failure."

Methods

"The pacing rate was then increased to 360 bpm for 10 days, and ELVD evolved to CHF with further cardiac enlargement and further decreased perfusion pressure together with clinical signs of fluid retention (ascites, pleural and pericardial effusion)."

"Since invasive measurement of arterial blood pressure demonstrated a hypotensive effect of VPI already in ELVD and a more sustained effect in advanced CHF, the pacing rate was not increased above 360 bpm in order to avoid symptomatic hypotension."

"The progressive model in the rabbit allows pacing rates up to and above 380 bpm without symptomatic hypotension At baseline (control), after being paced at 330 bpm for 10 days (ELVD) and at the end of the protocol (CHF), conscious arterial pressure was measured invasively via the medial ear artery and a 2D-guided M-mode echocardiogram was obtained."

Results

"In treated animals, left ventricular dilatation was attenuated, and in ELVD, the treated animals exhibited significantly smaller left ventricular enddiastolic diameters as compared to placebo ($p < 0.05$)."

"This increase was completely blunted in treated ELVD animals ($p < 0.05$ vs. placebo) and markedly attenuated in heart failure."

"These increases were markedly blunted in the treated group, and atrial mass index in the treated group was significantly smaller as compared to placebo both in ELVD ($p < 0.05$) and in heart failure ($p < 0.05$)."

"Total cardiac mass index was likewise significantly smaller in the treated animals with heart failure as compared to placebo ($p < 0.05$)."

"In treated animals, aldosterone was suppressed as compared to placebo both in ELVD ($p < 0.05$) and in heart failure."

"These increases were blunted in treated animals with ELVD and markedly attenuated in heart failure."

Discussion

"The current study was undertaken to assess the effects of combined inhibition of the RAS and NEP on cardiac remodelling in progressive, tachycardia-induced heart failure."

"The current study underscores the potential of early combined antagonism of the RAS and NEP on cardiac remodelling in heart failure."

"Early combined RAS and NEP inhibition had sustained effects on progressive experimental heart failure."

"We observed that increases in left atrial diameter which are normally seen with progressive heart failure were blunted in the treated group and this effect was sustained even in more advanced heart failure."

"The current data confirm previous studies which have addressed the concept of combined RAS and NEP inhibition (Lapointe and others [133]; Maki and others [134, 135]; Mishima and others [136]; Xu and others [137]) and extend these studies to the model of progressive, pacing-induced heart failure."

"We observed strong and sustained effects of combined RAS and NEP inhibition upon left ventricular gene expression."

Conclusion

"The current study demonstrates multiple beneficial effects of combined RAS and NEP inhibition in and upon the progression of tachycardia-induced heart failure in the rabbit."

"These effects include beneficial neurohumoral and haemodynamic changes as well as attenuated cardiac remodelling."

"These findings warrant that the pharmacological concept of combined RAS and NEP inhibition continues to be developed further."

Serum Angiotensin-Converting Enzyme 2 Concentration and Angiotensin-(1–7) Concentration in Patients with Acute Heart Failure Patients Requiring Emergency Hospitalization [138]

This is a machine-generated summary of:

Hisatake, Shinji; Kiuchi, Shunsuke; Kabuki, Takayuki; Oka, Takashi; Dobashi, Shintaro; Ikeda, Takanori: Serum angiotensin-converting enzyme 2 concentration and angiotensin-(1–7) concentration in patients with acute heart failure patients requiring emergency hospitalization [138].

Published in: Heart and Vessels (2016).
Link to original: https://doi.org/10.1007/s00380-016-0877-z

If you want to cite the papers, please refer to the original.
For technical reasons we could not place the page where the original quote is coming from.

Abstract-Summary "Serum ACE activity, ACE2, Ang-(1–7) concentration, plasma Ang II, aldosterone concentration, and plasma renin activity (PRA) were measured at the acute stage."

"We conducted a comparative study between patients with AHF and healthy volunteers."

"Patients with AHF showed lower serum ACE activity and plasma aldosterone concentration than healthy volunteers (12.3 vs. 15.1 IU/L, respectively; P = 0.01, 75.6 vs. 125.3 pg/mL, respectively; P = 0.000); there were no differences between the two groups in PRA and plasma Ang II concentration."

"Patients with AHF had a higher serum ACE2 concentration than healthy volunteers (7.9 vs. 4.8 ng/mL, respectively; P = 0.002), but their serum Ang-(1–7) concentration was significantly lower (2.4 vs. 3.1 ng/mL, respectively; P = 0.005)."

"Patients with AHF had a higher serum ACE2 concentration, lower serum Ang-(1–7) concentration, and lower serum ACE activity and plasma aldosterone concentrations than healthy volunteers, whereas PRA and plasma Ang II concentration were the same."

Introduction

"The existence of a new RAS cascade called the ACE2/Ang-(1–7)/Mas receptor axis has been established [139, 140]."

"Almost all reports about the ACE2/Ang-(1–7)/Mas receptor axis have been conducted using animals [20–50, 52–62, 64–103, 105, 106, 108–111, 113–117, 119–122, 124, 125, 127–130, 132–137, 139–141], and there are few reports about the dynamics of the ACE2/Ang-(1–7)/Mas receptor axis under various pathological conditions in clinical settings [56]."

"From the perspective of future medical treatment of cardiovascular disease, evaluating ACE2/Ang-(1–7)/Mas receptor axis dynamics in humans is of profound significance."

Methods

"At the acute stage of AHF, we collected venous blood transdermally from the upper limbs when patients were able to maintain a sitting posture for at least 30 min."

"Further, venous blood was also collected from healthy volunteers in the same way as that collected from the study patients."

"Serum concentrations of Ang-(1–7) was measured using ELISA kits (Peninsula Laboratories, LLC, San Carlos, CA) according to the manufacturer's instructions except for solid phase extraction (SPE)."

"We used the unpaired Student's t test to compare baseline characteristics of study patients and healthy volunteers."

"The unpaired Student's t test was used to compare serum ACE activity, ACE2, Ang-(1–7) concentration, as well as plasma Ang II, aldosterone concentration and PRA between the study patients and healthy volunteers."

"The multiple regression was used to analyze the influence of age, gender, blood pressure, estimated glomerular filtration rate (eGFR), hemoglobin A1c (HbA1c) and presence or absence of AHF to ACE2 and Ang-(1–7)."

Results

"There were differences between the two groups in terms of age, sex, height, or body mass index."

"There was no difference in systolic blood pressure between the two groups."

"Only the presence or absence of acute heart failure was a factor affecting the value of serum ACE2 concentration and serum Ang-(1–7) concentration."

"Patients with AHF showed lower serum ACE activity and plasma aldosterone concentration than healthy volunteers (12.3 vs. 15.1 IU/L, respectively; P = 0.01, 75.6 vs. 125.3 pg/mL, respectively; P = 0.000); there were no differences between the two groups in PRA and plasma Ang II concentration."

Discussion

"We measured circulatory system RAS and ACE 2/Ang-(1–7) in the blood from patients with AHF that required emergency hospitalization."

"There have been few reports on plasma renin activity, serum ACE activity, and plasma Ang II concentration in patients with AHF at the acute stage; however, there have been reports acknowledging the stimulation of PRA in heart failure cases [142]."

"Serum Ang-(1–7) concentrations were significantly lower in patients with AHF than in healthy volunteers."

"As previous reports on the measurement of Ang-(1–7) in the blood of living organisms have only examined healthy volunteers [143], the present study is the first report on the measurement of this protein in patients with AHF, making our findings extremely interesting."

"Because there was a significant difference in the age of healthy volunteers and patients with AHF, but we confirmed by multiple regression analysis that age had no influence on ACE2 and Ang-(1–7)."

Recombinant Human Angiotensin-Converting Enzyme 2 as a New Renin-Angiotensin System Peptidase for Heart Failure Therapy [144]

This is a machine-generated summary of:

Oudit, Gavin Y.; Penninger, Josef M.: Recombinant Human Angiotensin-Converting Enzyme 2 as a New Renin-Angiotensin System Peptidase for Heart Failure Therapy [144].

Published in: Current Heart Failure Reports (2011).

Link to original: https://doi.org/10.1007/s11897-011-0063-7

If you want to cite the papers, please refer to the original.

For technical reasons we could not place the page where the original quote is coming from.

Abstract-Summary "Angiotensin-converting enzyme 2 (ACE2) is a monocarboxypeptidase that metabolizes several peptides, including the degradation of angiotensin (Ang) II, a peptide with vasoconstrictive/proliferative effects, to generate Ang 1–7, which exerts vasodilatory/antiproliferative actions by acting through its receptor Mas."

"Human recombinant ACE2 also is a negative regulator of Ang II–induced myocardial hypertrophy, fibrosis, and diastolic dysfunction and suppresses pressure overload–induced heart failure."

"Due to its characteristics, the ACE2/Ang 1–7/Mas axis may represent new possibilities for developing novel therapeutic strategies for the treatment of hypertension and heart failure."

"This review summarizes the beneficial effects of ACE2 in heart disease and the potential use of human recombinant ACE2 as a novel therapy for heart failure."

Introduction

"The renin-angiotensin system (RAS) is a central regulator of cardiovascular and renal function and plays a key role in the pathophysiology of various cardiovascular disorders [145]."

"The RAS consists of a series of enzymatic reactions culminating in the generation of angiotensin (Ang) II in plasma as well as in various tissues, including the heart and kidneys."

"Angiotensin-converting enzyme 2 (ACE2) was discovered in 2000 [16, 146], and the functional importance of this enzyme has become unequivocal."

"ACE2 also plays a key role in kidney disease and reduces tubulointerstitial fibrosis and diabetic renal injury [147, 148]."

Biochemistry of Angiotensin-Converting Enzyme 2

"ACE2 can directly metabolize Ang II to generate Ang 1–7, but is also able to cleave Ang I to generate the inactive Ang 1–9 peptide [22, 146]."

"Analysis of angiotensin peptide processing in the intact heart showed that ACE2 is mainly responsible for Ang II to Ang 1–7 metabolism, while carboxypeptidase A generates Ang 1–9 from Ang I [23]."

"Increased Ang II levels result from the reduced hydrolysis of Ang II by ACE2."

"Increased plasma and tissue Ang II levels are likely a direct result of reduced metabolism of plasma Ang II in the absence of ACE2."

"ACE2 is predicted to antagonize the pressor, hypertrophic, and pro-oxidative effects of Ang II by decreasing the levels of Ang II due to increased degradation while directly promoting the formation of Ang 1–7 [24, 26, 149]."

Biochemical Characterization of Recombinant Human Angiotensin-Converting Enzyme 2

"The expression product was purified to homogeneity by applying a capture step on a DEAE Sepharose (GE Healthcare Life Sciences, Piscataway, NJ) anion exchanger resin."

"The eluted fractions containing the expression product were submitted to a polishing step on a Superdex 200 gel-filtration column (GE Healthcare Life Sciences) [24]."

"The expression product was compared to the commercially available ACE2 standard 933-ZN (R&D Systems, Inc., Minneapolis, MN)."

"Chemical and immunological properties of both products were almost identical, while rhACE2 showed a 93% enzymatic activity with Mca-APK-(Dnp)-OH substrate in comparison to rhACE2 standard 933-ZN."

Role of Angiotensin-Converting Enzyme 2 in Diastolic Dysfunction

"ACE2 negatively regulates the pathophysiological effects of a pressor and subpressor dose of Ang II on myocardial structure and function [24]."

"While loss of ACE2 increases Ang II levels, increased ACE2 action by the use of rhACE2 lowered Ang II and increased Ang 1–7 levels in vivo, providing definitive evidence for a key role of ACE2 in the metabolism of Ang II [24]."

"RhACE2 reduced the plasma and myocardial Ang II levels and increased plasma Ang 1–7 levels."

"In response to exogenous Ang II and pressure overload, ACE2 levels were decreased, thereby perpetuating the pathological effects of Ang II."

"The direct effect of Ang II on adult ventricular cardiomyocytes and cardiac fibroblasts were suppressed by rhACE2 in an Ang 1–7–dependent manner [24]."

"We proposed that ACE2 functions as a negative regulator of the RAS predominantly in the setting of increased Ang II, such as in heart disease."

Role of Angiotensin-Converting Enzyme 2 in Systolic Dysfunction

"ACE2-deficient mice also present increased plasma and heart Ang II levels in the heart leading to cardiac dysfunction, a phenotype that is critically dependent on the genetic background [27, 29]."

"ACE2 protein and activity are significantly augmented in failing human heart ventricles, resulting in an increased Ang 1–7–forming activity from Ang II conversion."

"Burrell and others [28] observed an increase in ACE2 expression in infarcted rat hearts after 28 days and in failing human hearts independently of AT_1R blockade."

"Increased production of superoxide, activation of matrix metalloproteinases, and pathological signaling lead to the severe adverse myocardial remodeling and dysfunction in ACE2 knockout mice [149]."

"Using the left anterior descending artery ligation model, we showed that ACE2 knockout mice had increased mortality with worsening heart function after MI [26]."

"In human HF, plasma ACE2 activity is increased and correlates with adverse clinical outcomes [31, 32]."

Vasoprotective Effects of Angiotensin-Converting Enzyme

"The in vitro biochemical activity of ACE2 supports its role as a potential regulator of blood pressure homeostasis via its modulation of the RAS as well as other regulatory peptide pathways [16, 22, 34, 146]."

"The potential role of ACE2 in essential hypertension is supported by our studies showing that ACE2 maps to quantitative trait loci on the X chromosome, which contributes to hypertension in a salt-induced model of hypertension (Sabra rats), spontaneous hypertensive rat (SHR), and SHR stroke-prone rats [35]."

"In these models of hypertension, ACE2 mRNA and protein levels were greatly reduced in association with increased blood pressure [35]."

"Based on in vitro biochemical data and in vivo findings, a reduction in ACE2 levels could lead to elevated Ang II levels, thus promoting increased blood pressure [24, 57]."

"These genetic data argue for a pathophysiological role of ACE2 in hypertension in these diet-induced and SHR models."

"Overexpression of ACE2 in the vasculature reduces blood pressure and improves endothelial function in hypertensive rats [38]."

Ang 1–7/Mas Axis in Heart Failure

"Ang 1–7 analogues or Mas receptor agonists can have potential as cardiovascular therapeutic agents."

"The relevance of the Ang 1–7/Mas axis in the heart is illustrated by recent findings with Mas-deficient mice."

"Mas-deficient mice exhibited a marked change of the extracellular matrix proteins to a profibrotic profile accompanied by cardiac dysfunction [150]."

"In adult cardiomyocytes, Ang 1–7 mediates antihypertrophic effects while also antagonizing Ang II–mediated activation of the NADPH oxidase [24, 151]."

"In an ACE2-deficient state, supplementation with Ang 1–7 suppressed the increased NADPH oxidase activity, resulting in reversal of pressure overload–induced HF [149]."

Enhancing Angiotensin-Converting Enzyme 2 Action as a Novel Therapy for Heart Failure

"There are alternate pathways for converting Ang I to Ang II that do not require ACE [152]."

"ACE-independent Ang II formation was found to be particularly robust in the heart, and this activity eventually was assigned to a serine proteinase belonging to the chymase family [152, 153]."

"A clinical consequence of these pathways where incomplete suppression of Ang II levels in plasma often is observed is seen in patients who take ACE inhibitors chronically [8, 15, 51, 63, 104, 107, 112, 154]."

"The generation of tissue Ang II by non–ACE-related enzymes such as chymase suggests that enhancing ACE2 action may indeed have a unique therapeutic role [24, 47]."

"One additional potential strategy can be to suppress the rate of cleavage of ACE2 from the surface of cardiac cells leading to retention of enzymatic activity, reduced Ang II, and increased Ang 1–7 within microenvironments of the heart."

Conclusions

"The novel role of ACE2 in hydrolyzing several other peptides, such as the apelin peptides and kinin metabolites, raises the possibility that peptide systems other than Ang II/Ang 1–7 may be responsible for the action of ACE2 on the cardiovascular system."

"Loss of ACE2 enhances the susceptibility to cardiovascular disease, including HF, while enhancing ACE2 action prevents adverse pathological remodeling and slows the progression to HF."

"As we move forward, any novel therapy aimed at enhancing ACE2 action will have to be tested against ACE inhibition, ARBs, and β-blockers, all of which have been shown to reduce the morbidity and mortality in patients with HF."

Bibliography

1. Elder DH, McAlpine-Scott J, Choy AM, Struthers AD, Lang CC (2013) Aortic valvular heart disease—is there a place for angiotensin-converting enzyme? Exp Rev Cardiovasc Ther 11(1):107–114
2. Khan MS, Fonarow GC, Khan H, Greene SJ, Anker SD, Gheorghiade M et al (2017) Renin-angiotensin blockade in heart failure with preserved ejection fraction: a systematic review and meta-analysis. ESC. Heart Fail 4:402–408
3. Weber KT (1997) Extracellular matrix remodeling in heart failure. A role for de novo angiotensin II generation. Circulation 96:4065–4082
4. Oliveros E, Oni E, Shahzad A, Kluger A, Lo K, Rangaswami J et al (2020) Benefits and risks of continuing angiotensin-converting enzyme inhibitors, angiotensin ii receptor antagonists, and mineralocorticoid receptor antagonists during hospitalizations for acute heart failure. Cardior Med 10:69–84
5. Gilstrap LG, Fonarow GC, Desai AS, Liang L, Matsouaka R, DeVore AD et al (2017) Initiation, continuation, or withdrawal of angiotensin-converting enzyme inhibitors/angiotensin receptor blockers and outcomes in patients hospitalized with heart failure with reduced ejection fraction. J Am Heart Assoc 6:e004675
6. Yoshioka K, Matsue Y, Yamaguchi T et al (2019) Safety and prognostic impact of early treatment with angiotensin-converting enzyme inhibitors or angiotensin receptor blockers in patients with acute heart failure. Am J Cardiovasc Drugs 19(6):597–605
7. Dalal J, Chandra P, Ray S et al (2023) Practical recommendations for the use of angiotensin receptor-neprilysin inhibitors (ARNI) in heart failure: insights from Indian cardiologists. Cardiol Ther 12:445–471
8. Nakada Y, Takahama H, Kanzaki H, Sugano Y, Hasegawa T, Ohara T, Amaki M, Funada A, Yoshida A, Yasuda S, Ogawa H, Anzai T (2015) The predictability of renin–angiotensin–aldosterone system factors for clinical outcome in patients with acute decompensated heart failure. Heart Vessel. 31(6):925–931. https://doi.org/10.1007/s00380-015-0688-7
9. Nishiyama K, Tsutamoto T, Kawahara C, Yamaji M, Sakai H, Yamamoto T, Fujii M, Horie M (2011) Relationship between biological variation in b-type natriuretic peptide and plasma renin concentration in stable outpatients with dilated cardiomyopathy. Circ J 75:1897–1904
10. Hobbs RE, Mills RM (2008) Endogenous b-type natriuretic peptide: a limb of the regulatory response to acutely decompensated heart failure. Clin Cardiol 31:407–412
11. Latini R, Masson S, Anand I, Salio M, Hester A, Judd D, Barlera S, Maggioni AP, Tognoni G, Cohn JN (2004) The comparative prognostic value of plasma neurohormones at baseline in patients with heart failure enrolled in val-heft. Eur Heart J 25:292–299
12. Tsutamoto T, Sakai H, Tanaka T, Fujii M, Yamamoto T, Wada A, Ohnishi M, Horie M (2007) Comparison of active renin concentration and plasma renin activity as a prognostic predictor in patients with heart failure. Circ J 71:915–921
13. de Boer RA, Schroten NF, Bakker SJ, Mahmud H, Szymanski MK, van der Harst P, Gansevoort RT, van Veldhuisen DJ, van Gilst WH, Hillege HL (2012) Plasma renin and outcome in the community: data from prevend. Eur Heart J 33:2351–2359
14. Teichholz LE, Kreulen T, Herman MV, Gorlin R (1976) Problems in echocardiographic volume determinations: echocardiographic–angiographic correlations in the presence of absence of asynergy. Am J Cardiol 37:7–11
15. Wang W, Bodiga S, Das SK, Lo J, Patel V, Oudit GY (2011) Role of ACE2 in diastolic and systolic heart failure. Heart Fail Rev 17:683–691. https://doi.org/10.1007/s10741-011-9259-x
16. Tipnis SR, Hooper NM, Hyde R, Karran E, Christie G, Turner AJ (2000) A human homolog of angiotensin-converting enzyme. Cloning and functional expression as a captopril-insensitive carboxypeptidase. J Biol Chem 275:33238–33243
17. Donoghue M, Hsieh F, Baronas E, Godbout K, Gosselin M, Stagliano N, Donovan M, Woolf B, Robison K, Jeyaseelan R, Breitbart RE, Acton S (2000) A novel angiotensin-converting

enzyme-related carboxypeptidase (ACE2) converts angiotensin I to angiotensin 1–9. Circ Res 87:E1–E9
18. Ishiyama Y, Gallagher PE, Averill DB, Tallant EA, Brosnihan KB, Ferrario CM (2004) Upregulation of angiotensin-converting enzyme 2 after myocardial infarction by blockade of angiotensin II receptors. Hypertension 43:970–976
19. Zhong JC, Ye JY, Jin HY, Yu X, Yu HM, Zhu DL, Gao PJ, Huang DY, Shuster M, Loibner H, Guo JM, Yu XY, Xiao BX, Gong ZH, Penninger JM, Oudit GY (2011) Telmisartan attenuates aortic hypertrophy in hypertensive rats by the modulation of ACE2 and profilin-1 expression. Regul Pept 166:90–97
20. Santos RA, Simoes E, Silva AC, Maric C, Silva DM, Machado RP et al (2003) Angiotensin-(1–7) is an endogenous ligand for the G protein-coupled receptor Mas. Proc Natl Acad Sci U S A 100(14):8258–8263. https://doi.org/10.1073/pnas.1432869100. This is one of the first papers describing that Mas receptor is a receptor for angotensin (1–7) to exert anti-diuretic actions and arterial relaxation response
21. Mercure C, Yogi A, Callera GE, Aranha AB, Bader M, Ferreira AJ, Santos RA, Walther T, Touyz RM, Reudelhuber TL (2008) Angiotensin(1-7) blunts hypertensive cardiac remodeling by a direct effect on the heart. Circ Res 103:1319–1326
22. Vickers C, Hales P, Kaushik V, Dick L, Gavin J, Tang J, Godbout K, Parsons T, Baronas E, Hsieh F, Acton S, Patane M, Nichols A, Tummino P (2002) Hydrolysis of biological peptides by human angiotensin-converting enzyme-related carboxypeptidase. J Biol Chem 277:14838–14843
23. Garabelli PJ, Modrall JG, Penninger JM, Ferrario CM, Chappell MC (2008) Distinct roles for angiotensin-converting enzyme 2 and carboxypeptidase A in the processing of angiotensins within the murine heart. Exp Physiol 93:613–621
24. Zhong J, Basu R, Guo D, Chow FL, Byrns S, Schuster M, Loibner H, Wang XH, Penninger JM, Kassiri Z, Oudit GY (2010) Angiotensin converting enzyme 2 suppresses pathological hypertrophy, myocardial fibrosis and cardiac dysfunction. Circulation 122:717–728
25. Bodiga S, Zhong JC, Wang W, Basu R, Lo J, Liu GC, Guo D, Holland SM, Scholey JW, Penninger JM, Kassiri Z, Oudit GY (2011) Enhanced susceptibility to biomechanical stress in ACE2 null mice is prevented by loss of the p47phox NADPH oxidase subunit. Cardiovasc Res 91:151–161
26. Kassiri Z, Zhong J, Guo D, Basu R, Wang X, Liu PP, Scholey JW, Penninger JM, Oudit GY (2009) Loss of angiotensin-converting enzyme 2 accelerates maladaptive left ventricular remodeling in response to myocardial infarction. Circ Heart Fail 2:446–455
27. Oudit GY, Kassiri Z, Patel MP, Chappell M, Butany J, Backx PH, Tsushima RG, Scholey JW, Khokha R, Penninger JM (2007) Angiotensin II-mediated oxidative stress and inflammation mediate the age-dependent cardiomyopathy in ACE2 null mice. Cardiovasc Res 75:29–39
28. Burrell LM, Risvanis J, Kubota E, Dean RG, MacDonald PS, Lu S, Tikellis C, Grant SL, Lew RA, Smith AI, Cooper ME, Johnston CI (2005) Myocardial infarction increases ACE2 expression in rat and humans. Eur Heart J 26:369–375
29. Gurley SB, Allred A, Le TH, Griffiths R, Mao L, Philip N, Haystead TA, Donoghue M, Breitbart RE, Acton SL, Rockman HA, Coffman TM (2006) Altered blood pressure responses and normal cardiac phenotype in ACE2-null mice. J Clin Invest 116:2218–2225
30. Yamamoto K, Ohishi M, Katsuya T, Ito N, Ikushima M, Kaibe M, Tatara Y, Shiota A, Sugano S, Takeda S, Rakugi H, Ogihara T (2006) Deletion of angiotensin-converting enzyme 2 accelerates pressure overload-induced cardiac dysfunction by increasing local angiotensin II. Hypertension 47:718–726
31. Epelman S, Shrestha K, Troughton RW, Francis GS, Sen S, Klein AL, Tang WH (2009) Soluble angiotensin-converting enzyme 2 in human heart failure: relation with myocardial function and clinical outcomes. J Card Fail 15:565–571. https://doi.org/10.1016/j.cardfail.2009.01.014
32. Wang Y, Moreira Mda C, Heringer-Walther S, Ebermann L, Schultheiss HP, Wessel N, Siems WE, Walther T (2010) Plasma ACE2 activity is an independent prognostic marker in Chagas' disease and equally potent as BNP. J Card Fail 16:157–163

33. Huentelman MJ, Grobe JL, Vazquez J, Stewart JM, Mecca AP, Katovich MJ, Ferrario CM, Raizada MK (2005) Protection from angiotensin II-induced cardiac hypertrophy and fibrosis by systemic lentiviral delivery of ACE2 in rats. Exp Physiol 90:783–790
34. Oudit GY, Crackower MA, Backx PH, Penninger JM (2003) The role of ACE2 in cardiovascular physiology. Trends Cardiovasc Med 13:93–101
35. Crackower MA, Sarao R, Oudit GY, Yagil C, Kozieradzki I, Scanga SE, Oliveira-dos-Santos AJ, da Costa J, Zhang L, Pei Y, Scholey J, Ferrario CM, Manoukian AS, Chappell MC, Backx PH, Yagil Y, Penninger JM (2002) Angiotensin-converting enzyme 2 is an essential regulator of heart function. Nature 417:822–828
36. Yamazato M, Yamazato Y, Sun C, Diez-Freire C, Raizada MK (2007) Overexpression of angiotensin-converting enzyme 2 in the rostral ventrolateral medulla causes long-term decrease in blood pressure in the spontaneously hypertensive rats. Hypertension 49:926–931
37. Feng Y, Xia H, Cai Y, Halabi CM, Becker LK, Santos RA et al (2010) Brain-selective overexpression of human angiotensinconverting enzyme type 2 attenuates neurogenic hypertension. Circ Res 106(2):373–382
38. Rentzsch B, Todiras M, Iliescu R, Popova E, Campos LA, Oliveira ML, Baltatu OC, Santos RA, Bader M (2008) Transgenic angiotensin-converting enzyme 2 overexpression in vessels of SHRSP rats reduces blood pressure and improves endothelial function. Hypertension 52:967–973
39. Zisman LS, Meixell GE, Bristow MR, Canver CC (2003) Angiotensin-(1-7) formation in the intact human heart: in vivo dependence on angiotensin II as substrate. Circulation 108:1679–1681
40. Zisman LS, Keller RS, Weaver B, Lin Q, Speth R, Bristow MR, Canver CC (2003) Increased angiotensin-(1–7)-forming activity in failing human heart ventricles: evidence for upregulation of the angiotensin-converting enzyme homologue ACE2. Circulation 108:1707–1712. https://doi.org/10.1161/01.CIR.0000094734.67990.99
41. Brosnihan KB, Li P, Tallant EA, Ferrario CM (1998) Angiotensin-(1-7): a novel vasodilator of the coronary circulation. Biol Res 31:227–234
42. Ren Y, Garvin JL, Carretero OA (2002) Vasodilator action of angiotensin-(1-7) on isolated rabbit afferent arterioles. Hypertension 39:799–802
43. Grobe JL, Mecca AP, Lingis M, Shenoy V, Bolton TA, Machado JM, Speth RC, Raizada MK, Katovich MJ (2007) Prevention of angiotensin II-induced cardiac remodeling by angiotensin-(1-7). Am J Physiol Heart Circ Physiol 292:H736–H742
44. De Mello WC, Ferrario CM, Jessup JA (2007) Beneficial versus harmful effects of angiotensin (1-7) on impulse propagation and cardiac arrhythmias in the failing heart. J Renin-Angiotensin-Aldosterone Syst 8:74–80
45. Urata H, Healy B, Stewart RW, Bumpus FM, Husain A (1990) Angiotensin II-forming pathways in normal and failing human hearts. Circ Res 66:883–890
46. Urata H, Kinoshita A, Misono KS, Bumpus FM, Husain A (1990) Identification of a highly specific chymase as the major angiotensin II-forming enzyme in the human heart. J Biol Chem 265:22348–22357
47. Wei CC, Hase N, Inoue Y, Bradley EW, Yahiro E, Li M, Naqvi N, Powell PC, Shi K, Takahashi Y, Saku K, Urata H, Dell'italia LJ, Husain A (2010) Mast cell chymase limits the cardiac efficacy of Ang I-converting enzyme inhibitor therapy in rodents. J Clin Invest 120:1229–1239
48. Jenne DE, Tschopp J (1991) Angiotensin II-forming heart chymase is a mast-cell-specific enzyme. Biochem J 276:567–568
49. Juillerat L, Nussberger J, Ménard J, Mooser V, Christen Y, Waeber B, Graf P, Brunner HR (1990) Determinants of angiotensin II generation during converting enzyme inhibition. Hypertension 16:564–572
50. Roig E, Perez-Villa F, Morales M, Jiménez W, Orús J, Heras M, Sanz G (2000) Clinical implications of increased plasma angiotensin II despite ACE inhibitor therapy in patients with congestive heart failure. Eur Heart J 21:53–57

51. Chamsi-Pasha MAR, Shao Z, Tang WH (2013) Wilson angiotensin-converting enzyme 2 as a therapeutic target for heart failure. Curr Heart Fail Rep 11:58–63. https://doi.org/10.1007/s11897-013-0178-0
52. Wang W, Bodiga S, Das SK, Lo J, Patel V, Oudit GY (2012) Role of ACE2 in diastolic and systolic heart failure. Heart Fail Rev 17(4–5):683–691
53. Keidar S, Gamliel-Lazarovich A, Kaplan M et al (2005) Mineralocorticoid receptor blocker increases angiotensin-converting enzyme 2 activity in congestive heart failure patients. Circ Res 97(9):946–953
54. Tikellis C, Bernardi S, Burns WC (2011) Angiotensin-converting enzyme 2 is a key modulator of the renin-angiotensin system in cardiovascular and renal disease. Curr Opin Nephrol Hypertens 20(1):62–68
55. Lazartigues E, Feng Y, Lavoie JL (2007) The two fACEs of the tissue renin-angiotensin systems: implication in cardiovascular diseases. Curr Pharm Des 13(12):1231–1245
56. Epelman S, Tang WH, Chen SY, Van Lente F, Francis GS, Sen S (2008) Detection of soluble angiotensin-converting enzyme 2 in heart failure: insights into the endogenous counter-regulatory pathway of the reninangiotensin-aldosterone system. J Am Coll Cardiol 52:750–754. https://doi.org/10.1016/j.jacc.2008.02.088
57. Wysocki J, Ye M, Rodriguez E, González-Pacheco FR, Barrios C, Evora K, Schuster M, Loibner H, Brosnihan KB, Ferrario CM, Penninger JM, Batlle D (2009) Targeting the degradation of angiotensin II with recombinant angiotensin-converting enzyme 2: prevention of angiotensin II-dependent hypertension. Hypertension 55:90–98
58. Gallagher PE, Ferrario CM, Tallant EA (2008) Regulation of ACE2 in cardiac myocytes and fibroblasts. Am J Physiol Heart Circ Physiol 295:H2373–H2379
59. Der Sarkissian S, Huentelman MJ, Stewart J, Katovich MJ, Raizada MK (2006) ACE2: a novel therapeutic target for cardiovascular diseases. Prog Biophys Mol Biol 91(1–2):163–198
60. Iwata M, Cowling RT, Yeo SJ, Greenberg B (2011) Targeting the ACE2-Ang-(1–7) pathway in cardiac fibroblasts to treat cardiac remodeling and heart failure. J Mol Cell Cardiol 51(4):542–547
61. Patel VB, Bodiga S, Fan D et al (2012) Cardioprotective effects mediated by angiotensin II type 1 receptor blockade and enhancing angiotensin 1–7 in experimental heart failure in angiotensin-converting enzyme 2-null mice. Hypertension 59(6):1195–1203
62. Masson R, Nicklin SA, Craig MA et al (2009) Onset of experimental severe cardiacfibrosis is mediated by overexpression of Angiotensin-converting enzyme 2. Hypertension 53(4):694–700
63. Tai C, Gan T, Zou L, Sun Y, Zhang Y, Chen W, Li J, Zhang J, Xu Y, Lu H, Xu D (2017) Effect of angiotensin-converting enzyme inhibitors and angiotensin II receptor blockers on cardiovascular events in patients with heart failure: a meta-analysis of randomized controlled trials. BMC Cardiovasc Disord 17(1):257. https://doi.org/10.1186/s12872-017-0686-z
64. Granger CB, McMurray JJ, Yusuf S et al (2003) Effects of candesartan in patients with chronic heart failure and reduced left-ventricular systolic function intolerant to angiotensin-converting-enzyme inhibitors: the CHARM-Alternative trial. Lancet 362:772–776
65. Havranek EP, Thomas I, Smith WB, Ponce GA, Bilsker M, Munger MA et al (1999) Dose-related beneficial long-term hemodynamic and clinical efficacy of irbesartan in heart failure. J Am Coll Cardiol 33(5):1174–1181
66. Granger CB, Ertl G, Kuch J, Maggioni AP, McMurray J, Rouleau JL et al (2000) Randomized trial of candesartan cilexetil in the treatment of patients with congestive heart failure and a history of intolerance to angiotensin-converting enzyme inhibitors. Am Heart J 139:609–617
67. Riegger GAJ, Bouzo H, Petr P, Münz J, Spacek R, Pethig H et al (1999) Improvement in exercise tolerance and symptoms of congestive heart failure during treatment with candesartan cilexetil. Circulation 100(22):2224–2230
68. Cohn JN, Tognoni G (2001) A randomized trial of the angiotensin-receptor blocker valsartan in chronic heart failure. N Engl J Med 345:1667–1675. https://doi.org/10.1056/NEJMoa010713

69. Matsumori A (2003) Assessment of response to candesartan in heart failure in Japan study I. Efficacy and safety of oral candesartan cilexetil in patients with congestive heart failure. Eur J Heart Fail 5:669–677
70. The Acute Infarction Ramipril Efficacy (AIRE) Study Group (1993) Effect of ramipril on mortality and morbidity of survivors of acute myocardial infarction with clinical evidence of heart failure. Lancet 342(8875):821–828
71. Swedberg K, Idanpaan-Heikkila U, Remes J (1987) Effects of enalapril on mortality in severe congestive heart failure. Results of the Cooperative North Scandinavian Enalapril Survival Study (CONSENSUS). N Engl J Med 316(23):1429–1435. https://doi.org/10.1056/NEJM198706043162301
72. Pfeffer MA, Braunwald E, Moyé LA et al (1992) Effect of captopril on mortality and morbidity in patients with left ventricular dysfunction after myocardial infarction: results of the survival and ventricular enlargement trial. N Engl J Med 327(10):669–677. https://doi.org/10.1056/NEJM199209033271001
73. Yusuf S, Pitt B, Davis CE, Hood WB, Cohn JN (1991) Effect of enalapril on survival in patients with reduced left ventricular ejection fractions and congestive heart failure. N Engl J Med 325(5):293–302. https://doi.org/10.1056/NEJM199108013250501
74. Kober L, Torp-Pedersen C, Carlsen JE, Bagger H, Eliasen P, Lyngborg K et al (1995) A clinical trial of the angiotensin-converting-enzyme inhibitor trandolapril in patients with left ventricular dysfunction after myocardial infarction. Trandolapril Cardiac Evaluation (TRACE) Study Group. N Engl J Med 333:1670–1676
75. Bulpitt CJ, Fletcher AE, Dössegger L, Neiss A, Nielsen T, Viergutz S (1998) Quality of life in chronic heart failure: cilazapril and captopril versus placebo. Heart 79(6):593–598
76. Widimský J, Uhlíř O, Kremer HJ, Jerie P (1995) Czech and Slovak spirapril intervention study (CASSIS). Eur J Clin Pharmacol 49(1–2):95–102
77. Chalmers JP, West MJ, Cyran J, De La Torre D, Englert M, Kramar M et al (1987) Placebo-controlled study of lisinopril in congestive heart failure: a multicentre study. J Cardiovasc Pharmacol 9:S89–S97
78. Colfer HT, Ribner HS, Gradman A, Hughes CV, Kapoor A, Laidlaw JC (1992) Effects of once-daily benazepril therapy on exercise tolerance and manifestations of chronic congestive heart failure. Am J Cardiol 70(3):354–358
79. Erhardt L, MacLean A, Ilgenfritz J, Gelperin K, Blumenthal M (1995) Fosinopril attenuates clinical deterioration and improves exercise tolerance in patients with heart failure. Eur Heart J 16(12):1892–1899
80. Brown EJ Jr, Chew PH, MacLean A, Gelperin K, Ilgenfritz JP, Blumenthal M (1995) Effects of fosinopril on exercise tolerance and clinical deterioration in patients with chronic congestive heart failure not taking digitalis. Am J Cardiol 75(8):596–600
81. Lechat P, Garnham SP, Desche P, Bounhoure JP (1993) Efficacy and acceptability of perindopril in mild to moderate chronic congestive heart failure. Am Heart J 126(3):798–806
82. Newman TJ, Maskin CS, Dennick LG, Meyer JH, Hallows BG, Cooper WH (1988) Effects of captopril on survival in patients with heart failure. Am J Med 84(3):140–144
83. Packer M, Califf RM, Konstam MA, Krum H, McMurray JJ, Rouleau JL, Swedberg K (2002) Comparison of omapatrilat and enalapril in patients with chronic heart failure. Circulation 106:920–926. https://doi.org/10.1161/01.cir.0000029801.86489.50
84. Cohn JN, Johnson G, Ziesche S, Cobb F, Francis G, Tristani F et al (1991) A comparison of enalapril with hydralazine–isosorbide dinitrate in the treatment of chronic congestive heart failure. N Engl J Med 325(5):303–310
85. Cosin-Aguilar J, Marrugat J, Sanz G, Massó J, Gil M, Vargas R et al (1999) Long-term results of the Spanish trial on treatment and survival of patients with predominantly mild heart failure. J Cardiovasc Pharmacol 33(5):733–740
86. Komajda M, Lutiger B, Madeira H, Thygesen K, Bobbio M, Hildebrandt P et al (2004) Tolerability of carvedilol and ACE-inhibition in mild heart failure. Results of CARMEN (Carvedilol ACE-Inhibitor Remodelling Mild CHF EvaluatioN). Eur J Heart Fail 6(4):467–475

87. Funck-Brentano C, Veldhuisen DJ, Ven LLM, Follath F, Goulder M, Willenheimer R (2011) Influence of order and type of drug (bisoprolol vs enalapril) on outcome and adverse events in patients with chronic heart failure: a post hoc analysis of the CIBIS-III trial. Eur J Heart Fail 13(7):765–772
88. Cowley AJ, McEntegart DJ, Hampton JR, Barnett DB, Bexton RS, Boyle R et al (1994) Long-term evaluation of treatment for chronic heart failure: a 1 year comparative trial of flosequinan and captopril. Cardiovasc Drug Ther 8(6):829–836
89. Dohmen HJ, Dunselman PH, Poole-Wilson PA (1997) Comparison of captopril and ibopamine in mild to moderate heart failure. Heart 78(3):285–290
90. Fonarow GC, Chelimsky-Fallick C, Stevenson LW, Luu M, Hamilton MA, Moriguchi JD et al (1992) Effect of direct vasodilation with hydralazine versus angiotensin-converting enzyme inhibition with captopril on mortality in advanced heart failure: the Hy-C trial. J Am Coll Cardiol 19(4):842–850
91. Rouleau JL, Pfeffer MA, Stewart DJ, Isaac D, Sestier F, Kerut EK et al (2000) Comparison of vasopeptidase inhibitor, omapatrilat, and lisinopril on exercise tolerance and morbidity in patients with heart failure: IMPRESS randomised trial. Lancet 356(9230):615–620
92. Northridge DB, Currie PF, Newby DE, McMurray JJ, Ford M, Boon NA, Dargie HJ (1999) Placebo-controlled comparison of candoxatril, an orally active neutral endopeptidase inhibitor, and captopril in patients with chronic heart failure. Eur J Heart Fail 1(1):67–72
93. Dickstein K, Kjekshus J (2002) Effects of losartan and captopril on mortality and morbidity in high-risk patients after acute myocardial infarction: the OPTIMAAL randomised trial. Lancet 360:752–760. https://doi.org/10.1016/S0140-6736(02)09895-1
94. Pitt B, Poole-Wilson PA, Segal R, Martinez FA, Dickstein K, Camm AJ et al (2000) Effect of losartan compared with captopril on mortality in patients with symptomatic heart failure: randomised trial—the Losartan Heart Failure Survival Study ELITE II. Lancet 355(9215):1582–1587
95. Pfeffer MA, McMurray JJV, Velazquez EJ et al (2003) Valsartan, captopril, or both in myocardial infarction complicated by heart failure, left ventricular dysfunction, or both. N Engl J Med 349:1893–1906. https://doi.org/10.1056/NEJMoa032292
96. McKelvie RS, Yusuf S, Pericak D, Avezum A, Burns RJ, Probstfield J et al (1999) Comparison of candesartan, enalapril, and their combination in congestive heart failure: randomized evaluation of strategies for left ventricular dysfunction (RESOLVD) pilot study. The RESOLVD Pilot Study Investigators. Circulation 100:1056–1064
97. van Vark LC, Bertrand M, Akkerhuis KM, Brugts JJ, Fox K, Mourad JJ, Boersma E (2012) Angiotensin-converting enzyme inhibitors reduce mortality in hypertension: a meta-analysis of randomized clinical trials of renin-angiotensin-aldosterone system inhibitors involving 158,998 patients. Eur Heart J 33:2088–2097
98. Cheng J, Zhang W, Zhang X, Han F, Li X, He X, Chen J (2014) Effect of angiotensin-converting enzyme inhibitors and angiotensin II receptor blockers on all-cause mortality, cardiovascular deaths, and cardiovascular events in patients with diabetes mellitus: a meta-analysis. JAMA Intern Med 174:773–785
99. Pitt B, Segal R, Martinez FA, Meurers G, Cowley AJ, Thomas I et al (1997) Randomised trial of losartan versus captopril in patients over 65 with heart failure (Evaluation of Losartan in the Elderly Study, ELITE). Lancet 349(9054):747–752
100. Dickstein K, Chang P, Willenheimer R et al (1995) Comparison of the effects of losartan and enalapril on clinical status and exercise performance in patients with moderate or severe chronic heart failure. J Am Coll Cardiol 26:438–445. https://doi.org/10.1016/0735-1097(95)80020-H
101. Willenheimer R, Helmers C, Pantev E, Rydberg E, Löfdahl P, Gordon A (2002) Safety and efficacy of valsartan versus enalapril in heart failure patients. Int J Cardiol 85:261–270. https://doi.org/10.1016/S0167-5273(02)00154-7
102. Lang RM, Elkayam U, Yellen LG, Krauss D, McKelvie RS, Vaughan DE et al (1997) Comparative effects of losartan and enalapril on exercise capacity and clinical status in patients with heart failure. J Am Coll Cardiol 30(4):983–991

103. Dunselman P (2001) Effects of the replacement of the angiotensin converting enzyme inhibitor enalapril by the angiotensin II receptor blocker telmisartan in patients with congestive heart failure: the replacement of angiotensin converting enzyme inhibition (REPLACE) investigators. Int J Cardiol 77(2):131–138
104. Sargento L, Simões AV, Longo S, Lousada N, dos Reis RP (2016) Treatment with optimal dose angiotensin-converting enzyme inhibitors/angiotensin receptor blockers has a positive effect on long-term survival in older individuals (aged >70 years) and octogenarians with systolic heart failure. Drugs Aging 33:675–683. https://doi.org/10.1007/s40266-016-0393-y
105. Barywani SB, Ergatoudes C, Schaufelberger M et al (2015) Does the target dose of neurohormonal blockade matter for outcome in systolic heart failure in octogenarians? Int J Cardiol 187:666–672
106. Heywood JT, Fonarow GC, Yancy CW et al (2010) Influence of renal function on the use of guideline-recommended therapies for patients with heart failure. Am J Cardiol 105:1140–1146
107. Kim H-J, Jo S-H, Lee M-H, Seo W-W, Choi J-O, Ryu K-H (2020) Effect of prescribing patterns of renin–angiotensin system blockers and beta-blockers on prognosis of heart failure. Adv Ther 37(9):3839–3849. https://doi.org/10.1007/s12325-020-01443-6
108. Ponikowski P, Voors AA, Anker SD, Bueno H, Cleland JGF, Coats AJS, Falk V, González-Juanatey JR, Harjola VP, Jankowska EA, Jessup M, Linde C, Nihoyannopoulos P, Parissis JT, Pieske B, Riley JP, Rosano GMC, Ruilope LM, Ruschitzka F, Rutten FH, van der Meer P (2016) 2016 ESC guidelines for the diagnosis and treatment of acute and chronic heart failure. Eur Heart J 37:2129–2200. https://doi.org/10.1093/eurheartj/ehw128
109. Yancy CW, Mariell Jessup C, Chair Biykem Bozkurt V et al (2017) Writing Group Members* 2017 ACC/AHA/HFSA focused update of the 2013 ACCF/AHA guideline for the management of heart failure ACC/AHA/HFSA focused update. Yancy et al. Selection of Writing Committee Members evidence review and evidence review committees class of recommendation and level of evidence. Circulation 136:137–161. https://doi.org/10.1161/CIR.0000000000000509
110. Nagai T, Yoshikawa T, Saito Y et al (2018) Clinical characteristics, management, and outcomes of Japanese patients hospitalized for heart failure with preserved ejection fraction—a report from the Japanese Heart Failure Syndrome With Preserved Ejection Fraction (JASPER) Registry. Circ J 82:1534–1545
111. Zheng SL, Chan FT, Nabeebaccus AA et al (2018) Drug treatment effects on outcomes in heart failure with preserved ejection fraction: a systematic review and meta-analysis. Heart 104:407–415
112. Dass B, Dimza M, Singhania G, Schwartz C, George J, Bhatt A, Radhakrishnan N, Bansari A, Bozorgmehri S, Mohandas R (2019) Renin–angiotensin–aldosterone system optimization for acute decompensated heart failure patients (ROAD-HF): rationale and design. Am J Cardiovasc Drugs 20:373–380. https://doi.org/10.1007/s40256-019-00389-7
113. Dries DL, Exner DV, Domanski MJ, Greenberg B, Stevenson LW (2000) The prognostic implications of renal insufficiency in asymptomatic and symptomatic patients with left ventricular systolic dysfunction. J Am Coll Cardiol 35:681–689
114. Belziti CA, Bagnati R, Ledesma P, Vulcano N, Fernández S (2010) Worsening renal function in patients admitted with acute decompensated heart failure: incidence, risk factors and prognostic implications. Rev Esp Cardiol 63:294–302. http://www.ncbi.nlm.nih.gov/pubmed/20196990. Accessed 6 Sep 2019
115. Vijayan A, Faubel S, Askenazi DJ, Cerda J, Fissell WH, Heung M, American Society of Nephrology Acute Kidney Injury Advisory Group et al (2016) Clinical use of the urine biomarker [TIMP-2] × [IGFBP7] for acute kidney injury risk assessment. Am J Kidney Dis 68:19–28
116. Djoussé L, Driver JA, Gaziano JM (2009) Relation between modifiable lifestyle factors and lifetime risk of heart failure. JAMA 302:394–400

117. Curtis LH, Whellan DJ, Hammill BG, Hernandez AF, Anstrom KJ, Shea AM et al (2008) Incidence and prevalence of heart failure in elderly persons, 1994–2003. Arch Intern Med 168:418–424
118. Valika AA, Gheorghiade M (2012) Ace inhibitor therapy for heart failure in patients with impaired renal function: a review of the literature. Heart Fail Rev 18:135–140. https://doi.org/10.1007/s10741-011-9295-6
119. Enseleit F, Hurlimann D, Luscher TF (2001) Vascular protective effects of angiotensin converting enzyme inhibitors and their relation to clinical events. J Cardiovasc Pharmacol 37(Suppl 1):S21–S30
120. Ljungman S, Kjekshus J, Swedberg K (1992) Renal function in severe congestive heart failure during treatment with enalapril (the Cooperative North Scandinavian Enalapril Survival Study [CONSENSUS] Trial). Am J Cardiol 70(4):479–487
121. Ruggenenti P, Remuzzi G (2011) Worsening kidney function in decompensated heart failure: treat the heart, don't mind the kidney. Eur Heart J 32(20):2476–2478
122. Hou FF et al (2006) Efficacy and safety of benazepril for advanced chronic renal insufficiency. N Engl J Med 354(2):131–140
123. Agarwal V, Briasoulis A, Messerli FH (2012) Effects of renin-angiotensin system blockade on mortality and hospitalization in heart failure with preserved ejection fraction. Heart Fail Rev 18:429–437. https://doi.org/10.1007/s10741-012-9329-8
124. Owan TE, Hodge DO, Herges RM, Jacobsen SJ, Roger VL, Redfield MM (2006) Trends in prevalence and outcome of heart failure with preserved ejection fraction. N Engl J Med 355:251–259
125. Desai AS, Lewis EF, Li R, Solomon SD, Assmann SF, Boineau R, Clausell N, Diaz R, Fleg JL, Gordeev I, McKinlay S, O'Meara E, Shaburishvili T, Pitt B, Pfeffer MA (2011) Rationale and design of the treatment of preserved cardiac function heart failure with an aldosterone antagonist trial: a randomized, controlled study of spironolactone in patients with symptomatic heart failure and preserved ejection fraction. Am Heart J 162(6):966–972.e910. https://doi.org/10.1016/j.ahj.2011.09.007
126. Yoshioka K, Matsue Y, Yamaguchi T, Kitai T, Kagiyama N, Okumura T, Kida K, Oishi S, Akiyama E, Suzuki S, Yamamoto M, Kuroda S, Matsumura A, Hirao K (2019) Safety and prognostic impact of early treatment with angiotensin-converting enzyme inhibitors or angiotensin receptor blockers in patients with acute heart failure. Am J Cardiovasc Drugs 19:597–605. https://doi.org/10.1007/s40256-019-00355-3
127. Gheorghiade M, Hall V, Lakier JB, Goldstein S (1989) Comparative hemodynamic and neurohormonal effects of intravenous captopril and digoxin and their combinations in patients with severe heart failure. J Am Coll Cardiol 13:134–142
128. Annane D, Bellissant E, Pussard E, Asmar R, Lacombe F, Lanata E et al (1996) Placebo-controlled, randomized, double-blind study of intravenous enalaprilat efficacy and safety in acute cardiogenic pulmonary edema. Circulation 94:1316–1324
129. Investigators S, Yusuf S, Pitt B, Davis CE, Hood WB Jr, Cohn JN (1992) Effect of enalapril on mortality and the development of heart failure in asymptomatic patients with reduced left ventricular ejection fractions. N Engl J Med 327:685–691
130. Sanam K, Bhatia V, Bajaj NS, Gaba S, Morgan CJ, Fonarow GC et al (2016) Renin-angiotensin system inhibition and lower 30-day all-cause readmission in medicare beneficiaries with heart failure. Am J Med 129:1067–1073
131. Birner C, Ulucan C, Bratfisch M, Götz T, Dietl A, Schweda F, Riegger GA, Luchner A (2012) Antihypertrophic effects of combined inhibition of the renin–angiotensin system (RAS) and neutral endopeptidase (NEP) in progressive, tachycardia-induced experimental heart failure. Naunyn Schmiedeberg's Arch Pharmacol 385:1117–1125. https://doi.org/10.1007/s00210-012-0791-6
132. Martin FL, Stevens TL, Cataliotti A, Schirger JA, Borgeson DD, Redfield MM et al (2005) Natriuretic and antialdosterone actions of chronic oral NEP inhibition during progressive congestive heart failure. Kidney Int 67(5):1723–1730

133. Lapointe N, Blais C, Adam A, Parker T, Sirois MG, Gosselin H et al (2002) Comparison of the effects of an angiotensin-converting enzyme inhibitor and a vasopeptidase inhibitor after myocardial infarction in the rat. J Am Coll Cardiol 39(10):1692–1698
134. Maki T, Nasa Y, Tanonaka K, Takahashi M, Takeo S (2003) Direct inhibition of neutral endopeptidase in vasopeptidase inhibitor-mediated amelioration of cardiac remodeling in rats with chronic heart failure. Mol Cell Biochem 254(1–2):265–273
135. Maki T, Nasa Y, Tanonaka K, Takahashi M, Takeo S (2003) Beneficial effects of sampatrilat, a novel vasopeptidase inhibitor, on cardiac remodeling and function of rats with chronic heart failure following left coronary artery ligation. J Pharmacol Exp Ther 305(1):97–105
136. Mishima T, Tanimura M, Suzuki G, Todor A, Sharov VG, Tanhehco EJ et al (2002) Effects of chronic neutral endopeptidase inhibition on the progression of left ventricular dysfunction and remodeling in dogs with moderate heart failure. Cardiovasc Drugs Ther 16(3):209–214
137. Xu J, Carretero OA, Liu Y, Yang F, Shesely EG, Oja-Tebbe N et al (2004) Dual inhibition of ACE and NEP provides greater cardioprotection in mice with heart failure. J Card Fail 10(1):83–89
138. Hisatake S, Kiuchi S, Kabuki T, Oka T, Dobashi S, Ikeda T (2016) Serum angiotensin-converting enzyme 2 concentration and angiotensin-(1–7) concentration in patients with acute heart failure patients requiring emergency hospitalization. Heart Vessel 32:303–308. https://doi.org/10.1007/s00380-016-0877-z
139. Santos RA, Ferreira AJ, Simões e Silva AC (2008) Recent advances in the angiotensin-converting enzyme 2-angiotensin (1-7)-Mas axis. Exp Physiol 93(5):519–527
140. Greenberg B (2008) An ACE in the hole alternative pathways of the renin angiotensin system and their potential role in cardiac remodeling. J Am Coll Cardiol 52:755–757
141. Ferrario CM, Chappell MC, Tallant EA, Brosnihan KB, Diz DI (1997) Counterregulatory actions of angiotensin-(1–7). Hypertension 30:535–541
142. Francis GS, Benedict C, Johnstone DE, Kirlin PC, Nicklas J, Liang CS, Kubo SH, Rudin-Toretsky E, Yusuf S (1990) Comparison of neuroendocrine activation in patients with left ventricular dysfunction with and without congestive heart failure. A substudy of the Studies of Left Ventricular Dysfunction (SOLVD). Circulation 82:1724–1729
143. Nussberger J, Brunner DB, Nyfeler JA, Linder L, Brunner HR (2001) Measurement of immunoreactive angiotensin-(1–7) heptapeptide in human blood. Clin Chem 47:726–729
144. Oudit GY, Penninger JM (2011) Recombinant human angiotensin-converting enzyme 2 as a new renin-angiotensin system peptidase for heart failure therapy. Curr Heart Fail Rep 8:176–183. https://doi.org/10.1007/s11897-011-0063-7
145. Zaman MA, Oparil S, Calhoun DA (2002) Drugs targeting the renin-angiotensin-aldosterone system. Nat Rev Drug Discov 1:621–636
146. Donoghue M, Hsieh F, Baronas E et al (2000) A novel angiotensin-converting enzyme-related carboxypeptidase (ACE2) converts angiotensin I to angiotensin 1–9. Circ Res 87:E1–E9
147. Oudit GY, Herzenberg AM, Kassiri Z, Wong D, Reich H, Khokha R, Crackower MA, Backx PH, Penninger JM, Scholey JW (2006) Loss of angiotensin-converting enzyme-2 leads to the late development of angiotensin II-dependent glomerulosclerosis. Am J Pathol 168:1808–1820
148. Zhong J, Guo D, Chen CB, Wang W, Schuster M, Loibner H, Penninger JM, Scholey JW, Kassiri Z, Oudit GY (2011) Prevention of angiotensin II-mediated renal oxidative stress, inflammation, and fibrosis by angiotensin-converting enzyme 2. Hypertension 57:314–322
149. Bodiga S, Zhong JC, Wang W et al (2011) Enhanced susceptibility to biomechanical stress in ACE2 null mice is prevented by loss of the p47(phox) NADPH oxidase subunit. Cardiovasc Res 91(1):151–161
150. Santos RA, Castro CH, Gava E et al (2006) Impairment of in vitro and in vivo heart function in angiotensin-(1-7) receptor MAS knockout mice. Hypertension 47:996–1002
151. Tallant EA, Ferrario CM, Gallagher PE (2005) Angiotensin-(1–7) inhibits growth of cardiac myocytes through activation of the Mas receptor. Am J Physiol Heart Circ Physiol 289(4):H1560–H1566

152. Urata H, Healy B, Stewart RW et al (1990) Angiotensin II-forming pathways in normal and failing human hearts. Circ Res 66:883–890
153. Urata H, Kinoshita A, Misono KS et al (1990) Identification of a highly specific chymase as the major angiotensin II-forming enzyme in the human heart. J Biol Chem 265:22348–22357
154. Juillerat L, Nussberger J, Menard J et al (1990) Determinants of angiotensin II generation during converting enzyme inhibition. Hypertension 16:564–572

Chapter 7
Immunomodulator Activity of ACE Inhibitors and Angiotensin Receptor Blockers in Hypertensive Patients

Mukesh Nandave

Introduction by the Editor

The strong association between autonomic and immune system plays a notable role in initiation of hypertension adding to cardiovascular pathology, organ damage and death. According to the reports there is a strong link between hypertension, pro-inflammatory cytokines, adaptive and innate immune systems [1]. Angiotensin converting enzyme (ACE) inhibitors are the most used anti-hypertensive agents. They prevent the conversion of angiotensin I to angiotensin II leading to vasodilation and reduced blood pressure. ACE inhibitors alter the ACE mediated degradation of bradykinin and substance P that can influence immune cell function as these proteins play significant role in inflammation [2]. Additionally, these proteins promote mast cell degranulation and release of chemokine followed by recruitment of other immune cells [3]. This is the fundamental mechanism that explains the link between ACE inhibitors and immune system modulation [4]. ACE2, which is homolog to ACE, converts angiotensin II to Ang-1-(1–7), a heptapeptide that activates Mas receptor and generates responses that are opposite in nature to angiotensin II. However, ACE inhibitors do not inhibit ACE2 like ACE because if smaller S2 pocket of active site [5]. Additionally, it is reported that ACE inhibitors increase the expression of ACE2 and conversion of angiotensin II to Ang-1(1–7) thus potentiating the anti-angiotensin II effects. Angiotension II produces pro-inflammatory action which is weakened by ACE inhibitors that reduces the levels of angiotensin II and increases the Ang-1(1–7) levels [6]. Moreover, increased ACE2 expression simultaneously increases the susceptibility of some pathogens such as SARS-CoV-2 that utilizes the ACE2 for the entry. However, there is limited data available on

M. Nandave (✉)
Department of Pharmacology, Delhi Pharmaceutical Sciences and Research University, New Delhi, Delhi, India

M. Nandave (ed.), *Angiotensin-converting Enzyme Inhibitors vs. Angiotensin Receptor Blockers*, https://doi.org/10.1007/978-981-97-7380-0_7

modification of ACE inhibitors indications in the prevention and treatment of COVID-19 [7, 8].

Angiotensin receptor blockers (ARBs) work by inhibiting renin angiotensin system (RAS) via the angiotensin II type 1 receptor (AT1R) blockage. Recent studies suggested that RAS is a complex system that not only controls water balance and blood pressure but also involved in the immune process. Immune cells (lymphocytic RAS) produce angiotensin II locally that act as cytokines and chemoattractant for T lymphocytes. Notably, In addition to AT1R which is antagonized by ARBs there is another receptor that have opposite action to AT1R called as angiotensin type 2 receptor (AT2R) that induces vasodilation by increasing the synthesis of nitric oxide. In an inflammatory condition, angiotensin II increases the AT1R receptor expression while the expression of AT2R remains the same thus potentiating inflammatory response. Receptors of angiotensin II are not only found to be present on endothelium but also found on the membranes of mammalian tissue and cells like endometrial stromal cells, lungs, T-lymphocytes or brain cells. Activation of AT1R leads to reactive oxygen species (ROS) production and enhances the inflammation by promoting pro-inflammatory signaling pathways. ARBs inhibit the AT1R mediated inflammatory responses by downregulating its expression. Some studies on cell culture and animals reported that ARBs also exert AT1R independent responses. Best example is PPAR induced anti-inflammatory pathways. According to the reports different sartans have different ability for the targeted receptor that depend on their affinity and interaction of their metabolite. Most experiments on ARBs is conducted on animals or cell culture so therefore mechanism on human body is still underexplored. However, it could be concluded that sartan modulates the immune system majorly by alleviating pro-inflammatory effects and thus reducing the risk of inflammation [8].

This chapter delves into the immunomodulatory properties of two widely prescribed antihypertensive agents, ACE inhibitors and ARBs. These agents are well known for the hypertension treatment; however, in recent years, they are attracting attention towards their potential to modify immune response. According to the study, auto-immune disease patients who are prescribed with ARBs for hypertension reported that they have observed the modification in symptoms associated with their immune disease. This chapter explores the mechanisms by which ACE inhibitors and ARBs modify the immune system and could be helpful in the treatment of auto-immune disease [9]. The immune modulation action of ACE inhibitors and ARBs primarily involves the reduction of cytokine secretion, reducing adhesion molecules expression. This chapter holds a considerable significance for the treatment of patients having co-morbidities marked inflammatory responses. Therefore, ACE inhibitors and ARBs have advantageous immune modulating properties that could be effective in patients with auto immune disorders, allergies or metabolic syndrome (Fig. 7.1).

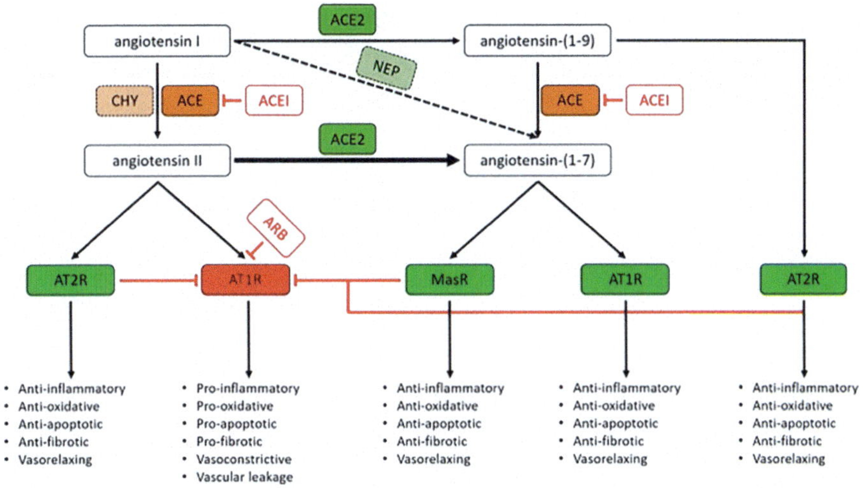

Fig. 7.1 Overview of major ACE and ACE2 substrates and products, the G-protein-coupled receptors (GPCRs) activated by these products, the biological consequences of the stimulation of these GPCRs and the mode of action of ACE inhibitors (*ACEI*) and angiotensin II type-1 receptor blockers (*ARB*). Besides ACE and ACE2, other proteolytic enzymes are also involved in the processing of renin-angiotensin system components, e.g. AngII can also be generated from AngI by chymase (*CHY*; secreted by mast cells) and Ang1–7 can be produced from AngI by neprilysin [also known as neutral endopeptidase (*NEP*)]. (Source: de Vries [10])

Machine Generated Summaries

Disclaimer: The summaries in this chapter were generated from Springer Nature publications using extractive AI auto-summarization: An extraction-based summarizer aims to identify the most important sentences of a text using an algorithm and uses those original sentences to create the auto-summary (unlike generative AI). As the constituted sentences are machine selected, they may not fully reflect the body of the work, so we strongly advise that the original content is read and cited. The auto generated summaries were curated by the editor to meet Springer Nature publication standards. To cite this content, please refer to the original papers.

Machine generated keywords: covid, sarscov, coronavirus, immune, respiratory, host, immune response, domain, inflammatory, cytokine, virus, ang, covid patient, host cell, spike protein.

COVID-19: Angiotensin-Converting Enzyme 2 (ACE2) Expression and Tissue Susceptibility to SARS-CoV-2 Infection [11]

This is a machine-generated summary of:

Beyerstedt, Stephany; Casaro, Expedito Barbosa; Rangel, Érika Bevilaqua: COVID-19: angiotensin-converting enzyme 2 (ACE2) expression and tissue susceptibility to SARS-CoV-2 infection [11].

Published in: European Journal of Clinical Microbiology & Infectious Diseases (2021).

Link to original: https://doi.org/10.1007/s10096-020-04138-6

If you want to cite the papers, please refer to the original.

For technical reasons we could not place the page where the original quote is coming from.

Abstract-Summary "Angiotensin-converting enzyme 2 (ACE2) is not only an enzyme but also a functional receptor on cell surfaces through which SARS-CoV-2 enters the host cells and is highly expressed in the heart, kidneys, and lungs and shed into the plasma."

"SARS-CoV-2 causes ACE/ACE2 balance disruption and RAAS activation, which leads ultimately to COVID-19 progression, especially in patients with comorbidities, such as hypertension, diabetes mellitus, and cardiovascular disease."

"ACE2 expression may have paradoxical effects, aiding SARS-CoV-2 pathogenicity, yet conversely limiting viral infection."

SARS-CoV-2 and ACE2

"Past outbreaks were also caused by highly pathogenic coronaviruses, including the acute respiratory syndrome coronavirus (SARS-CoV) in 2002 and the Middle East respiratory syndrome coronavirus (MERS-CoV) in 2012."

"The current outbreak, denominated coronavirus disease 2019 (COVID-19), is caused by the severe acute respiratory syndrome coronavirus 2 (SARS-CoV-2)."

"Wrapp and others [12] documented that SARS-CoV-2 RBD has ~ 10- to 20-fold higher affinity to hACE2 when compared to SARS-CoV RBD binding capacity."

"SARS-CoV-2 RBD binds to soluble hACE2 more strongly than SARS-CoV [13]."

"This enhanced affinity for hACE2 may contribute to SARS-CoV-2's higher infectivity, as COVID-19 is widespread worldwide and the number of cases is constantly increasing."

Angiotensin-Converting Enzyme 2 and Renin–Angiotensin–Aldosterone System

"The main axis of the RAAS is composed of ACE/angiotensin II (Ang II)/Ang II receptors AT1 and AT2."

"Chronic activation of RAAS is associated with Ang II/AT1 deleterious effects, exacerbating the inflammation, fibrosis, apoptosis, antidiuretic hormone (ADH) and aldosterone release, and ultimately water and sodium retention [14, 15] Discovered in 2000 [16] as an ACE homolog with distinguished function, ACE2 is an enzyme that catalyses the cleavage of Ang II into Ang (1-7), Ang I to Ang (1-9), and participates in the hydrolysis of other peptides."

"The ACE2/Ang (1–7)/Mas axis counterbalances the ACE/Ang II/AT1R axis and is an essential regulatory pathway of the RAAS."

"ACE2 regulates the ACE action by reducing the amount of Ang II and increasing Ang (1–7)."

"ACE2 downregulation promotes ACE/ACE2 imbalance and increases ACE/Ang II/AT1R axis pathological activation, leading to an increase in Ang II-mediated vasoconstriction and a decrease in Ang (1–7)-mediated vasodilation [15]."

ACE2 Distribution and COVID-19 Manifestations

"Zou and others [17] linked the ACE2 expression in different organs to their potential risk to SARS-CoV-2 infection."

"To note, stomach and liver samples had < 1% proportion of ACE2-positive cells, indicating that these tissues were considered as low risk for SARS-CoV-2 infection."

"The lower expression of ACE2, not only in nasal epithelium but also in bronchial epithelial cells in children, when compared to adults [18], may also explain the non-respiratory COVID-19 symptoms/clinical manifestations in the youngest."

"The oral cavity is also at potential risk for SARS-CoV-2 infection [19], as the oral mucosa also expresses ACE2, especially in tongue epithelial cells."

"ACE2 expression occurs in some sites of the digestive tract and, in fact, SARS-CoV-2's RNA was detected in faecal samples from COVID-19 patients [20]."

"In people with asthma, ACE-2 and TMPRSS2 gene expression in bronchial epithelial cells was not different from healthy individuals [21], which may explain the lack of association of asthma and COVID-19 severity."

Comorbidities and ACE/ACE2 Balance Disruption

"In line with the findings of cell type-specific expression in the other tissues, ACE and ACE2 protein expression revealed higher levels of ACE in either tubular or glomerular compartments, which was associated with a decrease in ACE2 expression in human kidney samples from individuals with type 2 diabetic kidney disease and hypertension [22]."

"Within the kidneys of patients with COVID-19, the cytopathic effects of SARS-CoV-2 in podocytes and proximal straight tubule cells may cause acute kidney injury, since these compartments express high levels of ACE2 and TMPRSS2 [23]."

"Differences in ACE2 bronchial epithelial expression between patients with chronic pulmonary disease who are overweight (mean BMI 29 kg/m^2) when compared to those not overweight (mean BMI 21 kg/m^2) may account for the higher rates of COVID-19 in obese individuals [24]."

"We may speculate, therefore, that in the COVID-19 setting, the downregulation of ACE2 induced by the SARS-CoV-2 may contribute to epicardial adipose tissue inflammation and ultimately to cardiac complications."

Monoclonal Antibody-Based Therapy Targeting the Spike Protein

"Investigation of antibodies with potent anti-SARS-CoV-2 neutralization activity that correlates with their competitive capacity with ACE2 for the receptor-binding domain (RBD) of the viral spike protein binding has important clinical implications."

"Other monoclonal antibodies, obtained from convalescent COVID-19 individuals, and with the capacity to recognize distinct epitopes of the RBD of the viral spike protein (CA1 and CB6), were equally potent to neutralize the SARS-CoV-2 in vitro [25]."

"After screening a large panel of human mAbs that target the spike protein, two antibodies, COV2-2196 and COV2-2130, recognized the non-overlapping epitopes on RBD and bound simultaneously to the S protein inducing virus neutralization in a synergistic manner [26]."

"IgG1 ab1, an antibody with high affinity and specificity to SARS-CoV-2 RBD and highly competitive with ACE2, prevented mice from disease burden by decreasing viral shedding in lung tissue when used prophylactically or therapeutically [27]."

ACE1/ACE2 Gene Polymorphisms

"Several studies have demonstrated strong association between ACE1-insertion/deletion (I/D) and COVID-19."

"A meta-analysis (48,758 healthy subjects from 30 different countries) significantly associated ACE1-I/D allele frequency ratio with the increase in the recovery rate, but not with mortality [28]."

"ACE1-I/D polymorphisms could explain the clinical course of COVID-19 among various ethnic populations."

"The frequency of the deletion allele among African Americans, Indians, and whites (0.59, 0.49, and 0.44, respectively) was also significantly different [29]."

"These findings could explain the differences in cardiovascular disease, in particular in African Americans, who exhibit the higher frequency of the deletion allele."

"The significance of the findings of ACE and ACE2 allele frequency ratio require further in vitro and functional studies to clarify their role in COVID-19 studies."

Conclusions

"ACE2 expression and its modulation by conditions and underlying comorbidities may increase tissue susceptibility to COVID-19."

"SARS-CoV-2 disrupts the ACE/ACE2 physiological balance and activates the Ang II/AT1R pathways, leading to severe complications of the disease."

"Strategies that target the overactivation of RAAS and its deleterious effects in COVID-19 setting deserve further investigation."

Involvement of Dopaminergic Signaling in the Cross Talk Between the Renin-Angiotensin System and Inflammation [30]

This is a machine-generated summary of:

Campos, Javier; Pacheco, Rodrigo: Involvement of dopaminergic signaling in the cross talk between the renin-angiotensin system and inflammation [30].

Published in: Seminars in Immunopathology (2020).

Link to original: https://doi.org/10.1007/s00281-020-00819-8

If you want to cite the papers, please refer to the original.

For technical reasons we could not place the page where the original quote is coming from.

Abstract-Summary "The interaction between the RAS and the dopaminergic system has been studied in the context of inflammation of the central nervous system (CNS), kidney, and intestine, where they exert antagonistic actions in the regulation of the immune system."

"We summarized, integrated, and discussed the cross talk of the dopaminergic system and the RAS in the regulation of inflammatory pathologies, including neurodegenerative disorders, such as Parkinson's disease."

"We also analyzed the impact of the commensal microbiota in the regulation of RAS and dopaminergic system and how it is involved in inflammatory disorders."

"We summarized the therapeutic approaches that have yielded positive results in preclinical or clinical studies regarding the use of drugs targeting the RAS and dopaminergic system for the treatment of inflammatory conditions."

"Further understanding of the molecular and cellular regulation of the RAS-dopaminergic cross talk should allow the formulation of new therapies consisting of novel drugs and/or repurposing already existing drugs, alone or in combination, for the treatment of inflammatory disorders."

Introduction

"Dopaminergic regulation of immunity is exerted by the stimulation of dopamine receptors expressed on immune cells, including dendritic cells [31–33], T cells [34–36], and B cells among other cellular types [37, 38]."

"It is noteworthy that high-affinity dopamine receptors (DRD3, DRD4, and DRD5), which are selectively stimulated by low dopamine concentrations (in the range of 20–500 nM), promote pro-inflammatory responses in the adaptive [35, 36, 39–42] and innate immune cells [31–33, 43]."

"The stimulation of low-affinity dopamine receptors (DRD1 and DRD2), which are exclusively stimulated by high dopamine levels (in the range of 1–10 μM), induces anti-inflammatory effects in the immune system [44, 45]."

"Dopamine is also involved in the regulation of blood pressure, renal function, cognition, and voluntary movements [46, 47], thus suggesting a potential communication between dopaminergic signaling and either local or systemic RAS."

Modulation of Inflammation by Dopamine and RAS

"Regarding the effect of the RAS and the dopaminergic system on kidney inflammation, it was recently shown that chronic kidney disease progression in humans is associated with increasing concentrations of urinary AngII and decreased levels of urinary dopamine, thus indicating a positive association of renal AngII concentration and a negative association of renal dopamine levels with inflammation and kidney dysfunction [48]."

"In the same direction, a recent study conducted with Sprague-Dawley rats fed with an overload of fructose shows that kidney inflammation and renal dysfunction involved an increased urinary expression of AngII followed by a decrease in urinary levels of dopamine [49]."

"These results indicate that gut homeostasis involves a reciprocal regulation between some components of the RAS and the dopaminergic system, which becomes dysregulated upon inflammation associated to IBD and ageing, resulting in increased pro-inflammatory signaling mediated by ATR1 and DRD3, and impaired anti-inflammatory signaling mediated by ATR2, DRD1, and DRD2."

Interaction Between RAS and Dopaminergic System in Neurogenerative Disorders

"A study addressing the role of the cross talk between the dopaminergic system and the RAS in the context of the gut-brain axis has demonstrated that gut inflammation induced in mice by the administration of DSS results in downregulation of DRD2 and ATR2 expression and increased expression of ATR1 in the nigrostriatal pathway."

"Using genetic and pharmacologic approaches, that study showed that DRD2 signaling in astrocytes induced the expression of the anti-inflammatory mediator αB-crystallin, which abolish the development of neuroinflammation and neurodegeneration in a mouse model of Parkinson's disease induced by 1-methyl-4-phenyl-1,2,3,6-tetrahydropyridine (MPTP) [50]."

"These findings indicate that signaling through low-affinity dopamine receptors and ATR2 expressed in glial cells attenuates neuroinflammation, whereas DRD3 and ATR1 promote neuroinflammation."

"Addressing the role of RAS in EAE, it has been shown an upregulation of AngII, ACE1, and ATR1 either in $CD4^+$ T-cells and monocytes infiltrating the CNS during the inflammatory process [51, 52]."

Intestinal Microbiota in the Modulation of RAS and its Role in Inflammatory and Metabolic Diseases

"Intestinal microbiota interacts with the organism by synthesizing metabolites, such as γ-aminobutyric acid (GABA) or short-chain fatty acids (SCFA), which exerts their effects by stimulating specific receptors expressed on the host cells [53]."

"Metabolites derived from commensal bacteria might stimulate their receptors expressed in innate and adaptive immune cells, strongly regulating the immune response of the host [53]."

"Another way by which gut microbiota might regulate host physiology is by degradation of proteins derived from the organism, yielding peptides with biological activity, including peptides derived from serum albumin, mucin, digestive enzymes, and debris protein derived from dying epithelial cells."

"To the direct production of metabolites that might affect host physiology, intestinal microbiota can also influence the production of key regulators of immunity, including dopamine and norepinephrine [54, 55]."

Conclusions and Projections

"Current evidence has shown a significant regulation of inflammation by RAS and dopaminergic system, as well as a complex interaction between both systems."

"The RAS and the dopaminergic system might trigger pro-inflammatory and anti-inflammatory outcomes systemically and in particular organs, including the kidney, the gut, and the brain."

"Further insight at the cellular and molecular level is needed in order to elucidate the detailed mechanisms of interaction by which changes on RAS or dopaminergic components control inflammation in the kidney, the gut, the brain, and systemically."

"The potential identification of heteromeric receptors conformed by protomers from different systems would open the possibility of development of new pharmacologic tools to be tested as therapeutic approaches for inflammatory disorders."

A Narrative Review of the Potential Pharmacological Influence and Safety of Ibuprofen on Coronavirus Disease 19 (COVID-19), ACE2, and the Immune System: A Dichotomy of Expectation and Reality [56]

This is a machine-generated summary of:

Smart, Lucinda; Fawkes, Neil; Goggin, Paul; Pennick, Graham; Rainsford, K. D.; Charlesworth, Bruce; Shah, Neil: A narrative review of the potential pharmacological influence and safety of ibuprofen on coronavirus disease 19 (COVID-19), ACE2, and the immune system: a dichotomy of expectation and reality [56].

Published in: Inflammopharmacology (2020).

Link to original: https://doi.org/10.1007/s10787-020-00745-z

If you want to cite the papers, please refer to the original.

For technical reasons we could not place the page where the original quote is coming from.

Abstract-Summary "This has been further conflicted by the initiation of studies to assess the efficacy of ibuprofen in improving outcomes in severe COVID-19 patients."

"The literature suggests that double-blind, placebo-controlled study results must be reported and carefully analysed for safety and efficacy in patients with COVID-19 before any recommendations can be made regarding the use of ibuprofen in such patients."

"Limited studies have suggested: (i) no direct interactions between ibuprofen and SARS-CoV-2 and (ii) there is no evidence to suggest ibuprofen affects the regulation of angiotensin-converting-enzyme 2 (ACE2), the receptor for COVID-19, in human studies."

"In vitro studies suggest ibuprofen may facilitate cleavage of ACE2 from the membrane, preventing membrane-dependent viral entry into the cell, the clinical significance of which is uncertain."

"In vitro evidence suggests that inhibition of the transcription factor nuclear factor-κB (NF-kB) by ibuprofen may have a role in reducing excess inflammation or cytokine release in COVID-19 patients."

"There is no evidence that ibuprofen will aggravate or increase the chance of infection of COVID-19."

Introduction

"Efforts to overcome the morbidity and mortality caused by this novel virus have been hampered by a lack of knowledge of the SARS-CoV-2 virus, particularly with regard to virulence, individual risk factors to host responses and appropriate treatment (Rokni and others [57])."

"It is becoming clear that the increased incidence of life-threatening cases caused by SARS-CoV-2 are, at least in part, a consequence of a cytokine storm in some individuals."

"The generation and analysis of evidence is essential to provide treatment recommendations, influence healthcare professionals' opinions and inform patient's self-care decisions during times of crisis."

"This article provides a safety and efficacy assessment of the pharmacological actions of ibuprofen and reviews the literature associated with ibuprofen's potential benefits and risks in relation to SARS-CoV-2 infection."

RAAS and Its Role in Inflammation

"Given the observation that system-wide imbalances in the ACE:ACE2 ratio favouring the pro-inflammatory ACE axis are commonly observed in certain disease states commonly comorbid in severe COVID-19, it could be hypothesised that immune dysregulation of the RAAS and associated increases in pro-inflammatory mediators in the lungs may play a central role in the pathophysiology of SARS-CoV-2, such as induction of acute lung injury (ALI) or ARDS—both of which are notable causes of death in critically ill patients suffering from COVID-19 (Wu and others [58])."

"Although small and with limited capacity for repeat, a cohort study of 12 SARS-CoV-2 patients demonstrated that circulating Ang II levels were markedly elevated compared to healthy controls, which was linearly correlated with viral load ($P = 0.035$) (Liu and others [59]), indicating that such downregulation of ACE2 could facilitate the multi-organ damage associated with viral infection."

RAAS, COVID-19 and Ibuprofen

"The mode of enhancement of the ACE2/Ang(1–7)/MasR axis by ibuprofen likely occurred via its direct inhibitory effects on the downstream pro-inflammatory mediators (e.g. NF-kB, COX2 & TGF-β1) of the ACE/Ang II/AT_1R axis."

"It could be hypothesised that ibuprofen may also indirectly impact the cleavage of ACE2 from the cell membrane, thus limiting viral infectivity, given that the circulating form of ACE2 lacks the membrane anchor used as the cell entry point for SARS-CoV-2."

"The clinical meaningfulness of the known effects of ibuprofen on cytokines (be it pro- or anti-inflammatory) are currently unknown in COVID-19 patients: the dose, timings of dose, severity of condition and the state of an individual's immune response are all potential determining factors and should be thoroughly assessed before conclusions can be drawn."

Discussion

"The literature contains strong evidence for the role of the RAAS, and in particular ACE2, in facilitating host cell infection, its downregulation thereof, and the consequential immune response triggered by the SARS-CoV-2 virus."

"To the interaction between SARS-CoV-2 and ACE2 in host cell infection, the literature also provides biological plausibility into how the RAAS could modulate the observed inflammatory response, recognising its physiological role as a key regulatory system of inflammation."

"It is certain that as more observational and epidemiological data are generated globally from infected patients, an enhanced understanding of the true situation surrounding ACE2 expression levels in the susceptibility to, and severity of, SARS-CoV-2 infection will be gained."

"This suggests ibuprofen to be a safe and effective anti-inflammatory in the instance of SARS-CoV-2 infection in properly selected patients with low risk of NSAID-related complications."

Conclusion

"This review explored the literature for any potential alteration of the risk/benefit profile in relation to SARS-CoV-2 infection."

"This is further confirmed by the analysis of observational data acquired from patient registries of SARS-CoV-2-positive patients in (i) Israel, which demonstrated that ibuprofen use was not associated with worse clinical outcomes compared with paracetamol or no antipyretic (Rinott and others [60]); (ii) Michigan, US, which demonstrated that NSAID use prior to admission was not associated with renal failure or increased mortality (Imam and others [61]); and (iii) individuals with rheumatic diseases who demonstrated that exposure to NSAIDs was not associated with increased risk of hospitalisation (Gianfrancesco and others [62])."

"There is no current evidence to suggest a mechanism by which ibuprofen exacerbates, aggravates, or increases the chance of infection with SARS-CoV-2."

Lower Serum Angiotensin-Converting Enzyme Level in Relation to Hyperinflammation and Impaired Antiviral Immune Response Contributes to Progression of COVID-19 Infection [63]

This is a machine-generated summary of:

Chen, Yuying; Huang, Da; Yuan, Wei; Chang, Jiang; Yuan, Zhize; Wu, Di; Han, Meifang; Luo, Xiaoping; Ning, Qin; Yan, Weiming: Lower Serum Angiotensin-Converting Enzyme Level in Relation to Hyperinflammation and Impaired Antiviral Immune Response Contributes to Progression of COVID-19 Infection [63].

Published in: Infectious Diseases and Therapy (2021).

Link to original: https://doi.org/10.1007/s40121-021-00513-8

If you want to cite the papers, please refer to the original.

For technical reasons we could not place the page where the original quote is coming from.

Abstract-Summary "We aimed to investigate the role of serum ACE in predicting the coronavirus disease 2019 (COVID-19) disease progression and the underlying mechanisms."

"We retrospectively enrolled 120 patients with confirmed COVID-19 who underwent serum ACE detection on admission."

"Patients with ACE level ≤33.5 U/L showed a higher cumulative virus RNA detection rate, elevated pro-inflammatory mediators levels, declined lymphocyte count, and decreased SARS-CoV-2-specific antibodies than those with ACE level >33.5 U/L. Lower serum ACE levels in relation to delayed virus elimination, hyper-inflammatory condition, and impaired host antiviral immune responses contribute to disease progression of COVID-19."

Introduction

"By acting as an endogenous counter-regulatory axis to the ACE axis, ACE2 converts Ang II into angiotensin 1–7 and exerts vasodilatory, anti-inflammatory, and anti-fibrotic effects via the Mas receptor [64, 65]."

"Besides being an RAS modulator, ACE2 was identified as the functional receptor for SARS-CoV-2 following the COVID-19 outbreak [66]."

"The latest research based on 136 patients with confirmed COVID-19 suggested that serum ACE level could serve as a marker to reflect the clinical condition of COVID-19 rather than an independent risk factor for disease severity [67]."

"120 patients with confirmed COVID-19 who underwent measurement of serum ACE levels on admission were retrospectively enrolled, to evaluate the potential role of serum ACE level in combination with other risk factors in predicting disease progression of COVID-19 and further investigate the possible mechanisms involved."

Methods

"Between January 13, 2020 and March 1, 2020, 120 patients with confirmed COVID-19 based on detection of SARS-CoV-2 RNA who were hospitalized at Tongji Hospital of Tongji Medical College, Huazhong University of Science and Technology and underwent detection of serum ACE levels on admission were enrolled in this retrospective study cohort."

"Real-time RT-PCR was performed using the following conditions: 50 °C for 10 min, 95 °C for 5 min, followed by 40 cycles of 95 °C for 10 s and 55 °C for

40 s. A cycle-count threshold value of <37 was defined as positive for SARS-CoV-2 RNA."

"Routine laboratory measurements including complete blood count, serum biochemical test (including liver and renal function, creatine kinase, LDH, and electrolytes), blood gas analysis, measurement of serum inflammatory mediators (CRP, ferritin, ESR, and PCT), myocardial enzyme spectrum analysis, and coagulation profile study were performed in the Department of Laboratory Medicine in Tongji Hospital according to the clinical requirement."

Results

"Although serum level of ACE has seldom been discussed as a risk factor for COVID-19 disease progression in the existing literature, significantly lower ACE levels were found in patients in the progressive than non-progressive group (mean 18.5 vs. 28.0 U/L, $P = 0.002$), suggesting its potential use as a biomarker of disease progression."

"According to vital signs recorded on the day of hospital admission, significantly higher respiratory rate and lower oxygen saturation were found in the progressive patients than the non-progressive patients (mean 24.9/min vs. 20.8/min, $P = 0.001$; and mean 90.4% vs. 96.0%, $P = 0.002$)."

"To further explore the possible mechanisms underlying the effect of ACE on COVID-19 disease progression, variations in the parameters reflecting inflammation and immune status were evaluated in patients with various levels of serum ACE."

Discussion

"In this real-world retrospective cohort of 120 patients with confirmed SARS-CoV-2 infection, comparison of the clinical and laboratory findings between patients with and without disease progression revealed that lower ACE level on admission correlated with higher incidence of disease progression."

"As shown in our results, an obviously diminished immune response to SARS-CoV-2 infection, as manifested by early significantly lower lymphocyte count, a marked decline in the total T cell, $CD4^+$ T cell, B cell, and NK cell counts as well as decreased IgG and IgM titers between two detections, was documented for patients with ACE ≤ 33.5 U/L. Such altered immunity was insufficient to eliminate the virus and has been considered a risk factor associated with COVID-19 disease progression [68–70]."

"The immune-mediated injury during SARS-CoV-2 infection, together with increased Ang II levels due to virus–host interactions and alternative formation pathways might contribute to the hyperinflammation in patients with COVID-19 with lower ACE level."

Conclusion

"In this retrospective real-world study, we identified that lower level of serum ACE on admission was an independent risk factor for higher incidence of COVID-19 disease progression, which might correlate with prolonged duration of viral shedding, excessive inflammation, and depressed immune response."

"This study may provide new insights into the clinical management of COVID-19 and enhance the rational allocation of medical resources."

Inflammation Triggered by SARS-CoV-2 and ACE2 Augment Drives Multiple Organ Failure of Severe COVID-19: Molecular Mechanisms and Implications [71]

This is a machine-generated summary of:

Iwasaki, Masae; Saito, Junichi; Zhao, Hailin; Sakamoto, Atsuhiro; Hirota, Kazuyoshi; Ma, Daqing: Inflammation Triggered by SARS-CoV-2 and ACE2 Augment Drives Multiple Organ Failure of Severe COVID-19: Molecular Mechanisms and Implications [71].

Published in: Inflammation (2020).

Link to original: https://doi.org/10.1007/s10753-020-01337-3

If you want to cite the papers, please refer to the original.

For technical reasons we could not place the page where the original quote is coming from.

Abstract-Summary "The widespread occurrence of severe acute respiratory syndrome coronavirus 2 (SARS-CoV-2) has led to a pandemic of coronavirus disease 2019 (COVID-19)."

"Massive cytokines including interleukin-6, nuclear factor kappa B (NFκB), and tumor necrosis factor alpha (TNFα) released from SARS-CoV-2-infected macrophages and monocytes lead inflammation-derived injurious cascades causing multi-organ injury/failure."

"This review summarizes the current evidence and understanding of the underlying mechanisms of SARS-CoV-2, ACE2 and inflammation co-mediated multi-organ injury or failure in COVID-19 patients."

Introduction

"Coronavirus disease-2019 (COVID-19) is a highly transmissible disease caused by severe acute respiratory syndrome coronavirus-2 (SARS-CoV-2)."

"Compared to the outbreaks of severe acute respiratory syndrome (SARS; 2002–2003; 774 deaths/8096 cases, case fatality rate (CFR) 9.6%) and Middle East respiratory syndrome (MERS; 2012–ongoing; 858 deaths/2494 cases, CFR 34.4%), the CFR of COVID-19 is relatively low (333,401 deaths/5,103,006 cases, CFR 6.5%) (recorded on May 23, 2020), but SARS-CoV-2 infection has caused the worst death toll worldwide [72]."

"A recent publication indicated that higher ACE2 concentrations led to increased vulnerability to SARS-CoV-2 infection in men compared to women, and that this finding was also associated with the higher incidence and fatality rate of COVID-19 in men [73]."

"This review aims to summarize the multi-organ injuries and failure and the underlying mechanisms of COVID-19 that are associated with SARS-CoV-2 infection via ACE2 entry route and beyond."

The Physiology of the Renin-Angiotensin System and ACE2

"The intracellular RAS is involved in the intracellular signaling pathways; Ang2 stimulates the production of reactive oxygen species (ROS) and nuclear factor kappa B (NFκB) via AT1R and the phosphatidylinositol-4,5-bisphosphate 3-kinase/protein kinase B (PI3K/Akt) pathway, leading to increases of proinflammatory cytokines such as IL-6, chemokines, and adhesion molecules in tissue-resident cells in the amplifying inflammatory cycle [74]."

"In a rheumatoid arthritis model, the ACE2/Ang-(1–7)/AT2R axis also provided an anti-inflammatory response by reducing the gene expressions of IL-1β and IL-6 and activating NFκB [75]."

"AT1R activation by Ang2 binding phosphonates ADAM17 via the intracellular mitogen-activated protein kinase (p38/MAPK) cellular signaling pathway facilitates the cleavage of ACE2 and tends to the ACE/Ang2/AT1R axis, leading to a positive feedback mechanism in the proinflammatory response [76]."

"ACE2 is expressed predominantly in the epithelial cells of the lung and intestine [77], suggesting that these organs may be the primary infected sites of SARS-CoV-2."

The Pathology of the Cytokine Storm

"The mIL-6R exists only on immune cells such as T cells, monocytes, macrophages, activated B cells, neutrophils, and osteoclasts [78], where the classic IL-6 signaling occurs following the anti-inflammatory bioreaction."

"The IL-6 trans-signaling leads to an immense effect due to the widespread presence of gp130 on both immune and non-immune cells and also due to the suppression of intracellular negative feedback by SOCS (suppressor of cytokine signaling) 3 via the Janus kinase-signal transducers and activators of transcription (JAK-STAT3) pathway in the immune cells [79]."

"Non-immune cells such as endothelial cells, smooth muscle cells, and fibroblasts are activated by NFκB and STAT3 and then release IL-7, which stimulates CD4-positive cells to release IL-6 and IL-17a, resulting in positive feedback to the non-immune cells in the IL-6 amplification cycle [80]."

"After N1H1 influenza infection, pulmonary endothelial cells secreted cytokines (IL-6, IFNα, IFNγ, and TNFα) and chemokines (CCL-2) and recruited innate immune cells (macrophages and natural killer cells) but not lymphocytes [81]."

The Mechanisms Underlying SARS-COV-2 Infection

"After virus attachment, the S1 protein of SARS-CoV-2 binds to ACE2 on the host cell membrane to enter the cell [82] after the activation of S1 protein ("cleavage") by host proteinase "priming.""

"Recent research revealed that furin cleaved the S1/S2 proteins of SARS-CoV-2 and was essential for virus fusion with the host membrane [83]."

"The triple expression of ACE2, TMPRSS2, and furin was detected in lung macrophages, kidney, adrenal stromal cells, intestine endocytes [84], and nasal epithelial cells [85], strongly suggesting that those organs are susceptible to SARS-CoV-2 infection."

"Viral S2 protein is activated by the proteolysis cleavage with the host cell's CatB/L in endosomes [86–88] or with TMPRSS2, CatB/L, and furin in the extracellular space [89], inducing viral envelope fusion to the host membrane and the release of the virus component."

"SARS-CoV-2 entry is facilitated by the host cells' ACE2, TMPRSS2, and furin, inducing the activation of A2R and the cytokine storm starting with IL-6 release."

Multi-Organ Dysfunction/Failure

"Two cohort studies showed that 19.7–27.8% of hospitalized COVID-19 patients exhibited myocardial injury as indicated by elevated hsTnI [90] and TnT [91]."

"Patient series with severe COVID-19 or non-survivors were more likely to have a higher prevalence of liver injury compared to mild cases and survivors [58, 92–95]."

"In a retrospective study, liver injury was detected in 35.4% of non-ICU patients with COVID-19 [93]."

"The liver biopsy of a COVID-19 patient revealed micro-vesicular steatosis and lobular and portal activity, suggesting that the injury was caused by either SARS-CoV-2 infection or drug-induced injury [92]."

"Neurological injuries including central nervous system (CNS) symptoms, peripheral nervous system (PNS) symptoms, and skeletal muscle injury symptoms have been observed in patients with mild to severe COVID-19 [92, 96–101]."

"The reported prevalence of the injuries among patients with COVID-19 include ARDS (81–100%) [92, 94, 95, 102], cardiac injury (28–77%) [92, 94, 95, 102], AKI (38–50%) [94, 95, 102], liver dysfunction (25–28%) [95, 102], coagulopathy (50–71%) [94, 103], hypoxic encephalopathy (20%) [92], and gastrointestinal hemorrhage (6–8%) [95, 102]."

Future Perspectives on Therapeutics and Ongoing Studies

"A comparison of remdesivir treatment (n = 155) and placebo (n = 78) for COVID-19 patients in China [104] (NCT04257656) was initiated for patients who exhibited severe disease within 14 days after symptom onset, but this double-blind placebo-controlled RCT was terminated early because there was no difference in clinical improvement between the remdesivir and placebo: hazard ratio (HR) 1.23, 95% confidence interval (CI), 0.87–1.75."

"Five placebo-controlled clinical studies have described the outcomes of chloroquine treatment for COVID-19 patients."

"A large retrospective single-center study of 12,594 patients showed no association between ARB/ACE-I use and the severity/mortality of COVID-19 (24.7% vs. 24.8%, 95% CI – 3.5–3.5) [105], as did another retrospective study (severity 32.9% vs. 30.7%, p = 0.65, mortality 27.3% vs. 33.0%, p = 0.34) [106]."

"Two retrospective studies with >100 hospitalized patients indicated that the use of an ARB/ACE-I had no correlation with clinical outcomes (HR 0.97, 95% CI 0.68–1.39; p = 0.88) [107] or the severity of COVID-19 symptoms [108]."

Conclusion

"This review has summarized the latest evidence regarding the mechanisms underlying COVID-19 and its associated multi-organ injuries and failure, plus the potential strategies for treatments to be studied/developed."

"Since SARS-CoV-2 binds to the host ACE2 with a subsequent release of proinflammatory cytokines, the primary infection and the characteristic symptoms can occur in the lungs and nasal airway where ACE2 and TMPRSS2 are strongly co-expressed, followed by vital organ injury due to a cytokine storm that is probably initiated by IL-6."

"Further clinical studies of the therapeutics for COVID-19 are urgently needed as antibody drugs and vaccines that can effectively cure the disease or tackle the SARS-CoV-2 pandemic are not yet available."

Rediscovering ACE: Novel Insights into the Many Roles of the Angiotensin-Converting Enzyme [109]

This is a machine-generated summary of:

Gonzalez-Villalobos, Romer A.; Shen, Xiao Z.; Bernstein, Ellen A.; Janjulia, Tea; Taylor, Brian; Giani, Jorge F.; Blackwell, Wendell-Lamar B.; Shah, Kandarp H.; Shi, Peng D.; Fuchs, Sebastien; Bernstein, Kenneth E.: Rediscovering ACE: novel insights into the many roles of the angiotensin-converting enzyme [109].

Published in: Journal of Molecular Medicine (2013).

Link to original: https://doi.org/10.1007/s00109-013-1051-z

If you want to cite the papers, please refer to the original.

For technical reasons we could not place the page where the original quote is coming from.

Abstract-Summary "Angiotensin-converting enzyme (ACE) is best known for the catalytic conversion of angiotensin I to angiotensin II."

"This review discusses recent studies examining the functional significance of ACE tissue-specific expression and the presence in ACE of two independent catalytic sites with distinct substrates and biological effects."

Introduction

"In part, these drugs are effective because ACE inhibitors prevent angiotensin II formation."

"To understand ACE, one must realize that ACE has many effects beyond angiotensin II production."

"The cloning of ACE revealed that the enzyme consists of two independent catalytic domains [110, 111]."

"Another important feature of ACE is the physical localization of high quantities of the enzyme on the surface of vascular endothelium, positioning ACE to produce angiotensin II in immediate juxtaposition to vascular smooth muscle [112, 113]."

"ACE in these and several other locations raise the question as to what are the local effects."

"We will focus on three topics: the local role of ACE in the kidney, novel insights into the function of each of the ACE catalytic domains, and studies on the role of ACE on the immune response."

The Phenotype of ACE Null Mice

"The multiple actions of ACE are demonstrated by the phenotype of mice null for all ACE expression [ACE knockout (KO) mice] [114, 115]."

"These hemodynamic and renal abnormalities are common to mice lacking either ACE, angiotensinogen, renin, or the AT_1 receptor (AT_1R), suggesting that the phenotype is caused by a lack of angiotensin II formation [116, 117]."

"ACE KO mice also have phenotypic abnormalities not seen in other models lacking renin-angiotensin system (RAS) components."

"The absence of ACE by germ cells induces male infertility, a phenotype not present in angiotensinogen KO mice [114, 115]."

"Further, analysis of rats treated with either an ACE inhibitor or an AT_1 receptor antagonist during only the first 2 weeks of life resulted in adult animals with widening of the renal papillary space and a reduction in the ability to concentrate urine, akin to the changes in ACE KO mice [118, 119]."

Importance of Endothelial ACE

"The conclusion from this and a variety of other studies is that while endothelial ACE is a major source of angiotensin II production, the plasticity of the RAS is such that changes in renin expression can compensate for remarkable alterations in both the tissue distribution and the tissue levels of ACE."

"The presence of other polymorphisms with significant effects on plasma ACE levels and their impact on blood pressure has been reported [120, 121]."

"A study conducted by Agerholm-Larsen in 2000 reported that in over 40 studies comprising 42,715 Caucasian subjects, plasma ACE was increased in the D/D genotype, but blood pressure, increased risk of myocardial infarction, coronary disease, or stroke was not associated with the polymorphism [122]."

"A mouse model that had about 75% normal plasma ACE activity (measured under substrate limiting conditions) but lacked all tissue-bound ACE was still highly deficient in overall ACE activity and presented with a reduced blood pressure equivalent to a complete ACE knockout mouse [123]."

The Important Role of Renal ACE

"The observation that the systemic knockout of either angiotensinogen, renin, ACE, or the AT_1 receptor results in a common phenotype consisting of renal arteriolar thickening, hypotension, juxtaglomerular cell hypertrophy, hypoplastic renal medulla and papilla, hydronephrosis, and the inability to concentrate urine has been used to support the concept that angiotensin II production is important in renal organogenesis [116, 117]."

"Normal renal development and renal function in these mouse models indicate that angiotensin II production by ACE from renal origin is thus not necessary to ensure proper organogenesis [124–126]."

"Because of the restricted expression of ACE to renal tissues, this model still had a profound reduction of total ACE protein including the lack of ACE on any tissues positioned to convert plasma angiotensin I to angiotensin II."

"A variety of experiments indicate that local ACE expression and angiotensin II generation within renal tissue is not sufficient to preserve normal kidney morphology and function in the setting of hypotension due to a systemic lack of ACE activity."

Renal ACE and Baseline Kidney Function

"The detailed physiologic study of specific functions of renal ACE has been complicated by the low blood pressure present in several ACE genetic models [127]."

"Mouse genetic models lacking renal ACE while maintaining normal blood pressure support the concept that, in normotensive animals, renal ACE is not critical for basal renal function."

"Further, a compound heterozygous mouse in which one ACE allele was null and a second ACE allele targeted ACE expression to the liver had a normal blood pressure, glomerular filtration rate (GFR), single nephron GFR, renal plasma flow, and renal concentrating ability [128]."

Renal ACE and Hypertension

"These findings suggest that intrarenal ACE has the capacity to increase local kidney angiotensin II levels and to induce hypertension even in the absence of systemic ACE."

"While previous data suggest that under physiological conditions both the systemic and intrarenal RAS work in a concerted manner to maintain homeostasis of blood pressure [129, 130], in certain pathological states, like the hypertension induced by angiotensin II infusion, there is an independent activation of the intrarenal RAS."

"ACE expression is not only increased during angiotensin II-induced hypertension but also in many other conditions where renal parenchymal function is compromised [131]."

"These studies showed that the absence of kidney ACE blunted the hypertension induced either by angiotensin II infusion or by nitric oxide synthesis inhibition."

"We found that the ACE within the kidney and the local, renal generation of angiotensin II work as master regulators of sodium transport along the nephron."

Function of the N- and C-Domains of ACE

"This was investigated in mouse models in which point mutations were introduced into the mouse genome, selectively inactivating the catalytic activity of either the ACE N- or C-domains [132, 133]."

"The N-KO mouse, lacking ACE N-domain activity, had renin and angiotensin I levels that were essentially identical to WT mice."

"The C-KO mouse, lacking C-domain activity, maintained a normal blood pressure only by elevating renin and by increasing seven-fold the plasma levels of angiotensin I. These data indicate that, at least under in vivo basal conditions, it is the ACE C-domain that is mainly responsible for the conversion of angiotensin I to angiotensin II."

"If the ACE C-domain is predominantly responsible for angiotensin II production, why has a catalytically active ACE N-domain been preserved over hundreds of millions of years?"

"Several studies implicate an ACE N-domain substrate as important in regulating the injury response."

ACE and Immunity

"Several lines of investigation have focused on potential roles of ACE in the immune response."

"Mouse experiments discussed below indicate that manipulation of myeloid cell ACE levels can have profound effects on the immune response."

"While a discussion of the complete effects of the ACE on the immune response are beyond this review, here we focus on studies indicating that enhanced ACE expression by myelomonocytic cells can markedly augment the immune response."

Cytokine Expression

"Equivalent cells derived from N-KO mice produce substantially higher levels of TNFα."

"While the precise biochemical differences giving rise to such exaggerated TNFα production by N-KO cells is not understood, it is known that a similar increase of TNFα production is observed in vivo in N-KO mice exposed to LPS."

"Further, increased TNFα production was found in peritoneal macrophages from N-KO mice made hypertensive by angiotensin II infusion."

"While these findings clearly show an effect of the ACE N-domain on cytokine production, what is not clear is whether this is a direct effect on the biochemistry of cytokine production or whether the biochemical milieu within the ACE N-KO mice somehow instructs macrophages along a developmental program leading to changes in differentiation state and an intrinsically higher inflammatory response to pro-inflammatory stimuli."

ACE and MHC Class I Peptide Processing

"ACE has been described as affecting another immune phenomenon, the processing of peptides displayed by major histocompatibility (MHC) class I molecules on the surface of cells [134, 135]."

"When WT mice were immunized with cells from a mouse that was an ACE KO, more than 20% of the $CD8^+$ T cells were activated and produced IFN-γ."

"These experiments suggested the very novel finding that the MHC class I peptide repertoire presented by a mouse null for ACE expression is sufficiently different from that of a WT mouse that the two animals recognize each other's tissues as foreign."

"In a second important control, a WT recipient mouse was immunized with cells from an ACE KO mouse."

"When the recipient WT mouse was immunized with ACE KO tissues and then challenged with WT cells (i.e., totally syngeneic cells) but from an animal treated with an ACE inhibitor, the WT recipient's T cells detected foreign epitopes, resulting in T cell activation and IFN-γ production."

The Genetic Overexpression of ACE in Myelomonocytic Cells

"ACE 10/10 mice have an enhanced innate and adaptive immune response that confers significant anti-tumoral and anti-bacterial protection [126, 136]."

"ACE 10/10 mice showed substantial anti-tumoral protection with tumors that averaged only one-sixth (1/6) the size of those in WT mice."

"When ACE 10/10 bone marrow was transplanted into WT mice, the recipient mice showed substantially increased protection against B16 melanoma, as compared to equivalent mice transplanted with WT bone marrow."

"When these mice were bred with the ACE 10/10 mice, the double mutants exhibited an anti-tumor immune response significantly better than angiotensinogen mice having WT ACE alleles."

"Further, ACE 10/10 mice treated with an ACE inhibitor displayed an anti-tumor response equivalent to ACE inhibitor treated WT mice; treatment of ACE 10/10 mice with an AT_1 receptor antagonist did not reduce the immune response."

"The immune protection conferred by the ACE 10 mutation extended beyond the anti-tumoral response."

Anti-Viral Memory Response

"When cells are infected with PyV, they will present this peptide on the cell surface bound to MHC class I. Many other viral peptides are also presented, but it is this peptide that will induce a strong $CD8^+$ T cell response."

"To investigate the immune response in ACE 10/10, we first infected female WT and ACE 10/10 mice with PyV. This causes a chronic, low-level infection [137]."

"For this experiment, we also used the vaccinia strain VV-LT which contains the LT359-368 PyV amino acid sequence against which the mice had previously been exposed during the original PyV infection."

"This is a chimeric vaccinia virus containing the critical MHC class I epitope from PyV. Four days after vaccinia infection, mouse ovary vaccinia viral titers were measured by a plaque assay."

"With VV-LT, six of the eight ACE 10/10 mice had no detectable vaccinia virus (lane 4)."

Conclusion

"ACE inhibitors were approved for human use in the early 1980s, but the enzyme was not cloned until 1988–1989."

"The combination of these two domains, relatively nonspecific substrate specificity, and wide tissue distribution have positioned ACE as an important enzyme in many different physiologic processes."

"Doctors routinely decrease ACE activity with ACE inhibitors."

"While ACE has been investigated for over 50 years, the modern understanding of this enzyme has motivated groups to synthesize and study ACE domain specific inhibitors [138, 139]."

Physiological Relevance of Angiotensin Converting Enzyme 2 as a Metabolic Linker and Therapeutic Implication of Mesenchymal Stem Cells in COVID-19 and Hypertension [140]

This is a machine-generated summary of:

Saha, Sarama; Chakrabarti, Sasanka; Singh, Praveen Kumar; Poddar, Jit; Satapathi, Soumitra; Saini, Surendra; Kakar, Sham S.; Roy, Partha: Physiological Relevance of Angiotensin Converting Enzyme 2 As a Metabolic Linker and Therapeutic Implication of Mesenchymal Stem Cells in COVID-19 and Hypertension [140].

Published in: Stem Cell Reviews and Reports (2020).

Link to original: https://doi.org/10.1007/s12015-020-10012-x

If you want to cite the papers, please refer to the original.

For technical reasons we could not place the page where the original quote is coming from.

Abstract-Summary "Severe acute respiratory syndrome corona virus – 2 (SARS-CoV-2) is a single stranded RNA virus and responsible for infecting human being."

"Some recently reported studies revealed that individuals of elderly age group and with pre-existing medical conditions such as hypertension, diabetes mellitus had severe consequences, even may lead to death."

"It is not clearly delineated whether hypertension itself or associated comorbidities or antihypertensive therapy contributes to the grave prognosis of COVID-19 infections."

"It has been reported that SARS-CoV-2 enters into the host cell through interaction between conserved residues of viral spike protein and angiotensin converting enzyme 2 (ACE2) receptor which is highly expressed in host's cardiac and pulmonary cells and finally transmembrane protease, serine-2 (TMPRSS2), helps in priming of the surface protein."

"Although various clinical trials are being conducted on renin-angiotensin-system inhibitor, till to date there is no standard treatment protocol approved for critically ill COVID-19 positive cases with pre-existing hypertension."

"Identification of future novel therapeutics in the form of mesenchymal stem cell either alone or in combination with pharmacological approach could be recommended for combating SARS-CoV-2 which might be dreadful to debilitating elderly people."

Epidemiology of COVID 19

"A novel corona virus which is responsible for ongoing outbreak of fatal acute respiratory tract infection was named as SARS-CoV-2 (Severe Acute Respiratory syndrome associated coronavirus) by International Committee on Taxonomy of Viruses (ICTV)."

"Human corona virus (CoV) was first reported in 1965 and belongs to the family coronaviridae."

"All identified human corona viruses belong to either alpha or beta genera and gamma and delta primarily include avian origin."

"New SARS COV 2 is a beta coronavirus from the subgenus Sarbecovirus [141]."

Physiological Relevance of ACE2

"It has two forms: (i) the full-length membrane bound ACE2 which has an extracellular domain acting as a receptor for the spike protein of SARS-COV-2, transmembrane domain and cytoplasmic domain which contains calmodulin binding site [142]; (ii) soluble form of ACE2 which circulates in the blood [143]."

"Although there is approximately 60% sequence similarity with the catalytic domain of ACE, the ACE inhibitors (ACEi) such as Lisiniopril, Ramipril do not attenuate the effect of ACE2 since the active sites differ [144]."

"ACEi does not seem to have direct effect on ACE2."

"The transmissibility of COVID-19 is primarily determined by specific interaction between conserved residues located on RBD of S protein and ACE2 receptor of host cell [141]."

Clinical Evidence

"Few recent studies conducted during the outbreak in China reported that approximately 20–30% of patients were vulnerable to develop severe consequences having distinctive co-morbidities such as diabetes mellitus (DM), hypertension, chronic obstructive pulmonary disease, cardiovascular and cerebrovascular diseases [102, 145, 146]."

"Bhandari and others [147] conducted a study on 21 COVID positive patients in North India, and reported that approximately 14% of participants had pre-existing hypertension and 10% had DM."

"From these studies it is obvious that most of the patients who were vulnerable to develop severe illness in the form of admission in ICU, required mechanical ventilation, or death as one of the outcomes for elderly age groups with distinctive co-morbidities having hypertension as common co-morbidity."

"With increase in duration of DM as well as in some cases, old people with hypertension need treatment with ACEi which may increase the expression of ACE2."

Biochemical Correlation with Severity of SARS-CoV-2 Infection

"Biochemical investigation reported a decrease in hemoglobin count whereas a significant increase in Ferritin, CRP and lactate dehydrogenase [148–150]."

"The non-structural proteins of coronavirus such as 1ab, ORF 10 and ORF 3a dissociates iron from hemoglobin giving rise to porphyrin."

"The decrease in hemoglobin content will lead to attenuation of oxygen exchange at alveolar level."

"In order to store the large amount of released iron, there will be rise in the level of ferritin [151]."

Comparison with Impact of Co-Morbidities in Middle East Respiratory Syndrome (MERS) and Severe Acute Respiratory Syndrome (SARS)

"Badawi and Ryoo [152] conducted a systematic analysis on 637 MERS-CoV positive cases and reported that approximately half of these populations had co-morbidities such as DM and hypertension who had a dreadful clinical outcome and even death accounting to 35% of positive cases."

"Kulcsar and others [153] developed a diabetic mice model which was prone to get infected with MERS-CoV. Following infection, the mice had severe consequences and delayed recovery compared to normal mice."

"Study, authors inferred that dysregulation of immune responses might contribute to the disease severity in MERS CoV positive cases with co-morbidities."

"Yang and others [154] conducted a study on 539 SARS positive cases with history of DM and concluded that diabetes is an independent determinant of morbidity and mortality of SARS patients."

Contradictory Evidence Related to ACEi and ARB

"The crucial effect of ACEi on cardiovascular system is produced by inhibiting the conversion of Ang I to Ang II resulting in decrease in plasma Ang II and attenuating the hydrolytic degradation of bradykinin."

"ACEi exhibits its vasodilatory and fibrinolytic effects through increase in blood level of bradykinin, prostaglandin and nitric oxide [155, 156]."

"ACEi had been documented to produce its anti-inflammatory, antifibrotic, antithrombotic and vasodilatory effects through the activation of ACE2/Ang(1–7)/MAS axis [157]."

"ACEi increases the expression of ACE2 as an acquired response to counterbalance the enhanced levels of Ang I and II."

Clinical Trial on ACEi/ARB and Human Recombinant ACE2

"A similar randomized control trial of Losartan (25 mg daily) is being conducted on 580 COVID-19 positive patients who do not require hospitalization (https://clinicaltrials.gov/ct2/show/NCT04311177)."

"2414 hypertensive COVID-19 positive patients were recruited."

"Two interventional clinical trials (NCT04375046 and NCT04382950) are going to be conducted by Kafrelsheikh University from May 2020 to determine whether alone Recombinant Bacterial ACE2 Receptors—Like Enzyme of B38-CAP or in combination with Aerosolized 13 cis-retinoic acid would be more effective than Recombinant Human ACE2 to control lung injury in COVID-19 positive patients."

"An interventional two arm pilot study (NCT04287686) had been launched by Guangzhou Medical University to determine the effect of recombinant human ACE2 in adult COVID-19 patients since February 2020."

"A pilot clinical trial (NCT01597635) was conducted on 44 acute lung injury patients to evaluate the safety and tolerability of recombinant human ACE2."

ACE2 as Therapeutic Target

"Hydroxycholoroquine which is commonly used for the treatment of malaria may be repurposed for preventing the entry of virus by inhibiting the glycosylation of host receptor and thus inhibiting the binding of spike protein of the virus to the active site of host receptor [94]."

"Umifenovir, an established drug for treatment and prophylaxis of influenza, is a promising repurposed drug for its action to interfere the interplay between S protein and ACE2 for SARS-CoV-2 viral entry as evidenced by in vitro studies [158, 159]."

"Camostatmesylate, an approved drug in Japan for the treatment of pancreatitis, showed a great hope by in vitro study with its inhibitory effect against host serine protease TMPRSS2 which helps in S protein priming to interact with ACE2 [159] and thus prevents entry of the virus into the host cell."

"The binding interface between Spike and ACE2 is targeted by Hesperidin to prevent entry of virus into the host cells [160]."

Therapeutic Importance of ACE2 and Mesenchymal Stem Cell (MSC)

"The lack of these MSC like cells may be responsible for delaying in recovery from lung injury resulting in severe outcome in patients with SARS-CoV-2 infection compared to healthy individuals."

"Liang and others [161] reported the outcome of a case study of human umbilical cord stem cell transplantation on 65 year old critically ill COVID-19 positive patient."

"RNA sequence analysis of transplanted MSCs confirmed the immunomodulatory property of MSCs because of expression of anti-inflammatory factors such as vascular endothelial growth factor and epidermal growth factor in MSCs and their ability to differentiate into AT2 (Angiotensin II receptor type 2) cells due to expression of surfactant proteins A and C. These studies indicated that MSC either alone or in combination with other pharmacological drugs could be recommended as a therapeutic intervention for the improvement of outcome of COVID-19 patients after further detailed patient sample analysis."

Mesenchymal Stem Cells and Cytokine Storm in COVID 19

"Cumulating evidence revealed that adult MSCs can influence the response of immune cells through various soluble factors such as transforming growth factor β1 (TGF β1), prostaglandin E 2 (PGE2), nitric oxide (NO), anti-inflammatory cytokine IL-10 and indole amine–pyrrole 2,3 dioxygenase (IDO) [162]."

"MSCs can reduce cytotoxicity by influencing cytokine release (IFN-γ) from NK cells through modulation of its proliferation which was induced by IL-2 and IL-15 [163]."

"These characteristic features of MSCs prompted the researchers to consider creatively the use of these cells for the treatment of COVID-19 patients with severe manifestations."

"Although most of the studies adopted intravenous mode of administration, one pilot study (NCT04276987) is being conducted on aerosol inhalation of the exosomes derived from allogenic adipose MSCs for the treatment of serious COVID-19 pneumonia patients [164]."

Future Prospects

"This information in future will help in the advancement of our knowledge about the cure and management of this virus infection in various ways."

"The study on structural details would provide relevant novel therapeutic target to encounter infection at the early stage and prevent the progression into a pandemic infection."

"All these aspects, there is an optimistic approach ahead which will help in the development of a novel drug for the treatment and management of SARS-CoV-2."

"To these aspects, the use of stem cell based therapies also appears to be a critical approach for the cure and management of this pandemic situation."

"A large cohort study using MSCs will provide the exact therapeutic potentiality of this stem cell based approach."

Conclusion

"Based on the findings presented in this review article, it is evident that although COVID-19 is not principally a metabolic or endocrine disorder, optimum regulation of plasma glucose and blood pressure are essential to avoid the obvious threat and enhanced risk of development of relevant complications such as heart failure and stroke in patients with COVID-19."

"Considering the lack of specific antiviral treatment for COVID-19 cases, in order to reduce the mortality, stem cell based therapy could be a novel therapeutic approach to decrease the severity of COVID-19 patients."

"It is speculated that a combined approach as depicted in this review will probably help in the cure and management of elderly patients with associated co-morbidities."

AAV8-Mediated Angiotensin-Converting Enzyme 2 Gene Delivery Prevents Experimental Autoimmune Uveitis by Regulating MAPK, NF-κB and STAT3 Pathways [165]

This is a machine-generated summary of:

Qiu, Yiguo; Tao, Lifei; Zheng, Shijie; Lin, Ru; Fu, Xinyu; Chen, Zihe; Lei, Chunyan; Wang, Jiaming; Li, Hongwei; Li, Qiuhong; Lei, Bo: AAV8-Mediated Angiotensin-Converting Enzyme 2 Gene Delivery Prevents Experimental Autoimmune Uveitis by Regulating MAPK, NF-κB and STAT3 Pathways [165].

Published in: Scientific Reports (2016).

Link to original: https://doi.org/10.1038/srep31912

If you want to cite the papers, please refer to the original.

For technical reasons we could not place the page where the original quote is coming from.

Abstract-Summary "With the discovery of the angiotensin-converting enzyme 2 (ACE2), a protective axis of RAS namely ACE2/Ang-(1–7)/Mas that counteracts the deleterious ACE/AngII/AT1R axis has been established."

"We investigated the hypothesis that enhancing the activity of the protective axis of RAS by subretinal delivery of an AAV8 (Y733F)-ACE2 vector would protect against the ocular inflammation in experimental autoimmune uveitis (EAU) mice through regulating the local immune responses."

"Our studies demonstrated that increased ACE2 expression exerts protective effects on inflammation in EAU mouse by modulating ocular immune responses, including the differentiation of Th1/Th17 cells and the polarization of M1/M2 macrophages; whereas the systemic immune responses appeared not affected."

"This proof-of-concept study suggests that activation of ocular ACE2/Ang-(1–7)/Mas axis with AAV gene transfer modulates local immune responses and may be a promising, long-lasting therapeutic strategy for refractory and recurrent uveitis, as well as other inflammatory eye diseases."

Introduction

"Increasing evidence have demonstrated that activation of this axis not only directly counterbalances the deleterious effects of the classical ACE/Ang II/AT1R axis, but also has a broad range of beneficial effects including ameliorating pathological conditions such as fibrosis and inflammation [166, 167]."

"ACE2/Ang-(1–7)/Mas axis acts as a negative regulator of the RAS and has become a vital therapeutic target in many inflammatory and autoimmune diseases, including type 1 diabetes [168], autoimmune myocarditis [169] and arthritis [170]."

"Oral delivery of ACE2/Ang-(1–7) bioencapsulated in plant cells conferred protection against ocular inflammation in EAU and EIU mice [171]."

"Enhancing the ACE2/Ang-(1–7)/Mas axis of the RAS may be a promising therapeutic approach for ocular inflammation."

"We hypothesize that over-expression of ACE2 attenuates the ocular local inflammation in EAU mouse by activating the protective ACE2/Ang-(1–7)/Mas axis and by inhibition of MAPK, NF-κB and STAT3 pathways."

Results

"To determine the effect of ACE2 over-expression on the local and systemic Th1/Th17 responses, retinas, spleens and draining lymph nodes (DLN) were collected to detect the mRNA levels of IFN-γ and IL-17."

"In the retina, the mRNA level of iNOS was increased in the AAV8-eGFP+EAU group, whereas, the level of Arginase-1 (Arg-1) was decreased compared with the ACE2 over-expression EAU eyes ($p < 0.05$)."

"The mRNA expressions of IL-6, IL-1β, TNF-α and MCP-1 were remarkably decreased and the level of IL-10 was increased in the AAV8-ACE2+EAU group."

"To further determine whether inhibition of the MAPK, NF-κB and STAT3 pathways is involved in the ACE2/Ang-(1–7)/Mas axis mediated protection in EAU eyes, phosphorylation level of p38 MAPK, ERK1/2, JNK, IκB-α and STAT3 in the retina were measured by Western blotting at the 14th day after immunization."

Discussion

"In line with the previous studies, we showed that activating the ACE2/Ang-(1–7)/Mas axis by over-expressing ACE2 resulted in a dramatic decrease of the typical Th1 and Th17 cytokines (IFN-γ and IL-17), indicating that enhancing ACE2 may ameliorate EAU by inhibiting local Th1 and Th17 responses."

"To the T cells, it has been shown that activation of ACE2/Ang-(1–7)/Mas axis reduces inflammatory responses in macrophages [172]."

"These result revealed that activating the local protective ACE2/Ang-(1–7)/Mas axis may be capable to regulate the polarization of classically activated M1 macrophage and the alternatively activated M2 macrophage in the eyes of EAU mice."

"We provide the first piece of evidence that the activation of ACE2 plays an anti-inflammatory role in ocular autoimmune inflammation by regulating the local immune responses and the protective effects are associated with the inhibition of MAPK, NF-κB and STAT3 pathways."

Materials and Methods

"To study whether the effect of AAV8-ACE2 was mediated by activating of Ang-(1–7)/Mas, osmotic mini-pumps (Alzet, Cupertino, CA, USA) filled with a selective Ang-(1–7) antagonist, A-779 (D-Ala7-ANG I/II/1–7) with the delivery rate of 125 μg $kg^{-1} \cdot h^{-1}$ (Bachem, Torrence, CA, USA) were implanted subcutaneously on the back between the shoulder blades and hips while animals were anesthetized by intraperitoneal injection with 75 mg/kg ketamine (Fujian Gutian pharmaceutical Co., Ltd, Ningde, Fujian, China) and 13.6 mg/kg xylazine (VEDCO Inc., St. Joseph, MO, USA)."

"Mice were immunized subcutaneously at the base of the tail and both thighs with 50 μg human IRBP 161–180 peptide in 100 μl PBS, emulsified 1:1 (vol/vol) in CFA (Sigma-Aldrich, St. Louis, MO, USA) supplemented with 1.0 mg/ml mycobacterium tuberculosis strain."

Relation of ACE2 with Co-morbidity Factors in SARS-CoV-2 Pathogenicity [173]

This is a machine-generated summary of:

Santra, Dipannita; Banerjee, Amrita; De, Subrata Kr.; Thatoi, Hrudayanath; Maiti, Smarajit: Relation of ACE2 with co-morbidity factors in SARS-CoV-2 pathogenicity [173].

Published in: Comparative Clinical Pathology (2023).

Link to original: https://doi.org/10.1007/s00580-023-03434-9

If you want to cite the papers, please refer to the original.

For technical reasons we could not place the page where the original quote is coming from.

Abstract-Summary "In the last 3 years of the pandemic situation, SARS-CoV-2 caused a significant number of deaths."

"Infection rates for symptomatic and asymptomatic patients are higher than that for death."

"Researchers explored that the major deaths are attributed to several comorbidity factors."

"The confounding factors and gender-associated infection/death rate are observed globally."

Introduction

"Certain comorbidities are associated with a strong ACE2 receptor expression and higher release of proprotein convertase that enhances the viral entry into the host cells."

"ACE2 receptor serves cellular entry point for COVID-19 to hook into and infect a wide range of human cells."

"ACE2 is a protein widely expressed at the surface of many cells and also acts as a cellular doorway for the SARS-CoV2 virus, which causes COVID-19."

"A decreased level of ACE2 secondary to SARS-CoV-2 infection followed by an increase in Ang II can exacerbate cardiovascular disease symptoms or promote further disease complications (Oudit and others [174]; Aksoy and others [175])."

"The level of ACE2 expression in the liver and kidney has been shown to increase when patients take ARB and ACEi medications, but these patients do not appear to have an increased risk of developing SARS-CoV-2 infection or suffering from severe disease."

ACE2 in Renin Angiotensin System

"RAS blockers increase angiotensin II, which is a substrate for ACE2."

"Following the initial entry of SARS-CoV-2 into the cells through ACE2, the virus further controls ACE2 expression, reducing the protective properties of the enzyme Ang II is transformed into Ang (1–7) and Ang-I into inactive Ang by ACE2 (1–9)."

"The unopposed action of Ang-II through its AT1 receptor is caused downregulation of ACE2."

"ACE-I/ARB may increase the amount of the soluble form of ACE2 and prevent the virus from entering the host cell."

"ARBs and ACE-Is both have differing effects on Ang-II, with the latter blocking its receptor while the former prevents its production (reduction in Ang-II levels) (no effect on levels of Ang-II)."

"ACE-I/ARB will protect against this organ damage by (1) possible upregulation of ACE2 activity, (2) reduced levels of Ang-II (by ACE-Is), and (3) inhibiting the ATI receptor of Ang-II."

Effect of ACE2 on Salt Balance

"It is believed that angiotensin-converting enzyme 2 (ACE2) balances off ACE by the breakdown of Ang II and producing Ang (1–7)."

"In mice, a high salt diet raised ACE2 activity in the urine, but a low salt diet lowered it (Wysocki and others [176])."

"Variations in salt intake alter Ang II activity largely via changes in renin release and plasma renin activity."

"Since Ang II is controlled by the enzyme ACE2, changes in ACE2 would be anticipated anytime ACE or Ang II levels fluctuate."

"It is likely that the rise in ACE2 levels is delayed or does not coincide with the rise in ACE activity, maintaining transiently high Ang II levels similar to those seen in participants after a low-salt diet."

"One would anticipate a decrease in ACE, followed by a fall in ACE2, if Ang II production reduces, as in a high-salt diet."

Effect of ACE2 on Hypertension

"It is theorized that an imbalance between the tissue's ACE and ACE2 proteins causes enhanced ACE2 expression to guard against increased blood pressure and ACE2 deficiency to exacerbate hypertension."

"Through negatively regulating the renin-angiotensin system, which includes the pressor-hypertrophic route of ANG II and the depressor-antiproliferative effects of Ang-(1–7) (Li and others [106]; Ferrario and others [157]), ACE2 adjusts blood pressure and maintains blood pressure homeostasis."

"Ang II is transformed by ACE2 into Ang (1–7), which works at the Mas receptor to lower blood pressure and lessen fibrosis and inflammation (South and others [177])."

"The main consequences of the ACE/Ang II/Ang II type 1 receptor pathway are countered by this, including vasoconstriction, sodium and water reabsorption, increased sympathetic nervous system tone, and increased oxidative stress, which results in inflammation and fibrosis (Masi and others [178])."

"These inhibitors boost the expression of the ACE2 receptor when administered in high doses, which increases SARS-CoV-2 infection (Fang and others [179])."

Effect of ACE2 on Diabetes

"For the treatment and prevention of diabetic nephropathy, a progressive condition characterized by proteinuria, thickening of the glomerular basement membrane, mesangial matrix expansion, and associated with chronic renal failure, ACE2 may be a significant target."

"In both mice and people with type 2 diabetes, there may be a correlation between decreased ACE2 expression in glomerular epithelial cells and increased ACE expression in diabetic kidney disease."

"Increased albuminuria and glomerular damage are brought on by ACE2 downregulation, which may also result in excessive Ang II buildup, particularly at the glomerular level (Ye and others [180])."

"Due to the glycosylation process, the expression of ACE2 is downregulated in diabetics, which may be a contributory factor for the severity of lung complications in comorbidity with SARS-CoV-2 invasion (Pal and Bhansali [181])."

"When ACE2 is overexpressed, it can break down Ang II and produce angiotensin 1–7, which has beneficial effects on COVID-19 (anti-fibrotic, anti-oxidant, anti-inflammatory, and vasodilatory)."

Effect of ACE2 on Cardiovascular Disease

"It is now recognized that there is a kind of RAS in which ACE2 degrades Ang II, the primary effectors of the traditional RAS, and generates Ang (1–7)."

"ACE2 is elevated in failing human hearts and atherosclerotic arteries, and its altered expression of cardiac and vascular disease in experimental models of CVD, and ACE2 is increased in failing human hearts and atherosclerotic vessels."

"ACE plays physiological functions through Ang II and AT1 receptors."

"Through the development of non-classical Ang (1–7) and Mas receptors, ACE2 acts the opposite functions to the ACE/Ang II/ATR1 axis (Santos and others [182]; Burns [183])."

"A protective mechanism against renal injury may be reflected by increased ACE2 expression, principally by tipping the scales in favor of vasoprotective Ang (1–7) from Ang II."

"There is mounting evidence that COVID-19 is associated with higher cardiovascular disease morbidity and death (CVD)."

Conclusions

"Compared to female patients with COVID-19, male patients had a much higher chance of dying."

"The risk of death linked with COVID-19 may be greatly decreased by implementing proper protection and interventions for COVID-19 patients in general, and in particular male patients with age 50 years who have comorbidities."

"There are a number of potential therapeutic strategies that can cure pregnancy difficulties brought on by COVID-19 infections and inhibit the binding of ACE2 and SARS-CoV-2 by employing recombinant ACE2 or by blocking the viral S-protein RBD (AzinheiraNobrega Cruz and others [184])."

"Pregnant women were more likely to seek hospitalization among reproductive women (15–44 years old) who tested positive for COVID-19 than nonpregnant women."

"The fact that older people are at higher risk of contracting COVID-19 infection may be related to their deteriorating immune systems, T-cell control, and declining CD4 counts (Liu and others [185])."

Bibliography

1. Marshall TG, Lee RE, Marshall FE (2006) Common angiotensin receptor blockers may directly modulate the immune system via VDR, PPAR and CCR2b. Theor Biol Med Model 3:1
2. Kostis WJ, Shetty M, Chowdhury YS, Kostis JB (2017) ACE inhibitor-induced angioedema: a review. Curr Hypertens Rep 20:1–7. https://doi.org/10.1007/s11906-018-0859-x
3. Hargreaves KM, Roszkowski MT, Swift JQ (1993) Bradykinin and inflammatory pain. Agents Actions 41:65–73
4. Byrd JB, Ram CVS, Lerma EV (2019) Pharmacologic treatment of hypertension, 4th edn. Elsevier Inc. https://doi.org/10.1016/B978-0-323-47871-7.00078-2
5. Ferrario CM, Jessup J, Chappell MC, Averill DB, Brosnihan KB, Tallant EA, Diz DI, Gallagher PE (2005) Effect of angiotensin-converting enzyme inhibition and angiotensin II receptor blockers on cardiac angiotensin-converting enzyme 2. Circulation 111:2605–2610. https://doi.org/10.1161/CIRCULATIONAHA.104.510461
6. Villalobos LA, Hipólito-Luengo ÁS, Ramos González M, Cercas E, Vallejo S, Romero A, Romacho T, Carraro R, Sánchez-Ferrer CF, Peiró C (2016) The angiotensin-(1-7)/mas axis counteracts angiotensin II-dependent and -independent pro-inflammatory signaling in human vascular smooth muscle cells. Front Pharmacol 7:1–10. https://doi.org/10.3389/fphar.2016.00482
7. Starr TN, Zepeda SK, Walls AC, Greaney AJ, Alkhovsky S, Veesler D, Bloom JD (2022) ACE2 binding is an ancestral and evolvable trait of sarbecoviruses. Nature 603:913–918. https://doi.org/10.1038/s41586-022-04464-z
8. Felkle D, Jarczyński M, Kaleta K, Zięba K, Nazimek K (2022) The immunomodulatory effects of antihypertensive therapy: a review. Biomed Pharmacother 153:113287
9. Higaki A, Caillon A, Paradis P et al (2019) Innate and innate-like immune system in hypertension and vascular injury. Curr Hypertens Rep 21:4
10. de Vries AAF (2020) Renin-angiotensin system inhibition in COVID-19 patients. Neth Heart J 28:396–405. https://doi.org/10.1007/s12471-020-01439-5
11. Beyerstedt S, Casaro EB, Rangel ÉB (2021) COVID-19: angiotensin-converting enzyme 2 (ACE2) expression and tissue susceptibility to SARS-CoV-2 infection. Eur J Clin Microbiol Infect Dis 40(5):905–919. https://doi.org/10.1007/s10096-020-04138-6
12. Wrapp D, Wang N, Corbett KS, Goldsmith JA, Hsieh C-L, Abiona O, Graham BS, McLellan JS (2020) Cryo-EM structure of the 2019-nCoV spike in the prefusion conformation. Science 367:1260
13. Tai W, He L, Zhang X, Pu J, Voronin D, Jiang S, Zhou Y, Du L (2020) Characterization of the receptor-binding domain (RBD) of 2019 novel coronavirus: implication for development of RBD protein as a viral attachment inhibitor and vaccine. Cell Mol Immunol 17:613–620

14. Silhol F, Sarlon G, Deharo JC, Vaïsse B (2020) Downregulation of ACE2 induces overstimulation of the renin–angiotensin system in COVID-19: should we block the renin–angiotensin system? Hypertens Res 43:854–856
15. Murray E, Tomaszewski M, Guzik TJ (2020) Binding of SARS-CoV-2 and angiotensin-converting enzyme 2: clinical implications. Cardiovasc Res 116:e87–e89
16. Tipnis SR, Hooper NM, Hyde R, Karran E, Christie G, Turner AJ (2000) A human homolog of angiotensin-converting enzyme. J Biol Chem 275:33238–33243
17. Zou X, Chen K, Zou J, Han P, Hao J, Han Z (2020) Single-cell RNA-seq data analysis on the receptor ACE2 expression reveals the potential risk of different human organs vulnerable to 2019-nCoV infection. Front Med 14:185–192
18. Saheb Sharif-Askari N, Saheb Sharif-Askari F, Alabed M, Temsah M-H, Al Heialy S, Hamid Q, Halwani R (2020) Airways expression of SARS-CoV-2 receptor, ACE2, and TMPRSS2 is lower in children than adults and increases with smoking and COPD. Mol Thera Methods Clin Dev 18:1–6
19. Xu H, Zhong L, Deng J, Peng J, Dan H, Zeng X, Li T, Chen Q (2020) High expression of ACE2 receptor of 2019-nCoV on the epithelial cells of oral mucosa. Int J Oral Sci 12:8
20. Amirian ES (2020) Potential fecal transmission of SARS-CoV-2: current evidence and implications for public health. Int J Infect Dis 95:363–370
21. Bradding P, Richardson M, Hinks TSC, Howarth PH, Choy DF, Arron JR, Wenzel SE, Siddiqui S (2020) ACE2, TMPRSS2, and furin gene expression in the airways of people with asthma-implications for COVID-19. J Allergy Clin Immunol 146:208–211
22. Mizuiri S, Ohashi Y (2015) ACE and ACE2 in kidney disease. World J Nephrol 4:74–82
23. Pan XW, Xu D, Zhang H, Zhou W, Wang LH, Cui XG (2020) Identification of a potential mechanism of acute kidney injury during the COVID-19 outbreak: a study based on single-cell transcriptome analysis. Intensive Care Med 46:1114–1116
24. Higham A, Singh D (2020) Increased ACE2 expression in the bronchial epithelium of COPD patients who are overweight. Obesity 28:1586–1589
25. Shi R, Shan C, Duan X, Chen Z, Liu P, Song J, Song T, Bi X, Han C, Wu L, Gao G, Hu X, Zhang Y, Tong Z, Huang W, Liu WJ, Wu G, Zhang B, Wang L, Qi J, Feng H, Wang F, Wang Q, Gao GF, Yuan Z, Yan J (2020) A human neutralizing antibody targets the receptor binding site of SARS-CoV-2. Nature 584:120–124
26. Zost SJ, Gilchuk P, Case JB, Binshtein E, Chen RE, Nkolola JP, Schäfer A, Reidy JX, Trivette A, Nargi RS, Sutton RE, Suryadevara N, Martinez DR, Williamson LE, Chen EC, Jones T, Day S, Myers L, Hassan AO, Kafai NM, Winkler ES, Fox JM, Shrihari S, Mueller BK, Meiler J, Chandrashekar A, Mercado NB, Steinhardt JJ, Ren K, Loo YM, Kallewaard NL, McCune BT, Keeler SP, Holtzman MJ, Barouch DH, Gralinski LE, Baric RS, Thackray LB, Diamond MS, Carnahan RH, Crowe JE Jr (2020) Potently neutralizing and protective human antibodies against SARS-CoV-2. Nature 584(7821):443–449
27. Li W, Chen C, Drelich A, Martinez DR, Gralinski LE, Sun Z, Schäfer A, Kulkarni SS, Liu X, Leist SR, Zhelev DV, Zhang L, Kim YJ, Peterson EC, Conard A, Mellors JW, Tseng CK, Falzarano D, Baric RS, Dimitrov DS (2020) Rapid identification of a human antibody with high prophylactic and therapeutic efficacy in three animal models of SARS-CoV-2 infection. Proc Natl Acad Sci U S A 117(47):29832–29838. https://doi.org/10.1073/pnas.2010197117
28. Hatami N, Ahi S, Sadeghinikoo A, Foroughian M, Javdani F, Kalani N, Fereydoni M, Keshavarz P, Hosseini A (2020) Worldwide ACE (I/D) polymorphism may affect COVID-19 recovery rate: an ecological meta-regression. Endocrine 68:479–484
29. Mathew J, Basheeruddin K, Prabhakar S (2001) Differences in frequency of the deletion polymorphism of the angiotensin-converting enzyme gene in different ethnic groups. Angiology 52(6):375–379
30. Campos J, Pacheco R (2020) Involvement of dopaminergic signaling in the cross talk between the renin-angiotensin system and inflammation. Semin Immunopathol 42(6):681–696. https://doi.org/10.1007/s00281-020-00819-8

31. Prado C, Bernales S, Pacheco R (2013) Modulation of T-cell mediated immunity by dopamine receptor d5. Endocr Metab Immune Disord Drug Targets 13(2):184–194
32. Prado C, Contreras F, Gonzalez H, Diaz P, Elgueta D, Barrientos M, Herrada AA, Lladser A, Bernales S, Pacheco R (2012) Stimulation of dopamine receptor D5 expressed on dendritic cells potentiates Th17-mediated immunity. J Immunol 188(7):3062–3070. https://doi.org/10.4049/jimmunol.1103096
33. Prado C, Gaiazzi M, Gonzalez H, Ugalde V, Figueroa A, Osorio-Barrios FJ, Lopez E, Lladser A, Rasini E, Marino F, Zaffaroni M, Cosentino M, Pacheco R (2018) Dopaminergic stimulation of myeloid antigen-presenting cells attenuates signal transducer and activator of transcription 3-activation favouring the development of experimental autoimmune encephalomyelitis. Front Immunol 9:571. https://doi.org/10.3389/fimmu.2018.00571
34. Cosentino M, Ferrari M, Kustrimovic N, Rasini E, Marino F (2015) Influence of dopamine receptor gene polymorphisms on circulating T lymphocytes: a pilot study in healthy subjects. Hum Immunol 76(10):747–752. https://doi.org/10.1016/j.humimm.2015.09.032
35. Franz D, Contreras F, Gonzalez H, Prado C, Elgueta D, Figueroa C, Pacheco R (2015) Dopamine receptors D3 and D5 regulate CD4(+)T-cell activation and differentiation by modulating ERK activation and cAMP production. J Neuroimmunol 284:18–29. https://doi.org/10.1016/j.jneuroim.2015.05.003
36. Osorio-Barrios F, Prado C, Contreras F, Pacheco R (2018) Dopamine receptor D5 signaling plays a dual role in experimental autoimmune encephalomyelitis potentiating Th17-mediated immunity and favoring suppressive activity of regulatory T-cells. Front Cell Neurosci 12:192. https://doi.org/10.3389/fncel.2018.00192
37. Papa I, Saliba D, Ponzoni M, Bustamante S, Canete PF, Gonzalez-Figueroa P, McNamara HA, Valvo S, Grimbaldeston M, Sweet RA, Vohra H, Cockburn IA, Meyer-Hermann M, Dustin ML, Doglioni C, Vinuesa CG (2017) TFH-derived dopamine accelerates productive synapses in germinal centres. Nature 547(7663):318–323. https://doi.org/10.1038/nature23013
38. Pacheco R, Prado CE, Barrientos MJ, Bernales S (2009) Role of dopamine in the physiology of T-cells and dendritic cells. J Neuroimmunol 216(1–2):8–19. https://doi.org/10.1016/j.jneuroim.2009.07.018
39. Gonzalez H, Contreras F, Prado C, Elgueta D, Franz D, Bernales S, Pacheco R (2013) Dopamine receptor d3 expressed on cd4+ t cells favors neurodegeneration of dopaminergic neurons during Parkinson's disease. J Immunol 190(10):5048–5056. https://doi.org/10.4049/jimmunol.1203121
40. Contreras F, Prado C, Gonzalez H, Franz D, Osorio-Barrios F, Osorio F, Ugalde V, Lopez E, Elgueta D, Figueroa A, Lladser A, Pacheco R (2016) Dopamine receptor D3 signaling on $CD4^+$ T cells favors Th1- and Th17-mediated immunity. J Immunol 196(10):4143–4149. https://doi.org/10.4049/jimmunol.1502420
41. Cosentino M, Fietta AM, Ferrari M, Rasini E, Bombelli R, Carcano E, Saporiti F, Meloni F, Marino F, Lecchini S (2007) Human $CD4^+$ $CD25^+$ regulatory T cells selectively express tyrosine hydroxylase and contain endogenous catecholamines subserving an autocrine/paracrine inhibitory functional loop. Blood 109(2):632–642
42. Wang W, Cohen JA, Wallrapp A, Trieu KG, Barrios J, Shao F, Krishnamoorthy N, Kuchroo VK, Jones MR, Fine A, Bai Y, Ai X (2019) Age-related dopaminergic innervation augments T helper 2-type allergic inflammation in the postnatal lung. Immunity 51(6):1102–1118. e1107. https://doi.org/10.1016/j.immuni.2019.10.002
43. Figueroa C, Gálvez-Cancino F, Oyarce C, Contreras F, Prado C, Valeria C, Cruz S, Lladser A, Pacheco R (2017) Inhibition of dopamine receptor D3 signaling in dendritic cells increases antigen cross-presentation to $CD8^+$ T-cells favoring anti-tumor immunity. J Neuroimmunol 303:99–107. https://doi.org/10.1016/j.jneuroim.2016.12.014
44. Torres-Rosas R, Yehia G, Pena G, Mishra P, del Rocio T-BM, Moreno-Eutimio MA, Arriaga-Pizano LA, Isibasi A, Ulloa L (2014) Dopamine mediates vagal modulation of the immune system by electroacupuncture. Nat Med 20(3):291–295. https://doi.org/10.1038/nm.3479

45. Yan Y, Jiang W, Liu L, Wang X, Ding C, Tian Z, Zhou R (2015) Dopamine controls systemic inflammation through inhibition of NLRP3 inflammasome. Cell 160(1–2):62–73. https://doi.org/10.1016/j.cell.2014.11.047
46. Pinoli M, Marino F, Cosentino M (2017) Dopaminergic regulation of innate immunity: a review. J Neuroimmune Pharm 12(4):602–623. https://doi.org/10.1007/s11481-017-9749-2
47. Beaulieu JM, Gainetdinov RR (2011) The physiology, signaling, and pharmacology of dopamine receptors. Pharmacol Rev 63(1):182–217. https://doi.org/10.1124/pr.110.002642
48. Matsuyama T, Ohashi N, Ishigaki S, Isobe S, Tsuji N, Fujikura T, Tsuji T, Kato A, Miyajima H, Yasuda H (2018) The relationship between the intrarenal dopamine system and intrarenal renin-angiotensin system depending on the renal function. Intern Med 57(22):3241–3247. https://doi.org/10.2169/internalmedicine.0994-18
49. Rukavina Mikusic NL, Kouyoumdzian NM, Uceda A, Del Mauro JS, Pandolfo M, Gironacci MM, Puyo AM, Toblli JE, Fernandez BE, Choi MR (2018) Losartan prevents the imbalance between renal dopaminergic and renin angiotensin systems induced by fructose overload. l-Dopa/dopamine index as new potential biomarker of renal dysfunction. Metabolism 85:271–285. https://doi.org/10.1016/j.metabol.2018.04.010
50. Shao W, Zhang SZ, Tang M, Zhang XH, Zhou Z, Yin YQ, Zhou QB, Huang YY, Liu YJ, Wawrousek E, Chen T, Li SB, Xu M, Zhou JN, Hu G, Zhou JW (2013) Suppression of neuroinflammation by astrocytic dopamine D2 receptors via alphaB-crystallin. Nature 494(7435):90–94. https://doi.org/10.1038/nature11748
51. Kawajiri M, Mogi M, Higaki N, Matsuoka T, Ohyagi Y, Tsukuda K, Kohara K, Horiuchi M, Miki T, Kira JI (2009) Angiotensin-converting enzyme (ACE) and ACE2 levels in the cerebrospinal fluid of patients with multiple sclerosis. Mult Scler 15(2):262–265. https://doi.org/10.1177/1352458508097923
52. Platten M, Youssef S, Hur EM, Ho PP, Han MH, Lanz TV, Phillips LK, Goldstein MJ, Bhat R, Raine CS, Sobel RA, Steinman L (2009) Blocking angiotensin-converting enzyme induces potent regulatory T cells and modulates TH1- and TH17-mediated autoimmunity. Proc Natl Acad Sci U S A 106(35):14948–14953. https://doi.org/10.1073/pnas.0903958106
53. Pacheco R (2019) Cross-talk between T-cells and gut-microbiota in neurodegenerative disorders. Neural Regen Res 14(12):2091–2092. https://doi.org/10.4103/1673-5374.262582
54. Asano Y, Hiramoto T, Nishino R, Aiba Y, Kimura T, Yoshihara K, Koga Y, Sudo N (2012) Critical role of gut microbiota in the production of biologically active, free catecholamines in the gut lumen of mice. Am J Physiol Gastrointest Liver Physiol 303(11):G1288–G1295. https://doi.org/10.1152/ajpgi.00341.2012
55. Diaz Heijtz R, Wang S, Anuar F, Qian Y, Bjorkholm B, Samuelsson A, Hibberd ML, Forssberg H, Pettersson S (2011) Normal gut microbiota modulates brain development and behavior. Proc Natl Acad Sci U S A 108(7):3047–3052. https://doi.org/10.1073/pnas.1010529108
56. Smart L, Fawkes N, Goggin P, Pennick G, Rainsford KD, Charlesworth B, Shah N (2020) A narrative review of the potential pharmacological influence and safety of ibuprofen on coronavirus disease 19 (COVID-19), ACE2, and the immune system: a dichotomy of expectation and reality. Inflammopharmacology 28(5):1141–1152. https://doi.org/10.1007/s10787-020-00745-z
57. Rokni M, Ghasemi V, Tavakoli Z (2020) Immune responses and pathogenesis of SARS-CoV-2 during an outbreak in Iran: comparison with SARS and MERS. Rev Med Virol 30:e2107. https://doi.org/10.1002/rmv.2107
58. Wu C et al (2020) Risk factors associated with acute respiratory distress syndrome and death in patients with coronavirus disease 2019 pneumonia in Wuhan, China. JAMA Intern Med 180(7):934–943. https://doi.org/10.1001/jamainternmed.2020.0994
59. Liu Y et al (2020) Clinical and biochemical indexes from 2019-nCoV infected patients linked to viral loads and lung injury. Sci China Life Sci 63:364–374. https://doi.org/10.1007/s11427-020-1643-8

60. Rinott E, Kozer E, Shapira Y, Bar-Haim A, Youngster I (2020) Ibuprofen use and clinical outcomes in COVID-19 patients. Clin Microbiol Infect 26(9):1259.e5–1259.e7. https://doi.org/10.1016/j.cmi.2020.06.003
61. Imam Z et al (2020) Older age and comorbidity are independent mortality predictors in a large cohort of 1305 COVID-19 patients in Michigan, United States. J Intern Med 288(4):469–476. https://doi.org/10.1111/joim.13119
62. Gianfrancesco M et al (2020) Characteristics associated with hospitalisation for COVID-19 in people with rheumatic disease: data from the COVID-19 global rheumatology Alliance physician-reported registry. Ann Rheum Dis 79:859. https://doi.org/10.1136/annrheumdis-2020-217871
63. Chen Y, Huang D, Yuan W, Chang J, Yuan Z, Wu D, Han M, Luo X, Ning Q, Yan W (2021) Lower serum angiotensin-converting enzyme level in relation to hyperinflammation and impaired antiviral immune response contributes to progression of COVID-19 infection. Infect Dis Ther 10(4):2431–2446. https://doi.org/10.1007/s40121-021-00513-8
64. Gaddam RR, Chambers S, Bhatia M (2014) ACE and ACE2 in inflammation: a tale of two enzymes. Inflamm Allergy Drug Targets 13:224–234
65. Danilczyk U, Eriksson U, Oudit GY, Penninger JM (2004) Physiological roles of angiotensin-converting enzyme 2. Cell Mol Life Sci 61:2714–2719
66. Wang Q, Zhang Y, Wu L et al (2020) Structural and functional basis of SARS-CoV-2 entry by using human ACE2. Cell 181:894–904
67. Zhu Z, Cai T, Fan L et al (2020) The potential role of serum angiotensin-converting enzyme in coronavirus disease 2019. BMC Infect Dis 20:883
68. Chen G, Wu D, Guo W et al (2020) Clinical and immunological features of severe and moderate coronavirus disease 2019. J Clin Invest 130:2620–2629
69. Tay MZ, Poh CM, Renia L, MacAry PA, Ng LFP (2020) The trinity of COVID-19: immunity, inflammation and intervention. Nat Rev Immunol 20(6):363–374. https://doi.org/10.1038/s41577-020-0311-8
70. Bermejo-Martin JF, Almansa R, Menéndez R, Mendez R, Kelvin DJ, Torres A (2020) Lymphopenic community acquired pneumonia as signature of severe COVID-19 infection. J Infect 80:e23–e24
71. Iwasaki M, Saito J, Zhao H, Sakamoto A, Hirota K, Ma D (2021) Inflammation triggered by SARS-CoV-2 and ACE2 augment drives multiple organ failure of severe COVID-19: molecular mechanisms and implications. Inflammation 44(1):13–34. https://doi.org/10.1007/s10753-020-01337-3
72. Wu Z, McGoogan JM (2020) Characteristics of and important lessons from the coronavirus disease 2019 (COVID-19) outbreak in China: summary of a report of 72314 cases from the Chinese Center for Disease Control and Prevention. JAMA 323(13):1239–1242. https://doi.org/10.1001/jama.2020.2648
73. Sama IE, Ravera A, Santema BT, van Goor H, Ter Maaten JM, Cleland JGF et al (2020) Circulating plasma concentrations of angiotensin-converting enzyme 2 in men and women with heart failure and effects of renin-angiotensin-aldosterone inhibitors. Eur Heart J 41(19):1810–1817
74. Fyhrquist F, Saijonmaa O (2008) Renin-angiotensin system revisited. J Intern Med 264(3):224–236. https://doi.org/10.1111/j.1365-2796.2008.01981.x
75. Terenzi R, Manetti M, Rosa I, Romano E, Galluccio F, Guiducci S, Ibba-Manneschi L, Matucci-Cerinic M (2017) Angiotensin II type 2 receptor (AT2R) as a novel modulator of inflammation in rheumatoid arthritis synovium. Sci Rep 7(1):13293. https://doi.org/10.1038/s41598-017-13746-w
76. Patel VB, Clarke N, Wang Z, Fan D, Parajuli N, Basu R, Putko B, Kassiri Z, Turner AJ, Oudit GY (2014) Angiotensin II induced proteolytic cleavage of myocardial ACE2 is mediated by TACE/ADAM-17: a positive feedback mechanism in the RAS. J Mol Cell Cardiol 66:167–176. https://doi.org/10.1016/j.yjmcc.2013.11.017

77. Hamming I, Timens W, Bulthuis ML, Lely AT, Navis G, van Goor H (2004) Tissue distribution of ACE2 protein, the functional receptor for SARS coronavirus. A first step in understanding SARS pathogenesis. J Pathol 203:631–637. https://doi.org/10.1002/path.1570
78. Rose-John S, Scheller J, Elson G, Jones SA (2006) Interleukin-6 biology is coordinated by membrane-bound and soluble receptors: role in inflammation and cancer. J Leukoc Biol 80(2):227–236. https://doi.org/10.1189/jlb.1105674
79. Naka T, Narazaki M, Hirata M, Matsumoto T, Minamoto S, Aono A, Nishimoto N et al (1997) Structure and function of a new STAT-induced STAT inhibitor. Nature 387(6636):924–929. https://doi.org/10.1038/43219
80. Murakami M, Harada M, Kamimura D, Ogura H, Okuyama Y, Kumai N, Okuyama A et al (2013) Disease-association analysis of an inflammation-related feedback loop. Cell Rep 3(3):946–959. https://doi.org/10.1016/j.celrep.2013.01.028
81. Teijaro JR, Walsh KB, Cahalan S, Fremgen DM, Roberts E, Scott F, Martinborough E, Peach R, Oldstone MB, Rosen H (2011) Endothelial cells are central orchestrators of cytokine amplification during influenza virus infection. Cell 146(6):980–991. https://doi.org/10.1016/j.cell.2011.08.015
82. Li F, Li W, Farzan M, Harrison SC (2005) Structure of SARS coronavirus spike receptor-binding domain complexed with receptor. Science 309(5742):1864–1868. https://doi.org/10.1126/science.1116480
83. Hoffmann M, Kleine-Weber H, Pohlmann S (2020) A multibasic cleavage site in the spike protein of SARS-CoV-2 is essential for infection of human lung cells. Mol Cell 78(4):779–784.e5. https://doi.org/10.1016/j.molcel.2020.04.022
84. Zhou L, Niu Z, Jiang X, Zhang Z, Zheng Y, Wang Z, Zhu Y, Gao L, Wang X, Sun Q (2020) Systemic analysis of tissue cells potentially vulnerable to SARS-CoV-2 infection by the protein-proofed single-cell RNA profiling of ACE2, TMPRSS2 and Furin proteases. bioRxiv. https://doi.org/10.1101/2020.04.06.028522
85. Wu C, Zheng S, Yu C, Zheng M (2020) Single-cell RNA expression profiling of ACE2, the putative receptor of Wuhan 2019-nCoV, in the nasal tissue. medRxiv. https://doi.org/10.1101/2020.02.11.20022228
86. Belouzard S, Chu VC, Whittaker GR (2009) Activation of the SARS coronavirus spike protein via sequential proteolytic cleavage at two distinct sites. Proc Natl Acad Sci U S A 106:5871–5876. https://doi.org/10.1073/pnas.0809524106
87. Millet JK, Whittaker GR (2015) Host cell proteases: critical determinants of coronavirus tropism and pathogenesis. Virus Res 202:120–134. https://doi.org/10.1016/j.virusres.2014.11.021
88. Simmons G, Gosalia DN, Rennekamp AJ, Reeves JD, Diamond SL, Bates P (2005) Inhibitors of cathepsin L prevent severe acute respiratory syndrome coronavirus entry. Proc Natl Acad Sci U S A 102(33):11876–11881. https://doi.org/10.1073/pnas.0505577102
89. Hoffmann M, Kleine-Weber H, Schroeder S, Kruger N, Herrler T, Erichsen S, Schiergens TS, Herrler G, Wu NH, Nitsche A, Muller MA, Drosten C, Pohlmann S (2020) SARS-CoV-2 cell entry depends on ACE2 and TMPRSS2 and is blocked by a clinically proven protease inhibitor. Cell 181:271–280. https://doi.org/10.1016/j.cell.2020.02.052
90. Shi S, Qin M, Shen B, Cai Y, Liu T, Yang F, Gong W et al (2020) Association of cardiac injury with mortality in hospitalized patients with COVID-19 in Wuhan, China. JAMA Cardiol 5(7):802–810. https://doi.org/10.1001/jamacardio.2020.0950
91. Guo T, Fan Y, Chen M, Wu X, Zhang L, He T, Wang H, Wan J, Wang X, Lu Z (2020) Cardiovascular implications of fatal outcomes of patients with coronavirus disease 2019 (COVID-19). JAMA Cardiol 5(7):811–818. https://doi.org/10.1001/jamacardio.2020.1017
92. Chen T, Wu D, Chen H, Yan W, Yang D, Chen G, Ma K et al (2020) Clinical characteristics of 113 deceased patients with coronavirus disease 2019: retrospective study. BMJ 368(m):1091. https://doi.org/10.1136/bmj.m1091
93. Huang C, Wang Y, Li X, Ren L, Zhao J, Hu Y, Zhang L, Fan G, Xu J, Gu X, Cheng Z, Yu T, Xia J, Wei Y, Wu W, Xie X, Yin W, Li H, Liu M, Xiao Y, Gao H, Guo L, Xie J, Wang G,

Jiang R, Gao Z, Jin Q, Wang J, Cao B (2020) Clinical features of patients infected with 2019 novel coronavirus in Wuhan, China. Lancet 395:497–506. https://doi.org/10.1016/s0140-6736(20)30183-5
94. Zhou F, Yu T, Du R, Fan G, Liu Y, Liu Z, Xiang J, Wang Y, Song B, Gu X, Guan L, Wei Y, Li H, Wu X, Xu J, Tu S, Zhang Y, Chen H, Cao B (2020) Clinical course and risk factors for mortality of adult inpatients with COVID-19 in Wuhan, China: a retrospective cohort study. Lancet 395:1054–1062. https://doi.org/10.1016/s0140-6736(20)30566-3
95. Zou X, Li S, Fang M, Hu M, Bian Y, Ling J, Yu S, Jing L, Li D, Huang J (2020) Acute physiology and chronic health evaluation II score as a predictor of hospital mortality in patients of coronavirus disease 2019. Crit Care Med 48(8):e657–e665. https://doi.org/10.1097/CCM.0000000000004411
96. Bernard-Valnet R, Pizzarotti B, Anichini A, Demars Y, Russo E, Schmidhauser M, Cerutti-Sola J, Rossetti AO, Du Pasquier R (2020) Two patients with acute meningoencephalitis concomitant with SARS-CoV-2 infection. Eur J Neurol 27(9):e43–e44. https://doi.org/10.1111/ene.14298
97. Lechien JR, Chiesa-Estomba CM, De Siati DR, Horoi M, Le Bon SD, Rodriguez A, Dequanter D et al (2020) Olfactory and gustatory dysfunctions as a clinical presentation of mild-to-moderate forms of the coronavirus disease (COVID-19): a multicenter European study. Eur Arch Otorrinolaringol 277(8):2251–2261. https://doi.org/10.1007/s00405-020-05965-1
98. Mao L, Jin H, Wang M, Hu Y, Chen S, He Q, Chang J et al (2020) Neurologic manifestations of hospitalized patients with coronavirus disease 2019 in Wuhan, China. JAMA Neurol 77(6):683–690. https://doi.org/10.1001/jamaneurol.2020.1127
99. Moriguchi T, Harii N, Goto J, Harada D, Sugawara H, Takamino J, Ueno M et al (2020) A first case of meningitis/encephalitis associated with SARS-Coronavirus-2. Int J Infect Dis 94:55–58. https://doi.org/10.1016/j.ijid.2020.03.062
100. Poyiadji N, Shahin G, Noujaim D, Stone M, Patel S, Griffith B (2020) COVID-19-associated acute hemorrhagic necrotizing encephalopathy: imaging features. Radiology 296(2):E119–E120. https://doi.org/10.1148/radiol.2020201187
101. Yin R, Feng W, Wang T, Chen G, Wu T, Chen D, Lv T, Xiang D (2020) Concomitant neurological symptoms observed in a patient diagnosed with coronavirus disease 2019. J Med Virol 92(10):1782–1784. https://doi.org/10.1002/jmv.25888
102. Yang X, Yu Y, Xu J, Shu H, Xia J, Liu H, Wu Y et al (2020) Clinical course and outcomes of critically ill patients with SARS-CoV-2 pneumonia in Wuhan, China: a single-centered, retrospective, observational study. Lancet Respir Med 8(5):475–481. https://doi.org/10.1016/S2213-2600(20)30079-5
103. Tang N, Li D, Wang X, Sun Z (2020) Abnormal coagulation parameters are associated with poor prognosis in patients with novel coronavirus pneumonia. J Thromb Haemost 18(4):844–847. https://doi.org/10.1111/jth.14768
104. Cheng Y, Luo R, Wang K, Zhang M, Wang Z, Dong L, Li J, Yao Y, Ge S, Xu G (2020) Kidney disease is associated with in-hospital death of patients with COVID-19. Kidney Int 97(5):829–838. https://doi.org/10.1016/j.kint.2020.03.005
105. Reynolds HR, Adhikari S, Pulgarin C, Troxel AB, Iturrate E, Johnson SB, Hausvater A et al (2020) Renin-angiotensin-aldosterone system inhibitors and risk of Covid-19. N Engl J Med 382(25):2441–2448. https://doi.org/10.1056/NEJMoa2008975
106. Li J, Wang X, Chen J, Zhang H, Deng A (2020) Association of renin-angiotensin system inhibitors with severity or risk of death in patients with hypertension hospitalized for coronavirus disease 2019 (COVID-19) infection in Wuhan, China. JAMA Cardiol 5(7):825–830. https://doi.org/10.1001/jamacardio.2020.1624
107. Tedeschi S, Giannella M, Bartoletti M, Trapani F, Tadolini M, Borghi C, Viale P (2020) Clinical impact of renin-angiotensin system inhibitors on in-hospital mortality of patients with hypertension hospitalized for coronavirus disease 2019. Clin Infect Dis 71(15):899–901. https://doi.org/10.1093/cid/ciaa492

108. Yang G, Tan Z, Zhou L, Yang M, Peng L, Liu J, Cai J et al (2020) Effects of angiotensin II receptor blockers and ACE (angiotensin-converting enzyme) inhibitors on virus infection, inflammatory status, and clinical outcomes in patients with COVID-19 and hypertension: a single-center retrospective study. Hypertension 76(1):51–58. https://doi.org/10.1161/HYPERTENSIONAHA.120.15143
109. Gonzalez-Villalobos RA, Shen XZ, Bernstein EA, Janjulia T, Taylor B, Giani JF, Blackwell WL, Shah KH, Shi PD, Fuchs S, Bernstein KE (2013) Rediscovering ACE: novel insights into the many roles of the angiotensin-converting enzyme. J Mol Med (Berl) 91(10):1143–1154. https://doi.org/10.1007/s00109-013-1051-z
110. Soubrier F, Alhenc-Gelas F, Hubert C et al (1988) Two putative active centers in human angiotensin I-converting enzyme revealed by molecular cloning. Proc Natl Acad Sci U S A 85(24):9386–9390
111. Bernstein KE, Martin BM, Edwards AS, Bernstein EA (1989) Mouse angiotensin-converting enzyme is a protein composed of two homologous domains. J Biol Chem 264:11945–11951
112. Erdos EG, Skidgel RA (1987) The angiotensin I-converting enzyme. Lab Investig 56:345–348
113. Ng KK, Vane JR (1967) Conversion of angiotensin I to angiotensin II. Nature 216(5117):762–766
114. Krege JH, John SW, Langenbach LL, Hodgin JB, Hagaman JR, Bachman ES, Jennette JC, O'Brien DA, Smithies O (1995) Male–female differences in fertility and blood pressure in ACE-deficient mice. Nature 375:146–148. https://doi.org/10.1038/375146a0
115. Esther CR Jr, Howard TE, Marino EM, Goddard JM, Capecchi MR, Bernstein KE (1996) Mice lacking angiotensin-converting enzyme have low blood pressure, renal pathology, and reduced male fertility. Lab Investig 74:953–965
116. Kim HS, Krege JH, Kluckman KD, Hagaman JR, Hodgin JB, Best CF, Jennette JC, Coffman TM, Maeda N, Smithies O (1995) Genetic control of blood pressure and the angiotensinogen locus. Proc Natl Acad Sci U S A 92:2735–2739
117. Takahashi N, Lopez ML, Cowhig JE Jr, Taylor MA, Hatada T, Riggs E, Lee G, Gomez RA, Kim HS, Smithies O (2005) Ren1c homozygous null mice are hypotensive and polyuric, but heterozygotes are indistinguishable from wild-type. J Am Soc Nephrol 16:125–132
118. Friberg P, Sundelin B, Bohman SO, Bobik A, Nilsson H, Wickman A, Gustafsson H, Petersen J, Adams MA (1994) Renin-angiotensin system in neonatal rats: induction of a renal abnormality in response to ACE inhibition or angiotensin II antagonism. Kidney Int 45:485–492
119. Guron G, Adams MA, Sundelin B, Friberg P (1997) Neonatal angiotensin-converting enzyme inhibition in the rat induces persistent abnormalities in renal function and histology. Hypertension 29:91–97
120. Zhu X, Bouzekri N, Southam L, Cooper RS, Adeyemo A, McKenzie CA, Luke A, Chen G, Elston RC, Ward R (2001) Linkage and association analysis of angiotensin I-converting enzyme (ACE)-gene polymorphisms with ACE concentration and blood pressure. Am J Hum Genet 68:1139–1148. https://doi.org/10.1086/320104
121. Levy D, DeStefano AL, Larson MG, O'Donnell CJ, Lifton RP, Gavras H, Cupples LA, Myers RH (2000) Evidence for a gene influencing blood pressure on chromosome 17. Genome scan linkage results for longitudinal blood pressure phenotypes in subjects from the Framingham heart study. Hypertension 36:477–483
122. Agerholm-Larsen B, Nordestgaard BG, Tybjaerg-Hansen A (2000) ACE gene polymorphism in cardiovascular disease: meta-analyses of small and large studies in whites. Arterioscler Thromb Vasc Biol 20:484–492
123. Esther CR, Marino EM, Howard TE, Machaud A, Corvol P, Capecchi MR, Bernstein KE (1997) The critical role of tissue angiotensin-converting enzyme as revealed by gene targeting in mice. J Clin Invest 99:2375–2385. https://doi.org/10.1172/jci119419
124. Cole J, Quach DL, Sundaram K, Corvol P, Capecchi MR, Bernstein KE (2002) Mice lacking endothelial angiotensin-converting enzyme have a normal blood pressure. Circ Res 90:87–92
125. Xiao HD, Fuchs S, Campbell DJ, Lewis W, Dudley SC Jr, Kasi VS, Hoit BD, Keshelava G, Zhao H, Capecchi MR et al (2004) Mice with cardiac-restricted angiotensin-converting

enzyme (ACE) have atrial enlargement, cardiac arrhythmia, and sudden death. Am J Pathol 165:1019–1032. https://doi.org/10.1016/S0002-9440(10)63363-9
126. Shen XZ, Li P, Weiss D, Fuchs S, Xiao HD, Adams JA, Williams IR, Capecchi MR, Taylor WR, Bernstein KE (2007) Mice with enhanced macrophage angiotensin-converting enzyme are resistant to melanoma. Am J Pathol 170:2122–2134
127. Traynor T, Yang T, Huang YG, Krege JH, Briggs JP, Smithies O, Schnermann J (1999) Tubuloglomerular feedback in ACE-deficient mice. Am J Phys 276:F751–F757
128. Hashimoto S, Adams JW, Bernstein KE, Schnermann J (2005) Micropuncture determination of nephron function in mice without tissue angiotensin-converting enzyme. Am J Physiol Renal Physiol 288:F445–F452. https://doi.org/10.1152/ajprenal.00297.2004
129. Imig JD, Navar GL, Zou LX, O'Reilly KC, Allen PL, Kaysen JH, Hammond TG, Navar LG (1999) Renal endosomes contain angiotensin peptides, converting enzyme, and AT(1A) receptors. Am J Phys 277:F303–F311
130. Ingert C, Grima M, Coquard C, Barthelmebs M, Imbs JL (2002) Contribution of angiotensin II internalization to intrarenal angiotensin II levels in rats. Am J Physiol Renal Physiol 283:F1003–F1010
131. Vio CP, Jeanneret VA (2003) Local induction of angiotensin-converting enzyme in the kidney as a mechanism of progressive renal diseases. Kidney Int Suppl 86:S57–S63
132. Fuchs S, Xiao HD, Cole JM, Adams JW, Frenzel K, Michaud A, Zhao H, Keshelava G, Capecchi MR, Corvol P et al (2004) Role of the N-terminal catalytic domain of angiotensin-converting enzyme investigated by targeted inactivation in mice. J Biol Chem 279:15946–15953. https://doi.org/10.1074/jbc.M400149200
133. Fuchs S, Xiao HD, Hubert C et al (2008) Angiotensin-converting enzyme C-terminal catalytic domain is the main site of angiotensin I cleavage in vivo. Hypertension 51(2):267–274
134. Sherman LA, Burke TA, Biggs JA (1992) Extracellular processing of peptide antigens that bind class I major histocompatibility molecules. J Exp Med 175:1221–1226
135. Eisenlohr LC, Bacik I, Bennink JR, Bernstein K, Yewdell JW (1992) Expression of a membrane protease enhances presentation of endogenous antigens to MHC class I-restricted T lymphocytes. Cell 71:963–972
136. Okwan-Duodu D, Datta V, Shen XZ, Goodridge HS, Bernstein EA, Fuchs S, Liu GY, Bernstein KE (2010) Angiotensin-converting enzyme overexpression in mouse myelomonocytic cells augments resistance to Listeria and methicillin-resistant Staphylococcus aureus. J Biol Chem 285:39051–39060. https://doi.org/10.1074/jbc.M110.163782
137. Swanson PA 2nd, Lukacher AE, Szomolanyi-Tsuda E (2009) Immunity to polyomavirus infection: the polyomavirus-mouse model. Semin Cancer Biol 19:244–251. https://doi.org/10.1016/j.semcancer.2009.02.003
138. Dive V, Georgiadis D, Matziari M, Makaritis A, Beau F, Cuniasse P, Yiotakis A (2004) Phosphinic peptides as zinc metalloproteinase inhibitors. Cell Mol Life Sci 61:2010–2019. https://doi.org/10.1007/s00018-004-4050-y
139. Redelinghuys P, Nchinda AT, Sturrock ED (2005) Development of domain-selective angiotensin I-converting enzyme inhibitors. Ann N Y Acad Sci 1056:160–175. https://doi.org/10.1196/annals.1352.035
140. Saha S, Chakrabarti S, Singh PK, Poddar J, Satapathi S, Saini S, Kakar SS, Roy P (2021) Physiological relevance of angiotensin converting enzyme 2 as a metabolic linker and therapeutic implication of mesenchymal stem cells in COVID-19 and hypertension. Stem Cell Rev Rep 17(1):132–143. https://doi.org/10.1007/s12015-020-10012-x
141. Lu R, Zhao X, Li J, Niu P, Yang B, Wu H, Wang W, Song H, Huang B, Zhu N, Bi Y (2020) Genomic characterisation and epidemiology of 2019 novel coronavirus: implications for virus origins and receptor binding. Lancet 395(10224):565–574
142. Lambert DW, Clarke NE, Hooper NM, Turner AJ (2008) Calmodulin interacts with angiotensin-converting enzyme-2 (ACE2) and inhibits shedding of its ectodomain. FEBS Lett 582(2):385–390

143. Batlle D, Wysocki J, Satchell K (2020) Soluble angiotensin-converting enzyme 2: a potential approach for coronavirus infection therapy? Clin Sci (Lond) 134:543–545. https://doi.org/10.1042/CS20200163
144. Tikellis C, Thomas MC (2012) Angiotensin-converting enzyme 2 (ACE2) is a key modulator of the renin angiotensin system in health and disease. Int J Pept 2012:256294. https://doi.org/10.1155/2012/256294
145. Guan WJ, Ni ZY, Hu Y, Liang WH, Ou CQ, He JX et al (2020) Clinical characteristics of coronavirus disease 2019 in China. N Engl J Med 382(18):1708–1720
146. Zhang JJ, Dong X, Cao YY, Yuan YD, Yang YB, Yan YQ, Akdis CA, Gao YD (2020) Clinical characteristics of 140 patients infected with SARS-CoV-2 in Wuhan, China. Allergy 75(7):1730–1741
147. Bhandari S, Bhargava A, Sharma S, Keshwani P, Sharma R, Banerjee S (2020) Clinical profile of covid-19 infected patients admitted in a tertiary care hospital in North India. J Assoc Physicians India 68:13–17
148. Co COC, Yu JRT, Laxamana LC, David-Ona DIA (2020) Intravenous thrombolysis for stroke in a COVID-19 positive Filipino patient, a case report. J Clin Neurosci 77:234–236
149. Avula A, Nalleballe K, Narula N, Sapozhnikov S, Dandu V, Toom S, Glaser A, Elsayegh D (2020) COVID-19 presenting as stroke. Brain Behav Immun 87:115–119
150. Abdulkadir TUNÇ, Ünlübaş Y, Alemdar M, Akyüz E (2020) Coexistence of COVID-19 and acute ischemic stroke report of four cases. J Clin Neurosci 77:227–229
151. Liu W, Li H (2020) COVID-19: attacks the 1-beta chain of hemoglobin and captures the porphyrin to inhibit human heme metabolism. ChemRxiv. https://doi.org/10.26434/chemrxiv.11938173.v7
152. Badawi A, Ryoo SG (2016) Prevalence of comorbidities in the Middle East respiratory syndrome coronavirus (MERS-CoV): a systematic review and meta-analysis. Int J Infect Dis 49:129–133
153. Kulcsar KA, Coleman CM, Beck SE, Frieman MB (2019) Comorbid diabetes results in immune dysregulation and enhanced disease severity following MERS-CoV infection. JCI Insight 4(20):e13774
154. Yang JK, Feng Y, Yuan MY, Yuan SY, Fu HJ, Wu BY, Sun GZ, Yang GR, Zhang XL, Wang L, Xu X (2006) Plasma glucose levels and diabetes are independent predictors for mortality and morbidity in patients with SARS. Diabet Med 23(6):623–628
155. Iyer SN, Yamada K, Diz DI, Ferrario CM, Chappell MC (2000) Evidence that prostaglandins mediate the antihypertensive actions of angiotensin-(1–7) during chronic blockade of the renin-angiotensin system. J Cardiovasc Pharmacol 36(1):109–117
156. Li P, Chappell MC, Ferrario CM, Brosnihan KB (1997) Angiotensin-(1–7) augments bradykinin-induced vasodilation by competing with ACE and releasing nitric oxide. Hypertension 29(1):394–398
157. Ferrario CM, Trask AJ, Jessup JA (2005) Advances in biochemical and functional roles of angiotensin-converting enzyme 2 and angiotensin-(1–7) in regulation of cardiovascular function. Am J Phys Heart Circ Phys 289(6):H2281–H2290
158. Kadam RU, Wilson IA (2017) Structural basis of influenza virus fusion inhibition by the antiviral drug arbidol. Proc Natl Acad Sci U S A 114(2):206–214
159. Khamitov RA, Loginova S, Shchukina VN, Borisevich SV, Maksimov VA, Shuster AM (2008) Antiviral activity of arbidol and its derivatives against the pathogen of severe acute respiratory syndrome in the cell cultures. Vopr Virusol 53(4):9–13
160. Wu C, Liu Y, Yang Y, Zhang P, Zhong W, Wang Y, Wang Q, Xu Y, Li M, Li X, Zheng M (2020) Analysis of therapeutic targets for SARS-CoV-2 and discovery of potential drugs by computational methods. Acta Pharm Sin B 10(5):766–788
161. Liang B, Chen J, Li T, Wu H, Yang W, Li Y, Li J, Yu C, Nie F, Ma Z, Yang M (2020) Clinical remission of a critically ill COVID-19 patient treated by human umbilical cord mesenchymal stem cells. Medicine (Baltimore) 99(31):e21429. https://doi.org/10.1097/MD.0000000000021429

162. Gao F, Chiu SM, Motan DAL, Zhang Z, Chen L, Ji HL, Tse HF, Fu QL, Lian Q (2016) Mesenchymal stem cells and immunomodulation: current status and future prospects. Cell Death Dis 7(1):e2062–e2062
163. Sotiropoulou PA, Perez SA, Gritzapis AD, Baxevanis CN, Papamichail M (2006) Interactions between human mesenchymal stem cells and natural killer cells. Stem Cells 24(1):74–85
164. Chrzanowski W, Kim SY, McClements L (2020) Can stem cells beat COVID-19: advancing stem cells and extracellular vesicles toward mainstream medicine for lung injuries associated with SARS-CoV-2 infections. Front Bioeng Biotechnol 8:554–561
165. Qiu Y, Tao L, Zheng S, Lin R, Fu X, Chen Z, Lei C, Wang J, Li H, Li Q, Lei B (2016) AAV8-mediated angiotensin-converting enzyme 2 gene delivery prevents experimental autoimmune uveitis by regulating MAPK, NF-κB and STAT3 pathways. Sci Rep 6:31912. https://doi.org/10.1038/srep31912
166. Simoes e Silva AC, Silveira KD, Ferreira AJ, Teixeira MM (2013) ACE2, angiotensin-(1–7) and Mas receptor axis in inflammation and fibrosis. Br J Pharmacol 169:477–492
167. Passos-Silva DG, Verano-Braga T, Santos RA (2013) Angiotensin-(1–7): beyond the cardio-renal actions. Clin Sci (Lond) 124:443–456
168. Yousif MH, Makki B, El-Hashim AZ, Akhtar S, Benter IF (2014) Chronic treatment with Ang-(1–7) reverses abnormal reactivity in the corpus cavernosum and normalizes diabetes-induced changes in the protein levels of ACE, ACE2, ROCK1, ROCK2 and omega-hydroxylase in a rat model of type 1 diabetes. J Diabetes Res 2014:142154
169. Sukumaran V et al (2011) Cardioprotective effects of telmisartan against heart failure in rats induced by experimental autoimmune myocarditis through the modulation of angiotensin-converting enzyme-2/angiotensin 1–7/mas receptor axis. Int J Biol Sci 7:1077–1092
170. da Silveira KD et al (2010) Anti-inflammatory effects of the activation of the angiotensin-(1–7) receptor, MAS, in experimental models of arthritis. J Immunol 185:5569–5576
171. Shil PK et al (2014) Oral delivery of ACE2/Ang-(1–7) bioencapsulated in plant cells protects against experimental uveitis and autoimmune uveoretinitis. Mol Ther 22:2069–2082
172. Souza LL, Costa-Neto CM (2012) Angiotensin-(1–7) decreases LPS-induced inflammatory response in macrophages. J Cell Physiol 227:2117–2122
173. Santra D, Banerjee A, De SK, Thatoi H, Maiti S (2023) Relation of ACE2 with co-morbidity factors in SARS-CoV-2 pathogenicity. Comp Clin Path 32(2):179–189. https://doi.org/10.1007/s00580-023-03434-9
174. Oudit GY, Kassiri Z, Jiang C, Liu PP, Poutanen SM, Penninger JM, Butany J (2009) SARS-coronavirus modulation of myocardial ACE2 expression and inflammation in patients with SARS. Eur J Clin Investig 39(7):618–625. https://doi.org/10.1111/j.1365-2362.2009.02153.x
175. Aksoy H, Karadag AS, Wollina U (2020) Angiotensin II receptors: impact for COVID-19 severity. Dermatol Ther 33(6):e13989. https://doi.org/10.1111/dth.13989. PMID: 32645228; PMCID: PMC7361069
176. Wysocki J, Garcia-Halpin L, Ye M, Maier C, Sowers K, Burns KD, Batlle D (2013) Regulation of urinary ACE2 in diabetic mice. Am J Physiol Renal Physiol 305(4):F600–F611. https://doi.org/10.1152/ajprenal.00600.2012. PMID:23761674; PMCID: PMC3891267
177. South AM, Shaltout HA, Washburn LK, Hendricks AS et al (2019) Fetal programming and the angiotensin-(1-7) axis: a review of the experimental and clinical data. Clin Sci 133:55–74. https://doi.org/10.1042/CS20171550
178. Masi S, Uliana M, Virdis A (2019) Angiotensin II and vascular damage in hypertension: role of oxidative stress and sympathetic activation. Vasc Pharmacol 115:13–17. https://doi.org/10.1016/j.vph.2019.01.004. PMID: 30707954
179. Fang L, Karakiulakis G, Roth M (2020) Are patients with hypertension and diabetes mellitus at increased risk for COVID-19 infection? Lancet Respir Med 8:e21. https://doi.org/10.1016/S2213-2600(20)30116-8
180. Ye M, Wysocki J, William J, Soler MJ, Cokic I, Batlle D (2006) Glomerular localization and expression of angiotensin-converting enzyme 2 and angiotensin-converting enzyme:

implications for albuminuria in diabetes. J Am Soc Nephrol 17(11):3067–3075. https://doi.org/10.1681/ASN.2006050423. PMID: 17021266

181. Pal R, Bhansali A (2020) COVID-19, diabetes mellitus and ACE2: the conundrum. Diabetes Res Clin Pract 162:108132. https://doi.org/10.1016/j.diabres.2020.108132. PMID: 32234504; PMCID: PMC7118535
182. Santos RA, Ferreira AJ, Verano-Braga T, Bader M (2013) Angiotensin-converting enzyme 2, angiotensin-(1–7) and Mas: new players of the renin–angiotensin system. J Endocrinol 216(2):R1–R17
183. Burns KD (2007) The emerging role of angiotensin-converting enzyme-2 in the kidney. Curr Opin Nephrol Hypertens 16(2):116–121. https://doi.org/10.1097/MNH.0b013e3280123c0e. PMID: 17293686
184. Azinheira Nobrega Cruz N, Stoll D, Casarini DE, Bertagnolli M (2021) Role of ACE2 in pregnancy and potential implications for COVID-19 susceptibility. Clin Sci (Lond) 135(15):1805–1824. https://doi.org/10.1042/CS20210284. PMID: 34338772; PMCID: PMC8329853
185. Liu PP, Blet A, Smyth D, Li H (2020) The science underlying COVID-19: implications for the cardiovascular system. Circulation 142(1):68–78. https://doi.org/10.1161/CIRCULATIONAHA.120.047549

Chapter 8
Role of ACE Inhibitors and Angiotensin Receptor Blockers in Peripheral Artery Disease

Mukesh Nandave

Introduction by the Editor

Peripheral artery disease (PAD) is a type of atherosclerotic vascular disease. PAD is increasing day by day and it increases the risk of cardiovascular disease and associated mortality. There is three to six times more chances of patient death with lower proximity PAD by cardiovascular event than those without PAD. However, PAD is frequently unnoticed and underdiagnosed despite its high prevalence. Most of the people are not aware of the symptoms or signs of PAD including critical limb ischemia, difficulty in walking, intermittent claudication. There is insufficient information regarding PAD associated cardiovascular events. Physical examination and medical history are the initial steps in the diagnosis of PAD. In a healthy individual, systolic blood pressure rises as it move down the arterial circulation thus it is higher lower limb comparison to upper limb. However, when there is a blockage in arteries systolic blood pressure downstream of blockage decreases which is directly proportional to severity of blockage. This principle is used in the PAD diagnosis, systolic pressure at ankle arteries is compared to brachial artery called ankle-brachial index (ABI). If the ABI value is above 1.40 then it is defined as reduced arterial flexibility and cannot be used in PAD diagnosis. In such cases toe-brachial index (TBI) is used, in which systolic pressure at first toe is compared to systolic pressure at brachial pressure. American Heart Association/American College of Cardiology (AHA/ACC) recommended resting ABI as primary method for diagnosis and management of PAD [1].

However, other medical conditions such as osteoarthritis, spinal stenosis, neuropathy have leg symptoms like PAD. These conditions mimics or co-exist with PAD. Therefore, diagnosis of PAD is a complex process [2].

M. Nandave (✉)
Department of Pharmacology, Delhi Pharmaceutical Sciences and Research University, New Delhi, Delhi, India

M. Nandave (ed.), *Angiotensin-converting Enzyme Inhibitors vs. Angiotensin Receptor Blockers*, https://doi.org/10.1007/978-981-97-7380-0_8

Hypertension is one of the key risk factor for the initiation of PAD. PAD signifies the progression of atherosclerosis which resulted from endothelial dysfunction. Several studies reported the significant function of Renin–angiotensin–aldosterone system (RAAS) in the development and progression of endothelial dysfunctional subsequently resulting in initiation of PAD. Angiotensin converting enzyme (ACE) inhibitors and angiotensin receptor blockers (ARBs) were found to improve endothelial function. ACE inhibitors were found to improve endothelial function by inhibiting the formation of angiotensin II as well as inhibition of kininase II resulting in increased level of endothelium dependent bradykinin. By inhibiting RAAS, ARBs and ACE inhibitors reduce the microalbuminuria which is a prominent marker for endothelial dysfunction. ACE inhibitors have been evaluated for the treatment of PAD in hypertensive patients with indications that these have better efficacy in PAD than any other anti-hypertensive agents. A HOPE trial (Heart Outcomes Prevention Analysis) compared the efficacy of ramipril with placebo cardiovascular disease patients but without heart failure which is characterized by reduced ejection fraction. This study involved 3099 PAD patients, subsequent analysis revealed that ramipril reduced the primary outcome of cardiovascular mortality, stroke, myocardial infarction in PAD patients similar to the patients without peripheral vascular disease [3]. The ONTARGET trial (Ongoing Telmisartan Alone and in Combination with Ramipril Global End Point Trial), this trial involves the comparison between telmisartan and ramipril or combination of ARBs and ACE inhibitors. However, there is no reduction in cardiovascular event related mortality, stroke or myocardial infarction cases was observed. Additionally, a greater number of adverse events were observed in the combination group [4]. Several other studies reported that ACE inhibitors and ARBs have shown decreased mortality rate in comparison to other anti-hypertensive agents. Therefore, European Society of Cardiology and AHA/ACC have recommended the ACE inhibitors and ARBs as a class II option in the treatment of PAD [5, 6]. The pre-specified subgroup analysis and post-hoc sub analysis of VALUE (Valsartan Antihypertensive Long-Term Use Evaluation) and ALLHAT (Antihypertensive and Lipid-Lowering Treatment to Prevent Heart Attack Trial) respectively reported that ACE inhibitors and ARBs did not produce the significant reduction in major cardiovascular events, myocardial infarction, and associated mortality in comparison to other anti-hypertensive agents in symptomatic PAD patients [7, 8]. Moreover, regulation of blood pressure play significant role in the management of PAD but it is still uncertain that ACE inhibitors and ARBs provide advantages in the treatment of PAD beyond blood pressure regulation.

However, few studies have evaluated the efficacy of anti-hypertensive agents for reducing the risk of PAD. There is a need to study the anti-hypertensive agents in the treatment and management of PAD. Moreover, this chapter explores the role of ACE inhibitors and ARBs in atherosclerosis, PAD, and other related disorders. This chapter discusses the probable mechanism behind the therapeutic efficacy of ACE inhibitors and ARBs in PAD and related cardiovascular disorders [9] (Fig. 8.1).

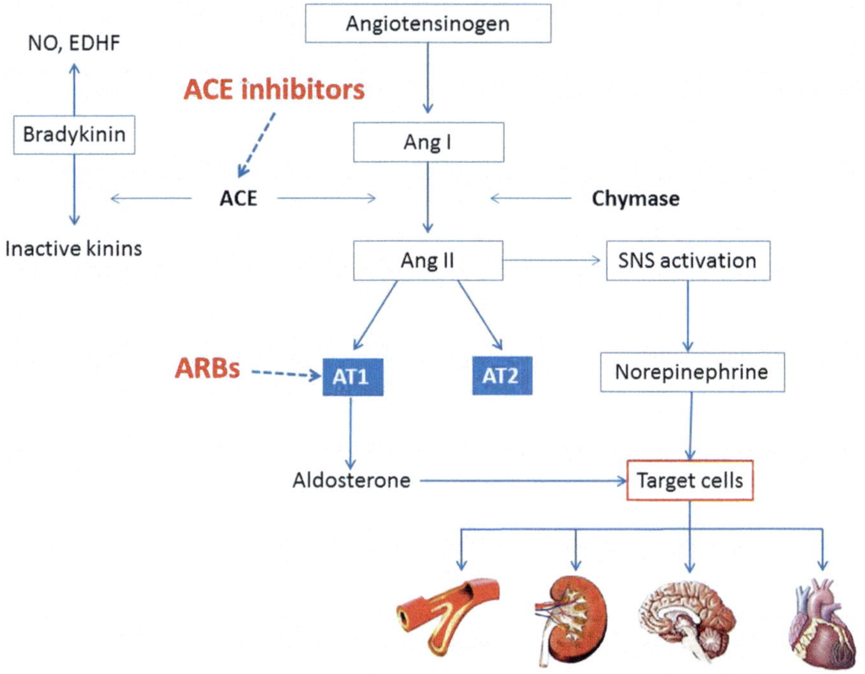

Fig. 8.1 The cascade of RAS systems, its components and effect on target organs, and the action point of ACE-inhibitors and ARBs. ACE angiotensin-converting enzyme, ARBs angiotensin receptor blockers AT1-receptor antagonists, AT1 angiotensin type 1 receptor subtype, AT2 angiotensin type 2 receptor subtype, EDHF endothelium-derived hyperpolarizing factor, NO nitric oxide, SNS sympathetic nervous system. (Source: Trimarco et al. [10])

Machine Generated Summaries

Disclaimer: The summaries in this chapter were generated from Springer Nature publications using extractive AI auto-summarization: An extraction-based summarizer aims to identify the most important sentences of a text using an algorithm and uses those original sentences to create the auto-summary (unlike generative AI). As the constituted sentences are machine selected, they may not fully reflect the body of the work, so we strongly advise that the original content is read and cited. The auto generated summaries were curated by the editor to meet Springer Nature publication standards. To cite this content, please refer to the original papers.

Machine generated keywords: ejection fraction, ejection, hfref, coronary, ami, cad, fraction, reduce ejection, lifestyle, registry, mmhg, acs, pci, failure reduce, discharge.

Renin–Angiotensin System Blockade and Risk of Heart Failure After Myocardial Infarction Based on Left Ventricular Ejection Fraction: A Retrospective Cohort Study [11]

This is a machine-generated summary of:

Cespón-Fernández, María; Raposeiras-Roubín, Sergio; Abu-Assi, Emad; Manzano-Fernández, Sergio; Flores-Blanco, Pedro; Barreiro-Pardal, Cristina; Castiñeira-Busto, María; Muñoz-Pousa, Isabel; López-Rodríguez, Elena; Caneiro-Queija, Berenice; Cobas-Paz, Rafael; Fernández-Barbeira, Saleta; Domínguez-Erquicia, Pablo; Domínguez-Rodríguez, Luis Manuel; López-Cuenca, Ángel; Gómez-Molina, Miriam; Baz-Alonso, José Antonio; Calvo-Iglesias, Francisco; Valdés-Chávarri, Mariano; Íñiguez-Romo, Andrés: Renin–Angiotensin System Blockade and Risk of Heart Failure After Myocardial Infarction Based on Left Ventricular Ejection Fraction: A Retrospective Cohort Study [11].

Published in: American Journal of Cardiovascular Drugs (2019).

Link to original: https://doi.org/10.1007/s40256-019-00343-7

If you want to cite the papers, please refer to the original.

For technical reasons we could not place the page where the original quote is coming from.

Abstract-Summary "The goal of this study was to determine the association between the use of angiotensin-converting enzyme inhibitors (ACEIs) and angiotensin II receptor blockers (ARBs) and follow-up heart failure (HF) according to left ventricular ejection fraction (LVEF) in patients with acute myocardial infarction (AMI)."

"ACEI/ARB use was not associated with fewer follow-up HF admissions in patients with LVEF >40% (univariate analysis: sub-hazard ratio [sHR] 1.10; 95% confidence interval [CI] 0.95–1.27; $p = 0.197$; IPW adjusting analysis: sHR 1.11; 95% CI 0.95–1.29; $p = 0.192$; PSM analysis: sHR 1.12; 95% CI 0.92–1.36; $p = 0.248$)."

"ACEI/ARB use was associated with a significant reduction in HF admission rates in patients with LVEF ≤ 40% (univariate analysis: HR 0.70; 95% CI 0.56–0.88; $p = 0.003$; IPW adjusting analysis: HR 0.64; 95% CI 0.50–0.83; $p = 0.001$; PSM analysis: HR 0.65; 95% CI 0.46–0.92; $p = 0.014$)."

"Among hospitalized survivors of AMI, the use of ACEIs/ARBs was associated with a lower risk of follow-up HF in patients with LVEF ≤ 40% but not in those with LVEF > 40%."

Introduction

"Considerable evidence exists for the prognostic benefits of angiotensin-converting enzyme inhibitors (ACEIs)/angiotensin II-receptor blockers (ARBs) in the prevention of HF after an AMI [12–16], especially in patients with reduced left ventricular ejection fraction (LVEF ≤ 40%) [17–19]."

"Knowledge is scarce about the real benefit of ACEIs/ARBs in patients with LVEF > 40%."

"Current guidelines only establish strong recommendations for the prescription of ACEIs/ARBs in patients with reduced LVEF."

"We analyzed the impact of post-AMI ACEI/ARB use in the development of HF according to LVEF using a contemporaneous population treated according to current recommendations."

Methods

"Using data from this registry (HF admissions during the 3-year period: 16.2 vs. 13.8% in patients treated vs. not treated with ACEIs/ARBs, respectively), we estimated that a sample size of 3220 patients would be sufficient to detect a significant difference in events with a 95% confidence level and 80% statistical power (assuming 15% missing follow-up data)."

"Trained physicians ascertained HF during follow-up by reviewing all medical attendances and hospital records for each patient and selected admissions in which HF was the primary diagnosis."

"We described baseline characteristics according to ACEI/ARB use and HF status using numbers and percentages for categorical data and mean ± standard difference for continuous data."

"Given important differences in key baseline characteristics between patients who did or did not receive ACEIs/ARBs, we complemented our study with a propensity score (PS) analysis."

Results

"CIF for HF admission was 5.4 per 100 person-years (95% CI 5.1–5.8) in patients receiving ACEIs/ARBs versus 4.6 per 100 person-years (95% CI 4.2–5.2) in those not receiving ACEIs/ARBs."

"ACEIs/ARBs were not associated with fewer follow-up HF admissions in patients with LVEF > 40% (univariate analysis: sHR 1.10; 95% CI 0.95–1.27; p = 0.197; IPW adjusting analysis: sHR 1.11; 95% CI 0.95–1.29; p = 0.192; PSM analysis: sHR 1.12; 95% CI 0.92–1.36; p = 0.248)."

"ACEI/ARB use was associated with a significant reduction in HF admission rate in patients with LVEF ≤ 40% (univariate analysis: HR 0.70; 95% CI 0.56–0.88;

p = 0.003; IPW adjusting analysis: HR 0.64; 95% CI 0.50–0.83; p = 0.001; PSM analysis: HR 0.65; 95% CI 0.46–0.92; p = 0.014)."

Discussion

"The main finding of our study, based on a contemporaneous population of patients with AMI, was that ACEI/ARB treatment was significantly associated with a lower number of HF admissions only in patients with LVEF $\leq$ 40%, not in patients with LVEF > 40%."

"The absence of benefit from ACEIs/ARBs in patients with LVEF > 40% in terms of hospitalization for HF is consistent with other non-contemporaneous studies such as the PREAMI [20] and APRES [21] trials."

"The role of ACEIs/ARBs in post-AMI HF admission has only rarely been specifically studied, especially in patients with LVEF > 40%."

"Our study showed that, despite improvements in coronary revascularization and treatment of AMI, ACEIs/ARBs remain useful in reducing post-AMI follow-up HF in patients with LVEF < 40%."

"This was the first study to directly evaluate the impact of ACEI/ARB prescriptions in HF admission according to LVEF post-AMI in the contemporary era, with high rates of revascularization and adjuvant optimal medical treatment."

Conclusion

"Our results indicate that post-AMI ACEI/ARB use is associated with fewer HF admissions in patients with LVEF $\leq$ 40% but not in those with LVEF > 40%."

"Further prospective randomized studies are needed to confirm the absence of benefit from ACEI/ARB treatment in reducing post-AMI HF admissions in patients with HF with preserved ejection fraction."

Effects of Angiotensin-Converting Enzyme Inhibitors and Angiotensin Receptor Blockers on Prothrombotic Processes and Myocardial Infarction Risk [22]

This is a machine-generated summary of:

Dézsi, Csaba András; Szentes, Veronika: Effects of Angiotensin-Converting Enzyme Inhibitors and Angiotensin Receptor Blockers on Prothrombotic Processes and Myocardial Infarction Risk [22].

Published in: American Journal of Cardiovascular Drugs (2016).

Link to original: https://doi.org/10.1007/s40256-016-0185-0

Copyright of the summarized publication:

Abstract-Summary "The authors highlight not only these relationships but also the potential protective effect of increased bradykinin levels and the inhibition of different angiotensin II (AT-II) receptors (AT2, AT4) against unfavorable prothrombotic influences, which—based on studies to date—decreases the risk of acute cardiovascular events."

"Comparisons are presented between the different effects of angiotensin-converting enzyme inhibitors and angiotensin receptor blockers on factors that influence thrombus formation and myocardial infarction risk."

Introduction

"Progressive coronary atherosclerosis is the main pathological base of ischemic heart disease, eventually resulting in overt disease."

"Two main forms of its manifestation are differentiated in clinical practice: stable coronary artery disease (SCAD) and acute coronary syndrome (ACS), which includes unstable angina (UA) pectoris and various forms of myocardial infarction (MI) such as ST-segment elevation myocardial infarction (STEMI) and non-ST-segment elevation myocardial infarction (NSTEMI) [23]."

"Most acute coronary events are underlain by rupture or erosion of plaques, which block the blood supply at given myocardial areas by thrombus formation."

"In patients who have experienced an acute MI (AMI), the incidence of plaque rupture (70–75%) is higher than that of plaque erosion (20–25%) [23, 24]."

Importance of Dawn and the Early Morning Hours and Roles of the Acute Risk Factors

"Plaque instability is determined mainly by a complex of inflammatory processes and immune system activation in the plaque, as well as thrombogenic factors in the circulating blood [25]."

"The development of ACS may be significantly determined by transient biological/physiological changes that follow a circadian rhythm and predominate in the early morning [26]."

"These changes acting on the short term are the 'acute risk factors' that represent the final impetus in the process leading to plaque instability and rupture, and may thereby increase the risk of CV events developing [27]."

"The effects of apparently unimportant changes such as these may be superposed to disorders already caused by chronic risk factors (e.g., the presence of unstable atherosclerotic plaques due to dyslipidemia and hypertension) and may initiate/enhance the triggered processes that lead to the acute events."

Relationship Between Hypertension and the Prothrombotic State

"Raised dawn and early morning blood pressure is one of the most significant acute risk factors that places a greater hemodynamic burden on the coronary circulation and is associated with the activation of several neurohumoral systems [27]."

"The morning surge in blood pressure represents the greatest danger, primarily for 'non-dipper' or 'extreme dipper' patients; in the former this is due to the pressure load that begins relatively early, at dawn, and lasts for 8–10 h, the latter because of the dangerously steep increase in blood pressure [28]."

"The levels of t-PA responsible for the initiation of fibrinolytic processes are also lowest in the critical dawn period and highest when the risk of developing CV events is the lowest [27, 29–31]."

"One may state that the well-known circadian rhythm of prothrombotic and other 'acute risk factors' may initiate processes, upon the effects of triggers, which together may increase the chance for plaque rupture in patients with a high CV risk."

Differences Between Angiotensin-Converting Enzyme Inhibitors and Angiotensin Receptor Blockers

"ACEIs and ARBs are the two most often used groups of RAAS inhibitors."

"If we compare the effects of perindopril (an ACEI with high tissue affinity), losartan, and telmisartan (ARBs) on the coagulative/prothrombotic factors (PAI-1, plasma fibrinogen, t-PA), we can see significant differences [32, 33]."

"Ferrari and colleagues [34, 35] compared the mechanisms of action of the two groups of RAAS and their effects on endothelial and vascular functions in detail."

"The results of ONTARGET also suggest ACEIs and ARBs have different effects and mechanisms of action: the risk of AMI showed a tendency to be lower in the ACEI ramipril group (relative risk [RR] 1.07; 95% confidence interval [CI] 0.94–1.22); although the mean systolic 24-h blood pressure was significantly (3%) lower in the ARB group, which can be regarded as clinically significant [36, 37]."

Conclusion

"Several studies have confirmed that ACEIs effectively reduce blood pressure, including in the critical night/morning period."

"The beneficial effects of ACEIs that reduce the risk of AMI have been demonstrated in several large studies."

"Not surprisingly, based on the results of studies with ACEIs and ARBs, both European (European Society of Cardiology [ESC]) and American (American College of Cardiology Foundation [ACCF]/American Heart Association [AHA]) guidelines prefer ACEIs for the prevention of recurring coronary events in patients after an AMI [38, 39]."

Comparative Effectiveness of Angiotensin II Receptor Blockers Versus Angiotensin-Converting Enzyme Inhibitors Following Contemporary Treatments in Patients with Acute Myocardial Infarction: Results from the Korean Working Group in Myocardial Infarction (KorMI) Registry [40]

This is a machine-generated summary of:

Song, Pil Sang; Seol, Sang-Hoon; Seo, Guang-Won; Kim, Dong-Kie; Kim, Ki-Hun; Yang, Jeong Hoon; Hahn, Joo-Yong; Gwon, Hyeon-Cheol; Ahn, Youngkeun; Jeong, Myung Ho; Song, Young Bin; Kim, Doo-Il; Other Korean Working Group in Myocardial Infarction (KorMI) Registry Investigators, None: Comparative Effectiveness of Angiotensin II Receptor Blockers Versus Angiotensin-Converting Enzyme Inhibitors Following Contemporary Treatments in Patients with Acute Myocardial Infarction: Results from the Korean Working Group in Myocardial Infarction (KorMI) Registry [40].

Published in: American Journal of Cardiovascular Drugs (2015).

Link to original: https://doi.org/10.1007/s40256-015-0140-5

If you want to cite the papers, please refer to the original.

For technical reasons we could not place the page where the original quote is coming from.

Abstract-Summary "A total of 8574 patients were selected from the prospective AMI registry, the Korean Working Group in Myocardial Infarction (KorMI) Registry, and divided into two groups on the basis of discharge prescription: ARB (n = 2281) or ACEI (n = 6293)."

"The study was also designed using propensity-score matching (1171 patients in the ARB vs. 2752 patients in the ACEI group)."

"The Cox model showed both the ARB and ACEI groups had similar risk of cardiac death or MI [adjusted hazard ratio (HR) for ARB 0.69, 95% confidence interval (CI) 0.38–1.25, $p = 0.22$]."

"After propensity-score matching, there was no significant difference in the incidence of cardiac death or MI between the groups (1.3% in the ARB group vs. 1.7% in the ACEI group, adjusted HR for ARB 0.68, 95% CI 0.38–1.23, $p = 0.21$)."

"In a broad spectrum of AMI patients with interventional and pharmacologic treatments, the short-term risk of cardiac death or MI was similar between ARB and ACEI groups."

Introduction

"According to the current American College of Cardiology/American Heart Association guidelines [41, 42], angiotensin-converting enzyme inhibitors (ACEIs) are reasonable for all patients with acute myocardial infarction (AMI) and no contraindications to their use."

"In the VALIANT trial, valsartan was non-inferior to captopril after AMI."

"The VALIANT trial investigators only enrolled patients with AMI that was complicated by heart failure, evidence of left ventricular (LV) systolic dysfunction, or both, and just about 35% of the patients underwent revascularization procedures."

"Results of the VALIANT and ONTARGET trials cannot be extrapolated to a broad spectrum of patients with AMI who underwent contemporary percutaneous coronary intervention (PCI), including patients with AMI and preserved LV systolic function, because the cardio-cerebrovascular protective effects of the two types of renin-angiotensin system blockers might be not identical in the different population [43]."

Methods

"The ARB and ACEI groups were matched by a greedy algorithm and the nearest available pair matching method among patients with an individual propensity score."

"Multivariate weighted Cox regression models adjusted for the available variables including all variables with univariate analysis $p < 0.05$ and ARB versus ACEI at discharge were used to assess the adjusted hazard ratio (HR) with a 95% confidence interval (CI) of the impact of ARB therapy on clinical outcomes in the propensity score-matched population."

"For subgroup analysis, patients were classified into low-, intermediate-, and high-risk groups according to the simple sum of the Global Registry of Acute Coronary Events (GRACE) scores [44]."

"The following variables were considered: age, history of congestive heart failure, history of MI, resting heart rate, systolic blood pressure, ST-segment depression, initial serum creatinine, elevated cardiac enzymes, and no in-hospital PCI (all variables included in the GRACE scores)."

Results

"Even when patients were divided into three risk strata according to the GRACE scoring system (a GRACE score below 88 was considered low risk, while scores between 89 and 118 and above 118 were assigned as intermediate- and high-risk categories, respectively) [44], there was no significant interaction between the use of an ARB versus ACEI and cardiac death or MI among each risk strata of the patients ($p_{interaction} = 0.28$)."

"Among the population of patients with preserved LV systolic function, no significant difference was observed in the incidences of the primary outcome between the two groups in both the overall (0.6% in the ARB group vs. 1.0% in the ACEI group, adjusted HR for ARB 0.61, 95% CI 0.29–1.29, p = 0.20) and propensity score-matched populations (1.0% in the ARB group vs. 1.5% in the ACEI group, adjusted HR for ARB 0.60, 95% CI 0.29–1.21, p = 0.15)."

Discussion

"This study is one of the largest non-randomized studies comparing the effect of two different blockers of the renin-angiotensin system, ARBs and ACEIs, on clinical outcomes in AMI patients undergoing contemporary PCI."

"No data are available on the comparative roles of ARBs and ACEIs in a broad spectrum of AMI patients treated with contemporary revascularization and secondary prevention therapies, including subjects with preserved LV systolic function."

"This signifies that ARBs and ACEIs have comparative effects on the clinical outcomes in a broad spectrum of patients with AMI after PCI."

"Considering that AMI patients are a heterogeneous group that includes variable risks of cardiac events, the establishment of the role of ARBs versus ACEIs in a broad spectrum of patients after AMI is very important."

"Large-scale randomized long-term trials are required to determine whether ARBs versus ACEIs made a difference in clinical outcomes in a broad spectrum of AMI patients treated with contemporary PCI."

Conclusions

"In a broad spectrum of AMI patients treated with contemporary interventional and pharmacologic therapies, the short-term risk of cardiac death or MI was similar in both the ARB and ACEI groups."

"Based on our analysis, ARBs could be regarded as a suitable option in a broad spectrum of patients with AMI after PCI."

"Further randomized trials are warranted to determine whether the findings of the present study could be generalized in this population."

Approaches for the Management of Resistant Hypertension in 2020 [45]

This is a machine-generated summary of:

Aronow, Wilbert S.: Approaches for the Management of Resistant Hypertension in 2020 [45].

Published in: Current Hypertension Reports (2020).

Link to original: https://doi.org/10.1007/s11906-019-1013-0

If you want to cite the papers, please refer to the original.

For technical reasons we could not place the page where the original quote is coming from.

Abstract-Summary "Resistant hypertension is diagnosed if the blood pressure (BP) is not controlled despite optimum doses of three first-line classes of antihypertensive drugs including a thiazide diuretic or if adequate BP control needs four or more antihypertensive drugs from different classes."

"Poor patient compliance, inadequate doses of antihypertensive drugs, poor office BP measurement technique, and having to pay for costs of drugs are factors associated with pseudoresistant hypertension."

"Secondary hypertension must be excluded and treated."

"Therapy of resistant hypertension includes improving compliance with use of medication, detection, and treatment of secondary hypertension, use of lifestyle measures, and treatment of obesity and other comorbidities."

"These patients should be treated with a loop diuretic such as furosemide every 12 h. If a fourth antihypertensive drug is needed to control blood pressure in persons treated with adequate doses of antihypertensive drugs from different classes including a thiazide-type diuretic, a mineralocorticoid receptor antagonist should be added to the therapeutic regimen."

"Further research is needed on investigational drugs and device therapy for treating resistant hypertension."

Introduction

"These hypertension guidelines recommend lifestyle measures plus blood pressure-lowering drugs for secondary prevention of recurrent cardiovascular disease events in persons with clinical cardiovascular disease (coronary heart disease, congestive heart failure, and stroke) and an average systolic blood pressure of 130 mmHg and higher or an average diastolic blood pressure of 80 mmHg and higher [46–48]."

"These guidelines recommend lifestyle measures plus blood pressure-lowering drugs for primary prevention of cardiovascular disease in persons with an estimated 10-year risk of atherosclerotic cardiovascular disease ≥10% [49] and an average systolic blood pressure of 130 mmHg and higher or an average diastolic blood pressure of 80 mmHg and higher [46, 50]."

"These guidelines recommend lifestyle measures plus blood pressure-lowering drugs for primary prevention of cardiovascular disease in persons with an estimated 10-year risk of atherosclerotic cardiovascular disease of < 10% [49] and an average systolic blood pressure of 140 mmHg and higher or an average diastolic blood pressure of 90 mmHg and higher [46, 50, 51]."

"The 2017 ACC/AHA hypertension guidelines recommend that the blood pressure should be lowered to less than 130/80 mmHg in persons with ischemic heart disease [46, 48, 52–57], in persons with heart failure with a decreased left ventricular ejection fraction [46, 58], in persons with heart failure with a preserved left ventricular ejection fraction [46, 58], in persons with chronic kidney disease [46, 59], in persons after renal transplantation [46], in persons with lacunar stroke [46, 60, 61], in persons with peripheral arterial disease [46, 47], in persons with diabetes mellitus [46, 62–65], in noninstitutionalized ambulatory community-dwelling persons older than 65 years of age [46, 52, 53], and for secondary stroke prevention [46, 66]."

Lifestyle Measures

"Lifestyle modification should be used in the treatment of hypertension [46, 67]."

"Weight reduction, consuming a diet rich in fruits, vegetables, and low-fat dairy products with less saturated fat and total fat, sodium reduction to not exceed 1.5 g daily, smoking cessation, regular aerobic physical activity, avoidance of excessive alcohol intake, avoidance of excessive caffeine, and avoidance of drugs which can increase blood pressure, including nonsteroidal anti-inflammatory drugs, glucocorticoids, and sympathomimetics, are recommended [46, 51, 67, 68]."

Drug Treatment of Primary Hypertension

"The 2017 ACC/AHA hypertension guidelines recommend for white and other non-black persons younger than 60 years of age with primary hypertension, the first antihypertensive drug should be an angiotensin-converting enzyme inhibitor or angiotensin receptor blocker, the second drug a thiazide diuretic (preferably chlorthalidone) or a calcium channel blocker, and if a third antihypertensive drug is needed, an angiotensin-converting enzyme inhibitor or angiotensin receptor blocker plus a thiazide diuretic plus a calcium channel blocker should be administered [46]."

"For white and other non-black persons aged 60 years of age and older with primary hypertension, the first antihypertensive drug should be a thiazide diuretic (preferably chlorthalidone) or a calcium channel blocker, and if a third antihypertensive drug is required, a thiazide diuretic plus a calcium channel blocker plus an angiotensin-converting enzyme inhibitor or angiotensin receptor blocker should be administered [46]."

Drug Treatment of Hypertension Associated with Comorbidities

"Patients with stable ischemic heart disease and hypertension should be treated with a beta blocker plus an angiotensin-converting enzyme inhibitor or angiotensin receptor blocker, and if a third antihypertensive drug is needed, a beta blocker plus an angiotensin-converting enzyme inhibitor or angiotensin receptor blocker plus a thiazide diuretic or a calcium channel blocker should be administered [46, 69–77]."

"Patients with hypertension and peripheral arterial disease should be treated with an angiotensin-converting enzyme or angiotensin receptor blocker or a calcium channel blocker or thiazide diuretic or beta blocker [46, 78]."

"Thiazide diuretics, angiotensin-converting enzyme inhibitors, angiotensin receptor blockers, and calcium channel blockers are effective antihypertensive drugs in patients with hypertension and diabetes mellitus and may be used as initial therapy [46, 79]."

"The prevalence of nonadherence to antihypertensive drug therapy in patients with treatment-resistant hypertension in a pooled analysis of 24 studies was 31.2% [80]."

Conclusion

"Poor patient compliance, inadequate doses of antihypertensive drugs, poor office blood pressure measurement technique, and having to pay for costs of drugs are factors associated with pseudoresistant hypertension."

"Factors contributing to resistant hypertension include obesity, a high-sodium, low-fiber diet, excess alcohol intake, physical inactivity, obstructive sleep apnea, use of cocaine, amphetamines, nonsteroidal anti-inflammatory drugs, oral contraceptive hormones, adrenal steroid hormones, sympathomimetic drugs (nasal decongestants and diet pills), erythropoietin, licorice, herbal supplements such as ephedra, progressive renal insufficiency, and inadequate diuretic therapy."

"Patient nonadherence to both lifestyle measures and antihypertensive drug therapy are major factors for treatment-resistant hypertension."

"Therapy of resistant hypertension includes improving compliance with use of medication, detection, and treatment of secondary hypertension, use of lifestyle measures, and treatment of obesity and other comorbidities."

"Further research is needed on investigational drugs and device therapy for treating resistant hypertension."

Comparison Between Beta-Blockers with Angiotensin-Converting Enzyme Inhibitors and Beta-Blockers with Angiotensin II Type I Receptor Blockers in ST-Segment Elevation Myocardial Infarction after Successful Percutaneous Coronary Intervention with Drug-Eluting Stents [81]

This is a machine-generated summary of:

Kim, Yong Hoon; Her, Ae-Young; Jeong, Myung Ho; Kim, Byeong-Keuk; Lee, Seung-Yul; Hong, Sung-Jin; Shin, Dong-Ho; Kim, Jung-Sun; Ko, Young-Guk; Choi, Donghoon; Hong, Myeong-Ki; Jang, Yangsoo: Comparison Between Beta-Blockers with Angiotensin-Converting Enzyme Inhibitors and Beta-Blockers with Angiotensin II Type I Receptor Blockers in ST-Segment Elevation Myocardial Infarction After Successful Percutaneous Coronary Intervention with Drug-Eluting Stents [81].

Published in: Cardiovascular Drugs and Therapy (2019).

Link to original: https://doi.org/10.1007/s10557-018-6841-7

If you want to cite the papers, please refer to the original.

For technical reasons we could not place the page where the original quote is coming from.

Abstract-Summary "We thought to compare 2-year major clinical outcomes between BB with ACEI and BB with ARB therapy in patients with STEMI after successful percutaneous coronary intervention (PCI) with drug-eluting stents (DES)."

"13,873 STEMI patients who underwent successful PCI with DES were enrolled and divided into two groups as the BB with ACEI group (n = 10,393) and the BB with ARB group (n = 3480)."

"Although the incidences of re-MI, TLR, and TVR were similar, the incidences of MACE (8.3% vs. 6.8%, log-rank p = 0.038, hazard ratio [HR] 1.210, 95% confidence interval [CI] 1.010–1.451, p = 0.039), all-cause death, CD, total revascularization, and non-TVR of the BB with ARB group were significantly higher than the BB with ACEI group after PSM."

"The combination BB with ACEI may be beneficial for reducing MACE in STEMI patients after successful PCI with DES than the BB with ARB."

Introduction

"The ACCF/AHA (American College of Cardiology Foundation/American Heart Association) [82] recommend that oral beta-blocker (BBs) should be initiated in the first 24 h and continued during and after hospitalization in patients with ST-segment elevation myocardial infarction (STEMI) and who do not have contraindications as a class 1 (level of evidence [LOE]: B) recommendation; an angiotensin-converting enzyme inhibitor(s) (ACEI) should be administrated for 24 h to all patients with STEMI without contraindications as a class 1 (LOE: A); and an angiotensin receptor blocker(s) (ARB) should be given to patients with STEMI who have indications for but are intolerant of ACEI (LOE: B)."

"Despite these beneficial roles of BB or ACEI/ARB in STEMI patients, limited data are available concerning long-term major clinical outcomes of combination therapy between BB with ACEI and BB with ARB therapy in patients with STEMI."

Material and Methods

"Triple combination (BB, ACEI, and ARB) was received (n = 127, 0.2%)."

"After discharge, the patients were recommended to stay on the same medications they received during hospitalization, including any kind of antiplatelet agent (aspirin, clopidogrel, ticagrelor and/or prasugrel), BB, ACEI, ARB and lipid lowering agents."

"The total duration of dual antiplatelet therapy (DAPT, the combination of aspirin [100 mg/day] and clopidogrel [75 mg/day]) was recommended for more than 12 months to patients who had undergone PCI."

"The major clinical endpoint was the occurrence of MACE defined as all-cause death, cardiac death (CD), recurrent myocardial infarction (re-MI), and total coronary revascularization during the 2-year follow-up period."

"Non-TVR was defined as a revascularization of any segment of the non-target coronary artery."

"Patients in the BB with ACEI group were then one-to-one matched to those in the BB with ARB group according to propensity scores with the nearest available pair matching method."

Results

"Even though the length of deployed stents were similar between the two groups, the number of deployed stents was higher in the BB with ARB group than BB with ACEI group (1.40 ± 0.72 mm vs. 1.37 ± 0.67 mm, $p = 0.018$) and the diameter of deployed stents were larger in the BB with ACEI group than the BB with ARB group (3.20 ± 0.38 mm vs. 3.18 ± 0.39 mm, p = 0.048)."

"At 1 year, the incidences of all-cause death (2.2% vs. 1.2%, p < 0.001) and CD (1.9% vs. 0.9%, p < 0.001) were significantly higher in the BB with ARB group compared with the BB with ACEI group."

"In all patients, the incidences of all-cause death, CD, total coronary revascularization, and TVR were significantly higher in the BB with ARB group compared with the BB with ACEI group."

Discussion

"After PSM analysis, our analysis showed that the following: (1) the cumulative incidence of MACE was higher in the BB with ARB group compared with the BB with ACEI group. (2) The cumulative incidences of all-cause death, CD, total coronary revascularization, and non-TVR were higher in the BB with ARB group than BB with ACEI group. (3) In addition, DM and MVD were significant predictors for non-TVR of PSM patients. (4) However, the cumulative incidences of re-MI, TLR, and TVR were not significantly different between the two groups."

"The results of this study may give some meaningful message to interventional cardiologist during or after PCI to select better combination between BB and ACEI or ARB to reduce the incidence of MACE."

"One of the meaningful messages of this study is that the combination of BB with ACEI reduced the incidence of non-TVR compared with the BB with ARB during 2-year follow-up period in STEMI patients after successful PCI."

Potential Uses of Sacubitril/Valsartan: Need for Data on Efficacy and Safety [83]

This is a machine-generated summary of:

Huet, Fabien; Akodad, Mariama; Kalmanovitch, Eran; Adda, Jerome; Agullo, Audrey; Batistella, Pascal; Roubille, Camille; Roubille, François: Potential Uses of Sacubitril/Valsartan: Need for Data on Efficacy and Safety [83].

Published in: American Journal of Cardiovascular Drugs (2018).

Link to original: https://doi.org/10.1007/s40256-018-0306-z

If you want to cite the papers, please refer to the original.

For technical reasons we could not place the page where the original quote is coming from.

Abstract-Summary "According to recent and promising studies, sacubitril/valsartan (SV) might be efficient in alternative indications in the area of HF with preserved left ventricular ejection fraction, chronic kidney disease, and so on."

Introduction

"Angiotensin-converting enzyme inhibitors (ACEis) and angiotensin receptor blockers (ARBs) have been the cornerstone for the treatment of heart failure (HF) with reduced ejection fraction (HFrEF) for decades [84]."

"The double-blind PARADIGM-HF trial demonstrated that sacubitril/valsartan (SV), an angiotensin receptor-neprilysin inhibitor (ARNi), was superior to enalapril in reducing the risks of cardiovascular death or HF-related hospitalization (relative risk reduction of 20%) in patients with chronic, stable HFrEF [85]."

"European and American medical guidelines recommended [84, 86] that SV should be prescribed as ACEi replacement in ambulatory HFrEF patients with remaining symptoms despite optimal medical treatment with an ACEi, beta-blocker, and mineralocorticoid receptor antagonist (MRA)."

"Several studies have suggested that SV might be useful in alternative indications such as hypertension, HF with preserved ejection fraction (HFpEF), post-myocardial infarction (post-MI), and chronic kidney disease (CKD)."

SV in Hypertension

"The combined therapy with calcium channel blockers (CCBs) and SV demonstrated a greater reduction in 24-h blood pressure and pulse pressure [87], which would be beneficial for patients with resistant hypertension."

"SV demonstrated to increase natriuresis and diuresis without effecting electrolyte balance, and is a better therapeutic option for patients with salt-sensitive hypertension."

"It was shown that SV is more effective than olmesartan in reducing blood pressure in elderly Asian patients with systolic hypertension [88]."

"In another multicenter, randomized, double-blind study comparing SV with valsartan, SV was associated with short-term increases in natriuresis and diuresis, superior blood pressure control, and significantly reduced NT-proBNP levels in Asian patients with salt-sensitive hypertension [89]."

"A recent review suggested that SV might be useful in resistant hypertension, salt-sensitive nocturnal hypertension, and Asian patients (highly dependent of salt intake) [90]."

Treating Arterial Stiffness to Prevent HFpEF

"To SV's positive effects of arterial pressure reduction, a preclinical study has highlighted SV's potential to reduce cardiac remodeling in a primary hypertensive rat model [91]."

"Consistently, a clinical trial comparing 57 SV-treated hypertension patients to 57 patients treated with olmesartan demonstrated a significant reduction of left ventricular (LV) hypertrophy, statistically independent of the blood pressure reduction, in those treated with SV [92]."

"SV's effects on large artery stiffness reduction might be able to reduce central aortic pressure, leading to a reduction in cardiac hypertrophy and fibrosis."

"The study will include patients aged >50 years with a left ventricular ejection fraction (LVEF) of $\geq$ 45% by echo and structural heart disease (left atrial enlargement or LV hypertrophy) with HF symptoms, requiring treatment with diuretics for HF at least 30 days prior to study entry, and elevated NT-proBNP."

Post-Myocardial Infarction

"Strong preclinical evidence supports SV's effectiveness in patients with MI [93–95]."

"No differences in fibrosis and hypertrophy between SV and ACEi treatments were observed, although SV significantly reduced the expression of post-MI hypertrophic markers [93]."

"SV significantly reduced inflammatory marker level (including interleukin-1β), renin-angiotensin aldosterone system (RAAS) activation, and extracellular matrix degradation in macrophages following acute MI, thus indicating SV's ability to reduce the risk of ventricular rupture in the acute phase [95]."

"The PARADISE-MI trial (NCT02924727) hypothesizes that SV may reduce cardiovascular morbidity and mortality in patients with MI, with evidence of LV systolic dysfunction and/or pulmonary congestion requiring intravenous treatment associated with the index MI event (and at least one risk factor)."

"It will include 4660 patients after an acute MI, and SV will be compared to ramipril."

SV to Prevent Chronic Kidney Disease

"According to several clinical trials, ACEis and ARBs reduce the risk of progression toward end-stage renal disease (ESRD) in diabetic patients with CKD, independent to their effect on arterial pressure reduction [96–99]."

"Preclinical studies applying these results to SV have shown promising results for SV in preterminal CKD [100–102], improving renal function and reducing several molecular markers of oxidative stress, inflammation and fibrosis."

"Although these results are encouraging, there are currently no clinical studies available to confirm these data, although the pending UK HARP-III study (International Standard Randomised Controlled Trial Number 11958993) will compare SV to irbesartan in order to evaluate the effect of SV on the reduction of glomerular filtration rate (GFR) and albuminuria after 12 months of therapy [103]."

"UK HARP-III has been designed on the fact that patients of the PARADIGM trial treated with SV had significantly lower rates of acute renal disease or hyperkalemia than the patients treated with enalapril."

SV, Diabetes and Other Endocrine Effects

"SV was also shown to have positive anti-diabetic effects in the PARADIGM-HF trial [85]."

"Patients with diabetes mellitus and HFrEF enrolled in PARADIGM-HF had greater long-term glycated hemoglobin (HbA_{1c}) reduction when treated with SV in comparison to enalapril [104]."

"Neprilysin's degradation of glucagon-like peptide-1 (GLP-1) receptor could explain the anti-hyperglycemic effects of SV [105]."

"The association of GLP-1 analogs and the reduction of neprilysin's degradation of endogenous GLP-1 by SV raises concerns for the risk of drug interaction in diabetic patients, including tachycardia, and altered neurocognitive functioning alterations due to increased neuroinflammation [105]."

"The effects of SV on lipid metabolism in obese patients are still being investigated."

Pitfalls, Safety, and Limits of SV

"It should be taken into consideration that NYHA class had no effect on death from cardiovascular causes ($p = 0.76$), but due to the fact patients with NYHA IV were under-represented in the PARADIGM trial (only 0.7% of the population) [85], initiation of SV in this fragile group of patients should be done with caution."

"Hyperkalemia was another adverse reaction reported in the PARADIGM trial, but in contrast to hypotension, potassium concentrations of > 6 mmol/L occurred significantly less frequently in patients treated with SV."

"A secondary analysis of the PARADIGM trial showed that the risk of hyperkalemia associated with use of MRAs was reduced by the SV group in comparison with the enalapril group (3.1 vs. 2.2 per 100 patient-years; hazard ratio 1.37; 95% CI 1.06–1.76; $p = 0.02$)."

Conclusion

"The effects of SV on cognitive function must be investigated to allow routine use of SV in populations with long survival expectancy."

"The incorporation of SV into the therapeutic arsenal for HF and hypertension relies on the cost-effectiveness of SV compared to enalapril, and several cost-effectiveness analysis suggested cost benefit [106]."

"One model predicted that although SV is costlier compared to enalapril, it is more effective over a life span (6.49 vs. 5.74 USD quality-adjusted life-years [QALYs]) in treating patients with HF."

"The cost-effectiveness of SV was highly dependent on duration of treatment, ranging from 249,411 USD per QALY at 3 years to 50,959 USD per QALY gained over a lifetime [107]."

"Another model predicted that SV decreased the number of hospitalizations (6.0% per year absolute reduction) and lifetime hospital costs by 8.0% (discounted) when compared with enalapril [108]."

Pathological Interactions Between the Endothelin-1 and the Angiotensin-Converting Enzyme Among Tunisian Coronary Patients [109]

This is a machine-generated summary of:

Chalghoum, Abdelkader; Noichri, Yosri; Dandana, Azza; Baudin, Bruno; Miled, Abdelhédi; Ferchichi, Salima: Pathological interactions between the endothelin-1 and the angiotensin-converting enzyme among Tunisian coronary patients [109].

Published in: BMC Cardiovascular Disorders (2016).

Link to original: https://doi.org/10.1186/s12872-016-0417-x

If you want to cite the papers, please refer to the original.

For technical reasons we could not place the page where the original quote is coming from.

Abstract-Summary "The aim of this study was to explore the endothelin-1 (ET-1) concentration and the angiotensin converting enzyme (ACE) activity among Tunisian patients with coronary heart disease, and to investigate the metabolic relationships between these two markers, … and to assess the possible relationship between them and the different risk factors."

"ET-1 concentration was determined by an analytical method (High Performance Chromatography, coupled by Mass Spectrometry), ACE activity was measured by a kinetic method for patients and healthy controls."

"A statistically significant increase of the ET-1 concentration was found among patients compared to healthy controls (15.2 ± 5.3 nM vs 7.1 ± 2.7 nM, p < 0,00001)."

"The study of the metabolic relationship between the ET-1 and ACE among coronary patients reveals other therapeutics targets."

Background

"Acute Coronary Syndrome (ACS) is classified among the major cause of mortality and morbidity in the western countries."

"The endothelin-1 (ET-1) and the hyperactivity of the angiotensin-converting enzyme (ACE) are classified among the coronary "unconventional risk factors" [110, 111]."

"Its peptide is strongly implicated in the ACS's genesis and complications by its vasoconstrictors, pro-oxidant and thrombotic effects [111, 112]. ACE (peptidyl-dipeptidase with zinc, EC, 3,4,15,1) is well known by its physiological role in the rennin angiotensin system by its role in angiotensin-I cleaving (an inactive decapeptide) to generate angiotensin II (a powerful vasoconstrictor) and its role in bradykinin hydrolysis (a potent vasodilatator)."

"Comes the aim of our study which is to quantify the serum concentrations of ET-1 and to measure the ECA serum activity in Tunisians coronary compared to controls subjects, investigate the impact of various risk factors on serum variation of these two parameters as well as the study of the correlation between these two vasoconstrictors."

Methods

"One hundred forty two healthy subjects (111 men and 31 women) middle-aged (56.8 ± 9.4 years) were considered as the control group."

"We were here between two choices: either having patients and "healthy subjects" holders of risk factors with a close age, or having a remarkable difference (not significant) of age and healthy controls without risk factors."

"The patients and healthy subjects signed a free and clear consent which explains the objectives of this work with an undertaking not to publish the names of participants, their personal data including test results (following the instructions of

Tunisian National Committee of Medical Ethics, consistent with the Declaration of Helsinki)."

"A collection of two tubes were made for each patient and witness: one tube without anticoagulant for determination lipid parameters, ET-1 concentration, and ACE activity and, the second one is heparinized tube for blood glucose."

Results

"Glucose, TC, LDL-C, and apolipoprotein B (Apo B) were significantly increased in patients compared to controls."

"Unlike apolipoprotein A1 concentration was significantly higher among control group compared to patients."

"A statistically significant elevation of the ET-1 concentration was observed among patients compared to healthy subjects."

Discussion

"Our study showed a statistically significant increase in the ET-1 values among patients compared to control subjects, which reflects its role not only in prolonged vasoconstriction but also in its atherogenic impact, its pro-oxidant effect (indirectly involved in the NADPH oxidase activation and radical oxygen species generation) and its pro-aggregating role (by his role in the thromboxane A2 synthesis) [112–115]."

"Vasoconstrictor and pro-oxidant effects accumulate in the pathophysiology of atherosclerosis and coronary syndromes [115–117]· The ET-1 concentration and the ACE activity dependent, in this study on gender, hypertension, smoking, obesity and dyslipidemia, unlike diabetes, Personal cardiovascular antecedents, alcohol and physical inactivity."

"The concentration and high activity in hypertensive compared with normotensive patients is explained by the vasoconstrictor effect of ET-1 and ECA and their roles in the sodium reabsorption."

Conclusion

"Our study shows the impact of the ET-1 higher concentration and the ACE higher activity in the ACS predisposition and pathophysiology, seen their vasoconstrictors, pro-oxidant and pro-aggregation roles."

"A thorough study of each component seems important to give other therapeutic targets (ET-1 inhibitors by analogy to ACE inhibitors …)."

"Besides to that, the study of molecular and genomics interactions between these two cardiovascular markers aim to elucidate the different metabolic cascades (activation and braking)."

Therapeutic Approach to Hypertension Urgencies and Emergencies During Acute Coronary Syndrome [118]

This is a machine-generated summary of:

Tocci, Giuliano; Figliuzzi, Ilaria; Presta, Vivianne; Miceli, Francesca; Citoni, Barbara; Coluccia, Roberta; Musumeci, Maria Beatrice; Ferrucci, Andrea; Volpe, Massimo: Therapeutic Approach to Hypertension Urgencies and Emergencies During Acute Coronary Syndrome [118].

Published in: High Blood Pressure & Cardiovascular Prevention (2018).

Link to original: https://doi.org/10.1007/s40292-018-0275-y

If you want to cite the papers, please refer to the original.

For technical reasons we could not place the page where the original quote is coming from.

Abstract-Summary "Uncontrolled hypertension is one of the most common determinant for the persistently high burden of cardiovascular (CV) disease, mostly including coronary artery disease (CAD) and hospital admissions due to acute coronary events."

"Markedly high blood pressure (BP) levels are also frequently observed during the acute phase of coronary syndromes (both ST-segment and non-ST-segment elevation myocardial infarction and unstable angina)."

"A sustained raise of BP levels above 180/110 mmHg associated with acute cardiac organ damage, i.e. myocardial ischemia, represents a condition of hypertension emergency and requires rapid hospital admission, prompt pharmacological therapies and non-pharmacological interventions, aimed at restoring coronary flow and preserve vital myocardium."

Introduction

"Effective and sustained BP reductions to the recommended therapeutic targets have demonstrated to significantly reduce the risk of developing coronary events, independently by age, gender and concomitant CV risk factors or comorbidities [119]."

"On the basis of the currently available evidence, the latest sets of European guidelines have proposed the BP targets of less than 140/90 mmHg in patients at very high CV risk, also including those with previous ACS or CAD, in order to reduce recurrent of coronary events and CV mortality [120]."

"Several observational studies performed in different European countries, including Italy, have consistently reported unexpectedly low rates of control of major CV risk factors, mostly including hypertension and dyslipidaemia, in high and very high risk individuals, thus highlighting the need for adopting preventing educational and therapeutic strategies aimed at achievement of multiple therapeutic targets in a setting of clinical practice [121–123]."

Pathoysiological Aspects of Blood Pressure Regulation During Acute Coronary Syndrome

"In physiological conditions, BP is mainly determined by peripheral resistances and cardiac output, which in turn are both regulated and contra-regulated by multiple, reciprocal and integrated factors [124]."

"During ACS left ventricular dysfunction may result in reduced cardiac output and extremely low BP levels (as defined by systolic BP less than 100 mmHg), thus producing peripheral vasoconstriction, symptomatic hypotension with reflex tachycardia and dyspnoea [125]."

"At cardiac level, marked BP elevation can be the trigger inducing myocardial ischemia, mostly in the presence of rapid and fast BP rise; at the same time, it can also produce and maintain a "vicious cycle" with deleterious consequences for both systolic and diastolic functions of the ventricles."

"Myocardial ischemia (i.e. low diastolic coronary flow) may induce rapid and reflex BP rise, which is expected to provide oxygen and other metabolites to dysfunctional myocardium."

Diagnostic Approach to Cardiac Hypertension Emergency

"This was due to the fact that: (1) angina can occur in the absence of clinically and angiographically evident CAD; (2) presence of left ventricular hypertrophy, a marker of cardiac organ damage which is frequently observed in hypertensive patients, can cause ST-segment alterations [126]."

"According to these algorithms, asymptomatic patients at low CV risk do not require further diagnostic investigation, whilst in symptomatic or asymptomatic patients at intermediate-risk, an exercise stress test should be performed [126–129]."

"In the presence of uninterpretable baseline ECG (i.e. du to left ventricular hypertrophy or branch block) or low-threshold positive exercise test, non-invasive imaging techniques, such as coronary angiography, may be considered for investigating CAD [126–129]."

"Asymptomatic hypertensive patients at high or very high CV risk should undergo stress myocardial scintigraphy and then coronary angiography, whilst symptomatic patients at high or very CV risk coronary angiography represents the gold standard [126–129]."

Therapeutic Approach to Cardiac Hypertension Emergency

"Prescription of beta-blockers (BBs) represents the first choice therapy in hypertensive patients with ACS, because of their favourable effects on reduced heart rate and myocardial oxygen consumption [120, 130, 131]."

"Intravenous BBs should be considered at clinical presentation in patients undergoing primary coronary interventions with no signs of acute heart failure or hypotension (systolic BP less than 100 mmHg) [120, 130, 131]."

"A meta-analysis of 17 clinical trials, performed with calcium channel blockers (CCBs) early administered during ST-segment elevation myocardial infarction (STEMI), showed no beneficial effect on death or re-infarction, with a trend of higher mortality for patients treated with nifedipine [132]."

"Nitrates are not routinely recommended in hypertensive patients with ACS, since there was no evidence of clinical benefit in a randomized controlled trial against placebo [120, 130, 131]."

Conclusions

"Uncontrolled hypertension is one of the most common determinant for CAD and hospital admissions due to acute coronary events."

"A sustained raise of BP levels above 180/110 mmHg associated with acute myocardial ischemia represents a condition of hypertension emergency and requires rapid hospital admission, prompt pharmacological therapies and non-pharmacological interventions, aimed at restoring coronary flow and preserve vital myocardium."

"During ACS BP levels should be rapidly monitored, excessive BP reductions must be avoided, and integrated pharmacological therapies with BBs and ACE inhibitors (or ARBs, if intolerant to ACE inhibition) should be early administered, aimed at reducing in-hospital CV mortality and preventing left ventricular dysfunction."

Adherence to Treatment, Safety, Tolerance, and Effectiveness of Perindopril/Amlodipine Fixed-Dose Combination in Greek Patients with Hypertension and Stable Coronary Artery Disease: A Pan-Hellenic Prospective Observational Study of Daily Clinical Practice [133]

This is a machine-generated summary of:

Liakos, Charalampos I.; Papadopoulos, Dimitrios P.; Kotsis, Vasilios T.: Adherence to Treatment, Safety, Tolerance, and Effectiveness of Perindopril/Amlodipine Fixed-Dose Combination in Greek Patients with Hypertension and

Stable Coronary Artery Disease: A Pan-Hellenic Prospective Observational Study of Daily Clinical Practice [133].

Published in: American Journal of Cardiovascular Drugs (2017).
Link to original: https://doi.org/10.1007/s40256-017-0232-5

If you want to cite the papers, please refer to the original.

For technical reasons we could not place the page where the original quote is coming from.

Abstract-Summary "Initiation of antihypertensive therapy with a two-drug fixed-dose combination (FDC) in a single tablet may be recommended in patients at high risk of cardiovascular events to improve adherence and effectiveness."

"This study assessed adherence to and the safety, tolerance, and effectiveness of the perindopril/amlodipine FDC in Greek patients with hypertension and stable coronary artery disease (CAD) over a 4-month period."

"A total of 1907 patients with hypertension and CAD (59.1% males) who had recently (≤2 weeks) commenced treatment with the perindopril/amlodipine FDC (5/5, 5/10, 10/5, or 10/10 mg) were studied at baseline and at 1 and 4 months."

"1607 (84.6%) patients received a constant treatment dose throughout the study."

"High adherence (MMAS score = 0) was reported by 1592 (83.6%), 1628 (85.7%), and 1477 (77.7%) patients at the second and the third visit and at both visits, respectively."

"Adverse reactions were reported by only 13 (0.7%) patients, were all minor, and did not result in treatment discontinuation."

"Office blood pressure (BP) was significantly decreased at the third visit (130.8 ± 8.4/78.2 ± 6.4 mmHg) compared with baseline (156.5 ± 15.0/89.9 ± 9.6 mmHg; $p < 0.001$), regardless of previous antihypertensive treatment."

"Patients with grade 1, 2, and 3 hypertension at baseline showed a reduction in BP of 19.3/9.4, 31.5/13.5, and 47.8/22.2 mmHg, respectively ($p < 0.001$)."

"The perindopril/amlodipine FDC is characterized by high adherence and effectiveness, regardless of previous treatment."

Introduction

"Patients with hypertension and stable coronary artery disease (CAD) are, by definition, at high risk for future cardiovascular (CV) events according to the 2013 European Society of Hypertension/European Society of Cardiology (ESH/ESC) guidelines for the management of arterial hypertension [120]."

"Monotherapy can effectively reduce BP in only a limited number of patients with hypertension, and most patients require the combination of at least two drugs to achieve BP control [120]."

"The 2013 ESH/ESC guidelines favor the combination of two antihypertensive drugs at fixed doses in a single tablet because reducing the number of daily pills improves adherence and increases the rate of BP control [120, 134, 135]."

"The main objective of this study was to record adherence to treatment with perindopril/amlodipine FDC in patients with essential arterial hypertension and stable CAD in routine clinical practice over a 4-month follow-up period."

Methods

"Demographic data (including sex and age), date of treatment initiation with perindopril/amlodipine FDC, previous treatment for hypertension, CV risk factors, comorbidities, and concomitant medications were recorded at baseline."

"Resting office BP and heart rate (HR), body mass index (BMI), and perindopril/amlodipine FDC dose were recorded at all three visits."

"Adherence to treatment, adverse reactions and/or events from treatment, and cause for discontinuation of treatment with perindopril/amlodipine FDC, if observed, were recorded at the second and the third visit."

"Stepwise binomial multiple logistic regression was used to investigate the relation of absolute adherence to treatment (dependent variable) with age, sex, baseline BMI, and baseline BP classification (independent variables)."

"Stepwise multiple linear regression tested the relation of office BP changes (SBP and DBP) between the first and the third visit (dependent variables) with age, sex, baseline BMI, baseline office BP (SBP and DBP, respectively), previous antihypertensive treatment (yes/no), and average adherence (independent variables)."

Results

"For the majority of patients who completed the study (n = 1607 [84.6%]) the dose of perindopril/amlodipine FDC treatment remained unchanged at all three visits (869 patients [45.7%] received 5/5 mg; 138 [7.3%] received 5/10 mg; 379 [19.9%] received 10/5 mg, and 221 [11.6%] received 10/10 mg, throughout the study)."

"Most patients were highly adherent to the perindopril/amlodipine FDC treatment during the study."

"A total of 1477 patients (77.7%; 95% CI 75.9–79.6) showed absolute adherence to the treatment (i.e., high adherence at both visits)."

"In patients receiving a constant dose of the FDC throughout the study, the mean BP decrease between the first and the third visit was 24.2/11.2 mmHg in those receiving 5/5 mg, 24.8/10.9 mmHg with 5/10 mg, 24.8/11.6 mmHg with 10/5 mg, and 31.6/13.3 mmHg with 10/10 mg."

Discussion

"This was a large-scale study evaluating the management of patients with hypertension at high risk of CV events and treated with the perindopril/amlodipine FDC, a common treatment option for hypertension with stable CAD in daily clinical private practice in Greece."

"Manolis and others [136] conducted a 6-month prospective observational study of 2231 patients with hypertension treated with perindopril/amlodipine FDC and found very good adherence to treatment (97.1% took the treatment "every day" or "quite often") and a low rate of premature treatment discontinuation due to adverse reactions (1.2%)."

"A study of similar design in 3888 patients with hypertension showed advantageous changes in metabolic parameters after treatment with the perindopril/amlodipine FDC (fasting blood glucose decreased by 5.5%, total cholesterol by 10.2%, and triglycerides by 15.4%) [137]."

"The administration of the triple combination perindopril/indapamide/amlodipine has been found effective and well-tolerated in high- and very high-risk patients with hypertension who have not reached target office BP values with previous treatment [138]."

Conclusions

"In Greek patients with hypertension and stable CAD, the perindopril/amlodipine FDC is a treatment option characterized by high adherence, tolerability, and efficacy and rare, minor side effects."

"The rapid and durable control of BP along with the limited adverse effects is probably key to the high adherence to this treatment."

"Treatment-induced peripheral edema is rare, even in warm countries such as Greece."

"The degree of BP reduction observed is associated with the severity of hypertension at baseline."

Efficacy of Zofenopril Vs. Irbesartan in Combination with a Thiazide Diuretic in Hypertensive Patients with Multiple Risk Factors Not Controlled by a Previous Monotherapy: A Review of the Double-Blind, Randomized "Z" Studies [139]

This is a machine-generated summary of:

Omboni, Stefano; Malacco, Ettore; Napoli, Claudio; Modesti, Pietro Amedeo; Manolis, Athanasios; Parati, Gianfranco; Agabiti-Rosei, Enrico; Borghi, Claudio: Efficacy of Zofenopril vs. Irbesartan in Combination with a Thiazide Diuretic in

Hypertensive Patients with Multiple Risk Factors not Controlled by a Previous Monotherapy: A Review of the Double-Blind, Randomized "Z" Studies [139].

Published in: Advances in Therapy (2017).

Link to original: https://doi.org/10.1007/s12325-017-0497-8

If you want to cite the papers, please refer to the original.

For technical reasons we could not place the page where the original quote is coming from.

Abstract-Summary "Combinations between an angiotensin converting enzyme (ACE) inhibitor or an angiotensin II receptor blocker (ARB) and hydrochlorothiazide (HCTZ) are among the recommended treatments for hypertensive patients uncontrolled by monotherapy."

"Four randomized, double-blind, parallel group studies with a similar design, including 1469 hypertensive patients uncontrolled by a previous monotherapy and with ≥ 1 cardiovascular risk factor, compared the efficacy of a combination of a sulfhydryl ACE inhibitor (zofenopril at 30 or 60 mg) or an ARB (irbesartan at 150 or 300 mg) plus HCTZ 12.5 mg."

"In the diabetic patients of the ZAMES study, no adverse effects of treatments on blood glucose and lipids as well as an improvement of renal function were observed."

"In patients with isolated systolic hypertension of the ZEUS study, a slight and similar improvement in renal function and small reductions in pulse wave velocity (PWV), augmentation index (AI), and central systolic BP were documented with both treatments."

"The fixed combination of zofenopril and HCTZ may have a relevant place in the treatment of high-risk or monotherapy-treated uncontrolled hypertensive patients requiring a more prompt, intensive, and sustained BP reduction, in line with the recommendations of current guidelines."

Introduction

"In the ZENITH study, both treatments had a similar positive effect on regression of cardiac and renal damage, whereas a larger proportion of patients showing carotid plaque regression was observed under zofenopril (31.6% vs. 16.1%; $p = 0.047$), particularly in the subgroup of patients taking the low dose of zofenopril (30 mg) plus HCTZ 12.5 mg (4.7% vs. 10.0% irbesartan 150 mg plus HCTZ 12.5 mg; $p = 0.043$)."

"In a subgroup of 93 elderly hypertensive patients of the ZEUS study, treatment with zofenopril or irbesartan was associated with small reductions in central SBP and arterial stiffness indices (pulse wave velocity or PWV and augmentation index or AI), which were similar between the two study drugs at any time point of the study, including the first 6 weeks when all patients were treated with the lowest dose of zofenopril or irbesartan combined with the thiazide diuretic."

Efficacy in Low Dose Subgroup

"In the subgroup of patients with moderate–severe hypertension (office BP ≥ 160 mmHg and DBP ≥ 100 mmHg) taking the lowest dose during the study, the zofenopril combination was associated with an antihypertensive response similar to that of the irbesartan combination (88.9% vs. 80.0%; $p = 0.596$)."

"In the patients of the ZEUS study maintaining the low drug doses throughout the study ($n = 77$), the magnitude of the daytime BP lowering was always slightly larger under zofenopril 30 mg plus HCTZ 12.5 mg than under irbesartan 150 mg plus HCTZ 12.5 mg [140]."

"For the low dose subgroup also the percentage of patients showing daytime SBP normalization (<135 mmHg) and daytime SBP response (SBP < 135 mmHg or reduction ≥ 10 mmHg) at study end was significantly larger under zofenopril (88.9% and 91.7%) than under irbesartan (73.2% and 78.0%; $p = 0.017$ and $p = 0.024$, respectively)."

Efficacy over 24 h

"As detailed in the publications of the individual "Z" studies, the good office BP control obtained with zofenopril and irbesartan was confirmed over 24 h by ABPM, which was available for 53% of patients included in primary endpoint analysis."

"In order to better assess the antihypertensive effect of the drugs over 24 h, we pooled individual ABPM data of the ZODIAC, ZENITH, and ZAMES studies, namely the "Z" studies with similar inclusion criteria (the ZEUS study included only isolated systolic hypertension or ISH patients, and selection of patients for study entry was based not only on office but also on ambulatory BP)."

"In the 561 patients of the pooled ABPM data analysis, the 24-h antihypertensive effect was similar between the two drugs, regardless of the dose employed: 24-h SBP was reduced by 7.6 (9.5, 5.7) mmHg under zofenopril and by 9.5 (11.2, 7.7) mmHg under irbesartan ($p = 0.155$), whereas DBP dropped by 5.5 (6.6, 4.4) mmHg and by 6.6 (7.6, 5.5) mmHg ($p = 0.170$)."

Long-Term Efficacy of the Combinations

"In the ZODIAC and ZENITH studies long-term follow-up of patients treated with high dose combination at study end was planned in order to collect more information on study drug efficacy and safety."

"In the ZODIAC study at the end of the 18 weeks of double-blind treatment, 229 patients among those receiving high dose combination treatment entered an open-label extension phase and were followed up for an additional 14 weeks."

"In the 223 patients of the ZENITH study receiving drug dose up-titration at the end of the 18 weeks of treatment and continuing the double-blind treatment for additional 30 weeks, no difference was observed in office BP response between the two treatment groups (28.6% zofenopril vs. 22.1% irbesartan; $p = 0.178$) [141]."

Tolerability of Both Drug Combinations

"Both drugs were well tolerated, with a very limited number of adverse events, which were well balanced between the two study arms (25.2% of patients receiving zofenopril and 21.9% receiving irbesartan; $p = 0.715$)."

"Only 66 patients (4.3%) were withdrawn from the studies because of an adverse event, 38 in the zofenopril (4.9%) and 28 in the irbesartan treatment group (3.6%; $p = 0.593$)."

"In the ZODIAC study, 6.3% of zofenopril-treated patients and 1.9% of irbesartan-treated patients reported a drug-related adverse event ($p = 0.172$) during the prolonged follow-up."

"Treatment-related adverse events occurred in 3.8%–3.5% of patients under the two study drugs ($p = 0.859$); of these patients four were definitely withdrawn from the extension phase (three taking zofenopril vs. one taking irbesartan; $p = 0.368$) [141]."

Limitations of this Review

"A major limitation of this review is that it reports mixed information from previous original publications and from new pooled data or subgroup analyses, particularly those based on ABPM data."

"In our review we briefly summarized the main results of the single studies, which helped introduce the reader to the secondary results which were available at the time of the original publications, but which were only outlined or even omitted for reasons of space."

"The current review gave us the possibility to add this information in order to provide a comprehensive presentation of all the available data of the "Z" studies."

Conclusions

"Zofenopril also showed some ancillary features which suggest that the fixed combination of this drug with HCTZ may have a particular place in the treatment of high-risk or monotherapy-treated uncontrolled hypertensive patients requiring a more prompt, intensive, and sustained BP reduction, in line with the recommendations of current guidelines [142, 143]."

"The effective BP reduction and the large proportion of responders in both treatment arms in the "Z" studies also support the findings of previous studies that, in most patients not responding to a single antihypertensive medication, combination treatment with two drugs may substantially increase the chance of response [144, 145]."

"Results of the large "Z" studies confirm that combination treatment between a drug acting on the RAAS and a thiazide diuretic should be among the preferred choices when monotherapies fail to lower BP to or below target levels, particularly in patients displaying multiple CV risk factors."

β-Blockers After Myocardial Infarction and 1-Year Clinical Outcome—A Retrospective Study [146]

This is a machine-generated summary of:

Hagsund, Tora; Olsson, Sven-Erik; Smith, J. Gustav; Madsen Hardig, Bjarne; Wagner, Henrik: β-blockers after myocardial infarction and 1-year clinical outcome—a retrospective study [146].

Published in: BMC Cardiovascular Disorders (2020).

Link to original: https://doi.org/10.1186/s12872-020-01441-0

If you want to cite the papers, please refer to the original.

For technical reasons we could not place the page where the original quote is coming from.

Abstract-Summary "Long term β-blocker therapy after myocardial infarction (MI) reduces mortality and recurrent MI but evidence for this treatment predates contemporary acute coronary care."

"β-blocker treatment is a key quality of care indicator in the Swedish national quality register for acute coronary care, RIKS-HIA."

"Between 2011 and 2015 a declining number of MI-patients discharged with a β-blocker from the coronary care unit (CCU) at Helsingborg and other hospitals was reported."

"MI-patients registered in RIKS-HIA discharged without β-blocker during 2011–2015 (no-β-group) and a control group (β-group) comprised of patients discharged with β-blocker treatment between January 1 to December 31, 2013, were matched by RIKS-HIA criteria for β-blocker use."

"The no-β-group included 141 patients, where 65.2% had a justified reason for non-β-blocker use."

"A majority of the patients in the no-β-group had a justified absence of a β-blocker."

"β-blocker treatment post-MI showed a trend towards fewer readmissions for MI."

Background

"According to current (2015) guidelines from European Society of Cardiology (ESC) for ST-Elevation Myocardial Infarction (STEMI) patients, long-term treatment with β-blockers is recommended to all patients without contraindications."

"According to American guidelines, continuation of treatment with β-blocker for 3 years is strongly recommended (Class I) for STEMI patients with normal left ventricular function."

"Regarding non-ST-Elevation Myocardial Infarction (NSTEMI) patients, the ESC guidelines recommends long-term β-blocker treatment in patients with an ejection fraction of < 40% [147]."

"In current (2015) treatment recommendation from the Swedish National board of Health and Welfare, long term treatment with a β-blocker post-MI is only recommended to patients with left ventricular systolic dysfunction (LVDF) [148]."

"The Swedish Society of Cardiology recommends β-blockers as long-term treatment in all patients with a history of acute coronary syndrome (ACS) and who are without contraindications [149]."

Methods

"The first patient group (no-β-group) comprised all MI patients who were discharged without a β-blocker, during 1 January 2011 to 1 January 2015."

"A control group (β-group) comprised all patients discharged with β-blocker treatment during 1st January 2013 to 31st December 2013."

"Patients eligible for β-blocker treatment was chosen based on RIKS-HIA's criteria for β-blocker treatment, (age < 80, discharged alive, absence of AV-block II or III and discharged with a diagnosis of a type 1 MI) [150]."

"In order to investigate similarities and differences between the no-β-group and β-group, relevant variables were selected and collected from the registries and from the patient's medical records."

"In the β-group, information was collected from the medical record regarding side effects attributable to β-blocker and whether treatment was terminated within a year."

Results

"Data from RIKS-HIA showed that of 1631 MI patients discharged from the CCU at Helsingborg hospital during the study period 1st of January 2011 to 1st of January 2015, 1155 patients met the criteria for β-blocker treatment."

"1155, a total of 171 patients (14.8%) were not prescribed a β-blocker."

"After reviewing the medical records, 24 of these patients (14.0%) turned out to be incorrectly registered as they did not meet the criteria for β-blocker treatment (n = 14) or were discharged with a β-blocker (n = 10)."

"There was a high prescription rate in both groups of the recommended secondary prevention related medications; statins, ASA and ADP receptor inhibitors."

Discussion

"When studying the correlation between lack of a β-blocker prescription and clinical outcome, our study showed that the patient group discharged without a β-blocker after MI had a significantly higher rate of readmissions for MI during 1 year after index event, compared with the patient group that was discharged with a β-blocker."

"The criteria for inclusion in the no-β-group (were patients <80 years, with a type-1 MI (i.e. STEMI and NSTEMI), discharged alive without a β-blocker and with absence of AV-block II-III, which differs from studies that only included patients with STEMI and who underwent PCI [151–156]."

"The main significant clinical differences between the groups, were likely associated with the absence or presence of β-blocker at discharge."

"The fact that the patient group characteristics in the present study differs from that in other observational studies on β-blockers post-MI might depend on the differences in inclusion criteria previously described."

Conclusion

"A majority of the patients in the no-β-group had a justified absence of a β-blocker."

"β-blocker treatment post-MI showed a trend to fewer readmissions for MI."

"As illustrated by this study, patient specific factors not visible in registry data affects whether a patient were prescribed a β-blocker post-MI or not."

Differential Prognostic Value of Resistin for Cardiac Death in Patients with Coronary Artery Disease According to the Presence of Metabolic Syndrome [157]

This is a machine-generated summary of:

Rallidis, Loukianos S.; Katsimardos, Andreas; Kosmas, Nikolaos; Rallidi, Taxiarchoula; Zapantiotis, Dimitrios; Varounis, Christos; Kountouri, Antonia: Differential prognostic value of resistin for cardiac death in patients with coronary artery disease according to the presence of metabolic syndrome [157].

Published in: Heart and Vessels (2021).

Link to original: https://doi.org/10.1007/s00380-021-01964-2

If you want to cite the papers, please refer to the original.

For technical reasons we could not place the page where the original quote is coming from.

Abstract-Summary "There are controversial data regarding the prognostic value of resistin in stable coronary artery disease (CAD) patients."

"We prospectively investigated the long-term prognostic value of resistin in patients with stable CAD."

"Follow-up data were obtained from 703 patients of whom 79 had a cardiac death (11.2%) and 205 (29.2%) met the secondary endpoints."

"Resistin levels could not predict cardiac death [HR 1.044; 95% CI 0.994–1.096; $p = 0.087$] neither secondary endpoints [HR 1.025; 95% CI 0.983–1.068; $p = 0.250$)."

"Among 298 patients (42.4%) with metabolic syndrome (MS) resistin levels were independently associated with cardiac death after adjustment for conventional risk factors [HR 1.121; 95% CI 1.045–1.204; $p = 0.002$)."

"Patients with resistin values ≥7.6 ng/mL (median level) had 2.8 times higher risk of cardiac death compared to those with resistin levels <7.6 ng/mL after adjustment for traditional risk factors and LVEF (HR 2.882; 95% CI 1.311–6.336; $p = 0.008$)."

"Resistin is independently associated with cardiac death in patients with stable CAD and MS."

Introduction

"Circulating resistin levels are higher in older patients and have been shown to increase by the effect of growth hormone, hyperglycemia, dexamethasone, androgens and inflammatory cytokines [tumor necrosis factor-a, interleukin (IL)-1, IL-6, and lipopolysaccharides]."

"Resistin has been shown to be involved in human atherosclerosis via multiple inflammatory and thrombosis pathways [158–160]."

"Due to its involvement in several metabolic pathways and its potential role in atherosclerosis pathophysiology, resistin could serve as a prognostic biomarker in patients with coronary artery disease (CAD)."

"The purpose of our study was to evaluate the prognostic value or resistin in a cohort of stable CAD patients."

Materials and Methods

"All patients were participants of the Lipoprotein-Associated phospholipasE A_2 in stable coronary aRTEry diSease (LAERTES) Study, as previously described [161] which is an ongoing prospective, hospital-based registry investigating risk factors and prognosis in patients with stable CAD."

"MS was defined as the presence at least 3 of 5 metabolic risk factors (waist circumference, high-density lipoprotein-cholesterol [HDL-C], triglycerides, blood pressure, fasting glucose) according to the NCEP/ATPIII [162]."

"Venous fasting blood samples were collected between 08:00 and 09:00 for the same day measurements of lipids and high sensitivity C-reactive protein (hsCRP), while the remaining serum was stored and frozen at – 80 °C until assayed."

"Serum levels of total cholesterol, HDL-C and triglycerides were measured enzymatically on an automatic analyser (Dimension RXL; Dade Behring, Marburg, Germany)."

"Unadjusted Kaplan–Meier survival curves illustrated the association between resistin levels and the incidence of cardiac death over time, and the log-rank test evaluated statistical significance."

Results

"Resistin levels could not predict cardiac death [HR 1.044; 95% CI 0.994–1.096; $p = 0.087$) neither secondary endpoints in the cohort of patients with CAD [HR 1.025; 95% CI 0.983–1.068; $p = 0.250$)."

"Resistin levels were higher in patients with MS compared to those without MS (7.6 [6.0–10.6] vs 6.8 [5.1–9.3] ng/mL, $p = 0.004$)."

"There was also a trend of higher resistin levels in patients with DM compared to those without DM but it did not reach statistical significance (7.3 [5.4–10.2] vs 6.9 [5.4–9.2] ng/mL, $p = 0.220$)."

"Resistin levels were independently associated with cardiac death in patients with MS after adjustment for conventional risk factors (age, DM, total cholesterol, hypertension, smoking and family history for premature CAD) [HR 1.121; 95% CI 1.045–1.204; p = 0.002)."

Discussion

"We found that resistin levels could not predict cardiac events, either cardiac death or the secondary endpoints, in the entire cohort of stable CAD patients."

"Of 176 post-ACS patients who were on statin treatment resistin levels were an independent marker of residual risk for recurrent coronary events during a mean period of 24-month follow-up [163]."

"Fontana and others reported an independent association between resistin levels and all cause or cardiovascular mortality in 359 patients with both CAD and DM [164]."

"Resistin was associated with homocysteine, an atherothrombotic risk factor which has been reported to be associated with cardiac death in CAD patients [165]."

"The strength of our study resides in the demonstration for the first time of the association of resistin with cardiac mortality in a homogeneous cohort of patients with stable CAD and MS with long follow-up."

Conclusion

"Resistin is independently associated with cardiac death in patients with stable CAD and MS."

"Larger prospective studies are required to replicate this finding and research work is mandatory to confirm the hypothesis that resistin serves as a link between insulin resistance and atherosclerosis."

Preliminary Results of the Acute Heart Failure Registry in the DELTA Region of Egypt (DELTA-HF): A Database and a Quality Initiative Project [166]

This is a machine-generated summary of:

Elasfar, Abdelfatah; Shaheen, Sherif; El-Sherbeny, Wafaa; Elsokkary, Hatem; Elhefnawy, Suzan; Al-Setiha, Mohammed: Preliminary results of the acute Heart Failure registry in the DELTA region of Egypt (DELTA-HF): a database and a quality initiative project [166].

Published in: The Egyptian Heart Journal (2019).

Link to original: https://doi.org/10.1186/s43044-019-0024-0

If you want to cite the papers, please refer to the original.

For technical reasons we could not place the page where the original quote is coming from.

Abstract-Summary "We aimed to describe the clinical characteristics and diagnostic and treatment options in patients with acute heart failure in the Delta region of Egypt and to explore the gap in the management in comparison to the international guidelines."

"DELTA-HF is a prospective observational cohort registry for all consecutive patients with acute heart failure (AHF) who were admitted to three tertiary care cardiac centers distributed in the Delta region of Egypt."

"A total of 220 patients (65.5% were males with a median age of 61.5 years and 50.9% had acute decompensation on top of chronic heart failure) was enrolled in our registry."

"The risk factors for heart failure included rheumatic valvular heart disease (10.9%), smoking (65.3%), hypertension (48.2%), diabetes mellitus (42.7%), and coronary artery disease (28.2%)."

"Exacerbating factors included infections (28.1%), acute coronary syndromes (25.5%), non-compliance to HF medications (19.6%), and non-compliance to diet (23.2%) in acute decompensated heart failure (ADHF) patients."

"None of our patients had been offered heart failure device therapy and only 50% were put on beta-blockers upon discharge."

"There is a clear gap in the management of patients with acute heart failure in the Delta region of Egypt with confirmed under-utilization of heart failure device therapy and under-prescription of guideline-directed medical therapies particularly beta-blockers."

Background

"In the USA, heart failure currently results in more than one million hospitalizations every year and the estimated 5-year mortality is approximately 50% [167]."

"Data about heart failure was only restricted to Western countries."

"New emerging data about heart failure came from some countries in the Middle East region including HEARTS and Gulf CARE registries [168, 169]."

"In Egypt, data about heart failure was very scarce till very recently when Egypt was included in the European heart failure survey about both acute and chronic heart failure [170]."

Methods

"DELTA-HF is a prospective cohort registry for all consecutive patients with AHF who were admitted to three tertiary care cardiac centers in the Delta region of Egypt within a period from April 2017 to May 2018, during which, data collection and short-term follow-up were done."

"We included only patients with AHF whether de novo or acute on top of chronic HF."

"We excluded patients who are less than 18 years of age, refused to give consent, and patients who were managed and discharged from the emergency department without hospital admission."

"For every patient, a standard case report form (CRF) has been filled out with an emphasis on clinical and demographic characteristics of included patients, course during hospital stay, and diagnostic and therapeutic options entertained prior to admission, during hospital stay and upon discharge."

"Verbal informed consent has been obtained from each included patient or his substitute decision maker."

Results

"A review of medical history showed that 50.9% were known as heart failure patients before, 48.2% had hypertension, 42.7% had diabetes mellitus, 56.3% had smoking history, 28.2% had coronary artery disease (15.5% had prior PCI, and 2.7% had prior CABG), and 10.9% had rheumatic heart disease (4.5% had prior percutaneous or surgical valve interventions)."

"Intravenous inotropic agents have been prescribed in 34.5% of patients, 41.8% had non-invasive respiratory ventilation (CPAP or BiPAP), 12.7% had invasive endotracheal intubation and mechanical ventilation, 38.2% had worsening of serum creatinine, 1.8% had renal replacement therapy (hemodialysis/ultrafiltration), 5.5% had blood transfusion, and 7.3% had ventricular tachyarrhythmias (VT and/or VF)."

"In acute decompensated heart failure (ADHF) patients' group, non-compliance to diet was an exacerbating factor in 23.2% of cases while it was 19.6% for non-compliance to medications."

Discussion

"Non-STEMI 2015 ESC guidelines recommend an immediate invasive strategy with intent to perform revascularization, irrespective of ECG or biomarker findings in patients with at least one very high-risk criterion (hemodynamic instability, cardiogenic shock, acute heart failure AHF, life-threatening arrhythmia, cardiac arrest, recurrent chest pain refractory to medical treatment, or dynamic ST changes particularly transient ST elevation) [131]."

"According to 2016 HF ESC guidelines, ICD is recommended to reduce the risk of sudden death and all-cause mortality in patients with symptomatic HF (NYHA classes II–III) and an LVEF ≤35% despite ≥3 months of optimal medical therapy (OMT), provided they are expected to survive substantially longer than 1 year with good functional status and they have ischemic heart disease "unless they had MI in previous 40 days" and dilated cardiomyopathy."

Conclusions

"There is a clear gap in the management of patients with heart failure in the Delta region of Egypt with confirmed very low use of NPs in the diagnosis and prognostication of heart failure, under-utilization of heart failure device therapy, low rate of coronary intervention, and under-prescription of guideline-directed medical therapies particularly beta-blockers."

"Limited resources and the lack of heart failure management programs are the main causes of this gap."

"We are planning to have a second phase of this registry with a bigger sample size and more hospitals representing the Delta region in Egypt."

Implementation of Cardiovascular Disease Prevention Guidelines in Clinical Practice—Can We Do Better? [171]

This is a machine-generated summary of:

Kotseva, Kornelia: Implementation of Cardiovascular Disease Prevention Guidelines in Clinical Practice—Can We Do Better? [171].

Published in: Current Treatment Options in Cardiovascular Medicine (2015).

Link to original: https://doi.org/10.1007/s11936-015-0415-9

If you want to cite the papers, please refer to the original.

For technical reasons we could not place the page where the original quote is coming from.

Abstract-Summary "There is considerable potential to raise the standard of cardiovascular prevention through more effective lifestyle intervention, control of other risk factors and appropriate use of cardioprotective medication."

"A more comprehensive multidisciplinary and professional approach accessible to both patients with established disease as well as those who are at high risk of developing CVD and provided in each country by existing or adapted 'prevention centres' is needed."

"Cardiovascular prevention requires an integrated family-based approach, involving multidisciplinary teams of health care professionals, adapted to medical and cultural settings in each country in order to achieve better lifestyles, risk factor control and adherence with cardioprotective medications in our patients with coronary disease and to reduce their risk of recurrent cardiovascular events and improve quality of life and survival."

Introduction

"The aim of the Joint European Societies (JES) guidelines on cardiovascular disease prevention is to improve the practice of cardiovascular prevention by encouraging the development of national guidance on cardiovascular disease prevention and its communication, implementation and evaluation through national societies in each country."

"Patients with coronary or other atherosclerotic cardiovascular disease, and those at high risk of developing CVD, have been defined as the highest clinical priorities for prevention."

"The 2012 Joint European Societies' guidelines defined the lifestyle and risk factor goals for patients with established CHD and people at high CVD risk as follows: stop smoking, make healthy food choices and be physically active, a body mass index (BMI) < 25 kg/m^2, blood pressure < 140/90 mmHg (<140/80 mmHg in patients with diabetes mellitus), LDL-cholesterol <1.8 mmol/L (<70 mg/dL) or at least 50% reduction in people at very high risk and < 2.5 mmol/L (<100 mg/dL) in people at high risk, glycated hemoglobin (HbA1C) < 7.0 mmol/L (<53 mmol/mol) in people with diabetes mellitus and appropriate use of cardioprotective drug therapies [172]."

Surveys Evaluating Guideline Implementations in Clinical Practice

"The results showed that a large majority of coronary patients did not achieve the guideline standards for secondary prevention with high prevalences of persistent smoking, unhealthy diets, physical inactivity and consequently most patients being overweight or obese with a high prevalence of diabetes [121, 173]."

"The results of EUROASPIRE IV are in accordance with earlier multinational surveys conducted in Europe, USA and other parts of the world, reporting high prevalences and an inadequate control of CVD risk factors in patients with CHD [174, 175]."

"The results of EUROASPIRE and other similar surveys conducted in EUROPE, USA or other parts of the world revealed that despite the compelling scientific evidence for prevention and rehabilitation following the development of coronary disease, a large majority of coronary patients are failing to achieve the lifestyle, risk factor and therapeutic targets set by the prevention guidelines."

Secondary Prevention or Cardiac Rehabilitation

"The meta-analysis of randomised trials of blood pressure-lowering medication in patients with coronary disease showed that the reduction of systolic blood pressure by 10 mmHg or diastolic blood pressure by 5 mmHg reduces CHD events (fatal and non-fatal) by about a quarter (RR 0.76; 95% CI 0.68–0.86) and stroke by about a third (RR 0.65; 95% CI 0.53–0.80) [71]."

"The following cardioprotective drug therapies shown to reduce morbidity and mortality in clinical trials in addition to drugs used for treatment of elevated blood pressure and glucose are recommended in the JES5 guidelines for CVD prevention: aspirin or other platelet-modifying drugs in all patients, beta-blockers in those after myocardial infarction, ACE inhibitors/ARBs in those with impaired left ventricular function and statins in all patients [172]."

"Recent data from the OASIS clinical trial of 18,809 patients with acute coronary syndromes showed that adherence to behavioural advice (diet, exercise and smoking cessation) after acute coronary syndrome was associated with a substantially lower risk of recurrent cardiovascular events [176]."

Conclusions

"The distinction between cardiac rehabilitation and secondary prevention is artificial, and the meta-analyses demonstrate, from different perspectives, the benefits of a comprehensive approach to reducing total cardiovascular risk."

"What is required is a comprehensive risk reduction approach to lifestyle, risk factor and therapeutic management to reduce total cardiovascular risk."

"A modern cardiovascular prevention program could be created by integrating 'cardiac rehabilitation' and 'secondary prevention' to deliver one comprehensive risk reduction service."

"This modern program will address lifestyle through a behavioural approach to smoking cessation, healthy eating, physical activity and weight management."

"All patients with acute coronary syndromes, or any other atherosclerotic disease, should have guaranteed access to a modern cardiovascular prevention program in every country."

Preventable Clinical and Psychosocial Factors Predicted Two out of Three Recurrent Cardiovascular Events in a Coronary Population [177]

This is a machine-generated summary of:

Sverre, E.; Peersen, K.; Weedon-Fekjær, H.; Perk, J.; Gjertsen, E.; Husebye, E.; Gullestad, L.; Dammen, T.; Otterstad, J. E.; Munkhaugen, J.: Preventable clinical and psychosocial factors predicted two out of three recurrent cardiovascular events in a coronary population [177].

Published in: BMC Cardiovascular Disorders (2020).

Link to original: https://doi.org/10.1186/s12872-020-01368-6

If you want to cite the papers, please refer to the original.

For technical reasons we could not place the page where the original quote is coming from.

Abstract-Summary "The relative importance of lifestyle, medical and psychosocial factors on the risk of recurrent major cardiovascular (CV) events (MACE) in coronary patients' needs to be identified."

"The main objective of this study is to estimate the association between potentially preventable factors on MACE in an outpatient coronary population from routine clinical practice."

"This prospective follow-up study of recurrent MACE, determine the predictive impact of risk factors and a wide range of relevant co-factors recorded at baseline."

"During a mean follow-up of 4.2 years from study inclusion (mean time from index event to end of study 5.7 years), 364 MACE occurred in 240 patients (21, 95% confidence interval, 19 to 24%), of which 39 were CV deaths."

"Preventable and potentially modifiable factors addressed accounted for 66% (95% confidence interval: 49 to 77%) of the risk for recurrent events."

"Coronary patients were at high risk of recurrent MACE."

"Potentially preventable clinical and psychosocial factors predicted two out of three MACE, which is why these factors should be targeted in coronary populations."

"Registered at ClinicalTrials.gov: NCT02309255."

Background

"Unhealthy lifestyle behaviour and low risk factor control is shown to contribute to the high risk of recurrent cardiovascular (CV) events observed in CHD patients [178, 179]."

"The relative importance of different determinants of long-term disease progression need to be studied further, since most previous studies are based on registries [178–180] with a limited number of clinical factors included."

"In the recent EuroAspire IV registry study, CV comorbidities, low education and depressive symptoms were strongly and significantly associated with CV death or non-fatal myocardial infarction (MI), stroke or heart failure in an outpatient population, whereas lifestyle factors and control of lipids and blood pressure (BP) were not [181]."

"The current prospective study aims to estimate the relative importance of preventable and potentially modifiable clinical and psychosocial factors associated with recurrent major adverse CV events (MACE) in an outpatient coronary population from routine clinical practice."

Methods

"We identified 1789 consecutive patients aged 18–80 years with a first or recurrent coronary event in 2011–2014 from the catchment areas of the Norwegian hospitals in Drammen and Vestfold."

"Data on recurrent CV events after baseline were collected from the patients` hospital medical records in 2018, after a mean follow-up of 4.2 years."

"Complete follow-up data were missing in only 14 (1.2%) patients who had moved out of the catchment area of the participating hospitals since study inclusion."

"Since patients with established CHD prior to inclusion were presumed to have different risk level and profile by study time, all analyses were stratified for prior CHD before the index event."

Results

"During a mean follow-up period of 4.2 (SD 0.4) years after study inclusion (mean time from index event to end of study was 5.7 (SD 0.9) years), 364 MACE events were observed in 240 (21 95% CI, 19–24%) patients, whereas 39 (3.4, 0.8% per year) died of CV causes."

"The risk of recurrent MACE was significantly higher in patients with CHD prior to the index event compared to those without (age adjusted RR = 2.37, 95% CI 1.84–3.07, $p < 0.001$)."

"Current smoking vs. never smoking (RR 1.24, 95% CI 1.01–1.53, $p = 0.048$) was also associated with MACE (data not shown)."

"In multi-adjusted sub-group analyses in patients with no CHD prior to the index event (n = 791), LDL-cholesterol (RR 1.38 per mmol/L increase, 95% CI 1.13–1.68, p = 0.002) was significantly associated with MACE."

Discussion

"Not taking statins, low or no physical activity and higher depression scores were the major potentially modifiable risk factors associated with MACE in multi-adjusted analysis."

"Low physical activity (<30 min 2–3 times/week) was also associated with MACE after adjusting for other CV risk factors, but the association became borderline significant (p = 0.071) after adjusting for CV comorbidity."

"Non-participation in CR was associated with MACE in analyses adjusted for age and CV risk factors."

"Not taking a statin was the strongest determinant of recurrent MACE, and remained significant after adjusting for other risk factors and CV comorbidities."

"Increasing waist circumference was significantly associated with MACE, but not when adjusted for other CV risk factors."

"In line with obesity, the effect of BP on MACE might have been partly modified through other risk factors like diabetes, CV comorbidity and increasing age."

Conclusions

"The risk of recurrent CV events remained high in an outpatient coronary population, particularly in the presence of CV comorbidity."

"Not taking statin therapy, insufficient physical activity, smoking, diabetes, higher depression scores and non-participation in CR were the major preventable and potentially modifiable factors associated with MACE."

"Potentially preventable clinical and psychosocial factors predicted two out of three MACE, and efforts that target the factors identified may reduce the incidence of recurrent CV events in outpatient coronary populations."

Long-Term Effects of Device-Guided Slow Breathing in Stable Heart Failure Patients with Reduced Ejection Fraction [182]

This is a machine-generated summary of:

Lachowska, Kamila; Bellwon, Jerzy; Narkiewicz, Krzysztof; Gruchała, Marcin; Hering, Dagmara: Long-term effects of device-guided slow breathing in stable heart failure patients with reduced ejection fraction [182].

Published in: Clinical Research in Cardiology (2018).

Link to original: https://doi.org/10.1007/s00392-018-1310-7

If you want to cite the papers, please refer to the original.

For technical reasons we could not place the page where the original quote is coming from.

Abstract-Summary "Slow breathing (SLOWB) alleviates symptoms of chronic heart failure (HF) but its long-term effects are unknown."

"We examined the acute and long-term impact of device-guided breathing on hemodynamics and prognostic parameters in HF patients with reduced ejection fraction (HFrEF)."

"Twenty-one patients with HFrEF (23.9 ± 5.8%, SD ± mean) on optimal medical therapy underwent blood pressure (BP), heart rate (HR), HR variability, 6-min walk test (6MWT), cardiopulmonary exercise testing (CPET), and echocardiography measurements before and 3 months after SLOWB home training (30 min daily)."

"Long-term SLOWB reduced office systolic BP ($P < 0.001$) but not central or ambulatory systolic BP."

"SLOWB reduced SDNN/RMSSD ratio ($P < 0.05$) after 3 months."

"No HF worsening, rehospitalisation or death occurred in group 1 out to 6-month follow-up."

"Two hospitalizations for HF decompensation and two deaths ensued in group 2 between 3- and 6-month follow-up."

Introduction

"Along with pharmacological approaches, surgical implantable electrical devices for the treatment of HF patients with reduced ejection fraction (HFrEF) improve symptoms, reduce the risk of death and all-cause mortality in primary and secondary prevention [183–186]."

"The use of slow breathing (SLOWB) technique has been shown to reduce dyspnoea, improve oxygen saturation and exercise tolerance in HF patients, acutely increase baroreflex gain and stability in patients with CV disease and a risk for sudden death [187–190]."

"Data from pilot studies of patients with systolic chronic HF have demonstrated the feasibility of device-guided SLOWB pacing with the use of the RESPeRATE, improvements in NYHA class and left ventricle ejection fraction (LVEF), reductions in pulmonary pressure [191, 192] and breathlessness [193]."

"Although the currently available results with paced breathing are promising in chronic HF and the mechanistic rationale for the use of SLOWB is apparent, not all HF patients seemed to respond to this behavioural technique [193]."

Methods

"On the second day, patients underwent echocardiography measurements and cardiopulmonary exercise testing (CPET)."

"On the third day of hospitalization, following the measurements of pulse wave velocity (PWV) and the assessment of the use of RESPeRATE® device patients were discharged home."

"Each patient underwent CPET three times over the duration of the study (at baseline, 3- and 6-month follow-up) using the Ergocard Exercise Testing System (Medisoft, Belgium)."

"Patients were asked not to perform intensive exercise for at least 48 h prior to test."

"On the first day, prior to 24-h ABPM and Holter ECG, patients underwent baseline continuous beat-to-beat measurements of BP, HR, respiration and saturation (ADInstruments, Dual Bio Amp; ADInstruments, Ltd. Oxford, UK) over a 20-min duration followed by a 15-min duration of SLOWB with the use of RESPeRATE device."

"All patients were asked to repeat all tests after 3 months of SLOWB home exercise during a 3-day hospitalization."

Results

"SLOWB significantly increased peak RER from baseline to 3-month (1.16 ± 0.08 vs 1.23 ± 0.14, $P < 0.05$) follow-up."

"No changes were observed in PVO_2 (14.3 ± 5.3 vs 13.4 ± 4.9 ml/kg/min, $P = 0.14$) and VE/Vco_2 slope (37.7 ± 7.4 vs 37.3 ± 8.7, $P = 0.84$) from baseline to 3-month follow-up."

"No patients experienced worsening, hospital admission or death for HF from baseline to 6-month follow-up (Group 1)."

Discussion

"The present study is the first to demonstrate the 6-month effects of device-guided SLOWB home training in stable patients with severe HFrEF, all of whom received evidence-based treatment including optimal multi-drug therapy, implementable devices and surgical procedures, if required."

"The major findings are that (1) acute SLOWB improves oxygen saturation and (2) long-term SLOWB home training increases cardiorespiratory capacity, functional performance and vagal activity in high-risk patients with severe HFrEF irrespective of the underlying aetiology (i.e. ischemic and nonischemic HF)."

"Our study suggests that SLOWB, with the use of RESPeRATE, if applied adequately (i.e. therapeutic breathing rate < 10 breaths/min achieved daily and synchronised with guiding tones as recommended in the RESPeRATE's built-in memory stores) can slow the progression of severe HFrEF in patients on optimal medical therapy, irrespective of the underlying aetiology of HF."

Cardiac Remodeling Following Reperfused Acute Myocardial Infarction Is Linked to the Concomitant Evolution of Vascular Function as Assessed by Cardiovascular Magnetic Resonance [194]

This is a machine-generated summary of:

Huttin, Olivier; Mandry, Damien; Eschalier, Romain; Zhang, Lin; Micard, Emilien; Odille, Freddy; Beaumont, Marine; Fay, Renaud; Felblinger, Jacques; Camenzind, Edoardo; Zannad, Faïez; Girerd, Nicolas; Marie, Pierre Y.: Cardiac remodeling following reperfused acute myocardial infarction is linked to the concomitant evolution of vascular function as assessed by cardiovascular magnetic resonance [194].

Published in: Journal of Cardiovascular Magnetic Resonance (2017).

Link to original: https://doi.org/10.1186/s12968-016-0314-6

If you want to cite the papers, please refer to the original.

For technical reasons we could not place the page where the original quote is coming from.

Abstract-Summary "Left ventricular (LV) remodeling following acute myocardial infarction (MI) is difficult to predict at an individual level although a possible interfering role of vascular function has yet to be considered to date."

"This study aimed to determine the extent to which this LV remodeling is influenced by the concomitant evolution of vascular function and LV loading conditions, as assessed by phase-contrast Cardiovascular Magnetic Resonance (CMR) of the ascending aorta."

"LV remodeling was: (i) assessed by the 6-month increase in end-diastolic volume (EDV) and/or ejection fraction (EF) and (ii) correlated with the indexed aortic stroke volume ($mL.m^{-2}$), determined by a CMR phase-contrast sequence, along with derived functional vascular parameters (total peripheral vascular resistance (TPVR), total arterial compliance index, effective arterial elastance)."

"At 6 months, most patients were under angiotensin enzyme converting inhibitors (86%) and beta-blockers (84%) and, on average, all functional vascular parameters were improved whereas blood pressure levels were not."

"LV remodeling following reperfused MI is strongly influenced by the variable decrease in systemic vascular resistance under standard care vasodilating medication."

"The CMR monitoring of vascular resistance may help to tailor these medications for improving vascular resistance and consequently, LV ejection fraction."

Background

"Aortic stroke volume (SV), along with derived functional vascular parameters, can also be assessed with phase-contrast CMR, independently of LV volume values and with an accuracy level that is not reached by Doppler techniques [195]."

"This vascular monitoring has yet to be investigated in the context of LV remodeling following reperfused acute MI and where patients are commonly referred to hypotensive medical regimens (angiotensin converting enzyme (ACE) inhibitors, beta-blockers)."

"These medications are indeed likely to influence blood pressure and vascular function and thereby, LV wall stress, a main stimulus for adverse LV remodeling [196]."

"In light of the above, the present study was aimed at determining the extent to which vascular function and LV loading conditions, assessed through an aortic phase-contrast CMR sequence, and their changes over time influences LV remodeling following reperfused MI."

Methods

"The study population was extracted from the single-center "REMI" (relation between aldosterone and cardiac REmodeling after Myocardial Infarction) cohort in which serial CMR and biomarker measurements were performed after reperfused acute MI [197, 198]."

"The MI area was analyzed on 8 to 10 short axis slices covering the LV volume and two vertical and horizontal long-axis slices, which were recorded with a T1-weighted segmented phase-sensitive inversion-recovery (PSIR) sequence 10 to 15 min after the injection of a gadolinium-labeled tracer (0.1 $mmol.kg^{-1}$ of body weight of Dotarem®, GUERBET, France) with the following parameters: 4.7/2.1 msec for TR/TE, a typical 250–350 msec inversion time adjusted to null the signal of the non-infarcted myocardium, 28–35 cm field-of-view, 192 × 128 matrix interpolated to 256 × 256, 8 mm slice-thickness and 20° flip angle."

Results

"An abnormally high TPVR (>40 mmHg.min.m^2.L^{-1}) was documented in as many as 56 patients at baseline (46%) and was still present in 27 (22%) at 6 months ($p < 0.001$)."

"The strongest multivariate correlates for the 6-month increase in EF were the concomitant change in TPVR ($p < 0.001$) and baseline EF ($p = 0.028$) (global $R^2 = 0.40$), while the strongest correlates for the 6-month increase in EDV were baseline stroke work ($p = 0.019$) and presence of microvascular obstruction at baseline ($p = 0.001$) (global $R^2 = 0.21$)."

"The two main observations are that i) the increase in EF was strongly linked to a concomitant decline in TPVR (6-month change in mmHg.min.m^2.L^{-1}, EDV−/EF−: +1 ± 8, EDV+/EF−: +3 ± 9, EDV−/EF+: −7 ± 6, EDV+/EF+: −15 ± 20, $p < 0.001$) and ii) the absence of EF improvement was associated with high persistent rates of abnormally high TPVR at 6 months (EDV−/EF−: 31%, EDV+/EF−: 38%, EDV−/EF+: 5%, EDV+/EF+: 13%, $p = 0.007$)."

Discussion

"Indexed stroke work, calculated by the product of mean BP and indexed SV, provides an indication of the aortic flow that can potentially be generated by the LV at sufficiently high pressure and has been indubitably recognized as a strong prognostic indicator in patients with severe MI and/or heart failure [199, 200]."

"The 6-month change in TPVR was selected as the strongest independent correlate of the concomitant enhancement in LV ejection fraction, together with the baseline level of ejection fraction, with these two variables accounting for up to 40% (corresponding to the R^2 value) of the significant increases in ejection fraction at 6 months."

"These SSFP-SV values were not used in our analyses in order to avoid their interdependence with the remodeling-related changes in LV volumes which were assessed with the same LV contours."

Conclusions

"The present study shows that LV remodeling following reperfused MI is linked to the concomitant evolution of loading conditions and particularly to the variable decrease in vascular resistance under standard care cardiovascular medication."

"It is likely that the non-invasive CMR monitoring of vascular resistance may help to tailor these medications in order to improve vascular resistance and consequently, LV ejection fraction."

Effects of SGLT2 Inhibitors on Cardiac Structure and Function [201]

This is a machine-generated summary of:

Novo, Giuseppina; Guarino, Tommaso; Di Lisi, Daniela; Biagioli, Paolo; Carluccio, Erberto: Effects of SGLT2 inhibitors on cardiac structure and function [201].

Published in: Heart Failure Reviews (2022).

Link to original: https://doi.org/10.1007/s10741-022-10256-4

If you want to cite the papers, please refer to the original.

For technical reasons we could not place the page where the original quote is coming from.

Abstract-Summary "In patients with HF and preserved EF, empagliflozin also showed favorable effects mainly related to the reduction of hospitalization for heart failure."

"These favorable effects are beyond the reduction of glycemic levels and mainly related to beneficial hemodynamic and anti-inflammatory effects of these drugs and improved cardiac energy metabolism."

SGLT2 Inhibitors and Heart Failure

"Starting from this background, recent studies reported the ability of dapaglifozin (DAPA-HF trial) [202] and of empaglifozin (EMPEROR-Reduced trial) [203] to reduce cardiovascular death and worsening heart failure in patients with HFrEF (left ventricular ejection fraction $\leq$ 40%) in addition to optimized medical therapy (GDT) and independently from glycemic status and presence of diabetes."

"Beyond patients with stable chronic HFrEF, a beneficial prognostic role of SGLT2 inhibitors has also been observed, in patients with recent worsening HF: indeed, in the SOLOIST-WHF trial, sotaglifozin, a dual SGLT1 and -2 inhibitor, proved to significantly reduce by 33% the risk of the composite end-point of cardiovascular death, HF hospitalizations, and urgent visits for HF, in a broad range of HF patients, including those with preserved ejection fraction (HFpEF) [204, 205]."

"Given the early reductions in HF hospitalization but not atherosclerosis-related events observed with SGLT2 inhibitors in the landmark trials, it is possible that the positive results on prognosis observed with these drugs might be related to early favorable hemodynamic effects on LV function rather than through modulation of atherothrombotic mechanisms [206, 207]."

Reverse Remodeling in Heart Failure

"Several studies have investigated the effects of SGLT2 inhibitors on LV remodeling with the aim to evaluate whether the beneficial prognostic effects of these drugs in HFrEF patients could have been mediated by a positive effect on LV volumes and shape."

"In this trial, non-diabetic HFrEF patients randomized to empagliflozin ($n = 40$) had a significant reduction of LV end-diastolic volume (-25.1 ± 26.0 ml vs. -1.5 ± 25.4 ml; $P < 0.001$) and LV end-systolic volume (-26.6 ± 20.5 ml vs. -0.5 ± 21.9 ml; $P < 0.001$) compared to placebo."

"A decrease in LV end-systolic and end-diastolic volume to a similar extent has also been reported by Lee and coworkers [208] in patients with type-2 diabetes and HFrEF enrolled in the SUGAR-DM-HF trial [Studies of Empagliflozin and Its Cardiovascular, Renal and Metabolic Effects in Patients with Diabetes Mellitus, or Prediabetes, and Heart Failure]."

Systolic Function

"Non-randomized studies in patients with normal systolic function at baseline failed to demonstrate a beneficial effect of SGLT2 inhibitors on LV EF [209–215]."

"The effects of SGLT2 inhibitors on LV systolic function become more evident in patients with HFrEF with or without diabetes mellitus."

"Studies evaluating GLS in patients with diabetes treated with SGLT2 inhibitors confirm that these drugs improve subclinical LV dysfunction and prevent LV function deterioration."

"Improved values of GLS, in the CMR study, resulted after treatment with empaglifozin ($10.2\% \pm 2.9\%$ at baseline vs $13.1\% \pm 4.1\%$ at follow-up, $p = 0.01$), in patients with type II diabetes mellitus patients [216]."

"In the setting of diabetic patients with HF, SGLT2 inhibitors mainly showed favorable results on longitudinal function; however, the results varied depending on the type of the studied population."

Structural and Functional Changes Induced by SGLT2 Inhibitor Therapy

"The possibility that the cardiovascular benefits of SGLT2 inhibition may be secondary to a reduction in LVM has been investigated by several studies."

"While the reduction in LVM in response to SGLT2 inhibitor therapy has been reported in other small and non-randomized studies in patients with type-2 diabetes with or without HF [210, 211, 215, 217], it has not been confirmed by other authors [209, 214]."

"Although it could be supposed that the regression of LVM might also be mediated by the hypotensive effect of SGLT2 inhibitors, in the EMPA-HEART trial, the change in 24-h ambulatory blood pressure was not associated with the change in LVM over the 6 months [218], suggesting that the observed reduction in LVM could be independent of blood pressure reduction and that other mechanisms may be involved in the LVM regression noted after empagliflozin exposure."

Diastolic Function

"An improvement of diastolic function with a reduction of left ventricular filling pressure on animal models [219] and humans was observed with SGLT2 inhibitor treatment."

"Higashikawa and others [220] investigated diastolic function after treatment with tofoglifozin, in elderly (≥65 years old) diabetic patients with HFpEF; all the main parameters evaluating diastolic function resulted improved, but no differences were found in LVEF."

"In diabetic patients treated with SGLT2 inhibitor dapaglifozin, during exercise stress, it was reported a significant reduction in right ventricular systolic pressure and in left ventricular filling pressure at 6-month follow-up compared to baseline, whether no changes in left ventricular systolic function was observed [221]."

"In the IDDIA trial, stress echocardiography detected a better diastolic function with lower left ventricular filling pressure (E/e') during stress, after a year of treatment."

Epicardial Adipose Tissue (EAT)

"Epicardial adipose tissue thickness is a real endocrine organ able to produce cytokines that can increase cardiovascular risk severity [222]."

"It can be easily assessed non-invasively through echocardiography and it can be used as a prognostic factor, also during SGLT2 inhibitor therapy."

"In diabetic patients, canaglifozin was associated with a reduction of epicardial adipose tissue thickness, demonstrating the multiple roles of these drugs on the total cardiovascular burden [223]."

Conclusions

"SGLT2 inhibitors became a cornerstone in the treatment of HFrEF thanks to their favorable effects demonstrated in reducing cardiovascular death and worsening heart failure (3–4); moreover, they reasonably could become recommended drugs for treating HFpEF [224]."

"These drugs seem to have favorable effects on cardiac remodeling and function."

"Studies demonstrated the effect of SGLT2 inhibitors in reducing LV mass and improving diastolic function [210, 215, 217, 225]."

"A gap in knowledge still exists regarding the effects of SGLT2 inhibitors on LV function and remodeling and on the mechanisms underlying these effects and it is desirable to fill it that large randomized clinical trial is carried out."

The Influence of Anti-hyperglycemic Drug Therapy on Cardiovascular and Heart Failure Outcomes in Patients with Type 2 Diabetes Mellitus [226]

This is a machine-generated summary of:

Asleh, Rabea; Sheikh-Ahmad, Mohammad; Briasoulis, Alexandros; Kushwaha, Sudhir S.: The influence of anti-hyperglycemic drug therapy on cardiovascular and heart failure outcomes in patients with type 2 diabetes mellitus [226].

Published in: Heart Failure Reviews (2017).

Link to original: https://doi.org/10.1007/s10741-017-9666-8

If you want to cite the papers, please refer to the original.

For technical reasons we could not place the page where the original quote is coming from.

Abstract-Summary "Patients with type 2 diabetes mellitus (DM) are at a substantially increased risk of heart failure (HF) and HF mortality."

"Despite the lack of evidence that tight glycemic control reduces the incidence of cardiovascular (CV) events, a growing body of evidence suggests that the choice of glucose-lowering agents may influence outcomes including HF."

"The sodium-glucose cotransporter 2 (SGLT2) inhibitors, empagliflozin and canagliflozin, have been recently shown to reduce the incidence of HF and cardiovascular mortality in patients with and without a history of HF."

"This review will summarize key findings of the impact of glucose-lowering agents on CV safety and HF-associated outcomes, present available data on the underlying mechanisms for the benefits of the SGLT2 inhibitors on HF, and discuss strategies to improve outcomes in patients with DM and high CV risk."

Introduction

"Diabetes mellitus (DM) is associated with a substantial increased risk of heart failure (HF), cardiovascular (CV) disease, and mortality [227]."

"HF has not been included within the primary endpoints in cardiovascular (CV) safety trials of glucose-lowering drug therapies."

"The focus on glycemic control effects of glucose-lowering agents has also added to the uncertainty of the impact of these agents on HF outcomes."

"In light of the implication of thiazolidinedione in fluid retention and associated HF exacerbation as well as the suggestive driven effect of some of the new glucose-lowering drugs on HF, most current trials do now include hospitalization for HF as a secondary endpoint."

Epidemiology

"According to the Framingham study, the risk of HF in DM patients is 2.4-fold higher in men and 5-fold higher in women as compared to non-DM individuals after adjustment for other risk factors including age, hypertension, obesity, dyslipidemia, and coronary artery disease [228]."

"In patients with DM, the prevalence of HF is greater than that of the general population, and as high as 22% of patients with DM over the age of 65 develop HF [229]."

"Among adult patients with DM, a 1% increase in hemoglobin A_{1C} levels is associated with an 8% increased risk of HF, independent of blood pressure, obesity, age and the presence of coronary artery disease, suggesting DM as an independent risk for incident HF [230]."

"DM patients have a 2–3-fold increased risk of developing HF after MI [231]."

Pathophysiology of Heart Failure in Diabetes

"The underlying pathophysiology of HF in DM is multifactorial but can largely be attributed to diabetic cardiomyopathy, hypertension, coronary artery disease, and extracellular fluid volume expansion [232]."

"Diabetic cardiomyopathy is manifested as abnormal cardiac structure and function in the absence of ischemic or hypertensive heart disease in individuals with DM."

"Insulin resistance, hyperinsulinemia, and hyperglycemia are central metabolic perturbations that accompany type 2 DM and are independently associated with the development of diabetic cardiomyopathy."

"Patients with HF develop marked insulin resistance that increases the risk of developing type 2 DM [233]."

Effects of Intensive Glucose-Lowering Therapies and Heart Failure

"The UKPDS was the first study to test the impact of long-term glycemic control on HF risk among patients with newly diagnosed diabetes, showing a log-linear relation with a 16% reduction in the risk of HF for each 1% reduction in hemoglobin A_{1C} level [234, 235]."

"Despite a significant risk reduction of MI and all-cause mortality events in the 10-year UKPDS follow-up [236], there was no association between tight glycemic control and risk reduction of HF hospitalization or HF mortality (HR 0.93, 95% CI 0.63–1.38, P = NS)."

"The ACCORD [237], ADVANCE [238], and VADT [239] trials enrolling nearly 25,000 patients have shown that intensive blood-glucose lowering had no effect on HF-associated events (ADVANCE: HR 0.95, 95% CI 0.86–1.21, ACCORD: HR 1.18, 95% CI, 0.93–1.49; P = NS)."

"The VADT was the only study included HF incidence as a primary endpoint showing no effect of tight glycemic control on risk of HF (HR 0.93, 95% CI 0.67–1.29, P = NS)."

Differential Effects of Anti-Hyperglycemic Drug Classes on Heart Failure Outcomes

"A study from Cleveland Clinic included 20,540 DM patients treated either with metformin, thiazolidinedione, or a sulphonylurea found that patients who received metformin were at lower HF risk than those treated with a sulphonylurea (adjusted HR 0.76, 95% CI 0.64–0.91; P = 0.003) [240]."

"After a 3.8-year follow-up, the rate of primary endpoint (composite of CV death, nonfatal MI and nonfatal stroke) was significantly lower among patients with liraglutide than those with placebo (HR 0.87, 95% CI 0.78–0.97; P = 0.01 for superiority)."

"A growing body of evidence from recent clinical trials supports a remarkable improvement in CV outcomes including hospitalization for HF with SGLT2 inhibitors among high-risk patients with type 2 DM and established CV disease."

"Compared with other glucose-lowering drugs, use of SGLT2 inhibitors was associated with decreased risk of CV mortality, MACE, and hospitalization for HF in over 90,000 patients with type 2 DM [241]."

Clinical Implications and Future Strategies of Care

"Because most patients with type 2 DM develop CV disease and are frequently encountered in cardiology practice, it is essential to consider initiation and titration of new glucose-lowering drugs that have been demonstrated to exert CV benefits."

"As diabetologists participate in reducing CV outcomes in the DM population by prescribing statins and anti-hypertensive medications to high-risk patients, cardiologist should also be aware of the potential benefits of the newly investigated anti-hyperglycemic drugs that have favorable CV effects in such patients."

"Identifying new patients with DM will enable an earlier initiation of new therapies that have CV advantages."

"Metformin is the first-line therapy in the majority of DM patients, but strategies may be changed in the future toward using new therapies that not only lower blood glucose but also reduce CV risk."

Conclusions

"DM is associated with a substantial increased risk of incident CV disease including incident HF, HF hospitalization, and CV death."

"One RCT on glargine indicated CV safety by showing neutral effects on both HF and MACE."

"Of the impact of the three major DPP-4 inhibitors on HF, saxagliptin showed an increased risk of hospitalization for HF in the whole study cohort, alogliptin was associated with higher rates of new hospitalizations for HF, while sitagliptin had a neutral effect."

"These promising findings may provide a new therapeutic strategy to reduce the risk and slow progression of HF among patients with DM and high CV risk."

"Future studies will further clarify the impact of SGLT2 inhibitors on risk and progression of HF and future large-scale clinical trials will address the therapeutic benefit of these drugs in patients with low CV risk, in non-DM individuals and in patients with established HF."

Impact of Sacubitril/Valsartan on Lipid Parameters in Patients with Heart Failure with Reduced Ejection Fraction [242]

This is a machine-generated summary of:

Barman, Hasan Ali; Tanyolaç, Selim; Dogan, Omer; Bal, Erdem; Atıcı, Adem; Özyıldırım, Serhan; Yiğit, Zerrin: Impact of Sacubitril/Valsartan on Lipid Parameters in Patients with Heart Failure with Reduced Ejection Fraction [242].

Published in: Clinical Drug Investigation (2022).

Link to original: https://doi.org/10.1007/s40261-022-01161-7

If you want to cite the papers, please refer to the original.

For technical reasons we could not place the page where the original quote is coming from.

Abstract-Summary "This study aims to investigate the long-term impact of the sacubitril/valsartan combination on lipid parameters in patients with heart failure with reduced ejection fraction."

"Single-center retrospective cross-sectional study, data of patients using sacubitril/valsartan because of heart failure with reduced ejection fraction were collected."

"A total of 192 patients with a functional capacity New York Heart Association II–V, and who were using sacubitril/valsartan because of heart failure with reduced ejection fraction, were included in this study."

"Sacubitril/valsartan in patients with heart failure with reduced ejection fraction, independent of statin use, may cause a decrease in total cholesterol and triglyceride levels and an improvement in high-density lipoprotein cholesterol levels."

Introduction

"Previous studies have reported the relative contribution of risk factors to the development of HF, and they have shown that hypertension, coronary artery disease, diabetes mellitus, and dyslipidemia are strongly associated with the development of HF [12–14]."

"Statins commonly used in the treatment of dyslipidemia have been shown to reduce adverse events associated with HF in primary and secondary prevention studies on patients with HF with and without coronary artery disease [243]."

"Sacubitril/valsartan, an angiotensin receptor-neprilysin inhibitor, has been shown to significantly reduce cardiovascular mortality, hospitalizations, and all-cause mortality in HF with reduced ejection fraction (HFrEF) [85]."

"Considering the underlying etiology of coronary artery disease and comorbid conditions such as diabetes, hypertension, and hyperlipidemia in two-thirds of the patients with HF, the metabolic effects of the molecule used in treatment are also important."

"Although the positive effects of angiotensin receptor blockers on lipids are known, there are not enough studies on the sacubitril/valsartan combination."

Patients and Methods

"One hundred and ninety-two patients with a functional capacity New York Heart Association II–IV, and who were using sacubitril/valsartan because of HFrEF between February 2016 and March 2018, were included in this study."

"The lipid levels in these patients were measured at 3-month intervals."

"The New York Heart Association functional classification was used to describe the severity of symptoms and exercise intolerance, and two cardiologists classified patients with HF according to the severity of their symptoms."

"The changes in the lipid levels in the patients were tested using an analysis of variance and/or Friedman analysis in repeated measurements according to the distribution of the data."

"The patients were compared by dividing them into two groups according to whether they used statins."

"TC, HDL-C, TG, and NT-proBNP levels over 3 years were compared with baseline levels in the statin-using and statin-free groups."

Results

"There were fewer female patients and a lower mean age in the statin-using group: 30 out of 102 patients in the statin-using group were female (29%), and 41 out of 90 patients in the statin-free group were female (45%), which was a statistically significant difference ($p = 0.021$)."

"While the mean age of patients in the statin-using group was 64.3 ± 7.9 years, the mean age of patients in the statin-free group was 68.0 ± 11.4 years, which was a statistically significant difference ($p = 0.009$)."

"The decrease in these levels was statistically significant ($p < 0.001$)."

"The decrease in TC and TG levels was statistically significant compared to baseline levels ($p < 0.001$)."

"NT-proBNP levels decreased every year, which was statistically significant ($p < 0.05$)."

Discussion

"We investigated the changes in lipid levels in patients with HFrEF who received sacubitril/valsartan treatment during a long-term follow-up."

"The main results of this study are as follows: (1) the use of sacubitril/valsartan in patients with HFrEF, independent of statin use, decreased TC and TG levels; (2) the use of sacubitril/valsartan in patients with HFrEF, independent of statin use, increased HDL-C levels; and (3) the use of sacubitril/valsartan in patients with HFrEF decreased NT-proBNP levels."

"Of the PARAGON-HF study, which included patients with HF with preserved ejection fraction, a significant decrease in TG levels and a slight increase in HDL and low-density lipoprotein levels were found with sacubitril/valsartan treatment [244]."

"The use of sacubitril/valsartan in patients with HFrEF, independent of statin use, resulted in a decrease in TC and TG levels, and an increase in HDL-C levels."

Conclusions

"The use of sacubitril/valsartan in patients with HFrEF, independent of statin use, resulted in a decrease in TC and TG levels and an improvement in HDL-C levels."

"Large randomized clinical trials are needed to confirm the beneficial clinical and metabolic effects of sacubitril/valsartan."

From Clinical Trials to Bedside: The Use of Antihypertensives in Aged Individuals. Part 1: Evaluation and Evidence of Treatment Benefit [245]

This is a machine-generated summary of:

MacLaughlin, Eric J.; Ernst, Michael E.: From Clinical Trials to Bedside: the Use of Antihypertensives in Aged Individuals. Part 1: Evaluation and Evidence of Treatment Benefit [245].

Published in: Current Hypertension Reports (2019).

Link to original: https://doi.org/10.1007/s11906-019-0987-y

If you want to cite the papers, please refer to the original.

For technical reasons we could not place the page where the original quote is coming from.

Abstract-Summary "In part 1, we discuss the evaluation of the aged hypertensive patient and review the clinical trial evidence for treatment benefit of hypertension in the elderly."

"Elderly patients with suspected hypertension need careful evaluation of their blood pressure, as errors in measurement technique, inaccurate devices, or overreliance on office blood pressure readings may lead to under- or over-treatment, thereby increasing risks of adverse medication effects and/or cardiovascular events."

"Key prospective hypertension trials such as HYVET and SPRINT, which were focused in mostly healthy, community-dwelling elderly cohorts, have unequivocally demonstrated benefits of lowering blood pressure in reducing cardiovascular events in the very elderly."

"Hypertension is a major modifiable risk factor and the benefits of treatment in lowering cardiovascular events are realized for most individuals, even at advanced ages."

Introduction

"While benefits observed in clinical trials predominately populated with younger and middle-aged individuals would generally be expected to extend to older individuals sharing the same disease processes, advancing age produces a heterogenous spectrum of phenotypes ranging from robust to frail, and the approach to management of hypertension in older individuals must reflect these individualized considerations."

"Because there is no consensus definition for "elderly," "aged," or "older" individuals with respect to hypertension (although generally, clinical trials have recognized subjects aged 60–79 years as "old" and those 80 years and older as "very old"), this review is written with attention to the biologic or phenotype of the aged hypertensive rather than restricted to an exclusive chronological age categorization."

"Issues addressed in this review are most likely to be commonly encountered in those aged 75 years and older, as these are the widely heterogenous group for which the risks and benefits of treatment are finely balanced and individualization of treatment is most warranted."

Pathophysiology of the Aging Hypertensive and Implications for Treatment

"Blood pressure patterns in older individuals are predominated by the high prevalence of isolated systolic hypertension, characterized by the increase in systolic blood pressure accompanied by a fall in diastolic blood pressure, and a widening of pulse pressure [246]."

"Because all antihypertensives have the potential to lower both systolic and diastolic blood pressure, the drop in diastolic blood pressure in older individuals can adversely impact coronary blood flow."

"In younger individuals, coronary artery blood flow is enhanced by the boost in central aortic pressure provided by the reflected arterial wave in diastole [247]."

"As this boost is lost in older adults, those with underlying coronary ischemia may be particularly susceptible to the effects of antihypertensives in lowering the diastolic blood pressure."

"Epidemiologic observations of a U-shaped curve showing higher mortality in older persons with lower blood pressure further complicate treatment decisions in elderly [248]."

Importance of Appropriate Blood Pressure Measurement in Older Adults

"Appropriate blood pressure measurement and monitoring for the diagnosis and management of hypertension, while important for all patients with high blood pressure, is critical in aged individuals."

"Older patients with high blood pressure typically have isolated systolic hypertension and widened pulse pressure due to increased arterial stiffening."

"Another aspect when considering blood pressure measurement in older patients, particularly those with increased levels of frailty, is an assessment for possible orthostatic hypotension."

"Detection of white coat hypertension (WCH), which is when blood pressure readings in the office setting are elevated but not outside the clinic setting [249], while critical in all patients with hypertension, is particularly noteworthy in older individuals."

"Masked hypertension (MH), which is when blood pressure is normal in the clinic setting but elevated outside the clinic and is associated with a significant increase in the risk of CV events [249], is common in the elderly."

Evidence for Treatment Benefit in Aged Hypertensives

"SPRINT was designed to assess if intensive BP lowering (SBP < 120 mmHg) was more effective in reducing CV outcomes than standard BP lowering (SBP < 140 mmHg) in patients who had a SBP of > 130 mmHg and either had CVD or were at high-risk of ASCVD [250]."

"SPRINT was stopped early after a mean follow-up of 3.26 years due a 25% decrease risk in the primary composite outcome of MI, other ACS, stroke, HF, or death from CV causes (NNT = 61) and 27% decrease in all-cause mortality (NNT = 90) associated with intensive BP lowering."

"Results of the SPRINT Memory and Cognition IN Decreased hypertension (SPRINT MIND) study found that while intensive BP lowering did not result in a statistically significant reduction in the primary outcome of adjudicated probable dementia, it was associated with a reduced risk of mild cognitive impairment (MCI; 19%, $p = 0.01$) and MCI plus probable dementia (15%, $p = 0.02$) [251]."

Conclusion

"Hypertension is widely prevalent in older patients, with most developing high blood pressure as they advance in age."

"Older patients have a higher risk of hypotension and adverse effects of treatment compared with younger hypertensive individuals."

"Out-of-office measurements can be beneficial to assess patients with, or at risk for, high blood pressure, and monitoring of therapy."

"Data from well-done randomized controlled trials have unequivocally demonstrated that treating high blood pressure, even in the very elderly, decreases the risk of adverse cardiovascular events."

Bibliography

1. Bevan GH, White Solaru KT (2020) Evidence-based medical management of peripheral artery disease. Arterioscler Thromb Vasc Biol 40(3):541–553
2. Campia U, Gerhard-Herman M, Piazza G, Goldhaber SZ (2019) Peripheral artery disease: past, present, and future. Am J Med 132(10):1133–1141
3. Yusuf S, Sleight P, Pogue J, Bosch J, Davies R, Dagenais G, Heart Outcomes Prevention Evaluation Study Investigators (2000) Effects of an angiotensin-converting-enzyme inhibitor, ramipril, on cardiovascular events in high-risk patients. N Engl J Med 342:145–153. https://doi.org/10.1056/NEJM200001203420301
4. Yusuf S, Teo KK, Pogue J, Dyal L, Copland I, Schumacher H, Dagenais G, Sleight P, Anderson C, ONTARGET Investigators (2008) Telmisartan, ramipril, or both in patients at high risk for vascular events. N Engl J Med 358:1547–1559. https://doi.org/10.1056/NEJMoa0801317
5. Aboyans V, Ricco JB, Bartelink MEL, Björck M, Brodmann M, Cohnert T, Collet JP, Czerny M, De Carlo M, Debus S, Espinola-Klein C, Kahan T, Kownator S, Mazzolai L, Naylor AR, Roffi M, Röther J, Sprynger M, Tendera M, Tepe G, Venermo M, Vlachopoulos C, Desormais I, ESC Scientific Document Group (2018) 2017 ESC guidelines on the diagnosis and treatment of peripheral arterial diseases, in collaboration with the European Society for Vascular Surgery (ESVS): document covering atherosclerotic disease of extracranial carotid and vertebral, mesenteric, renal, upper and lower extremity arteries. Endorsed by: the European Stroke Organization (ESO). The Task Force for the Diagnosis and Treatment of Peripheral Arterial Diseases of the European Society of Cardiology (ESC) and of the European Society for Vascular Surgery (ESVS). Eur Heart J 39(9):763–816. https://doi.org/10.1093/eurheartj/ehx095
6. Gerhard-Herman MD, Gornik HL, Barrett C, Barshes NR, Corriere MA, Drachman DE, Fleisher LA, Fowkes FG, Hamburg NM, Kinlay S et al (2017) 2016 AHA/ACC guideline on the management of patients with lower extremity peripheral artery disease: executive summary: a report of the American College of Cardiology/American Heart Association task force on clinical practice guidelines. Circulation 135:e686–e725
7. Zanchetti A, Julius S, Kjeldsen S, McInnes GT, Hua T, Weber M, Laragh JH, Plat F, Battegay E, Calvo-Vargas C et al (2006) Outcomes in subgroups of hypertensive patients treated with regimens based on valsartan and amlodipine: an analysis of findings from the VALUE trial. J Hypertens 24:2163–2168. https://doi.org/10.1097/01.hjh.0000249692.96488.46
8. Piller LB, Simpson LM, Baraniuk S, Habib GB, Rahman M, Basile JN, Dart RA, Ellsworth AJ, Fendley H, Probstfield JL et al (2014) ALLHAT Collaborative Research Group. Characteristics and long-term follow-up of participants with peripheral arterial disease during ALLHAT. J Gen Intern Med 29:1475–1483. https://doi.org/10.1007/s11606-014-2947-1
9. Clement DL (2009) Treatment of hypertension in patients with peripheral arterial disease: an update. Curr Sci Inc 11:271–276
10. Trimarco B, Santoro C, Pepe M et al (2017) The benefit of angiotensin AT1 receptor blockers for early treatment of hypertensive patients. Intern Emerg Med 12:1093–1099. https://doi.org/10.1007/s11739-017-1713-x
11. Cespón-Fernández M, Raposeiras-Roubín S, Abu-Assi E, Manzano-Fernández S, Flores-Blanco P, Barreiro-Pardal C, Castiñeira-Busto M, Muñoz-Pousa I, López-Rodríguez E, Caneiro-Queija B, Cobas-Paz R, Fernández-Barbeira S, Domínguez-Erquicia P, Domínguez-Rodríguez LM, López-Cuenca Á, Gómez-Molina M, Baz-Alonso JA, Calvo-Iglesias F, Valdés-Chávarri M, Íñiguez-Romo A (2019) Renin-angiotensin system blockade and risk of heart failure after myocardial infarction based on left ventricular ejection fraction: a retrospective cohort study. Am J Cardiovasc Drugs 19(5):487–495. https://doi.org/10.1007/s40256-019-00343-7
12. Fourth International Study of Infarct Survival Collaborative Group. ISIS-4 (1995) A randomized factorial trial assessing oral captopril, oral mononitrate, and intravenous magnesium sulphate in 58,050 patients with suspected acute myocardial infarction. Lancet 345:669–685

13. GISSI-3: Gruppo Italiano per lo Studio della Sopravvivenza nell'infarto Miocardico (1994) Effects of lisinopril and transdermal glyceryl trinitrate singly and together on 6-week mortality and ventricular function after acute myocardial infarction. Lancet 343(8906):1115–1122
14. Pfeffer MA, Braunwald E, Moyé LA et al (1992) Effect of captopril on mortality and morbidity in patients with left ventricular dysfunction after myocardial infarction: results of the survival and ventricular enlargement trial. N Engl J Med 327(10):669–677. https://doi.org/10.1056/NEJM199209033271001
15. Kober L, Torp-Pedersen C, Carlsen JE, Bagger H, Eliasen P, Lyngborg K et al (1995) A clinical trial of the angiotensin-converting-enzyme inhibitor trandolapril in patients with left ventricular dysfunction after myocardial infarction. Trandolapril Cardiac Evaluation (TRACE) Study Group. N Engl J Med 333:1670–1676
16. Cleland JG, Erhardt L, Murray G, Hall AS, Ball SG (1997) Effect of ramipril on morbidity and mode of death among survivors of acute myocardial infarction with clinical evidence of heart failure. A report from the AIRE Study Investigators. Eur Heart J 18(1):41–51
17. Granger CB, McMurray JJ, Yusuf S et al (2003) Effects of candesartan in patients with chronic heart failure and reduced left-ventricular systolic function intolerant to angiotensin-converting-enzyme inhibitors: the CHARM-Alternative trial. Lancet 362:772–776
18. Dagenais GR, Yusuf S, Bourassa MG, Yi Q, Bosch J, Lonn EM et al (2001) Effects of ramipril on coronary events in high-risk persons: results of the Heart Outcomes Prevention Evaluation Study. Circulation 104(5):522–526
19. Yusuf S, Pitt B, Davis CE, Hood WB, Cohn JN (1991) Effect of enalapril on survival in patients with reduced left ventricular ejection fractions and congestive heart failure. N Engl J Med 325(5):293–302. https://doi.org/10.1056/NEJM199108013250501
20. The PREAMI Investigators (2006) Effect of angiotensin-converting enzyme inhibition with perindopril on left ventricular remodeling and clinical outcome. Results of the Randomized Perindopril and Remodeling in Elderly with Acute Myocardial Infarction (PREAMI) study. Arch Intern Med 166:659–666
21. Kjøller-Hansen L et al (2000) The angiotensin-converting enzyme inhibition post revascularization study (APRES). J Am Coll Cardiol 35:881–888
22. Dézsi CA, Szentes V (2016) Effects of angiotensin-converting enzyme inhibitors and angiotensin receptor blockers on prothrombotic processes and myocardial infarction risk. Am J Cardiovasc Drugs 16(6):399–406. https://doi.org/10.1007/s40256-016-0185-0
23. Willerson JT, Holmes DR Jr (eds) (2015) Coronary heart disease syndromes: pathophysiology and clinical recognition. In: Coronary artery disease. Springer, London. pp 365–407
24. Virmani R, Kolodgie FD, Burke AP et al (2000) Lessons from sudden coronary death: a comprehensive morphological classification scheme for atherosclerotic lesions. Arterioscler Thromb Vasc Biol 20(5):1262–1275
25. Santos-Gallego CG, Picatoste B, Badimón JJ (2014) Pathophysiology of acute coronary syndrome. Curr Atheroscler Rep 16(401):1–9. PMID: 24504549
26. Bentzon JF, Otsuka F, Virmani R, Falk E (2014) Mechanisms of plaque formation and rupture. Circ Res 114:1852–1866
27. Tofler GH, Muller JE (2006) Triggering of acute cardiovascular disease and potential preventive strategies. Circulation 114:1863–1872
28. White WB (2007) Clinical assessment of early morning blood pressure in patients with hypertension. Prev Cardiol 10:210–214
29. Feng DL, Tofler GH (1995) Diurnal physiologic processes and circadian variation of acute myocardial infarction. J Cardiovasc Risk 2(6):494–498
30. Takeda N, Maemura K (2011) Circadian clock and cardiovascular disease. J Cardiol 57(3):249–256
31. Angleton P, Chandler WL, Schmer G (1989) Diurnal variation of tissue-type plasminogen activator and its rapid inhibitor (PAI-1). Circulation 79:101–106

32. Fogari R, Mugellini A, Zoppi A et al (2002) Losartan and perindopril effects on plasma plasminogen activator inhibitor-1 and fibrinogen in hypertensive type 2 diabetic patients. Am J Hypertens 15(4 Pt 1):316–320
33. Remková A, Kratochvílová H, Ďurina J (2008) Impact of the therapy by renin–angiotensin system targeting antihypertensive agents perindopril versus telmisartan on prothrombotic state in essential hypertension. J Human Hypertens 22:338–345
34. Ferrari R, Boersma E (2013) The impact of ACE inhibition on all-cause and cardiovascular mortality in contemporary hypertension trials: a review. Expert Rev Cardiovasc Ther 11:705–717. https://doi.org/10.1586/erc.13.42
35. Ferrari R (2013) RAAS inhibition and mortality in hypertension. Glob Cardiol Sci Pract 3:269–278
36. Investigators O, Yusuf S, Teo KK, Pogue J, Dyal L, Copland I et al (2008) Telmisartan, ramipril, or both in patients at high risk for vascular events. N Engl J Med 358(15):1547–1559
37. Mancia G, Parati G, Bilo G et al (2012) Ambulatory blood pressure values in the Ongoing Telmisartan Alone and in Combination with Ramipril Global Endpoint Trial (ONTARGET). Hypertension 60(6):1400–1406
38. Task Force on the management of ST-segment elevation acute myocardial infarction of the European Society of Cardiology (ESC), Steg PG, James SK, Atar D, Badano LP, Blomstrom-Lundqvist C et al (2012) ESC guidelines for the management of acute myocardial infarction in patients presenting with ST-segment elevation. Eur Heart J 33(20):2569–2619
39. O'Gara PT et al (2012) 2013 ACCF/AHA guideline for the management of ST-elevation myocardial infarction: executive summary. Circulation 127:529–555
40. Song PS, Seol SH, Seo GW, Kim DK, Kim KH, Yang JH, Hahn JY, Gwon HC, Ahn Y, Jeong MH, Song YB, Kim DI, Other Korean Working Group in Myocardial Infarction Registry Investigators (2015) Comparative effectiveness of angiotensin II receptor blockers versus angiotensin-converting enzyme inhibitors following contemporary treatments in patients with acute myocardial infarction: results from the Korean Working Group in Myocardial Infarction (KorMI) Registry. Am J Cardiovasc Drugs 15(6):439–449. https://doi.org/10.1007/s40256-015-0140-5
41. O'Gara PT, Kushner FG, Ascheim DD et al (2013) 2013 ACCF/AHA guideline for the management of ST-elevation myocardial infarction: a report of the American College of Cardiology Foundation/American Heart Association task force on practice guidelines. Circulation 127:362–425
42. Amsterdam EA, Wenger NK, Brindis RG, Casey DE Jr, Ganiats TG, Holmes DR Jr, Jaffe AS, Jneid H, Kelly RF, Kontos MC, Levine GN, Liebson PR, Mukherjee D, Peterson ED, Sabatine MS, Smalling RW, Zieman SJ (2014) 2014 AHA/ACC guideline for the management of patients with non ST-elevation acute coronary syndromes: a report of the American College of Cardiology/American Heart Association task force on practice guidelines. J Am Coll Cardiol 64:S0735–S1097
43. Ferrari R, Rosano GM (2013) Not just numbers, but years of science: putting the ACE inhibitor—ARB meta-analyses into context. Int J Cardiol 166:286–288
44. Eagle KA, Lim MJ, Dabbous OH, Pieper KS, Goldberg RJ, Van de Werf F, Goodman SG, Granger CB, Steg PG, Gore JM, Budaj A, Avezum A, Flather MD, Fox KA (2004) A validated prediction model for all forms of acute coronary syndrome: estimating the risk of 6-month postdischarge death in an international registry. JAMA 291:2727–2733
45. Aronow WS (2020) Approaches for the management of resistant hypertension in 2020. Curr Hypertens Rep 22(1):3. https://doi.org/10.1007/s11906-019-1013-0
46. Whelton PK, Carey RM, Aronow WS, Casey DE Jr, Coillins KJ, Dennison Himmelfarb C et al (2018) 2017 ACC/AHA/AAPA/ABC/ACPM/AGS/APhA/ASH ASPC/NMA/PCNA guideline for the prevention, detection, evaluation and management of high blood pressure in adults. A report of the American College of Cardiology/American Heart Association task force on clinical practice guidelines. J Am Coll Cardiol 71:e127–e248. These guidelines discuss the management of resistant hypertension

47. Thompson AM, Hu T, Eshelbrenner CL, Reynolds K, He J, Bazzano LA (2011) Antihypertensive treatment and secondary prevention of cardiovascular disease events among persons without hypertension: a meta-analysis. JAMA 305:913–922
48. Czernichow S, Zanchetti A, Turnbull F, Barzi F, Ninomiya KAP et al (2011) The effects of blood pressure reduction and of different blood pressure-lowering regimens on major cardiovascular events according to baseline blood pressure: meta-analysis of randomized trials. J Hypertens 29:4–16
49. Goff DC Jr, Lloyd-Jones DM, Bennett G, Coady S, D'Agostino RB Sr, Gibbons R et al (2014) 2013 ACC/AHA guideline on the assessment of cardiovascular risk: a report of the American College of Cardiology/American Heart Association task force on practice guidelines. J Am Coll Cardiol 63:2935–2959
50. Blood Pressure-Lowering Treatment Trialists' Collaboration (2014) Blood pressure-lowering treatment based on cardiovascular risk: a meta-analysis of individual patient data. Lancet 384:591–598
51. Chobanian AV, Bakris GL, Black HR, Cushman WC, Green LA, Izzo JL Jr et al (2003) The seventh report of the Joint National Committee on prevention, detection, evaluation, and treatment of high blood pressure. The JNC 7 report. JAMA 289:2560–2572
52. Wright JT Jr, Williamson JD, Whelton PK, Snyder JK, Sink KM, Rocco MV et al (2015) A randomized trial of intensive versus standard blood-pressure control. N Engl J Med 373:2103–2116
53. Williamson JD, Supiano MA, Applegate WB, Berlowitz DR, Campbell RC, Chertow GM et al (2016) Intensive vs standard blood pressure control and cardiovascular disease outcomes in adults aged ≥75 years. A randomized clinical trial. JAMA 315:2673–2682
54. Bundy JD, Li C, Stuchlik P, Bu X, Kelly TN, Mills KT et al (2017) Systolic blood pressure reduction and risk of cardiovascular disease and mortality: a systematic review of cardiovascular disease and mortality: a systematic review and network meta-analysis. JAMA Cardiol 2:775–781
55. Oparil S, Lewis CE (2016) Should patients with cardiovascular risk factors receive intensive treatment of hypertension to <120/80 mm target? A protagonist view from the SPRINT trial (Systolic Blood Pressure Intervention trial). Circulation 134:1308–1310
56. Aronow WS (2017) Managing hypertension in the elderly: what is different, what is the same? Curr Hypertens Rep 19:67. https://doi.org/10.1007/s11906-017-0764-8
57. Rochlani Y, Khan MH, Aronow WS (2017) Managing hypertension in patients aged 75 years and older. Curr Hypertens Rep 19:88. https://doi.org/10.1007/s11906-017-0785-3
58. Yancy CW, Jessup M, Bozkurt B, Butler J, Casey DE Jr, Colvin MM et al (2017) 2017 ACC/AHA/HFSA focused update of the 2013 ACCF/AHA guideline for the management of heart failure. A report of the American College of Cardiology /American Heart Association task force on clinical practice guidelines and the Heart Failure Society of America. Developed in collaboration with the American Academy of Family Physicians, the American College of Chest Physicians, and International Society for Heart and Lung Transplantation. J Am Coll Cardiol 70:776–803
59. Upadhyay A, Earley A, Haynes SM, Uhlig K (2011) Systematic review: blood pressure target in chronic kidney disease and proteinuria as an effect modifier. Ann Intern Med 154:541–548
60. SPS3 Study Group, Benavente OR, Coffey CS, Conwit R, Hart RG, McClure LA et al (2013) Blood-pressure targets in patients with recent lacunar stroke: the SPS3 randomised trial. Lancet 382:507–515
61. Oparil S (2016) SPS3 evidence supports intensive blood pressure control. Circulation 133:552–554
62. Emdin CA, Rahimi K, Neal B, Callender T, Perkovic V, Patel A (2015) Blood pressure lowering in type 2 diabetes: a systematic review and meta-analysis. JAMA 313:603–615
63. Margolis KL, O'Connor PJ, Morgan TM, Buse JB, Cohen RM, Cushman WC et al (2014) Outcomes of combined cardiovascular risk factor management strategies in type 3 diabetes: the ACCORD randomized trial. Diabetes Care 37:1721–1728

64. Soliman EZ, Byington RP, Bigger JT, Evans G, Okin PM, Goff DC Jr et al (2015) Effect of intensive blood pressure lowering on left ventricular hypertrophy in patients with diabetes mellitus: Action to Control Cardiovascular Risk in Diabetes Blood Pressure Trial. Hypertension 66:1123–1129
65. Aronow WS (2016) Orthostatic hypotension in diabetics in the ACCORD (Action to Control Cardiovascular Risk in Diabetes) blood pressure trial. Hypertension 68:851–852
66. Wang WT, You LK, Chiang CE, Sung SH, Chuang SY, Cheng HM et al (2016) Comparative effectiveness of blood pressure-lowering drugs in patients who have already suffered from stroke: traditional and Bayesian network meta-analysis of randomized trials. Medicine 95:e3302
67. Aronow WS (2017) Lifestyle measures for treating hypertension. Arch Med Sci 13:1241–1243. This paper discusses lifestyle measures for treating hypertension
68. Ojji DB, Mayosi B, Francis V, Badri M, Cornelius V, Smythe W et al (2019) Comparison of drug therapies for lowering blood pressure in black Africans. N Engl J Med 380:2429–2439
69. Aronow WS, Fleg JL, Pepine CJ, Artinian NT, Bakris G, Brown AS et al (2011) ACCF/AHA 2011 expert consensus document on hypertension in the elderly: a report of the American College of Cardiology Foundation task force on clinical expert consensus documents. Developed in collaboration with the American Academy of Neurology, American Geriatrics Society, American Society for Preventive Cardiology, American Society of Hypertension, American Society of Nephrology, Association of Black Cardiologists, and European Society of Hypertension. J Am Coll Cardiol 57:2037–2114. These guidelines discuss management of resistant hypertension
70. Rosendorff C, Lackland DT, Allison M, Aronow WS, Black HR, Blumenthal RS et al (2015) AHA/ACC/ASH scientific statement. Treatment of hypertension in patients with coronary artery disease: a scientific statement from the American Heart Association, American College of Cardiology, and American Society of Hypertension. J Am Coll Cardiol 65:1998–2038
71. Law MR, Morris JK, Wald NJ (2009) Use of blood pressure lowering drugs in the prevention of cardiovascular disease: meta-analysis of 147 randomised trials in the context of expectations from prospective epidemiological studies. BMJ 338:b1665
72. Aronow WS (2010) Current role of beta blockers in the treatment of hypertension. Expert Opin Pharmacother 11:2599–2607
73. The CAPRICORN Investigators (2001) Effect of carvedilol on outcome after myocardial infarction in patients with left-ventricular dysfunction: the CAPRICORN randomised trial. Lancet 357:1385–1390
74. Freemantle N, Cleland J, Young P, Mason J, Harrison J (1999) Beta blockade after myocardial infarction: systematic review and meta regression analysis. BMJ 318:1730–1737
75. HOPE (Heart Outcomes Prevention Evaluation) Study Investigators (2000) Effects of an angiotensin-converting-enzyme inhibitor, ramipril, on cardiovascular events in high-risk patients. N Engl J Med 342:145–153
76. Fox KM, EURopean trial On reduction of cardiac events with Perindopril in stable coronary Artery disease Investigators (2003) Efficacy of perindopril in reduction of cardiovascular events among patients with stable coronary artery disease: randomised, double-blind, placebo-controlled, multicentre trial (the EUROPA study). Lancet 362(9386):782–788
77. Pfeffer MA, Braunwald E, Moye LA, Basta L, Brown EJ Jr, Cuddy TE et al (1992) Effect of captopril on mortality and morbidity in patients with left ventricular dysfunction after myocardial infarction. Results of the survival and ventricular enlargement trial. N Engl J Med 327:669–677
78. Bavry AA, Anderson RD, Gong Y, Denardo SJ, Cooper-Dehoff RM, Handberg EM et al (2010) Outcomes among hypertensive patients with concomitant peripheral and coronary artery disease: findings from the INternational VErapamil-SR/Trandolapril STudy. Hypertension 55:48–53
79. Turnbull F, Neal B, Algert C, Chalmers J, Chapman N, Cutler J et al (2005) Effects of different blood pressure-lowering regimens on major cardiovascular events in individuals with and

without diabetes mellitus: results of prospectively designed overviews of randomized trials. Arch Intern Med 165:1410–1419
80. Durand H, Hayes P, Morrissey EC, Newell J, Casey M, Murphy AW et al (2017) Medication adherence among patients with apparent treatment-resistant hypertension: systematic review and meta-analysis. J Hypertens 35:2346–2357. An analysis of 24 studies showed that the prevalence of nonadherence to drug therapy is 31.2% in patients with resistant hypertension
81. Kim YH, Her AY, Jeong MH, Kim BK, Lee SY, Hong SJ, Shin DH, Kim JS, Ko YG, Choi D, Hong MK, Jang Y (2019) Comparison between beta-blockers with angiotensin-converting enzyme inhibitors and Beta-blockers with angiotensin II type I receptor blockers in ST-segment elevation myocardial infarction after successful percutaneous coronary intervention with drug-eluting stents. Cardiovasc Drugs Ther 33(1):55–67. https://doi.org/10.1007/s10557-018-6841-7
82. American College of Emergency Physicians; Society for Cardiovascular Angiography and Interventions, O'Gara PT, Kushner FG, Ascheim DD, Casey DE Jr, Chung MK et al (2013) 2013 ACCF/AHA guideline for the management of ST-elevation myocardial infarction: a report of the American College of Cardiology Foundation/American Heart Association task force on practice guidelines. J Am Coll Cardiol 61:e78–e140
83. Huet F, Akodad M, Kalmanovitch E, Adda J, Agullo A, Batistella P, Roubille C, Roubille F (2019) Potential uses of sacubitril/valsartan: need for data on efficacy and safety. Am J Cardiovasc Drugs 19(1):1–10. https://doi.org/10.1007/s40256-018-0306-z
84. Ponikowski P, Voors AA, Anker SD, Bueno H, Cleland JGF, Coats AJS et al (2016) 2016 ESC guidelines for the diagnosis and treatment of acute and chronic heart failure. Eur J Heart Fail 18:891–975
85. McMurray JJV, Packer M, Desai AS et al (2014) Angiotensin–neprilysin inhibition versus enalapril in heart failure. N Engl J Med 371:993–1004. https://doi.org/10.1056/NEJMoa1409077
86. Yancy CW, Jessup M, Bozkurt B, Butler J, Casey DE, Colvin MM et al (2016) 2016 ACC/AHA/HFSA focused update on new pharmacological therapy for heart failure: an update of the 2013 ACCF/AHA guideline for the management of heart failure: a report of the American College of Cardiology/American Heart Association task force on clinical practice guidelines and the Heart Failure Society of America. J Am Coll Cardiol 68:1476–1488
87. Wang J-G, Yukisada K, Sibulo A, Hafeez K, Jia Y, Zhang J (2017) Efficacy and safety of sacubitril/valsartan (LCZ696) add-on to amlodipine in Asian patients with systolic hypertension uncontrolled with amlodipine monotherapy. J Hypertens 35:877–885
88. Supasyndh O, Wang J, Hafeez K, Zhang Y, Zhang J, Rakugi H (2017) Efficacy and safety of sacubitril/valsartan (LCZ696) compared with olmesartan in elderly Asian patients (≥ 65 years) with systolic hypertension. Am J Hypertens 30:1163–1169
89. Wang T-D, Tan R-S, Lee H-Y, Ihm S-H, Rhee M-Y, Tomlinson B et al (1979) Effects of sacubitril/valsartan (LCZ696) on natriuresis, diuresis, blood pressures, and NT-proBNP in salt-sensitive hypertension. Hypertension 2017(69):32–41
90. Kario K (2018) The sacubitril/valsartan, a first-in-class, angiotensin receptor neprilysin inhibitor (ARNI): potential uses in hypertension, heart failure, and beyond. Curr Cardiol Rep 20:1–8. https://doi.org/10.1007/s11886-018-0944-4
91. Trivedi RK, Polhemus DJ, Li Z, Yoo D, Koiwaya H, Scarborough A et al (2018) Combined angiotensin receptor-neprilysin inhibitors improve cardiac and vascular function via increased NO bioavailability in heart failure. J Am Heart Assoc 7:e008268
92. Schmieder RE, Wagner F, Mayr M, Delles C, Ott C, Keicher C et al (2017) The effect of sacubitril/valsartan compared to olmesartan on cardiovascular remodelling in subjects with essential hypertension: the results of a randomized, double-blind, active-controlled study. Eur Heart J 38:3308–3317
93. Kompa AR, Lu J, Weller TJ, Kelly DJ, Krum H, von Lueder TG et al (2018) Angiotensin receptor neprilysin inhibition provides superior cardioprotection compared to angiotensin

converting enzyme inhibition after experimental myocardial infarction. Int J Cardiol 258:192–198
94. von Lueder TG, Wang BH, Kompa AR, Huang L, Webb R, Jordaan P et al (2015) Angiotensin receptor neprilysin inhibitor LCZ696 attenuates cardiac remodeling and dysfunction after myocardial infarction by reducing cardiac fibrosis and hypertrophy. Circ Heart Fail 8:71–78
95. Ishii M, Kaikita K, Sato K, Sueta D, Fujisue K, Arima Y et al (2017) Cardioprotective effects of LCZ696 (sacubitril/valsartan) after experimental acute myocardial infarction. JACC Basic Transl Sci 2:655–668
96. Lewis EJ, Hunsicker LG, Bain RP, Rohde RD (1993) The effect of angiotensin converting enzyme inhibition on diabetic nephropathy. The Collaborative Study Group. N Engl J Med 329:1456–1462
97. Yusuf S, Dagenais G, Pogue J, Bosch J, Sleight P (2000) Vitamin E supplementation and cardiovascular events in high-risk patients. The Heart Outcomes Prevention Evaluation Study Investigators. N Engl J Med 342:154–160
98. Blood Pressure Lowering Treatment Trialists' Collaboration (2003) Effects of different blood-pressure-lowering regimens on major cardiovascular events: results of prospectively designed overviews of randomized trials. Lancet 362:1527–1535
99. Lewis EJ, Hunsicker LG, Clarke WR et al (2001) Renoprotective effect of the angiotensin-receptor antagonist irbesartan in patients with nephropathy due to type 2 diabetes. N Engl J Med 345:851–860
100. Jing W, Vaziri ND, Nunes A, Suematsu Y, Farzaneh T, Khazaeli M et al (2017) LCZ696 (sacubitril/valsartan) ameliorates oxidative stress, inflammation, fibrosis and improves renal function beyond angiotensin receptor blockade in CKD. Am J Transl Res 9:5473–5484
101. Suematsu Y, Jing W, Nunes A, Kashyap ML, Khazaeli M, Vaziri ND et al (2018) LCZ696 (sacubitril/valsartan), an angiotensin-receptor neprilysin inhibitor, attenuates cardiac hypertrophy, fibrosis, and vasculopathy in a rat model of chronic kidney disease. J Card Fail 24:266–275
102. Ushijima K, Ando H, Arakawa Y, Aizawa K, Suzuki C, Shimada K et al (2017) Prevention against renal damage in rats with subtotal nephrectomy by sacubitril/valsartan (LCZ696), a dual-acting angiotensin receptor-neprilysin inhibitor. Pharmacol Res Perspect 5(4):e00336. https://doi.org/10.1002/prp2.336
103. UK Harp-III Collaborative Group (2017) Randomized multicentre pilot study of sacubitril/valsartan versus irbesartan in patients with chronic kidney disease: United Kingdom Heart and Renal Protection (HARP)-III-rationale, trial design and baseline data. Nephrol Dial Transpl 32:2043–2051
104. Seferovic JP, Claggett B, Seidelmann SB et al (2017) Effect of sacubitril/valsartan versus enalapril on glycaemic control in patients with heart failure and diabetes: a post-hoc analysis from the PARADIGM-HF trial. Lancet Diabetes Endocrinol 5(5):333–340. https://doi.org/10.1016/S2213-8587(17)30087-6
105. Packer M (2018) Augmentation of glucagon-like peptide-1 receptor signalling by neprilysin inhibition: potential implications for patients with heart failure. Eur J Heart Fail 20(6):973–977
106. Rodgers JE (2017) Sacubitril/valsartan: the newest addition to the toolbox for guideline-directed medical therapy of heart failure. Am J Med 130:635–639
107. King JB, Shah RU, Bress AP, Nelson RE, Bellows BK (2016) Cost-effectiveness of sacubitril–valsartan combination therapy compared with enalapril for the treatment of heart failure with reduced ejection fraction. JACC Heart Fail 4:392–402
108. Ademi Z, Pfeil AM, Hancock E, Trueman D, Haroun RH, Deschaseaux C et al (2017) Cost-effectiveness of sacubitril/valsartan in chronic heart-failure patients with reduced ejection fraction. Swiss Med Wkly 147:w14533
109. Chalghoum A, Noichri Y, Dandana A, Baudin B, Miled A, Ferchichi S (2016) Pathological interactions between the endothelin-1 and the angiotensin-converting enzyme among

Tunisian coronary patients. BMC Cardiovasc Disord 16(1):244. https://doi.org/10.1186/s12872-016-0417-x

110. Jordan W, Reinbacher A, Cohrs S, Grunewald RW, Mayer G, Rüther E et al (2005) Obstructive sleep openea: plasma endothelin-1 precursor but not endothelin-1 levels are elevated and decline with nasal continues positive airway pressure. Peptides 26:1654–1660
111. Yanagisawa M, Inoue A, Ishikawa T, Kasuya Y, Kimura S, Kumagaye S et al (1988) Primary structure, synthesis, and biological activity of rat endothelin, an endothelium-derived vasoconstrictor peptide. Proc Natl Acad Sci 85:6964–6967
112. Walczak M, Fedorowicz A, Chłopicki S, Szymura-Oleksiak J (2010) Determination of endothelin-1 in rats using a high-performance liquidchromatography coupled to electrospray tandem mass spectrometry. Talanta 82:710–718
113. Yanagisawa M, Masaki T (1989) Endothelin, a novel endothelium-derived peptide. Pharmacological activities, regulation and possible roles in cardiovascular control. Biochem Pharmacol 38(12):1877–1883
114. Demacker PN, Veerkamp MJ, Bredie SJ, Marcovina SM, de Graaf J, Stalenhoef AF (2000) Comparison of the measurement of lipids and lipoproteins versus essay of apolipoprotein B for estimation of coronary heart disease: a study in familial combined hyperlipemia. Atherosclerosis 153:483–490
115. Zhao W, Zhao D, Yan R, Sun Y (2009) Cardiac oxidative stress and remodeling following infraction: role of NADPH oxidase. Cardiovasc Path 18:156–166
116. Akif M, Masuyer G, Schwager SL, Bhuyan BJ, Mugesh G, Isaac RE et al (2011) Structural characterization of angiotensin 1 converting enzyme in complex with a selenium analogue of captopril. FEBS J 278:3644–3650
117. Baudin B (2002) New aspects on angiotensin-converting enzyme: from gene to disease. Clin Chem Lab Med 40:256–265
118. Tocci G, Figliuzzi I, Presta V, Miceli F, Citoni B, Coluccia R, Musumeci MB, Ferrucci A, Volpe M (2018) Therapeutic approach to hypertension urgencies and emergencies during acute coronary syndrome. High Blood Press Cardiovasc Prev 25(3):253–259. https://doi.org/10.1007/s40292-018-0275-y
119. Ettehad D, Emdin CA, Kiran A, Anderson SG, Callender T, Emberson J, Chalmers J, Rodgers A, Rahimi K (2016) Blood pressure lowering for prevention of cardiovascular disease and death: a systematic review and meta-analysis. Lancet 387:957–967
120. Mancia G, Fagard R, Narkiewicz K, Redon J, Zanchetti A, Bohm M, Christiaens T, Cifkova R, De Backer G, Dominiczak A, Galderisi M, Grobbee DE, Jaarsma T, Kirchhof P, Kjeldsen SE, Laurent S, Manolis AJ, Nilsson PM, Ruilope LM, Schmieder RE, Sirnes PA, Sleight P, Viigimaa M, Waeber B, Zannad F (2014) 2013 ESH/ESC guidelines for the management of arterial hypertension. The task force for the management of arterial hypertension of the European Society of Hypertension (ESH) and of the European Society of Cardiology (EGC). J Hypertens 31:1281–1357
121. Kotseva K, Wood D, De Bacquer D, De Backer G, Ryden L, Jennings C et al (2016) EUROASPIRE IV: a European Society of Cardiology survey on the lifestyle, risk factor and therapeutic management of coronary patients from 24 European countries. Eur J Prev Cardiol 23(6):636–648
122. Borghi C, Tubach F, De Backer G, Dallongeville J, Guallar E, Medina J et al (2016) Lack of control of hypertension in primary cardiovascular disease prevention in Europe: results from the EURIKA study. Int J Cardiol 01(218):83–88
123. Figliuzzi I, Presta V, Citoni B, Miceli F, Simonelli F, Battistoni A et al (2018) Achievement of multiple therapeutic targets for cardiovascular disease prevention: retrospective analysis of real practice in Italy. Clin Cardiol 41(6):788–796. https://doi.org/10.1002/clc.22955
124. Beevers G, Lip GY, O'Brien E (2001) ABC of hypertension: the pathophysiology of hypertension. BMJ 322(7291):912–916
125. Khalid L, Dhakam SH (2008) A review of cardiogenic shock in acute myocardial infarction. Curr Cardiol Rev 4(1):34–40

126. Chin D, Battistoni A, Tocci G, Passerini J, Parati G, Volpe M (2012) Non-invasive diagnostic testing for coronary artery disease in the hypertensive patient: potential advantages of a risk estimation-based algorithm. Am J Hypertens 25(12):1226–1235
127. Volpe M, Trimarco B, Battistoni A, Mancia G, Italian Society of Hypertension (2013) Clinical management of coronary heart disease in hypertension: practical recommendations from the Italian Society of Hypertension (SIIA). High Blood Press Cardiovasc Prev. 20(3):129–134
128. Radico F, Cicchitti V, Zimarino M, De Caterina R (2014) Angina pectoris and myocardial ischemia in the absence of obstructive coronary artery disease: practical considerations for diagnostic tests. JACC Cardiovasc Interv 7(5):453–463
129. Dowsley T, Al-Mallah M, Ananthasubramaniam K, Dwivedi G, McArdle B, Chow BJ (2013) The role of noninvasive imaging in coronary artery disease detection, prognosis, and clinical decision making. Can J Cardiol 29(3):285–296
130. Ibanez B, James S, Agewall S, Antunes MJ, Bucciarelli-Ducci C, Bueno H et al (2018) 2017 ESC guidelines for the management of acute myocardial infarction in patients presenting with ST-segment elevation. Eur Heart J 39:119–177
131. Roffi M, Patrono C, Collet JP et al (2016) 2015 ESC guidelines for the management of acute coronary syndromes in patients presenting without persistent ST-segment elevation: task force for the management of acute coronary syndromes in patients presenting without persistent ST-segment elevation of the European Society of Cardiology (ESC). Eur Heart J 37(3):267–315
132. Held PH, Yusuf S, Furberg CD (1989) Calcium channel blockers in acute myocardial infarction and unstable angina: an overview. BMJ 299(6709):1187–1192
133. Liakos CI, Papadopoulos DP, Kotsis VT (2017) Adherence to treatment, safety, tolerance, and effectiveness of perindopril/amlodipine fixed-dose combination in Greek patients with hypertension and stable coronary artery disease: a Pan-Hellenic prospective observational study of daily clinical practice. Am J Cardiovasc Drugs 17(5):391–398. https://doi.org/10.1007/s40256-017-0232-5
134. Gupta AK, Arshad S, Poulter NR (2010) Compliance, safety, and effectiveness of fixed-dose combinations of antihypertensive agents: a meta-analysis. Hypertension 55:399–407
135. Claxton AJ, Cramer J, Pierce C (2001) A systematic review of the association between dose regimens and medication compliance. Clin Ther 23:1296–1310
136. Manolis A, Grammatikou V, Kallistratos M, Zarifis J, Tsioufis K (2015) Blood pressure reduction and control with fixed-dose combination perindopril/amlodipine: a Pan-Hellenic prospective observational study. J Renin-Angiotensin-Aldosterone Syst 16:930–935
137. Nádházi Z, Dézsi CA (2016) The results of ACES (Antihypertensive Combinations' Long Term Efficacy Comparing Study): analysis of metabolic effects of antihypertensive combination therapies. Clin Drug Investig 36:819–827
138. Tóth K, Investigators PIANIST (2014) Antihypertensive efficacy of triple combination perindopril/indapamide plus amlodipine in high-risk hypertensives: results of the PIANIST study (Perindopril-Indapamide plus AmlodipiNe in high rISk hyperTensive patients). Am J Cardiovasc Drugs 14:137–145
139. Omboni S, Malacco E, Napoli C, Modesti PA, Manolis A, Parati G, Agabiti-Rosei E, Borghi C (2017) Efficacy of zofenopril vs. irbesartan in combination with a thiazide diuretic in hypertensive patients with multiple risk factors not controlled by a previous monotherapy: a review of the double-blind, randomized "Z" studies. Adv Ther 34(4):784–798. https://doi.org/10.1007/s12325-017-0497-8
140. Modesti PA, Omboni S, Taddei S et al (2016) Zofenopril or irbesartan plus hydrochlorothiazide in elderly patients with isolated systolic hypertension untreated or uncontrolled by previous treatment: a double-blind, randomized study. J Hypertens 34:576–587
141. Malacco E, Omboni S, Parati G (2015) Blood pressure response to zofenopril or irbesartan each combined with hydrochlorothiazide in high-risk hypertensives uncontrolled by monotherapy: a randomized, double-blind, controlled, parallel group, noninferiority trial. Int J Hypertens 2015:139465

142. Mancia G, Fagard R, Narkiewicz K et al (2014) 2013 ESH/ESC practice guidelines for the management of arterial hypertension. Blood Press 23:3–16
143. Weber MA, Schiffrin EL, White WB et al (2014) Clinical practice guidelines for the management of hypertension in the community: a statement by the American Society of Hypertension and the International Society of Hypertension. J Clin Hypertens (Greenwich) 16:14–26
144. Wald DS, Law M, Morris JK, Bestwick JP, Wald NJ (2009) Combination therapy vs. monotherapy in reducing blood pressure: meta-analysis on 11,000 participants from 42 trials. Am J Med 122:290–300
145. Law MR, Wald NJ, Morris JK, Jordan RE (2003) Value of low dose combination treatment with blood pressure lowering drugs: analysis of 354 randomised trials. BMJ 326:1427
146. Hagsund T, Olsson SE, Smith JG, Madsen Hardig B, Wagner H (2020) β-Blockers after myocardial infarction and 1-year clinical outcome—a retrospective study. BMC Cardiovasc Disord 20(1):165. https://doi.org/10.1186/s12872-020-01441-0
147. Roffi M, Patrono C, Collet J-P, Mueller C, Valgimigli M, Andreotti F et al (2016) 2015 ESC guidelines for the management of acute coronary syndromes in patients presenting without persistent ST-segment elevation. Task force for the management of acute coronary syndromes in patients presenting without persistent ST-segment elevation of the European Society of Cardiology (ESC). Eur Heart J 37(3):267–315
148. Socialstyrelsen (2015) Nationella riktlinjer för hjärtsjukvård. p 120
149. Koul S, Hagström E, Smith G (2015) Akut kranskärlssjukdom Rekommendationer för bedömning, behandling och sekundärprevention [Internet]. Svenska Kardiologföreningen. p 34. http://www.cardio.se/nationella-riktlinjer
150. SWEDEHEART (2016) Hur tas RIKS-HIA:s kvalitetsindex fram? [2016 May]. http://www.ucr.uu.se/swedeheart/index.php/nyheter/137-hur-tas-riks-hias-kvalitetsindex-fram
151. Ozasa N, Kimura T, Morimoto T, Hou H, Tamura T, Shizuta S et al (2010) Lack of effect of oral beta-blocker therapy at discharge on long-term clinical outcomes of ST-segment elevation acute myocardial infarction after primary percutaneous coronary intervention. Am J Cardiol 106(9):1225–1233
152. Yang JH, Hahn JY, Song YB, Choi SH, Choi JH, Lee SH et al (2014) Association of beta-blocker therapy at discharge with clinical outcomes in patients with ST-segment elevation myocardial infarction undergoing primary percutaneous coronary intervention. JACC Cardiovasc Interv 7(6):592–601
153. Bao B, Ozasa N, Morimoto T, Furukawa Y, Nakagawa Y, Kadota K et al (2013) Beta-blocker therapy and cardiovascular outcomes in patients who have undergone percutaneous coronary intervention after ST-elevation myocardial infarction. Cardiovasc Interv Ther 28(2):139–147
154. Kernis SJ, Harjai KJ, Stone GW, Grines LL, Boura JA, O'Neill WW et al (2004) Does beta-blocker therapy improve clinical outcomes of acute myocardial infarction after successful primary angioplasty? J Am Coll Cardiol 43(10):1773–1779
155. Konishi M et al (2011) Additive effects of β-blockers on renin-angiotensin system inhibitors for patients after acute myocardial infarction treated with primary coronary revascularization. Circ J 75:1982–1991
156. Nakatani D et al (2013) Impact of beta blockade therapy on long-term mortality after ST-segment elevation acute myocardial infarction in the percutaneous coronary intervention era. Am J Cardiol 111:457–464
157. Rallidis LS, Katsimardos A, Kosmas N, Rallidi T, Zapantiotis D, Varounis C, Kountouri A (2022) Differential prognostic value of resistin for cardiac death in patients with coronary artery disease according to the presence of metabolic syndrome. Heart Vessel 37(5):713–719. https://doi.org/10.1007/s00380-021-01964-2
158. Langheim S, Dreas L, Veschini L, Maisano F, Foglieni C, Ferrarello S, Sinagra G, Zingone B, Alfieri O, Ferrero E, Maseri A, Ruotolo G (2010) Increased expression and secretion of resistin in epicardial adipose tissue of patients with acute coronary syndrome. Am J Physiol Heart Circ Physiol 298(3):H746–H753

159. Calabro P, Samudio I, Willerson JT, Yeh ETH (2004) Resistin promotes smooth muscle cell proliferation through activation of extracellular signal-regulated kinase 1/2 and phosphatidylinositol 3-kinase pathways. Circulation 110:3335–3340
160. Calabrò P, Cirillo P, Limongelli G, Maddaloni V, Riegler L, Palmieri R, Pacileo G, De Rosa S, Pacileo M, De Palma R, Golino P, Calabrò R (2011) Tissue factor is induced by resistin in human coronary artery endothelial cells by the NF-κB-dependent pathway. J Vasc Res 48:59–66
161. Rallidis LS, Tellis CC, Lekakis J, Rizos I, Varounis C, Charalampopoulos A, Zolindaki M, Dagres N, Anastasiou-Nana M, Tselepis A (2012) Lipoprotein-associated phospholipase A2 bound on high-density lipoprotein is associated with lower risk for cardiac death in stable coronary artery disease patients. J Am Coll Cardiol 60:2053–2060
162. Grundy SM, Cleeman JI, Daniels SR, Donato KA, Eckel RH, Franklin BA, Gordon DJ, Krauss RM, Savage PJ, Smith SC Jr, Spertus JA, Costa F, American Heart Association, National Heart, Lung, and Blood Institute (2005) Diagnosis and management of the metabolic syndrome: an American Heart Association/National Heart, Lung, and Blood Institute scientific statement. Circulation 112:2735–2752
163. Khera AV, Qamar A, Murphy SA, Cannon CP, Sabatine MS, Rader DJ (2015) On-statin resistin, leptin, and risk of recurrent coronary events after hospitalization for an acute coronary syndrome (from the Pravastatin or Atorvastatin Evaluation and Infection Therapy-Thrombolysis in Myocardial Infarction 22 Study). Am J Cardiol 116:694–698
164. Fontana A, Spadaro S, Copetti M, Spoto B, Salvemini L, Pizzini P, Frittitta L, Mallamaci F, Pellegrini F, Trischitta V, Menzaghi C (2015) Association between resistin levels and all-cause and cardiovascular mortality: a new study and a systematic review and meta-analysis. PLoS One 10(3):e0120419
165. Rallidis LS, Kosmas N, Rallidi T, Pavlakis G, Kiouri E, Zolindaki M (2020) Homocysteine is an independent predictor of long-term cardiac mortality in patients with stable coronary artery disease in the era of statins. Coron Artery Dis 31:152–156
166. Elasfar A, Shaheen S, El-Sherbeny W, Elsokkary H, Elhefnawy S, Al-Setiha M (2019) Preliminary results of the acute heart failure registry in the DELTA region of Egypt (DELTA-HF): a database and a quality initiative project. Egypt Heart J 71(1):27. https://doi.org/10.1186/s43044-019-0024-0
167. Heidenreich PA, Albert NM, Allen LA, Bluemke DA, Butler J, Fonarow GC, Ikonomidis JS, Khavjou O, Konstam MA, Maddox TM, Nichol G, Pham M, Piña IL, Trogdon JG, American Heart Association Advocacy Coordinating Committee; Council on Arteriosclerosis, Thrombosis and Vascular Biology; Council on Cardiovascular Radiology and Intervention; Council on Clinical Cardiology; Council on Epidemiology and Prevention; Stroke Council (2013) Forecasting the impact of heart failure in the United States: a policy statement from the American Heart Association. Circ Heart Fail 6:606–619
168. Alhabib KF, Elasfar AA, Alfaleh H et al (2014) Clinical features, management, and short- and long-term outcomes of patients with acute decompensated heart failure: phase I results of the HEARTS database methods and results. Eur J Heart Fail 16:462. https://doi.org/10.1002/ejhf.57
169. Sulaiman K, Panduranga P, Al-Zakwani I et al (2015) Clinical characteristics, management, and outcomes of acute heart failure patients: observation from the Gulf acute heart failure registry (Gulf CARE). Eur J Heart Fail 17(4):374–384. https://doi.org/10.1002/ejhf.245
170. Hassanein M, Abdelhamid M, Ibrahim B et al (2015) Clinical characteristics and management of hospitalized and ambulatory patients with heart failure–results from ESC heart failure long-term registry–Egyptian cohort. ESC Hear Fail 2(3):159–167
171. Kotseva K (2015) Implementation of cardiovascular disease prevention guidelines in clinical practice—can we do better? Curr Treat Options Cardiovasc Med 17(12):58. https://doi.org/10.1007/s11936-015-0415-9
172. Perk J, De Backer G, Gohlke H, Graham I, Reiner Z, Verschuren M, Albus C, Benlian P, Boysen G, Cifkova R, Deaton C, Ebrahim S, Fisher M, Germano G, Hobbs R, Hoes A,

Karadeniz S, Mezzani A, Prescott E, Ryden L, Scherer M, Syvänne M, Scholte op Reimer WJ, Vrints C, Wood D, Zamorano JL, Zannad F, European Association for Cardiovascular Prevention and Rehabilitation (EACPR), ESC Committee for Practice Guidelines (CPG) (2012) European guidelines on cardiovascular disease prevention in clinical practice (version 2012). The Fifth Joint Task Force of the European Society of Cardiology and Other Societies on Cardiovascular Disease Prevention in Clinical Practice (constituted by representatives of nine societies and by invited experts). Eur Heart J 33(13):1635–1701

173. Kotseva K, Rydén L, De Backer G, De Bacquer D, Wood D (2015) EURObservational Research Programme: EUROASPIRE survey of cardiovascular prevention and diabetes in 24 countries in Europe. Eur Heart J 36:950–955
174. Mehta RH, Bhatt DL, Steg PG et al (2008) REACH Registry Investigators. Modifiable risk factors control and its relationship with 1 year outcomes after coronary artery bypass surgery: insights from the REACH registry. Eur Heart J 29:3052–3060
175. Tang L, Patao C, Chuang J, Wong ND (2013) Cardiovascular risk factor control and adherence to recommended lifestyle and medical therapies in persons with coronary heart disease (from the National Health and Nutrition Examination Survey 2007-2010). Am J Cardiol 112:1126–1132
176. Chow CK, Jolly S, Rao-Melacini P, Fox KAA, Anand SS, Yusuf S (2010) Association of diet, exercise, and smoking modification with risk of early cardiovascular events after acute coronary syndromes. Circulation 121:750–758
177. Sverre E, Peersen K, Weedon-Fekjær H, Perk J, Gjertsen E, Husebye E, Gullestad L, Dammen T, Otterstad JE, Munkhaugen J (2020) Preventable clinical and psychosocial factors predicted two out of three recurrent cardiovascular events in a coronary population. BMC Cardiovasc Disord 20(1):61. https://doi.org/10.1186/s12872-020-01368-6
178. Ek A, Ekblom O, Hambraeus K, Cider A, Kallings LV, Borjesson M (2019) Physical inactivity and smoking after myocardial infarction as predictors for readmission and survival: results from the SWEDEHEART-registry. Clin Res Cardiol 108(3):324–332
179. Bhatt DL, Eagle KA, Ohman EM, Hirsch AT, Goto S, Mahoney EM, Wilson PW, Alberts MJ, D'Agostino R, Liau CS et al (2010) Comparative determinants of 4-year cardiovascular event rates in stable outpatients at risk of or with atherothrombosis. JAMA 304(12):1350–1357
180. Jernberg T, Hasvold P, Henriksson M, Hjelm H, Thuresson M, Janzon M (2015) Cardiovascular risk in post-myocardial infarction patients: nationwide real world data demonstrate the importance of a long-term perspective. Eur Heart J 36(19):1163–1170
181. De Bacquer D, De Smedt D, Kotseva K, Jennings C, Wood D, Ryden L, Gyberg V, Shahim B, Amouyel P, Bruthans J et al (2019) Incidence of cardiovascular events in patients with stabilized coronary heart disease: the EUROASPIRE IV follow-up study. Eur J Epidemiol 34(3):247–258
182. Lachowska K, Bellwon J, Narkiewicz K, Gruchała M, Hering D (2019) Long-term effects of device-guided slow breathing in stable heart failure patients with reduced ejection fraction. Clin Res Cardiol 108(1):48–60. https://doi.org/10.1007/s00392-018-1310-7
183. Ponikowski P, Voors AA, Anker SD, Bueno H, Cleland JGF, Coats AJS, Falk V, González-Juanatey JR, Harjola VP, Jankowska EA, Jessup M, Linde C, Nihoyannopoulos P, Parissis JT, Pieske B, Riley JP, Rosano GMC, Ruilope LM, Ruschitzka F, Rutten FH, van der Meer P (2016) 2016 ESC guidelines for the diagnosis and treatment of acute and chronic heart failure. Eur Heart J 37:2129–2200. https://doi.org/10.1093/eurheartj/ehw128
184. Buckert D, Cieslik M, Tibi R, Radermacher M, Rasche V, Bernhardt P, Hombach V, Rottbauer W, Wohrle J (2018) Longitudinal strain assessed by cardiac magnetic resonance correlates to hemodynamic findings in patients with severe aortic stenosis and predicts positive remodeling after transcatheter aortic valve replacement. Clin Res Cardiol 107(1):20–29. https://doi.org/10.1007/s00392-017-1153-7
185. Bleiziffer S, Bosmans J, Brecker S, Gerckens U, Wenaweser P, Tamburino C, Linke A, Investigators AS (2017) Insights on mid-term TAVR performance: 3-year clinical

and echocardiographic results from the CoreValve ADVANCE study. Clin Res Cardiol 106(10):784–795. https://doi.org/10.1007/s00392-017-1120-3
186. Rother J, Achenbach S, Trobs M, Blachutzik F, Nef H, Marwan M, Schlundt C (2016) Comparison of standard- and high-dose intracoronary adenosine for the measurement of coronary fractional flow reserve (FFR). Clin Res Cardiol 105(12):1003–1010. https://doi.org/10.1007/s00392-016-1010-0
187. Fu M, Ahrenmark U, Berglund S, Lindholm CJ, Lehto A, Broberg AM, Tasevska-Dinevska G, Wikstrom G, Agard A, Andersson B, All investigators of the HRHFs (2017) Adherence to optimal heart rate control in heart failure with reduced ejection fraction: insight from a survey of heart rate in heart failure in Sweden (HR-HF study). Clin Res Cardiol 106(12):960–973. https://doi.org/10.1007/s00392-017-1146-6
188. Bernardi L, Spadacini G, Bellwon J, Hajric R, Roskamm H, Frey AW (1998) Effect of breathing rate on oxygen saturation and exercise performance in chronic heart failure. Lancet 351(9112):1308–1311. https://doi.org/10.1016/S0140-6736(97)10341-5
189. Bernardi L, Porta C, Spicuzza L, Bellwon J, Spadacini G, Frey AW, Yeung LY, Sanderson JE, Pedretti R, Tramarin R (2002) Slow breathing increases arterial baroreflex sensitivity in patients with chronic heart failure. Circulation 105(2):143–145
190. Muller D, Remppis A, Schauerte P, Schmidt-Schweda S, Burkhoff D, Rousso B, Gutterman D, Senges J, Hindricks G, Kuck KH (2017) Clinical effects of long-term cardiac contractility modulation (CCM) in subjects with heart failure caused by left ventricular systolic dysfunction. Clin Res Cardiol 106(11):893–904. https://doi.org/10.1007/s00392-017-1135-9
191. Parati G, Malfatto G, Boarin S, Branzi G, Caldara G, Giglio A, Bilo G, Ongaro G, Alter A, Gavish B, Mancia G (2008) Device-guided paced breathing in the home setting: effects on exercise capacity, pulmonary and ventricular function in patients with chronic heart failure: a pilot study. Circ Heart Fail 1(3):178–183. https://doi.org/10.1161/CIRCHEARTFAILURE.108.772640
192. Kawauchi TS, Umeda IIK, Braga LM, Mansur AD, Rossi-Neto JM, Sousa AGDR, Hirata MH, Cahalin LP, Nakagawa NK (2017) Is there any benefit using low-intensity inspiratory and peripheral muscle training in heart failure? A randomized clinical trial. Clin Res Cardiol 106(9):676–685. https://doi.org/10.1007/s00392-017-1089-y
193. Ekman I, Kjellstrom B, Falk K, Norman J, Swedberg K (2011) Impact of device-guided slow breathing on symptoms of chronic heart failure: a randomized, controlled feasibility study. Eur J Heart Fail 13(9):1000–1005. https://doi.org/10.1093/eurjhf/hfr090
194. Huttin O, Mandry D, Eschalier R, Zhang L, Micard E, Odille F, Beaumont M, Fay R, Felblinger J, Camenzind E, Zannad F, Girerd N, Marie PY (2017) Cardiac remodeling following reperfused acute myocardial infarction is linked to the concomitant evolution of vascular function as assessed by cardiovascular magnetic resonance. J Cardiovasc Magn Reson 19(1):2. https://doi.org/10.1186/s12968-016-0314-6
195. Lotz J, Meier C, Leppert A, Galanski M (2002) Cardiovascular flow measurement with phase-contrast MR imaging: basic facts and implementation. Radiographics 22:651–671
196. Pfeffer MA, Braunwald E (1990) Ventricular remodeling after myocardial infarction. Experimental observation and clinical implications. Circulation 81:1161–1172. https://doi.org/10.1161/01.CIR.81.4.1161
197. Huttin O, Petit MA, Bozec E, Eschalier R, Juillière Y, Moulin F, Lemoine S, Selton-Suty C, Sadoul N, Mandry D, Beaumont M, Felblinger J, Girerd N, Marie PY (2015) Assessment of left ventricular ejection fraction calculation on long-axis views from cardiac magnetic resonance imaging in patients with acute myocardial infarction. Medicine (Baltimore) 94(43):e1856
198. Huttin O, Zhang L, Lemarié J, Mandry D, Juillière Y, Lemoine S, Micard E, Marie PY, Sadoul N, Girerd N, Selton-Suty C (2015) Global and regional myocardial deformation mechanics of microvascular obstruction in acute myocardial infarction: a three dimensional speckle-tracking imaging study. Int J Cardiovasc Imaging 31(7):1337–1346

199. Jeger RV, Lowe AM, Buller CE, Pfisterer ME, Dzavik V, Webb JG, Hochman JS, Jorde UP, Investigators SHOCK (2007) Hemodynamic parameters are prognostically important in cardiogenic shock but similar following early revascularization or initial medical stabilization: a report from the SHOCK trial. Chest 132(6):1794–1803
200. Cotter G, Moshkovitz Y, Kaluski E, Milo O, Nobikov Y, Schneeweiss A, Krakover R, Vered Z (2003) The role of cardiac power and systemic vascular resistance in the pathophysiology and diagnosis of patients with acute congestive heart failure. Eur J Heart Fail 5(4):443–451
201. Novo G, Guarino T, Di Lisi D, Biagioli P, Carluccio E (2023) Effects of SGLT2 inhibitors on cardiac structure and function. Heart Fail Rev 28(3):697–707. https://doi.org/10.1007/s10741-022-10256-4
202. McMurray JJV, Solomon SD, Inzucchi SE, Køber L, Kosiborod MN, Martinez FA, Ponikowski P, Sabatine MS, Anand IS, Bělohlávek J, Böhm M, Chiang CE, Chopra VK, de Boer RA, Desai AS, Diez M, Drozdz J, Dukát A, Ge J, Howlett JG, Katova T, Kitakaze M, Ljungman CEA, Merkely B, Nicolau JC, O'Meara E, Petrie MC, Vinh PN, Schou M, Tereshchenko S, Verma S, Held C, DeMets DL, Docherty KF, Jhund PS, Bengtsson O, Sjöstrand M, Langkilde AM, DAPA-HF Trial Committees and Investigators (2019) Dapagliflozin in patients with heart failure and reduced ejection fraction. N Engl J Med 381(21):1995–2008. https://doi.org/10.1056/NEJMoa1911303. Epub 2019 Sep 19. PMID: 31535829
203. Packer M, Anker SD, Butler J, Filippatos G, Pocock SJ, Carson P, Januzzi J, Verma S, Tsutsui H, Brueckmann M, Jamal W, Kimura K, Schnee J, Zeller C, Cotton D, Bocchi E, Böhm M, Choi DJ, Chopra V, Chuquiure E, Giannetti N, Janssens S, Zhang J, Gonzalez Juanatey JR, Kaul S, Brunner-La Rocca HP, Merkely B, Nicholls SJ, Perrone S, Pina I, Ponikowski P, Sattar N, Senni M, Seronde MF, Spinar J, Squire I, Taddei S, Wanner C, Zannad F, EMPEROR-Reduced Trial Investigators (2020) Cardiovascular and renal outcomes with empagliflozin in heart failure. N Engl J Med 383(15):1413–1424. https://doi.org/10.1056/NEJMoa2022190. Epub 2020 Aug 28. PMID: 32865377
204. Bhatt DL, Szarek M, Steg PG, Cannon CP, Leiter LA, McGuire DK, Lewis JB, Riddle MC, Voors AA, Metra M, Lund LH, Komajda M, Testani JM, Wilcox CS, Ponikowski P, Lopes RD, Verma S, Lapuerta P, Pitt B, SOLOIST-WHF Trial Investigators (2021) Sotagliflozin in patients with diabetes and recent worsening heart failure. N Engl J Med 384(2):117–128. https://doi.org/10.1056/NEJMoa2030183. Epub 2020 Nov 16. PMID: 33200892
205. Perkovic V, Jardine MJ, Neal B, Bompoint S, Heerspink HJL, Charytan DM, Edwards R, Agarwal R, Bakris G, Bull S, Cannon CP, Capuano G, Chu PL, de Zeeuw D, Greene T, Levin A, Pollock C, Wheeler DC, Yavin Y, Zhang H, Zinman B, Meininger G, Brenner BM, Mahaffey KW, CREDENCE Trial Investigators (2019) Canagliflozin and renal outcomes in type 2 diabetes and nephropathy. N Engl J Med 380(24):2295–2306. https://doi.org/10.1056/NEJMoa1811744. Epub 2019 Apr 14. PMID: 30990260
206. Abraham WT, Lindenfeld J, Ponikowski P, Agostoni P, Butler J, Desai AS, Filippatos G, Gniot J, Fu M, Gullestad L, Howlett JG, Nicholls SJ, Redon J, Schenkenberger I, Silva-Cardoso J, Störk S, Krzysztof Wranicz J, Savarese G, Brueckmann M, Jamal W, Nordaby M, Peil B, Ritter I, Ustyugova A, Zeller C, Salsali A, Anker SD (2021) Effect of empagliflozin on exercise ability and symptoms in heart failure patients with reduced and preserved ejection fraction, with and without type 2 diabetes. Eur Heart J 42(6):700–710. https://doi.org/10.1093/eurheartj/ehaa943. PMID: 33351892
207. Nassif ME, Windsor SL, Tang F, Khariton Y, Husain M, Inzucchi SE, McGuire DK, Pitt B, Scirica BM, Austin B, Drazner MH, Fong MW, Givertz MM, Gordon RA, Jermyn R, Katz SD, Lamba S, Lanfear DE, LaRue SJ, Lindenfeld J, Malone M, Margulies K, Mentz RJ, Mutharasan RK, Pursley M, Umpierrez G, Kosiborod M (2019) Dapagliflozin effects on biomarkers, symptoms, and functional status in patients with heart failure with reduced ejection fraction: the DEFINE-HF trial. Circulation 140(18):1463–1476. https://doi.org/10.1161/CIRCULATIONAHA.119.042929. Epub 2019 Sep 16 PMID: 31524498
208. Lee MMY, Brooksbank KJM, Wetherall K, Mangion K, Roditi G, Campbell RT, Berry C, Chong V, Coyle L, Docherty KF, Dreisbach JG, Labinjoh C, Lang NN, Lennie V,

McConnachie A, Murphy CL, Petrie CJ, Petrie JR, Speirits IA, Sourbron S, Welsh P, Woodward R, Radjenovic A, Mark PB, McMurray JJV, Jhund PS, Petrie MC, Sattar N (2021) Effect of empagliflozin on left ventricular volumes in patients with type 2 diabetes, or prediabetes, and heart failure with reduced ejection fraction (SUGAR-DM-HF). Circulation 143(6):516–525. https://doi.org/10.1161/CIRCULATIONAHA.120.052186. Epub 2020 Nov 13. PMID: 33186500; PMCID: PMC7864599

209. Cohen ND, Gutman SJ, Briganti EM, Taylor AJ (2019) Effects of empagliflozin treatment on cardiac function and structure in patients with type 2 diabetes: a cardiac magnetic resonance study. Intern Med J 49(8):1006–1010. https://doi.org/10.1111/imj.14260. PMID: 30784160
210. Matsutani D, Sakamoto M, Kayama Y, Takeda N, Horiuchi R, Utsunomiya K (2018) Effect of canagliflozin on left ventricular diastolic function in patients with type 2 diabetes. Cardiovasc Diabetol 17(1):73. https://doi.org/10.1186/s12933-018-0717-9. PMID: 29788955; PMCID: PMC5963148
211. Soga F, Tanaka H, Tatsumi K, Mochizuki Y, Sano H, Toki H, Matsumoto K, Shite J, Takaoka H, Doi T, Hirata KI (2018) Impact of dapagliflozin on left ventricular diastolic function of patients with type 2 diabetic mellitus with chronic heart failure. Cardiovasc Diabetol 17(1):132. https://doi.org/10.1186/s12933-018-0775-z. PMID: 30296931; PMCID: PMC6174555
212. Lan NSR, Yeap BB, Fegan PG, Green G, Rankin JM, Dwivedi G (2021) Empagliflozin and left ventricular diastolic function following an acute coronary syndrome in patients with type 2 diabetes. Int J Cardiovasc Imaging 37(2):517–527. https://doi.org/10.1007/s10554-020-02034-w. Epub 2020 Sep 21 PMID: 32959096
213. Tanaka H, Soga F, Tatsumi K, Mochizuki Y, Sano H, Toki H, Matsumoto K, Shite J, Takaoka H, Doi T, Hirata KI (2020) Positive effect of dapagliflozin on left ventricular longitudinal function for type 2 diabetic mellitus patients with chronic heart failure. Cardiovasc Diabetol 19(1):6. https://doi.org/10.1186/s12933-019-0985-z. PMID: 31910853; PMCID: PMC6947966
214. Hsu JC, Wang CY, Su MM, Lin LY, Yang WS (2019) Effect of empagliflozin on cardiac function, adiposity, and diffuse fibrosis in patients with type 2 diabetes mellitus. Sci Rep 9(1):15348. https://doi.org/10.1038/s41598-019-51949-5. PMID: 31653956; PMCID: PMC6814842
215. Hwang IC, Cho GY, Yoon YE, Park JJ, Park JB, Lee SP, Kim HK, Kim YJ, Sohn DW (2020) Different effects of SGLT2 inhibitors according to the presence and types of heart failure in type 2 diabetic patients. Cardiovasc Diabetol 19(1):69. https://doi.org/10.1186/s12933-020-01042-3. PMID: 32466760; PMCID: PMC7254690
216. Thirunavukarasu S, Jex N, Chowdhary A, Hassan IU, Straw S, Craven TP, Gorecka M, Broadbent D, Swoboda P, Witte KK, Cubbon RM, Xue H, Kellman P, Greenwood JP, Plein S, Levelt E (2021) Empagliflozin treatment is associated with improvements in cardiac energetics and function and reductions in myocardial cellular volume in patients with type 2 diabetes. Diabetes 70(12):2810–2822. https://doi.org/10.2337/db21-0270. Epub 2021 Oct 5. PMID: 34610982; PMCID: PMC8660983
217. Brown AJM, Gandy S, McCrimmon R, Houston JG, Struthers AD, Lang CC (2020) A randomized controlled trial of dapagliflozin on left ventricular hypertrophy in people with type two diabetes: the DAPA-LVH trial. Eur Heart J 41(36):3421–3432. https://doi.org/10.1093/eurheartj/ehaa419. PMID: 32578850; PMCID: PMC8202417
218. Verma S, Mazer CD, Yan AT, Mason T, Garg V, Teoh H, Zuo F, Quan A, Farkouh ME, Fitchett DH, Goodman SG, Goldenberg RM, Al-Omran M, Gilbert RE, Bhatt DL, Leiter LA, Jüni P, Zinman B, Connelly KA (2019) Effect of empagliflozin on left ventricular mass in patients with type 2 diabetes mellitus and coronary artery disease: the EMPA-HEART CardioLink-6 Randomized Clinical Trial. Circulation 140(21):1693–1702. https://doi.org/10.1161/CIRCULATIONAHA.119.042375. Epub 2019 Aug 22 PMID: 31434508
219. Cappetta D, De Angelis A, Ciuffreda LP, Coppini R, Cozzolino A, Miccichè A, Dell'Aversana C, D'Amario D, Cianflone E, Scavone C, Santini L, Palandri C, Naviglio S, Crea F, Rota M,

Altucci L, Rossi F, Capuano A, Urbanek K, Berrino L (2020) Amelioration of diastolic dysfunction by dapagliflozin in a non-diabetic model involves coronary endothelium. Pharmacol Res 157:104781. https://doi.org/10.1016/j.phrs.2020.104781. Epub 2020 Apr 28 PMID: 32360273

220. Higashikawa T, Ito T, Mizuno T, Ishigami K, Kohori M, Mae K, Usuda D, Takagi S, Sangen R, Saito A, Iguchi M, Kasamaki Y, Fukuda A, Kanda T, Okuro M (2020) Effects of tofogliflozin on cardiac function in elderly patients with diabetes mellitus. J Clin Med Res 12(3):165–171. https://doi.org/10.14740/jocmr4098. Epub 2020 Mar 2. PMID: 32231752; PMCID: PMC7092764
221. Kayano H, Koba S, Hirano T, Matsui T, Fukuoka H, Tsuijita H, Tsukamoto S, Hayashi T, Toshida T, Watanabe N, Hamazaki Y, Geshi E, Murakami M, Aihara K, Kaneko K, Yamada H, Kobayashi Y, Shinke T (2020) Dapagliflozin influences ventricular hemodynamics and exercise-induced pulmonary hypertension in type 2 diabetes patients—a randomized controlled trial. Circ J 84(10):1807–1817. https://doi.org/10.1253/circj.CJ-20-0341. Epub 2020 Sep 12 PMID: 32921680
222. Rosito GA, Massaro JM, Hoffmann U, Ruberg FL, Mahabadi AA, Vasan RS, O'Donnell CJ, Fox CS (2008) Pericardial fat, visceral abdominal fat, cardiovascular disease risk factors, and vascular calcification in a community-based sample: the Framingham Heart Study. Circulation 117(5):605–613. https://doi.org/10.1161/CIRCULATIONAHA.107.743062. Epub 2008 Jan 22 PMID: 18212276
223. Yagi S, Hirata Y, Ise T, Kusunose K, Yamada H, Fukuda D, Salim HM, Maimaituxun G, Nishio S, Takagawa Y, Hama S, Matsuura T, Yamaguchi K, Tobiume T, Soeki T, Wakatsuki T, Aihara KI, Akaike M, Shimabukuro M, Sata M (2017) Canagliflozin reduces epicardial fat in patients with type 2 diabetes mellitus. Diabetol Metab Syndr 4(9):78. https://doi.org/10.1186/s13098-017-0275-4. PMID: 29034006; PMCID: PMC5628447
224. Anker SD, Butler J, Filippatos G, Ferreira JP, Bocchi E, Böhm M, Brunner-La Rocca HP, Choi DJ, Chopra V, Chuquiure-Valenzuela E, Giannetti N, Gomez-Mesa JE, Janssens S, Januzzi JL, Gonzalez-Juanatey JR, Merkely B, Nicholls SJ, Perrone SV, Piña IL, Ponikowski P, Senni M, Sim D, Spinar J, Squire I, Taddei S, Tsutsui H, Verma S, Vinereanu D, Zhang J, Carson P, Lam CSP, Marx N, Zeller C, Sattar N, Jamal W, Schnaidt S, Schnee JM, Brueckmann M, Pocock SJ, Zannad F, Packer M, EMPEROR-Preserved Trial Investigators (2021) Empagliflozin in heart failure with a preserved ejection fraction. N Engl J Med 385(16):1451–1461. https://doi.org/10.1056/NEJMoa2107038. Epub 2021 Aug 27. PMID: 34449189
225. Rau M, Thiele K, Hartmann NK, Schuh A, Altiok E, Möllmann J, Keszei AP, Böhm M, Marx N, Lehrke M (2021) Empagliflozin does not change cardiac index nor systemic vascular resistance but rapidly improves left ventricular filling pressure in patients with type 2 diabetes: a randomized controlled study. Cardiovasc Diabetol 20(1):6. https://doi.org/10.1186/s12933-020-01175-5. PMID: 33413355; PMCID: PMC7791833
226. Asleh R, Sheikh-Ahmad M, Briasoulis A, Kushwaha SS (2017) The influence of antihyperglycemic drug therapy on cardiovascular and heart failure outcomes in patients with type 2 diabetes mellitus. Heart Fail Rev 23(3):445–459. https://doi.org/10.1007/s10741-017-9666-8
227. Whiting DR, Guariguata L, Weil C, Shaw JIDF (2011) Diabetes atlas: global estimates of the prevalence of diabetes for 2011 and 2030. Diabetes Res Clin Pract 94(3):311–321. https://doi.org/10.1016/j.diabres.2011.10.029
228. Dei Cas A, Fonarow GC, Gheorghiade M, Butler J (2015) Concomitant diabetes mellitus and heart failure. Curr Probl Cardiol 40(1):7–43. https://doi.org/10.1016/j.cpcardiol.2014.09.002
229. Bertoni AG, Hundley WG, Massing MW, Bonds DE, Burke GL, Goff DC (2004) Heart failure prevalence, incidence, and mortality in the elderly with diabetes. Diabetes Care 27(3):699–703. https://doi.org/10.2337/diacare.27.3.699
230. Metra M, Zacà V, Parati G, Agostoni P, Bonadies M, Ciccone M, Cas AD, Iacoviello M, Lagioia R, Lombardi C, Maio R, Magrì D, Musca G, Padeletti M, Perticone F, Pezzali N, Piepoli M, Sciacqua A, Zanolla L, Nodari S, Filardi PP, Dei Cas L, Heart Failure Study

Group of the Italian Society of Cardiology (2011) Cardiovascular and noncardiovascular comorbidities in patients with chronic heart failure. J Cardiovasc Med 12(2):76–84. https://doi.org/10.2459/JCM.0b013e32834058d1
231. Stone PH, Muller JE, Hartwell T, York BJ, Rutherford JD, Parker CB, Turi ZG, Strauss HW, Willerson JT, Robertson T, Braunwald E, Jaffe AS (1989) The effect of diabetes mellitus on prognosis and serial left ventricular function after acute myocardial infarction: contribution of both coronary disease and diastolic left ventricular dysfunction to the adverse prognosis. The MILIS study group. J Am Coll Cardiol 14(1):49–57. https://doi.org/10.1016/0735-1097(89)90053-3
232. Jia G, Whaley-Connell A, Sowers JR (2018) Diabetic cardiomyopathy: a hyperglycaemia- and insulin-resistance-induced heart disease. Diabetologia 61(1):21–28. https://doi.org/10.1007/s00125-017-4390-4
233. Doehner W, Rauchhaus M, Ponikowski P, Godsland IF, von Haehling S, Okonko DO, Leyva F, Proudler AJ, Coats AJS, Anker SD (2005) Impaired insulin sensitivity as an independent risk factor for mortality in patients with stable chronic heart failure. J Am Coll Cardiol 46(6):1019–1026. https://doi.org/10.1016/j.jacc.2005.02.093
234. UK Prospective Diabetes Study (UKPDS) Group (1998) Effect of intensive blood-glucose control with metformin on complications in overweight patients with type 2 diabetes (UKPDS 34). Lancet 352:854–865
235. Stratton IM, Adler AI, Neil HA et al (2000) Association of glycaemia with macrovascular and microvascular complications of type 2 diabetes (UKPDS 35): prospective observational study. BMJ 321:405–412
236. Holman RR, Paul SK, Bethel MA, Matthews DR, Neil HAW (2008) 10-year follow-up of intensive glucose control in type 2 diabetes. N Engl J Med 359(15):1577–1589. https://doi.org/10.1056/NEJMoa0806470
237. Friedewald WT, Buse JB, Bigger JT et al (2008) Effects of intensive glucose lowering in type 2 diabetes. N Engl J Med 358:2545–2559
238. Patel A, MacMahon S, Chalmers J et al (2008) Intensive blood glucose control and vascular outcomes in patients with type 2 diabetes. N Engl J Med 358(24):2560–2572. https://doi.org/10.1056/NEJMoa0802987
239. Duckworth W, Abraira C, Moritz T, Reda D, Emanuele N, Reaven PD, Zieve FJ, Marks J, Davis SN, Hayward R, Warren SR, Goldman S, McCarren M, Vitek ME, Henderson WG, Huang GD, VADT Investigators (2009) Glucose control and vascular complications in veterans with type 2 diabetes. N Engl J Med 360(2):129–139. https://doi.org/10.1056/NEJMoa0808431
240. Pantalone KM, Kattan MW, Yu C, Wells BJ, Arrigain S, Jain A, Atreja A, Zimmerman RS (2009) The risk of developing coronary artery disease or congestive heart failure, and overall mortality, in type 2 diabetic patients receiving rosiglitazone, pioglitazone, metformin, or sulfonylureas: a retrospective analysis. Acta Diabetol 46(2):145–154. https://doi.org/10.1007/s00592-008-0090-3
241. Birkeland KI, Jørgensen ME, Carstensen B, Persson F, Gulseth HL, Thuresson M, Fenici P, Nathanson D, Nyström T, Eriksson JW, Bodegård J, Norhammar A (2017) Cardiovascular mortality and morbidity in patients with type 2 diabetes following initiation of sodium-glucose co-transporter-2 inhibitors versus other glucose-lowering drugs (CVD-REAL Nordic): a multinational observational analysis. Lancet Diabetes Endocrinol 5(9):709–717. https://doi.org/10.1016/S2213-8587(17)30258-9
242. Barman HA, Tanyolaç S, Dogan O, Bal E, Atıcı A, Özyıldırım S, Yiğit Z (2022) Impact of sacubitril/valsartan on lipid parameters in patients with heart failure with reduced ejection fraction. Clin Drug Investig 42(6):533–540. https://doi.org/10.1007/s40261-022-01161-7
243. Preiss D, Campbell RT, Murray HM et al (2015) The effect of statin therapy on heart failure events: a collaborative meta-analysis of unpublished data from major randomized trials. Eur Heart J 36(24):1536–1546

244. Selvaraj S, Claggett BL, Packer M, Zannad F, Anand IS, Pieske B et al (2021) Effects of sacubitril/valsartan on serum lipids in heart failure with preserved ejection fraction. J Am Heart Assoc 10(17):e022069
245. MacLaughlin EJ, Ernst ME (2019) From clinical trials to bedside: the use of antihypertensives in aged individuals. Part 1: evaluation and evidence of treatment benefit. Curr Hypertens Rep 21(11):82. https://doi.org/10.1007/s11906-019-0987-y
246. Franklin SS, Gustin W, Wong ND, Larson MG, Weber MA, Kannel WB et al (1997) Hemodynamic patterns of age-related changes in blood pressure. The Framingham Heart Study. Circulation 96(1):308–315
247. O'Rourke MF (2002) From theory into practice: arterial haemodynamics in clinical hypertension. J Hypertens 20(10):1901–1915
248. Lv YB, Gao X, Yin ZX, Chen HS, Luo JS, Brasher MS et al (2018) Revisiting the association of blood pressure with mortality in oldest old people in China: community based, longitudinal prospective study. BMJ 361:k2158. In this large cohort of 144,403 participants aged 80 years and older, systolic blood pressure trajectories showed an accelerated decline in the last 2 years of life which did not appear due to intensification of antihypertensive therapy. This suggests that epidemiological associations of low systolic BP with higher mortality may be due to reverse causation bias
249. Whelton PK, Carey RM, Aronow WS, Casey DE Jr, Collins KJ, Dennison Himmelfarb C et al (2018) 2017 ACC/AHA/AAPA/ABC/ACPM/AGS/APhA/ASH/ASPC/NMA/PCNA guideline for the prevention, detection, evaluation, and management of high blood pressure in adults: a report of the American College of Cardiology/American Heart Association task force on clinical practice guidelines. Hypertension 71(6):e13–e115
250. Sprint Research Group, Wright JT Jr, Williamson JD, Whelton PK, Snyder JK, Sink KM et al (2015) A randomized trial of intensive versus standard blood-pressure control. N Engl J Med 373(22):2103–2116
251. SPRINT MIND Investigators for the SPRINT Research Group (2019) Effect of intensive vs standard blood pressure control on probable dementia: a randomized clinical trial. JAMA 321(6):553–561. This sub-study of SPRINT found that treating to an intensive SBP goal of < 120 mmHg was associated with a decreased risk of mild cognitive impairment and the combined rate of mild cognitive impairment or probable dementia. While there was no decrease in the primary cognitive outcome of adjudicated dementia, it is important to note that this outcome was likely underpowered as SPRINT was stopped early and there were fewer cases of dementia than expected
252. Grover S, Bell G, Lincoff M, Jeorg L, Madsen PL, Huang S, Leow S, Figtree G, Chakrabarty A, Leong DP, Woodman RJ, Selvanayagam JB (2015) Utility of CMR markers of myocardial injury in predicting LV functional recovery: results from PROTECTION AMI CMR Substudy. Heart Lung Circ 24(9):891–897
253. Hamirani YS, Wong A, Kramer CM, Salerno M (2014) Effect of microvascular obstruction and intramyocardial hemorrhage by CMR on LV remodeling and outcomes after myocardial infarction: a systematic review and meta-analysis. JACC Cardiovasc Imaging 7(9):940–952
254. Bolognese L, Neskovic AN, Parodi G, Cerisano G, Buonamici P, Santoro GM, Antoniucci D (2002) Left ventricular remodeling after primary coronary angioplasty: patterns of left ventricular dilation and long-term prognostic implications. Circulation 106:2351–2357

Chapter 9
Role of ACE Inhibitors and Angiotensin Receptor Blockers in Covid19 Patients

Mukesh Nandave

Introduction by the Editor

COVID-19 is caused by SARS-CoV virus and has resulted into significant morbidity and mortality worldwide since it was first identified in China's Wuhan. It is well known that SARS-CoV binds to angiotensin converting enzyme-2 (ACE2) present on the outer surface of the cell membrane to enter into the host [1]. When the host is exposed to the virus, CoVs bind to the cells expressing specific ACE2 receptors with the help of spike protein. With the onset of COVID-19, ACE2 expression is down-regulated however its role in developing lung injury in patients with SARS-CoV infection is disputable. Few experimental data demonstrate that severe lung injury and fibrosis in SARS-CoV animal models is mainly mediated by Ang-II inflammation [2]. The reduced ACE2 expression prior to SARS-CoV-2 infection elevates local concentration of Ang-II in the lungs and causes severe lung injury. SARS-CoV epidemic data also suggested that ACE2 dependent SARS-CoV-2 infection may decrease ACE2 expression in heart, promoting severe heart injury [2].

Angiotensin-II receptor blockers (ARBs) and angiotensin-converting enzyme inhibitors (ACEs) are considered as first line therapy in the hypertension treatment and diabetes. The effects of ACEs inhibitors and ARBs in COVID-19 patients are highly controversial. Some of the studies with strong methodologies have discussed the issue but biases still exist. Some of the animal studies have reported ACE inhibitors and ARBs associated upregulation of ACE2 expression [1, 3, 4]. However, limited clinical data is available on the ACE inhibitors and ARBs associated variations in ACE2 level in plasma [1, 5]. Notably COVID-19 patients with other co-morbidities such as hypertension, cardiovascular diseases and diabetes are found to

M. Nandave (✉)
Department of Pharmacology, Delhi Pharmaceutical Sciences and Research University, New Delhi, Delhi, India

M. Nandave (ed.), *Angiotensin-converting Enzyme Inhibitors vs. Angiotensin Receptor Blockers*, https://doi.org/10.1007/978-981-97-7380-0_9

have more risk of adverse clinical outcome like mortality [6, 7]. It might be possible that hypertension or cardiovascular patients who are taking ACE inhibitors and ARBs are more at risk of SARS-CoV-2 infection and adverse clinical outcomes [1, 8]. However, some of the studies have suggested that ACE inhibitors and ARBs associated increased ACE2 expression could protect the lungs of COVID-19 patients against damage [9]. Some Researchers have supported the idea that restoring the ACE1/ACE2 balance with ARBs or ACEIs could exert a protective role and attenuate lung tissue damage in SARS-CoV-2 pneumonia [2]. Additionally, discontinuing the ACE inhibitors and ARBs therapy in patients who are at higher risk of SARS-CoV-2 infection can produce negative consequences. Despite the limited conclusive data, some professional bodies have recommended continuation of ACE inhibitors and ARBs in COVID-19 patients [1]. Based on currently available evidence, it could be concluded that increased ACE2 levels can have protective effect on kidney, heart and lungs which is facilitated by the administration of ACE inhibitors/ARBs. This mechanism supports the data on ACE inhibitors/ARBs associated with reduced mortality risk in COVID-19 patients [10].

It is necessary that researchers should explore the association between the administration of ACE inhibitors/ARBs and increased mortality or adverse clinical outcomes such as like mechanical ventilation, ICU admission as well as SARS-CoV-2 positivity extent. Systematic review studied association between ACE inhibitors/ARBs with SARS-Cov-2 in users and non-users, but there were several limitations in that study. The authors did not report the severity of SARS-CoV-2 in patients who are using ACE inhibitors/ARBs and non-users. Notably, this review included the data from pre-print articles that are non-peer reviewed therefore raising concern over their reliability [11].

A meta-analysis reported that usage of ACE inhibitors/ARBs in COVID-19 patients slightly increase the risk of severe clinical outcomes such as mechanical ventilation, ICU admission or death but these results were not statistically significant. When same parameters were analyzed in hypertensive COVID-19 patients, the risk of severe outcomes was found to be decreased. Interestingly, no difference was observed in risk between ACE inhibitors/ARBs users and non-users. This analysis stats that administration of ACE inhibitors/ARBs in hypertensive COVID-19 patients has no significant difference in risk of severe outcomes as compared to patients who are not using these medications [10].

Therefore, this chapter explores the debatable data over the administration of ACE inhibitors and ARBs in hypertensive patients suffering from COVID-19. This also discusses the possibility of the risk to catch SARS-CoV-2 infection in patients taking ACE inhibitors and ARBs (Fig. 9.1).

Machine Generated Summaries

Disclaimer: The summaries in this chapter were generated from Springer Nature publications using extractive AI auto-summarization: An extraction-based summarizer aims to identify the most important sentences of a text using an algorithm and

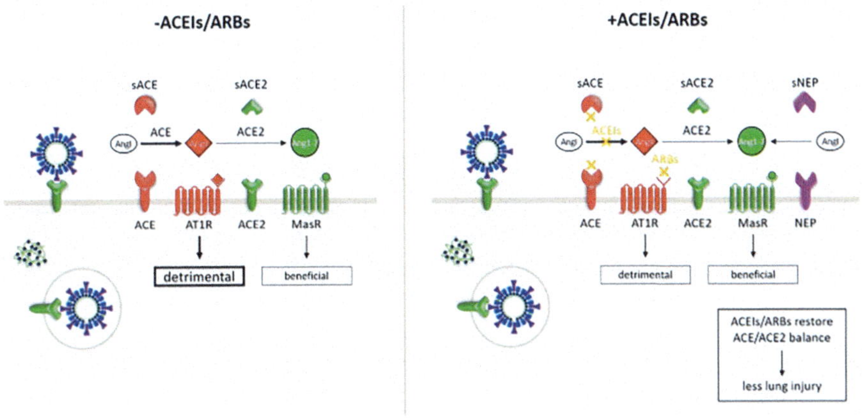

Fig. 9.1 Schematic representation of hypothesis 1. ACE inhibitors (*ACEIs*) and angiotensin II type-1 receptor blockers (*ARBs*) alleviate COVID-19 by inhibiting the harmful ACE/AngII/AT1R axis, which gained dominance due to SARS-CoV-2-induced downregulation of ACE2. (Source: de Vries [12])

uses those original sentences to create the auto-summary (unlike generative AI). As the constituted sentences are machine selected, they may not fully reflect the body of the work, so we strongly advise that the original content is read and cited. The auto generated summaries were curated by the editor to meet Springer Nature publication standards. To cite this content, please refer to the original papers.

Machine generated keywords: covid, sarscov, virus, respiratory, coronavirus, infection, covid patient, covid infection, lung, severe, ace receptor, pneumonia, ace, ras, angii.

Use of Angiotensin-Converting Enzyme Inhibitors and Angiotensin II Receptor Blockers in Context of COVID-19 Outbreak: A Retrospective Analysis [13]

This is a machine-generated summary of:

Xu, Jiuyang; Huang, Chaolin; Fan, Guohui; Liu, Zhibo; Shang, Lianhan; Zhou, Fei; Wang, Yeming; Yu, Jiapei; Yang, Luning; Xie, Ke; Huang, Zhisheng; Huang, Lixue; Gu, Xiaoying; Li, Hui; Zhang, Yi; Wang, Yimin; Hayden, Frederick G.; Horby, Peter W.; Cao, Bin; Wang, Chen: Use of angiotensin-converting enzyme inhibitors and angiotensin II receptor blockers in context of COVID-19 outbreak: a retrospective analysis [13].

Published in: Frontiers of Medicine (2020).

Link to original: https://doi.org/10.1007/s11684-020-0800-y

If you want to cite the papers, please refer to the original.

For technical reasons we could not place the page where the original quote is coming from.

Abstract-Summary "The possible effects of angiotensin-converting enzyme inhibitors (ACEIs) or angiotensin II receptor blockers (ARBs) on COVID-19 disease severity have generated considerable debate."

"Patients on anti-hypertensive treatment with or without ACEI/ARB were compared on their clinical characteristics and outcomes."

"Among the 101 patients with a history of hypertension and taking at least one anti-hypertensive medication, 40 patients were receiving ACEI/ARB as part of their regimen, and 61 patients were on antihypertensive medication other than ACEI/ARB."

"We observed no statistically significant differences in percentages of in-hospital mortality (28% vs. 34%, P = 0.46), ICU admission (20% vs. 28%, P = 0.37) or invasive mechanical ventilation (18% vs. 26%, P = 0.31) between patients with or without ACEI/ARB treatment."

"Further multivariable adjustment of age and gender did not provide evidence for a significant association between ACEI/ARB treatment and severe COVID-19 outcomes."

Outcomes in Patients with COVID-19 Infection Taking ACEI/ARB [14]

This is a machine-generated summary of:

Rico-Mesa, Juan Simon; White, Averi; Anderson, Allen S.: Outcomes in Patients with COVID-19 Infection Taking ACEI/ARB [14].

Published in: Current Cardiology Reports (2020).

Link to original: https://doi.org/10.1007/s11886-020-01291-4

If you want to cite the papers, please refer to the original.

For technical reasons we could not place the page where the original quote is coming from.

Abstract-Summary "Severe acute respiratory syndrome coronavirus 2 (SARS-CoV-2) is the virus responsible for the aggressive coronavirus disease (COVID-19) pandemic."

"Investigators have stipulated that COVID-19 patients receiving angiotensin-converting-enzyme inhibitors (ACEI) may be subject to poorer outcomes."

"Worse outcomes appear to be more prevalent in patients with hypertension and diabetes mellitus (DM), possibly due to overexpression of angiotensin-converting enzyme 2 (ACE2) receptor in airway alveolar epithelial cells."

"Investigators suspect that SARS-CoV-2 uses the ACE2 receptor to enter the lungs in a mechanism similar to SARS-CoV. Several hypotheses have been proposed to date regarding the net effect of ACEI/ARB on COVID-19 infections."

"Positive effects include ACE2 receptor blockade, disabling viral entry into the heart and lungs, and an overall decrease in inflammation secondary to ACEI/ARB."

"Negative effects include a possible retrograde feedback mechanism, by which ACE2 receptors are upregulated."

"Even though physiological models of SARS-CoV infection show a theoretical benefit of ACEI/ARB, these findings cannot be extrapolated to SARS-CoV-2 causing COVID-19."

Introduction

"Severe acute respiratory syndrome coronavirus 2 (SARS-CoV-2) is the virus responsible for COVID-19, a global pandemic with catastrophic consequences for healthcare systems and populations around the world."

"SARS-CoV-2 shares similarities with SARS-CoV, the virus responsible for the 2002–2003 SARS epidemic, and Middle Eastern respiratory syndrome coronavirus (MERS), the virus responsible for MERS [15]."

"Following the SARS epidemic, researchers extensively investigated the pathophysiologic mechanisms of SARS-CoV infection, including the interaction of the virus with the heart and lungs."

"Based on these studies, researchers believe that the angiotensin-converting enzyme 2 (ACE2) receptor, located on alveolar epithelial cells, serves as a high affinity receptor and co-transporter for SARS-CoV-2 to enter the lungs [16]."

Background

"The renin-angiotensin-aldosterone system (RAAS) maintains plasma sodium concentration via feedback from blood pressure, baroreceptors, and sodium and potassium levels."

"Angiotensin II stimulates vasoconstriction, cardiovascular response, and aldosterone and ADH production; this ultimately increases blood pressure and body fluid volume through sodium, potassium, and free water resorption [16]."

"Discovered in 2000, ACE2 receptor appears to counter-regulate RAAS activation by degrading angiotensin II [17]."

COVID-19 and Comorbidity

"Three separate studies identified hypertension and DM as highly prevalent among COVID-19 patients: A. According to Yang and others, among 52 critically ill patients, DM was present in 17% of cases [18]. B. According to Guan and others, among 1099 patients, DM was present in 16.2% of cases and hypertension was present in 23.7% of cases [19]. C. According to Zhang and others, among 140 hospitalized patients, DM was present in 12% of cases and hypertension was present in 30% of cases [20]."

"While both hypertension and DM are treated with ACEI and ARB, medication use was not assessed in any of the three aforementioned studies, leading to an inconclusive hypothesis."

"One study to date has analyzed the effect of ACEI and ARB use on the COVID-19 population."

"SARS-CoV-2 was recently associated with cardiac injury, defined by a troponin > 28 pg/ml or electrocardiogram/echocardiogram abnormalities, in 12% of patients from a COVID-19 cohort."

Pros and Cons of ACE Inhibition

"The etiology of cardiac damage in patients with COVID-19 is unclear, but ACE2 receptors may play a role, given the high affinity of SARS-CoV for ACE2 receptors [8]."

"A recent commentary published in the Lancet Respiratory Medicine hypothesizes that the use of ACE2 receptor increasing drugs is at higher risk for severe COVID-19 infection."

"This ACE2 receptor upregulation results in increased binding sites for SARS-CoV-2, leading to preferential COVID-19 infection."

"Li and others, for example, proposed that ACEI inhibition of ACE may stimulate a negative feedback (given the lack of angiotensin II, upregulating ACE2 receptors and decreasing overall inflammation [21])."

"Recent findings also demonstrate that patients on the ARB olmesartan had increased secretion of urinary ACE2, likely from an upregulation mechanism, although unclear [22]."

"Given the contradictory hypotheses, rapidly evolving nature of the disease, and social media-related hysteria, several cardiology associations (HFSA/ACC/AHA and ESC Hypertension Council) released an official statement regarding the continuation of ACEI and ARB for COVID-19 patients [23]."

Conclusions

"There is a lack of scientific evidence and clinical data to support discontinuing ACE/ARB use in patients with COVID-19 and co-existing heart failure, hypertension, or ischemic heart disease."

"The well-studied reduction in mortality conferred by ACE/ARB use and the beneficial effects for patients with diabetes, chronic kidney disease, and proteinuria or albuminuria currently outweigh the theoretical risks."

"As the COVID-19 pandemic continues to rapidly evolve and affect more patients with cardiovascular comorbidities, further research is needed to clarify the accuracy of existing hypotheses."

Renin–Angiotensin System Modulation and Outcomes in Patients Hospitalized for Interstitial SARS-CoV2 Pneumonia: A Cohort Study [24]

This is a machine-generated summary of:

Landolfo, Matteo; Maino, Alberto; Di Salvo, Emanuela; Fiorini, Giulia; Peterlana, Dimitri; Borghi, Claudio: Renin–angiotensin system modulation and outcomes in patients hospitalized for interstitial SARS-CoV2 pneumonia: a cohort study [24].

Published in: Internal and Emergency Medicine (2022).

Link to original: https://doi.org/10.1007/s11739-022-02929-7

If you want to cite the papers, please refer to the original.

For technical reasons we could not place the page where the original quote is coming from.

Abstract-Summary "We performed a cohort study on consecutive patients admitted for COVID-19 pneumonia at the Internal Medicine Unit of Sant'Orsola-Malpighi Hospital in Bologna, Italy."

"Patients with chronic use of RAS modulation were compared with those without for the composite outcome of in-hospital mortality or ICU admission."

"Of the 268 patients enrolled in the study, 93 (35%, mean age 68 ± 13 years, 67% males) were treated with RASi (58% ACEIs and 42% ARBs)."

"There were no meaningful differences between the RASI and no RASI group regarding clinical and laboratory parameters at admission."

"One hundred eight patients (40%) were admitted to ICU during hospitalization due to severe respiratory failure, and 24 (9%) died."

"The risk of in-hospital death or ICU admission was lower in the RASI group than in the non-RASI group (age and sex-adjusted HR 0.57, 95% CI 0.37–0.8), even after adjustment for several comorbidities (fully adjusted HR 0.44, 95% CI 0.26–0.74)."

"Seven (7.5%) patients died in the RASi group vs. 17 (9.7%) in the non-RASi group, leading to a non-statistically significant mortality risk reduction (fully adjusted HR 0.69, 95% CI 0.18–1.90)."

"The lower risk in the RASi group was primarily related to ARBs use compared to ACEIs (HR 0.5, 95% CI 0.28–0.92 and HR 0.82, 95% CI 0.51–1.32, respectively)."

"Our study showed an inverse association between the chronic use of RASi and COVID-19 pneumonia severity (either ICU admissions or in-hospital death), even when significant comorbidities are considered."

Introduction

"Experimental data were consistent with RAS inhibitors (RASi) increasing the expression of the ACE2 receptors, somehow favoring the SARS-CoV2 binding and entry into the respiratory epithelium."

"They supported that restoring the ACE1/ACE2 balance with angiotensin-receptor blockers (ARBs) or angiotensin-converting enzyme inhibitors (ACEIs) could exert a protective role and attenuate lung tissue damage in SARS-CoV pneumonia [25, 26]."

"The principal limitations of these studies concerned the heterogeneous study population, unknown reasons for RASi discontinuation, variability of outcomes, the lack of data regarding previous RASi exposure and the potential difference between angiotensin-converting enzyme inhibitors (ACEIs) and angiotensin-receptor blockers (ARBs) [27]."

"We aimed to evaluate further the impact of chronic RASi exposure in hospitalized patients with COVID-19-related pneumonia, to investigate its association with the severity of the disease and outcome."

Methods

"We enrolled a cohort of consecutive patients admitted at the Internal Medicine Unit of the Sant'Orsola-Malpighi Hospital in Bologna (Italy) for SARS-CoV2 interstitial pneumonia during the second pandemic wave, from January 2021 to May 2021."

"Respiratory support with low-flow oxygen (nasal cannula or Venturi mask) was given according to the single patient need and to keep arterial oxygen saturation above 90%."

"The study primary outcome is a composite of in-hospital mortality and ICU admission for severe respiratory failure, whichever occurred first."

"Hazard ratios, as surrogates of risk ratios, obtained by Cox-regression models, were used to compare patients with chronic RASi treatment and patients without for the composite outcome and mortality."

"For the composite outcome, patients were followed until ICU admission or in-ward death (before ICU), whichever occurred first."

"For the analysis of mortality, patients were followed until in-hospital death (before or after ICU admission)."

Results

"94 (82%) were admitted to the ICU (of which nine died), whereas 22 subjects (mean age 84 ± 6 years) were not considered eligible for ICU admission because of severe comorbidities."

"Regarding in-hospital mortality, of the 24 deaths observed, seven (7.5%) occurred in the RASi group, whereas 17 (9.7%) in the non-RASi group, leading to a not statistically significant mortality risk reduction in the RASi group compared with the non-RASi group (age and sex-adjusted HR 0.46, CI 95% 0.18–1.20; fully adjusted HR 0.59, CI 95% 0.18–1.90)."

"Besides, the lower risk of death or ICU admission in the RASi group was primarily related to ARBs use compared to ACEIs (HR for the composite outcome 0.5, 95% CI 0.28–0.92 and HR 0.82, 95% CI 0.51–1.32, respectively)."

Discussion

"Our study was designed to assess the impact of the prosecution of chronic RASi, either ACEIs or ARBs, on COVID-19 severity in a carefully selected population of patients admitted for various degrees of respiratory failure due to SARS-CoV2 interstitial pneumonia confirmed by HRCT findings of interstitial lung disease."

"In recent studies on COVID-19 patients with HF, in which poorer outcomes are expected and in which the pre-existing lung fluid handling and gas diffusion process impairment can be worsened by the superimposed infection, chronic treatment with RASi agents was not associated with less respiratory involvement, increased risk of death or better outcomes [28, 29]."

"The presence of an inverse association between chronic RASi exposure and COVID-19 pneumonia severity should be considered from the perspective that the benefit might also be related to the effect of continuing RASi on the underlying disease."

Beneficial Effects of Angiotensin II Receptor Blockers on Mortality in Patients with COVID-19: A Retrospective Study from 2019 to 2020 in China [30]

This is a machine-generated summary of:

Xu, Ke; He, Wu; Yu, Bo; Zhong, Kaineng; Zhou, Da; Wang, Dao Wen: Beneficial Effects of Angiotensin II Receptor Blockers on Mortality in Patients with COVID-19: A Retrospective Study from 2019 to 2020 in China [30].

Published in: Cardiovascular Drugs and Therapy (2023).

Link to original: https://doi.org/10.1007/s10557-023-07494-5

If you want to cite the papers, please refer to the original.

For technical reasons we could not place the page where the original quote is coming from.

Abstract-Summary "This multicenter retrospective study investigated whether ACEI/ARB administration was beneficial in patients with COVID-19 and CVDs."

"In the multivariate Cox regression model, after adjusting for age, gender, comorbidities, and in-hospital medications, ARB use was associated with lower all-cause mortality (adjusted HR, 0.53; 95% CI, 0.38–0.73; P < 0.001)."

"After propensity score-matched analysis, the adjusted HR for the use of ARB associated with all-cause mortality was 0.62 (95% CI, 0.40–0.88; P = 0.02)."

"Further subgroup analyses found that the adjusted HRs for the use of ARB associated with all-cause mortality were 0.52 (95% CI, 0.30–0.89; P = 0.016), 0.37 (95% CI, 0.21–0.64; P < 0.001), 0.42 (95% CI, 0.28–0.64; P < 0.001), and 0.55 (95% CI, 0.37–0.84; P = 0.005) in patients with heart failure, diabetes, and hypercholesterolemia, and severe COVID-19, respectively."

"ARB administration was significantly associated with a lower risk of all-cause mortality in patients with COVID-19 and CVDs."

Introduction

"Many risk factors contributing to the death of patients with COVID-19 have been studied and identified, including older age, male sex, obesity, diabetes, and hypertension, all of which are associated with higher severity rates and mortality [31, 32]."

"Some small-scale studies found an association between the use of ACEIs/ARBs and a lower risk of mortality in patients with COVID-19 and hypertension [33–35]."

"It is still thought that the use of RAAS inhibitors in patients may lead to an increase in ACE2 levels, which may contribute to the development of infection, even though most studies found that treatment with ACEI/ARB is harmless in patients with COVID-19 [36]."

"In light of this, our study aimed to determine the association between ARB use and the risk of all-cause mortality in patients with COVID-19 and CVDs and to provide more evidence for the use of ARBs to treat patients with COVID-19."

Methods

"All patients with COVID-19, according to the China and WHO interim guidelines, from 138 hospitals in Hubei Province were screened; those who died or were discharged between December 29, 2019 (i.e., when the first patients were admitted) and August 31, 2021, were included in our study."

"Those aged <18 years and lacking important basic information, laboratory test results, treatment information, and reverse transcriptase–polymerase chain reaction results for SARS-CoV-2 were excluded."

"The collected information included age, sex, comorbidities, exposure history, oxygen support during hospitalization, vital signs (temperature, respiratory rate, pulse rate, and systolic and diastolic blood pressures), serum laboratory tests (including routine blood tests, blood chemical variables, procalcitonin, and coagulation function tests), therapeutic strategy during hospitalization, and outcomes."

"Patients who were unable to take medication because of hypotension or mechanical ventilation without nasal feeding and those who discontinued treatment were included in our study classified into the no treatment group."

Results

"After adjusting for age, gender, comorbidities, and in-hospital medications (such as metformin and statins), the use of ARBs was associated with lower all-cause mortality (adjusted HR, 0.54; 95% CI, 0.39–0.74; $P < 0.001$)."

"The adjusted HR for the use of ARBs associated with all-cause mortality was 0.62 (95% CI, 0.40–0.88; $P = 0.02$), which indicated that the use of ARBs was related to the lower risk of all-cause mortality, consistent with the result of K–M curve analysis ($P = 0.001$)."

"The above results indicate that there was a strong association between the use of ARBs and a lower risk of all-cause mortality by the multivariate Cox regression model, K–M curves, and propensity score-matched analysis."

"The data suggest that there was a significantly lower risk of all-cause mortality in the ARB group than in the non-ARB group among patients with heart failure, diabetes, hypercholesterolemia, or severe COVID-19."

Discussion

"A study from nine hospitals in Hubei Province in 2020 showed that among hospitalized patients with COVID-19 and coexisting hypertension, inpatient use of ACEIs/ARBs was associated with a lower risk of all-cause mortality than ACEIs/ARBs nonusers [33]."

"The European Society of Cardiology (ESC) guidance for the diagnosis and management of CVDs during the COVID-19 pandemic, published in 2022, suggests that despite much early speculation of a link between the use of ACEIs or

ARBs and increased risk from COVID-19, a series of clinical studies across the world have shown no increased risk of COVID-19 or the risk of developing severe complications or death from COVID-19 in patients taking ACEIs or ARBs, when compared to the risk in patients taking other antihypertensive drugs [37]."

"Our study collected clinical data in the early stages of the pandemic in Hubei Province, conducted an epidemiological analysis, and determined that the use of ARBs in patients with COVID-19 and CVDs contributed to a good prognosis."

Conclusion

"ARB treatment was significantly associated with a lower risk of all-cause mortality in patients with COVID-19 and CVDs."

"This strong association generally considers the different types of comorbidities."

"AT receptor blockers are recommended for the treatment of patients with COVID-19 and CVDs."

Neither ACEIs nor ARBs Are Associated with Respiratory Distress or Mortality in COVID-19 Results of a Prospective Study on a Hospital-Based Cohort [38]

This is a machine-generated summary of:

Anzola, Gian Paolo; Bartolaminelli, Clara; Gregorini, Gina Alessandra; Coazzoli, Chiara; Gatti, Francesca; Mora, Alessandra; Charalampakis, Dimitrios; Palmigiano, Andrea; De Simone, Michele; Comini, Alice; Dellaglio, Erica; Cassetti, Salvatore; Chiesa, Maurizio; Spedini, Francesca; d'Ottavi, Patrizia; Savio, Maria Cristina: Neither ACEIs nor ARBs are associated with respiratory distress or mortality in COVID-19 results of a prospective study on a hospital-based cohort [38].

Published in: Internal and Emergency Medicine (2020).

Link to original: https://doi.org/10.1007/s11739-020-02500-2

If you want to cite the papers, please refer to the original.

For technical reasons we could not place the page where the original quote is coming from.

Abstract-Summary "Considerable concern has emerged for the potential harm in the use of angiotensin-converting enzyme inhibitors (ACEIs) and angiotensin receptor inhibitors (ARBs) in COVID-19 patients, given that ACEIs and ARBs may increase the expression of ACE2 receptors that represent the way for coronavirus 2 to entry into the cell and cause severe acute respiratory syndrome."

"Assess the effect of ACEI/ARBs on outcome in COVID-19 patients."

"A total of 431 patients consecutively presenting at the Emergency Department and found to be affected by COVID-19 were assessed."

"Outcome variables were NO, MILD, SEVERE respiratory distress (RD) operationally defined and DEATH."

"Distribution of antihypertensive treatment was: ACEIs 77/221 (35%), ARBs 63/221 (28%), OTHER than ACEIs or ARBs 64/221 (29%)."

"The proportion of patients taking ACEIs, ARBs or OTHERs who developed MILD or SEVERE RD was 43/77 (56%), 33/53 (52%), 39/64 (61%) and 19/77 (25%), 16/63 (25%) and 16/64 (25%), respectively, with no statistical difference between groups."

"ACEIs and ARBs do not promote a more severe outcome of COVID-19."

Introduction and Aim of the Study

"In early December 2019, a new pathogen, later identified as a novel enveloped RNA betacoronavirus, that is currently been named severe acute respiratory syndrome coronavirus (SARS-CoV-2), gave rise to an outbreak of pneumonia that started from Wuhan in the Chinese province of Hubei and spread across a large territory of the country infecting more than 80,000 subjects in less than a couple of months [39]."

"Despite being probably less lethal than SARS, which had a reported case fatally rate of 43.3% (32.2–52.4) in patients aged 60 years or older [40], current coronavirus disease 19 (COVID-19) is not at all a benign disease."

"Partly to help solving this issue, we undertook a prospective study aimed at assessing the clinical characteristics, with particular emphasis on the type of antihypertensive medication, of all consecutive patients presenting at the Emergency Department of a Community Hospital in Gavardo, in the neighborhood of Brescia in Lombardia (Italy), and found to be positive for SARS-CoV-2 infection."

Material and Method

"The place of recruitment was the Emergency Department of the Hospital of Gavardo, situated in the neighborhood of Brescia in Lombardia and belonging to the Local Health Authority (LHA) ASST Garda."

"Clinical severity was categorized as: NO respiratory distress (NO RD = Sat."

"Due to the often dramatic clinical emergency, some variables were incompletely assessed in a non-significant proportion of patients except for BMI that was available in only 195/431 (45%)."

"The prevalence of each categorical variable and the means of continuous variables were calculated in patients with NO, MILD or SEVERE RD and in deceased subjects."

"Single comparisons were performed with Chi-square test or Fisher's exact test when appropriate on categorical variables and with independent sample t test (if normally distributed) or with Mann–Whitney U test on continuous variables."

"Variables that had proved significant on univariate analysis were entered multivariate binomial logistic regression analyses to identify independent predictors of MILD RD, SEVERE RD and DEATH."

Results

"Some variables were able to discriminate also MILD from SEVERE RD: these were age (67 ± 13 vs. 78 ± 11), CVD (18% vs. 42%), creatinine (1.04 ± 0.46 vs. 1.71 ± 1.26) and CRP (96 ± 70 vs. 152 ± 83)."

"Two ROC curves were fitted to CRP and creatinine values with SEVERE RD as outcome of interest."

"For CRP, the threshold value of 77.5 correctly identified 87% of SEVERE RD cases with 11.8% of false positives, whereas for creatinine the threshold value of 1.05 was less efficient as it picked up only 69.6% of cases with 8.8% of false positives."

"Three multivariate logistic regression analyses were performed, with MILD RD, SEVERE RD and DEATH as dependent variables and taking as covariates those that had turned significant predictors in univariate analysis."

"Age and CRP were independent predictor of MILD RD, SEVERE RD and DEATH, AST only of MILD RD and creatinine of SEVERE RD and DEATH."

Discussion

"The main finding was that there was not even the least hint that ACEIs or ARBs behave differently from OTHERs in terms of increased frequency of worse outcomes."

"In univariate analyses, the relative risk of MILD RD and SEVERE RD increased by a factor of 2–16 with age, male gender, BMI, hypertension, renal failure and CVD, in agreement with most earlier reports [39, 41–46]."

"CRP was the single most powerful predictor of outcome, linearly increasing from NO RD to MILD RD to SEVERE RD in a way that allowed the establishment of a threshold for SEVERE RD, with a good tradeoff of 87% sensitivity and 88.8% specificity."

"We studied prospectively a cohort of consecutive Emergency Department patients found to have COVID-19 and were able to assess the relationship between ACEI and ARB use and the severity of the disease."

"Although many clinical variables had an individual effect on outcome, age, creatinine and CRP were the only independent predictors of SEVERE RD and DEATH."

Angiotensin Enzyme Inhibitors and Angiotensin Receptor Blockers as Protective Factors in COVID-19 Mortality: A Retrospective Cohort Study [47]

This is a machine-generated summary of:

Yahyavi, Ashkan; Hemmati, Nima; Derakhshan, Pegah; Banivaheb, Behrooz; Karimi Behnagh, Arman; Tofighi, Rozhin; TehraniYazdi, Alireza; Kabir, Ali: Angiotensin enzyme inhibitors and angiotensin receptor blockers as protective factors in COVID-19 mortality: a retrospective cohort study [47].

Published in: Internal and Emergency Medicine (2020).

Link to original: https://doi.org/10.1007/s11739-020-02523-9

If you want to cite the papers, please refer to the original.

For technical reasons we could not place the page where the original quote is coming from.

Abstract-Summary "Targeting the renin-angiotensin system is proposed to affect mortality due to coronavirus disease 2019 (COVID-19)."

"We aimed to compare the mortality rates in COVID-19 patients who received angiotensin-converting enzyme inhibitors or angiotensin receptor blockers (ACEIs/ARBs) and those who did not."

"The mortality frequency was higher in patients with a history of underlying diseases (22.4% vs 12.7%, P value <0.001)."

"The mortality rate in patients who received ACEIs/ARBs were higher than non-receivers (29.3% vs. 19.5%, P value = 0.013, OR = 1.3, 95% CI 1.1, 1.7) in the univariate analysis."

"The use of ACEIs/ARBs was a protective factor against mortality in the model when adjusted for underlying conditions, length of stay, age, gender, and ICU admission (P value < 0.001, OR = 0.5, 95% CI 0.3, 0.7)."

"ACEIs/ARBs are protective factors against mortality in COVID-19 patients with HTN, and these agents can be considered potential therapeutic options in this disease."

"The survival probability is higher in ACEIs/ARBs receivers than non-receivers."

Introduction

"Several medications have been proposed, one of which is based on targeting the angiotensin-converting enzyme 2 (ACE2) receptor with special recombinant molecules [48]."

"Studies have revealed that based on the biochemical and crystal structure of severe acute respiratory syndrome coronavirus (SARS-CoV), this virus's surface glycoprotein exhibits a high affinity for the human ACE2 receptor."

"Overexpression of the ACE2 receptor was associated with aggravated disease in animal models and, by facilitating the virus's entry, it resulted in increased damage to the lung tissue."

"The vast distribution of ACE2 receptors on the surface of various types of cells throughout the body also explains the possible cause behind multi-organ failure in severe cases [49, 50]."

"Targeting the ACE/angiotensin II/angiotensin I receptor (ACE/AngII/ATIR) is proposed as a novel management strategy in patients suffering from HTN."

"Angiotensin-converting enzyme inhibitors (ACEIs) and angiotensin receptor blockers (ARBs) are capable of targeting the ACE/AngII/ATIR signaling pathway, as well as impacting the ACE/Ang receptor expression [51]."

Methods

"In this retrospective cohort study, patients diagnosed with COVID-19 (according to World Health Organization interim guidance [52]), admitted to 17 referral hospitals affiliated to Iran University of medical sciences (IUMS) between February 20th and April 4th were enrolled."

"Whenever a patient is admitted to a hospital, the data (personal information, diagnosis, discharge information, all services, and administered medications) are captured in real-time."

"Recorded data included demographic variables, underlying comorbidities including DM, HTN, chronic kidney disease (CKD), chronic pulmonary diseases (CPD), malignancies, cardiovascular diseases (CVD), chronic use of immunosuppressive medications, intensive care unit (ICU) admission, length of hospital stay (LOS) and clinical outcomes (death/recovery)."

"As of immunosuppressant medications, all patients who received any of the drugs in the following classes chronically were included: calcineurin inhibitors, anti-proliferative agents, mammalian target of rapamycin inhibitors, and steroids."

"All the patients had a history of receiving these medications both before and during hospitalization."

Results

"The frequency of chronic use of immunosuppressants, DM, ICU admission, CKD, CPD, mortality (22.3% vs. 17.8%, P value = 0.030, OR = 1.3, 95% CI 1.0, 1.7) and gender was higher among ARBs receivers when excluding patients who received ACEIs."

"The rate of all underlying conditions was higher in ACEIs/ARBs receivers except for malignancy (P value = 0.348)."

"A logistic regression model was designed with mortality as the dependent variable and ACEIs/ARBs administration, CVD, CKD, CPD, DM, malignancy, and chronic use of immunosuppressants, age, gender, ICU admission, LOS, CCBs, diuretics, and beta-blockers as independent variables."

"These variables included ACEIs/ARBs administration, CVD, CKD, CPD, DM, malignancy, chronic use of immunosuppressants, ICU admission, gender, age, CCBs, beta-blockers, and diuretics."

"Patients with a history of ACEIs/ARBs administration had a lower risk of mortality than non-receivers (HR = 0.7, 95% CI 0.6, 0.9, P value = 0.008)."

Discussion

"A study with a small sample size suggested that ACEIs/ARBs can improve the clinical outcome of COVID-19 patients with HTN [53]."

"The results of our study demonstrate that by adjusting for underlying diseases, ICU admission, and demographic characteristics, medications that affect the RAS system (ACEIs and ARBs) became protective factors of mortality."

"Although these rates were higher, all except LOS shown to be independent risk factors of mortality in COVID-19 patients, the mortality rate of ACEIs receivers did not differ with non-receivers when excluding patients who received ARBs."

"Administration of ACEIs/ARBs was shown to be a protective factor (OR = 0.3) although it was not statistically significant, probably due to the sample size being small, in a recent study by Yang and others [54]. In another study by Peng Zhang and others, in-hospital administration of ACEIs/ARBs in patients with concurrent HTN and COVID-19 was found to lower mortality risk in these cases (hazard ratio = 0.4) [33]."

"Our findings are also in accordance with the results of these mentioned studies, which suggest ACEIs/ARBs as potential therapeutic options in all COVID-19 patients."

Conclusion

"Administration of ACEIs/ARBs in COVID-19 patients with concurrent HTN will result in improved clinical outcomes, and these medications can be potential therapeutic options and increase the survival probability in these cases."

"Other anti-HTN medications did not have a protective effect on mortality."

"COVID-19 patients with a history of chronic immunosuppressant administration, malignancy, CPD, CVD, DM, HTN, and CKD were found to have an increased risk of mortality."

The Effect of ACE Inhibitors and ARBs on Outcomes in Hospitalized Patients with COVID-19 [55]

This is a machine-generated summary of:

Najafi, Narges; Davoudi, Alireza; Izadyar, Hamideh; Alishahi, Abbas; Mokhtariani, Armaghan; Soleimanpourian, Bahareh; Tabarrayi, Mina; Moosazadeh, Mahmood; Daftarian, Zahra; Ahangarkani, Fatemeh: The effect of ACE inhibitors and ARBs on outcomes in hospitalized patients with COVID-19 [55].

Published in: Irish Journal of Medical Science (2022).

Link to original: https://doi.org/10.1007/s11845-022-03096-6

If you want to cite the papers, please refer to the original.

For technical reasons we could not place the page where the original quote is coming from.

Abstract-Summary "The effects of ACEIs and ARBs on outcomes of COVID-19 patients were evaluated."

"The incidence of moderate and severe forms of COVID-19 was significantly higher in patients taking ACEI/ARB drugs (P-value = 0.012)."

"Patients taking ACEI/ARB drugs (P-value = 0.034), patients with hypertension (P-value = 0.011), and patients with dyslipidemia (P-value = 0.011) experienced more severe forms of COVID-19."

"There was an association between increased length of hospital stay and dyslipidemia (P-value = 0.033) and the use of ACEI/ARB drugs (P-value = 0.041), while no correlation was found between other parameters in univariate linear regression analysis as well as multivariate linear regression."

"ACEI/ARB drugs put COVID-19 patients at high risk for moderate to severe forms of COVID-19 and higher length of hospital stay."

Background

"ACEI and ARBs can help restore the balance between ACE1 and ACE2 and have beneficial effects in controlling COVID-19 [56, 57]."

"Several animal studies have also confirmed the protective effect of ARBs against COVID-19 by increasing ACE2 levels [58–60]."

"The effect of the use of ACEI and ARBs and the increase in ACE2 expression in the pathogenicity of the COVID-19 is not known."

"The virus may enter the cell due to increased ACE2 expression following the use of ACEI and ARBs."

"Despite the contradictory effects of ACEI and ARBs, there is no evidence to discontinue the routine use of these drugs in COVID-19 patients, and it is recommended to continue their routine usage [60–62]."

"Considering the contradictory opinions about the use of ACEI and ARBs in patients with hypertension and the high prevalence of hypertension among individuals in Iran [63], in this study, the influence of ACE inhibitors and ARBs in the outcome of COVID-19 patients was evaluated."

Methods

"In a cross-sectional study, we evaluated the medical records of all patients over 18 years old who were hospitalized with COVID-19 in Razi Hospital (an infectious disease referral center in Mazandaran province in north of Iran)."

"Data documented in the patient's health record were collected from hospitalized COVID-19 patients from February 20 to May 21, 2020."

"Demographics data included age, sex, and body mass index (BMI); clinical features such as underlying diseases and severity of diseases and both ACE (including losartan and valsartan) and ARB (including captopril and enalapril) medications were recorded."

"The outcomes of COVID-19 were compared between patients receiving pretreatment ACE inhibitors or ARBs and those who did not receive these drugs."

"Univariate linear regression was performed to evaluate the association between ACEI/ARB using status, demographic characteristics and existing comorbidities with adverse outcomes of COVID-19."

Results

"The mean length of hospital stay of patients taking ACEI/ARBs was longer, but there was no statistically significant relationship (P-value = 0.108)."

"Patients, 29 (22%) were taking ACEI/ARB drugs with a mean length of stay in the ICU (5.37 ± 4.09 days vs. 5.78 ± 5.2 days) (P-value = 0.311)."

"Ordinal logistic regression analysis on parameters including age, sex, BMI, ACEI/ARB usage status, and underlying diseases showed that patients taking ACEI/ARB drugs (adjusted odds ratios [adjOR] 1.253, 95% CI (1.017–1.543), P-value = 0.034), patients with hypertension (adjOR 0.786, 95% CI (0.653-0.947), P-value = 0.011), and patients with dyslipidemia (adjOR 1.289, 95% CI (1.061-1.565), P-value = 0.011) experienced the severe form of COVID-19 more than other patients."

Discussions

"An important finding of our study was that the use of ACEI/ARBs could increase the severity of COVID-19 infection, but no significant relationship was found between the length of hospital stay in the ICU, the need for ICU hospitalization, and the need for mechanical ventilation."

"In the study of Braude and others, patients with hypertension taking ACEI/ARB medications regardless of age, other comorbidities, and COVID-19 severity had decreased hospital stay lengths compared to other patients [64]."

"Similar to our results, in Mehta and others's study on the relationship between ACEI/ARB use and ICU hospitalization in COVID-19 patients, ICU hospitalization rates were higher in patients receiving ACEI, but no association was found between ARB use and ICU hospitalization [1]."

"Several studies have found the use of ACEI/ARBs in patients with COVID-19 to have no influence on mortality [56, 65, 66]."

Conclusion

"We concluded that ACE and ARB drugs put COVID-19 patients at high risk for moderate to severe forms of infection."

"ACE and ARB users' mean length of hospital stay was higher than those of non-ACE/ARB users."

"These drugs did not significantly affect specific outcomes of COVID-19, such as the need for admission to ICU, length of ICU stay, ventilation, and mortality."

Association Between Angiotensinogen (AGT), Angiotensin-Converting Enzyme (ACE) and Angiotensin-II Receptor 1 (AGTR1) Polymorphisms and COVID-19 Infection in the Southeast of Iran: A Preliminary Case-Control Study [67]

This is a machine-generated summary of:

Kouhpayeh, Hamid Reza; Tabasi, Farhad; Dehvari, Mohammad; Naderi, Mohammad; Bahari, Gholamreza; Khalili, Tahereh; Clark, Courtney; Ghavami, Saeid; Taheri, Mohsen: Association between angiotensinogen (AGT), angiotensin-converting enzyme (ACE) and angiotensin-II receptor 1 (AGTR1) polymorphisms and COVID-19 infection in the southeast of Iran: a preliminary case-control study [67].

Published in: Translational Medicine Communications (2021).

Link to original: https://doi.org/10.1186/s41231-021-00106-0

If you want to cite the papers, please refer to the original.

For technical reasons we could not place the page where the original quote is coming from.

Abstract-Summary "The disease is caused by severe acute respiratory syndrome coronavirus-2 (SARS-CoV--2) infection, targeting angiotensin-converting enzyme-2 (ACE2) receptor for cell entry."

"We aimed to evaluate the association between AGT rs699 C > T, ACE rs4646994 I/D, and AGTR1 rs5186 C > A variants and the risk of COVID-19 infection and the severity in a sample of the southeast Iranian population."

"Genotyping of the ACE gene rs4646994, and AGT rs699, and AGTR1 rs5186 polymorphisms was performed by polymerase chain reaction (PCR) and PCR-restriction fragment length polymorphism (PCR-RFLP), respectively."

"Our results showed that the II genotype of ACE rs4646994 and the I allele decreased the risk of COVID-19 infection."

"We found that the TC genotype and C allele of AGT rs699 increased the risk of COVID-19 infection."

"The AGTR1 rs5186 was not associated with COVID-19 infection."

"These findings suggest that ACE rs4646994 and AGT rs699 polymorphisms increase the risk of COVID-19 infection in a southeast Iranian population."

Introduction

"Angiotensin II receptor 1 (AGTR1) may drive COVID-19 pathology: AGTR1 is G-protein coupled receptor (GPCR), mediates signaling and most functions of angiotensin-II that generated by the angiotensin-I converting enzyme (ACE1) [68, 69]."

"Previous evidence regarding SARS-CoV infection, mediated by ACE-2, which highly express in pulmonary tissue, indicates that binding SARS virus results in a decrease in ACE2 activity and expression [70], leading to an increase in angiotensin-II level [71]."

"Further, downregulated ACE2 decreases peptides converted from angiotensin-II to counteract its effects, including pro-apoptotic properties [72], inflammation, and fibrosis [73, 74], all of which are the basis of COVID-19 pathobiology."

"Angiotensin-II exerts its effects via AGTR1, encoded by the AGTR1 gene on chromosome 3q24."

"Given the current evidence regarding the potential implication of angiotensin-related signaling cascade in COVID-19 [72, 73], we investigate the association between AGT rs699 C > T, ACE rs4646994 indel, and AGTR1 rs5186 C > A variants and the risk of COVID-19 infection in a sample of the southeast Iranian population."

Materials and Methods

"The sample population for this case-control study comprised 258 COVID-19 subjects who tested positive for SARS-CoV-2 infection using real-time reverse transcription polymerase chain reaction (RT-PCR) technique and 246 healthy control subjects with similar geographic and ethnic backgrounds."

"Samples were collected in Bu-Ali Sina Hospital, designated as a specialized center for infectious disease in Zahedan, from May 2020 through September 2020, in which the original SARS-CoV-2 was dominant."

"Further, the control group comprised individuals who tested negative to COVID-19 by RT-PCR method AND clinical diagnostic criteria, which finally ruled out the disease."

"Severe cases were defined as patients with a positive RT-PCR result for COVID-19, and clinical signs comply with severe pneumonia plus one of the following conditions: $SpO_2 < 90\%$ on room air or respiratory rate > 30 breath/min or sign of severe respiratory distress."

"The non-severe case was defined as patients with a positive RT-PCR in the absence of any criteria for severe disease."

Results

"Although there were no differences regarding sex between severe and non-severe cases ($p = 0.31$), patients with severe disease had significantly higher age than non-severe patients ($p = 0.003$)."

"Genotyping of AGT rs699 revealed a remarkable difference between COVID-19 positive patients and healthy controls; TC genotype (OR = 8.43, 95% CI = 4.99–14.24, $p < 0.001$, TC vs. TT) as well as C allele (OR = 2.25, 95% CI = 1.71–2.96, $p < 0.001$, C vs. T) increased the risk of COVID-19 infection."

"ACE rs4646994 showed a significant association with non-severe disease in recessive model (OR = 0.42, 95%CI = 0.18–0.99, $p = 0.03$, II vs DD + ID)."

"The C allele of AGTR1 rs5186 was a significant association with non-severe disease (OR = 0.51, 95%CI = 0.29–0.90, $p = 0.01$, C vs. A)."

Discussion

"Our result showed that ACE indel and ATG rs699 is associated with susceptibility to COVID-19 infection; however, we did not observe any association between these polymorphisms and the risk of severe disease, but the age and prevalence of diabetes and hypertension in patients with severe disease were remarkably higher than patients with a non-severe disease."

"Patients with underlying diabetes and hypertension show a decreased ACE2 expression state, associated with increased angiotensin-II and a pro-inflammatory condition [75]."

"Our results suggest ACE rs4646994 and AGT rs699 are associated with the risk of COVID-19 infection and may be used as predictive biomarkers, for instabce the diagnosis of patients at higher risk for developing COVID-19 infection."

"We found that ACE rs4646994 I allele and AGT C allele are associated with decreased and increased risk of COVID-19 infection, respectively."

Angiotensin-Converting Enzyme Inhibitors (ACEI) or Angiotensin Receptor Blockers (ARBs) May Be Safe for COVID-19 Patients [76]

This is a machine-generated summary of:

Wang, Wenjun; Zhao, Xiaohui; Wei, Wei; Fan, Weiwang; Gao, Kai; He, Shengxiu; Zhuang, Xijing: Angiotensin-converting enzyme inhibitors (ACEI) or angiotensin receptor blockers (ARBs) may be safe for COVID-19 patients [76].

Published in: BMC Infectious Diseases (2021).

Link to original: https://doi.org/10.1186/s12879-021-05821-5

If you want to cite the papers, please refer to the original.

For technical reasons we could not place the page where the original quote is coming from.

Abstract-Summary "To investigate the effects of angiotensin-converting enzyme inhibitor (ACEI) and angiotensin receptor blockers (ARBs) administration to hypertension patients with the coronavirus disease 2019 (COVID-19) induced pneumonia."

"We did a comparative analysis of various parameters such as the pneumonia progression, length-of-stay in the hospital, and the level of alanine aminotransferase (ALT), serum creatinine (Cr), and creatine kinase (CK) between the day when these patients were admitted to the hospital and the day when the treatment ended."

"There was no significant difference in the usage of drug treatment of COVID-19 between groups A and B ($p > 0.05$)."

"All patients were cured and discharged after treatment, and no recurrence of COVID-2019 induced pneumonia occurred after the discharge."

"There was also no significant difference in other general parameters between the patients of the groups A and B on the day of admission to the hospital ($p > 0.05$)."

"The ALT, CK, and Cr levels did not significantly differ between groups A and B on the day of admission and the day of discharge ($p > 0.05$)."

"To treat the hypertension patients with COVID-19 caused pneumonia, anti-hypertensive drugs (ACEs and ARBs) may be used according to the relative guidelines."

Background

"Coronavirus disease 2019 (COVID-19), caused by a novel coronavirus (SARS-CoV-2), began in Wuhan, Hubei province, China in December 2019."

"Similar to the SARS viruse, the SARS-CoV-2 infect alveolar cells via binding to the S-receptor binding domain and angiotensin-converting enzyme (ACE) 2 receptor and causes a series of pathological changes in the patients [77–83]."

"Previous studies on SARS-CoV have shown that the elevation of AngII contributes to the occurrence and aggravation of acute pneumonia, and that SARS-CoV infection induces a decrease in the expression of tissue ACE 2 [84]."

"We evaluated the therapeutic effect of an ACEI and ARBs on 67 inpatients with hypertension and COVID-19 caused pneumonia in the Raytheon Mountain Hospital in Wuhan between February 12, 2020 and March 30, 2020 and report their disease progression and recovery status."

Methods

"The data included in this study were collected from COVID-19 patients hospitalized in A4, A8, A13, and B1 wards of Raytheon Mountain Hospital in Wuhan from February 18, 2020 to March 30, 2020."

"The parameters measured in this study included age, gender, comorbidities, the severity classification and recovery status of COVID-19 induced pneumonia, COVID-19 medication, the medication used for hypertension, length-of-stay in the hospital, and serum level of ALT, Cr, and CK on the day of admission in the hospital (beginning of treatment) and the day of discharge from the hospital (end of the treatment)."

"Baseline data included age, gender, underlying disease, serum biochemical markers, and COVID-19 testing during the first 3 days after admission."

"The data at discharge time included the data of the last medical record within one week before the discharge, including the drugs used for COVID-19, serum level of alanine aminotransferase (ALT), serum creatinine (Cr), creatine kinase (CK), disease changes and clinical outcome."

Results

"Among the COVID-19 patients who met the diagnostic criteria of the 2018 Chinese guidelines for the management of hypertension [85], 67 patients were included (14 in A4, 13 in A8, 24 in A13 and 16 in B1), accounting for 33.17% of the total number of patients in A4, A8, A13 and B1.Among 67 patients, there were 33 males and 34 females."

"During the treatment, one patient in group A and three patients in group B progressed from the mild pneumonia stage to severe pneumonia stage."

"At the end of their stay in the hospital, all the patients recovered and tested negative for COVID-19 by nucleic acid detection test."

"No patients had the recurrence of COVID-19 induced pneumonia after discharge."

Discussion

"Some physicians in our hospital also stopped the use of ACEIs and/or ARBs drugs in COVID-19 patients."

"Some studies showed that ARBs or ACEIs induces the expression of ACE2 [86]; however, whether the upregulated expression of ACE2 causes an increased risk of infection with SARS-CoV-2 and/or a deterioration in the progression of COVID-19, is unknown."

"Most studies investigating whether ARBs/ACEIs aggravate COVID-19 induced pneumonia have indicated that inhibition of the RAAS system upregulates the expression of ACE2 and alleviates viral pneumonia [87]."

"Although this study might suffer from the limitation of a smaller sample size number of patients, it still provides evidence that ACEs/ARBs do not increase the aggravation risk of COVID-19 pneumonia."

"To treat hypertension patients with COVID-19 induced pneumonia, antihypertensive drugs such as ACEs and ARBs may be used in accordance with the relative guidelines."

Renin–Angiotensin System Inhibitors and Mortality in Patients with COVID-19 [88]

This is a machine-generated summary of:

Rossi, Luca; Malagoli, Alessandro; Biagi, Andrea; Zanni, Alessia; Sticozzi, Concetta; Comastri, Greta; Pannone, Luigi; Gandolfi, Stefano; Vergara, Pasquale; Villani, Giovanni Quinto: Renin–angiotensin system inhibitors and mortality in patients with COVID-19 [88].

Published in: Infection (2020).

Link to original: https://doi.org/10.1007/s15010-020-01550-0

If you want to cite the papers, please refer to the original.

For technical reasons we could not place the page where the original quote is coming from.

Abstract-Summary "Association of renin–angiotensin system inhibitors with risk of death in patients with hypertension (HTN) and coronavirus disease 2019 (COVID-19) is not well characterized."

"The aim of this study was to evaluate the outcomes of patients with HTN and COVID-19 with respect to different chronic antihypertensive drug intake."

"We performed a retrospective, observational study from a large cohort of patients with HTN and with a laboratory-confirmed severe acute respiratory syndrome coronavirus 2 infection admitted to the Emergency Rooms (ER) of the Piacenza Hospital network from February 21, 2020 to March 20, 2020."

"There were 1050 patients admitted to the ERs of the Piacenza Hospital network with COVID-19."

"Of them, 248 patients were chronically treated with ACEi, 181 with ARBs, and 161 with other drugs (O-drugs) including beta blockers, diuretics and calcium-channel inhibitors."

"During a follow-up of 38 days (IQR 7.0–46.0), 256 patients (43.4%) died, without any difference stratifying for antihypertensive drugs."

"In patients with HTN and COVID-19, neither ACEi nor ARBs were independently associated with mortality."

Introduction

"Angiotensin-Converting Enzyme inhibitors (ACEi) and Angiotensin-Receptor Blockers (ARBs) are a group of pharmaceuticals that have different effects on angiotensin II, the primary substrate of the angiotensin-converting enzyme 2 (ACE2), commonly applied in the treatment of hypertension (HTN)."

"The potential bridge between SARS-CoV-2 pathophysiology and ACEi/ARBs effects derives from evidences showing that SARS-CoV-2 uses ACE2 receptor to enter in human alveolar epithelial cells [89]."

"Use of ACEIs and ARBs might upregulate ACE2 expression, thus increasing patient susceptibility to viral host cell entry."

"The purpose of the present study was to evaluate the association of ACEi and ARBs with risk of death in patients with HTN and COVID-19."

Methods

"This was a retrospective observational study performed at Piacenza Hospital Network, including 3 Hospitals in Piacenza Province, Italy ('Guglielmo da Saliceto' Piacenza Hospital, Castel San Giovanni Hospital and Fiorenzuola d'Arda Hospital); the Hospital network is referral for 287 152 inhabitants."

"All consecutive patients with laboratory-confirmed COVID-19 infection admitted to the Emergency Rooms (ER) of the Piacenza Hospital network from February 21, 2020 to March 20, 2020 and HTN were enrolled in the study."

"Clinical data are routinely collected during ER access and hospitalization in Piacenza Hospital network on a shared electronic medical record."

"Due to the retrospective nature of the study, no sample size calculation was a priori performed; sample size was equal to patients admitted to ERs of the Piacenza Hospital network."

"ANOVA and Bonferroni post hoc test for multiple comparisons were performed to estimate differences between groups stratified by the antihypertensive drug treatment."

"Log-rank test was used to compare survival times of patients stratified by the antihypertensive drug treatment."

Results

"The median time from illness onset to hospital admission was 7 days (IQR 3–10)."

"Non-survivor patients were older [72.9 years old (IQR 64.1–80.2) vs 79.5 years old (IQR 73.9–84.8), $p < 0.001$] and showed more comorbidities compared to survivors."

"Underlying diseases were present in nearly half of patients, with hyperlipidemia being the most common, followed by diabetes, cardiovascular disease, chronic kidney disease and stroke."

"240 (40.7%) patients had 3 or more coexisting medical conditions, without significant differences between groups."

"All 90 patients treated in the outpatient setting were alive."

"159 patients on ACEi were successfully matched with 163 patients on ARBs and 149 on O-Drugs."

"After matching, no significant differences in mortality were found between ACEi, ARBs, and O-drugs groups (log-rank test: p = 0.102)."

Discussion

"Data showed that RAS inhibitors were not associated with an increased mortality of COVID-19 in patient with HTN."

"Uncertainties have been raised on the use antihypertensive drugs that modulate the RAS in patient at risk for COVID-19; it has been suggested that they could act as a potential risk factor for poor outcome in COVID-19 patients by up-regulating ACE2."

"ACE2 has been found to be protective in a number of different lung injury models and it seems reasonable that RAS inhibitors should increase ACE2 level in human lungs [90, 91]."

"On the basis of this detrimental effect, some experts have postulated that use of ACEi/ARBs could increase risk for or severity of COVID-19, suggesting the withdrawal of these drugs [92]."

"Data regarding the effects of RAS inhibitors on lung-specific expression of ACE2 are lacking."

Clinical Implications

"Despite the theoretical uncertainties regarding whether RAS inhibition may influence the infectivity of SARS-CoV-2, there are few available evidences about switching from a RAS inhibitor to another antihypertensive therapy in patients with known or suspected COVID-19."

"Changes in antihypertensive drug treatment require dose titration and potentially exposes patients to the side effects related to the new regimen; the risk of SARS-CoV-2 exposure related to the transient lockdown interruption for face-to-face visits should not be neglected."

"Several Specialty Societies strongly recommended to continue RAS inhibitors in patients in otherwise stable condition who are at risk for, are being evaluated for, or have COVID-19."

Strengths and Limitations

"This study was a retrospective observational analysis of data from a Hospital Network of a single Province in Italy."

"It is plausible that the effects of ACEi/ARBs may be different among patients in ethnically or geographically diverse populations."

"Since the study was underpowered to detect any differential effect between ACEi and ARBs, future bigger observational studies and on-going prospective randomized trials are advisable to fully elucidate possible protective effects of those drug treatments [93–96]."

Conclusions

"In patients with hypertension, Angiotensin-Converting Enzyme inhibitors and Angiotensin-Receptor Blockers are not associated with mortality of COVID-19."

"Our data confirm Specialty Societal recommendations, suggesting that treatment with renin–angiotensin system inhibitors should not be discontinued or replaced with other antihypertensive drugs because of COVID-19."

Impact of In-Hospital Discontinuation with Angiotensin Receptor Blockers or Converting Enzyme Inhibitors on Mortality of COVID-19 Patients: A Retrospective Cohort Study [97]

This is a machine-generated summary of:

de Abajo, Francisco J.; Rodríguez-Miguel, Antonio; Rodríguez-Martín, Sara; Lerma, Victoria; García-Lledó, Alberto: Impact of in-hospital discontinuation with angiotensin receptor blockers or converting enzyme inhibitors on mortality of COVID-19 patients: a retrospective cohort study [97].

Published in: BMC Medicine (2021).

Link to original: https://doi.org/10.1186/s12916-021-01992-9

If you want to cite the papers, please refer to the original.

For technical reasons we could not place the page where the original quote is coming from.

Abstract-Summary "We aimed to assess whether the in-hospital discontinuation of ARBs or ACEIs, in real-life conditions, was associated with a reduced risk of death as compared to their continuation and also to compare head-to-head the continuation of ARBs with the continuation of ACEIs."

"We identified outpatient users of ACEIs/ARBs and divided them in two cohorts depending on treatment discontinuation/continuation at admission."

"Out of 625 ACEI/ARB users, 340 (54.4%) discontinued treatment."

"The in-hospital mortality rates were 27.6% and 27.7% in discontinuation and continuation cohorts, respectively (HR=1.01; 95%CI 0.70–1.46)."

"No difference in mortality was observed between ARB and ACEI discontinuation (28.6% vs. 27.1%, respectively), while a significantly lower mortality rate was found among patients who continued with ARBs (20.8%, N = 125) as compared to those who continued with ACEIs (33.1%, N = 136; p = 0.03)."

"The discontinuation of ACEIs/ARBs at admission did not improve the in-hospital survival."

"The continuation with ARBs was associated with a trend to a reduced mortality as compared to their discontinuation and to a significantly lower mortality risk as compared to the continuation with ACEIs, particularly in high-risk patients."

Background

"Promptly, in the first weeks of May, three large epidemiological studies were published supporting the lack of association between the outpatient use of RASIs and risk of COVID-19 [65, 66, 68–75, 77–87, 89–96, 98, 99]."

"According to this, several observational studies have reported a protective effect of inpatient use of RASIs on mortality as compared to non-use (or non-RASI use) in COVID-19 patients [1, 33–37, 39–46, 48–54, 56–66, 68–75, 77–87, 89–96, 98–101]."

"No study has carried out a head-to-head comparison of in-hospital use of these drugs in COVID-19 patients admitted to the hospital."

"The present research was aimed (1) to quantify the magnitude of RASI discontinuation at admission in seven hospitals from the Autonomous Community of Madrid, Spain; (2) to compare in real-life conditions the in-hospital mortality in patients in whom ACEIs or ARBs were discontinued with those in whom RASIs were continued; and (3) to perform a head-to-head comparison between in-hospital use of ACEIs and ARBs regarding mortality in admitted patients for COVID-19."

Methods

"We excluded those in whom the continuation or discontinuation of RASI treatment could not be properly assessed at admission, including patients transferred to another hospital from the emergency department (ED) and patients who presented the outcome (death or admission to the intensive care unit (ICU)) or were discharged within the first 3 days of hospital admission."

"We proceeded as follows: (1) A binary logistic model was constructed to estimate the propensity score (PS) of RASI discontinuation conditioned on baseline co-morbidities, outpatient treatments, hospital of admission, date of admission (in three periods of equal length), severity score at admission, presence of pneumonia, and treatments prescribed in the first 3 days of hospitalization (including antihypertensive drugs, chloroquine/hydroxychloroquine, and antivirals, the latter two prescribed per protocol for most admitted COVID-19 patients) [102]; (2) Then, we built a Cox proportional hazards model which included the exposure and the estimated PS as a flexible function (restricted cubic splines with 5 knots accounting for 5th, 25th, 50th, 75th, and 95th percentiles) to compute the PS-adjusted hazard ratios (HRs) and their 95% confidence intervals (95%CI); we preferred to use a flexible function instead of simple PS adjustment due to the lack of a linear relationship between PS and the outcome) [103]; (3) We also estimated the controlled direct effect of RASI discontinuation on outcomes by including in the PS-adjusted Cox model the potential mediators (those associated with the exposure, as well as the outcome, controlling for the exposure [103]: systemic corticosteroids, anticoagulants, and immunomodulators when death was the outcome and immunomodulators and anticoagulants when the outcome was death plus ICU admission)."

Results

"In 141 of them, we were unable to assess the continuation of RASIs (59 patients were directly admitted to the ICU: 47 from the ED and 12 from other hospitals; 44 were transferred from the ED to another hospital; 38 had the event—death or ICU admission—or were discharged within the first 3 days of admission); and in 53, the intention-to-discontinue was uncertain (22 presented a sole prescription in days 1 and 31 in days 2 or 3)."

"ICU admission was similar in both groups (5.6% vs. 6.0% for patients who discontinued and continued with RASIs, respectively), as well as the median hospital stay (11 vs. 10 days)."

"Among patients in whom RASIs were discontinued, 94 (27.6%) died in-hospital whereas 79 (27.7%) died among patients in whom RASIs were continued, which yielded a PS-adjusted HR of 1.01 (95%CI 0.71–1.46) that was not modified after controlling for potential mediators (MC-HR=1.01; 95%CI 0.70–1.46)."

Discussion

"The main findings of the present study are as follows: (1) RASIs were discontinued in around half of the patients admitted to hospital for COVID-19 during March 2020; (2) the discontinuation rate increased over time, being particularly notorious since March 11; (3) the discontinuation of RASIs as a group was not associated with an increased or decreased risk of in-hospital death or ICU admission, but the results disaggregated by ARBs and ACEIs were not homogeneous; and (4) the continuation of treatment with ARBs was associated with a significantly lower all-cause mortality than the continuation of treatment with ACEIs."

"The results from two randomized clinical trials in which regular users of RASIs who were admitted to hospital for COVID-19 were assigned to discontinuation or continuation arms, have been reported (BRACE-CORONA [104] and REPLACE COVID [105] trials) and both found no difference in the mortality rates, supporting our results."

Conclusions

"The discontinuation of RASIs at hospital admission was common place in the first wave of COVID-19 pandemic in Spain, influenced by the widely spread hypothesis that postulated a more severe disease in patients treated with these drugs."

"Our results show that the discontinuation of these drugs at admission did not improve the in-hospital survival."

"We found that the discontinuation of treatment with ARBs was associated with a trend to an increased mortality risk as compared to their continuation."

"The continuation with ARBs was associated to a significantly lower mortality risk as compared to the continuation with ACEIs, particularly evident in high-risk subgroups."

Renin-Angiotensin-System Inhibition in the Context of Corona Virus Disease-19: Experimental Evidence, Observational Studies, and Clinical Implications [106]

This is a machine-generated summary of:

Triposkiadis, Filippos; Starling, Randall C.; Xanthopoulos, Andrew; Butler, Javed; Boudoulas, Harisios: Renin-angiotensin-system inhibition in the context of corona virus disease-19: experimental evidence, observational studies, and clinical implications [106].

Published in: Heart Failure Reviews (2020).

Link to original: https://doi.org/10.1007/s10741-020-10022-4

If you want to cite the papers, please refer to the original.

For technical reasons we could not place the page where the original quote is coming from.

Abstract-Summary "While the potential for benefit with the use of renin-angiotensin-aldosterone system inhibitors (RAASi) and the risks from stopping them is more evident, potential harm by RAASi may also be caused by the increase in the activity of the ACE2 receptor, the inefficient counter regulatory axis in the lungs in which the proinflammatory prolyloligopeptidase (POP) is the main enzyme responsible for the conversion of deleterious angiotensin (ANG) II to protective ANG [1–7] and the proinflammatory properties of ACE2(+) cells infected with SARS-CoV-2."

Lung Renin Angiotensin System

"The traditional view is that some of renin-angiotensin system intermediate products may be processed in alternative ways by ACE2, establishing a second axis through ACE2/ANG [1–7]/Mas receptor which counteracts the effects of the classical axis [107]."

"Recent evidence suggests that prolyloligopeptidase (POP) is the main enzyme responsible for the conversion of deleterious ANG II to protective ANG [1–7] in the circulation and lungs, whereas ACE2 contributes to ANG [1–7] formation in the kidney [108]."

"It is questionable whether an efficient ACE2/ANG [1–7]/Mas axis is operative in the lungs."

ACE2 and Coronavirus Entry

"The major entry of SARS-CoV-2 is via the respiratory system where it readily affects differentiated cells that express more ACE2 [109]."

"The type II transmembrane serine proteases TMPRSS2 and ADAM17 (a disintegrin and metalloproteinase) promote SARS-CoV entry by ACE2 cleavage, promotes viral uptake, and SARS-S cleavage, resulting in activation of the viral S protein, which in turn fuses with cell membrane [110]."

"The attachment of the viruses to cell surface ACE2 protects them from immune surveillance mechanisms and provides the virus access to the host cell system, an environment not just to sustain and proliferate, but also to mutate and modify host evasion mechanisms."

"The precise relationship, however, between ACE2 levels and activity, viral infectivity, and severity of infection, is incompletely understood."

ACE2 and Lung Inflammatory Injury

"Prior to COVID-19 pandemic, it was suggested that ACE2 dysregulation is implicated in acute inflammatory lung injury (ILI) by inducing an imbalance in the RAS."

"High levels of PICs were expressed in the SARS-CoV-infected ACE2(+) cells, but not in the uninfected cells suggesting that cells infected by SARS-CoV produce elevated levels of PICs which may cause immuno-mediated damage to the lungs resulting in ILI [111]."

"Similar were the findings in a recent study [112] which used gene set enrichment analysis (GSEA) and showed that the high expression of ACE2 is related to innate immune responses, adaptive immune responses, B cell regulation, and cytokine secretion, as well as an enhanced cytokine-induced inflammatory response."

"It has been postulated that the immune system dysfunction involved in the high expression of ACE2 may be related to the development of the hyperinflammatory response in COVID-19 [112]."

Effect of RAAS Inhibitors on ACE

"Professional scientific societies recommend the unrestricted prescription of RAASi during the COVID-19 pandemic."

"In a recent statement of the European Medicinal Agencies (EMA), it is emphasized (10 June 2020 EMA/284513/2020): "Recent observational studies of angiotensin converting enzyme (ACE) inhibitors and angiotensin receptor blockers (ARBs, also called sartans) have not shown an effect of these medicines on the risk of becoming infected with severe acute respiratory syndrome coronavirus 2 (the virus causing COVID-19) and do not indicate a negative impact on the outcome for patients with COVID-19 disease."

"EMA therefore reiterates its previous advice that patients should continue to use ACE inhibitors or ARBs as advised by their doctors"."

Research in the COVID-19 Era: The Lack of Randomized Studies

"Further, members of scientific societies are under pressure and feel that they have an obligation to provide answers, even when such answers are not available."

"Answering the question whether RAASi are safe in the COVID-19 context is crucial."

"Some questions about therapy cannot wait for RCTs to be conducted (e.g., RAASi safety in the COVID-19 context) and scientific societies feel that they have an obligation to make recommendations based on observational studies (OSs)."

"OSs, however, do not provide the final answer."

Clinical Implications

"In our current practice when it comes to prescribe a RAASi in the COVID-19 context, we base our decision on the following premises: (a) COVID-19 is a pandemic responsible for millions of infections and hundreds of thousands deaths worldwide;

(b) COVID-19 is due to SARS-CoV-2 which binds and enters host cells through the ACE2 receptor; (c) the protective ACE2/ANG [1–7]/Mas axis may not be efficiently operative in the lungs; (d) RAASi may increase the tissue expression of ACE2; (e) lethal complications of COVID-19 are more common in diseases frequently treated with RAASi such as hypertension, other cardiovascular disease, and diabetes; (f) confounding cannot be corrected even after application of multiple adjustment techniques; (g) RAASi had proved lifesaving in the pre COVID-19 era; (h) RCTs testing the efficacy and safety of RAASi in the COVID-19 era are lacking; and (i) considering that RCTs are lacking we must follow the trail to the next best external evidence and work from there [113]."

Conclusion

"Evidence regarding the efficacy and safety of RAASi in the COVID-19 context is based on OSs, which have provided useful information in the past but have also led to errors even after application of multiple adjustment techniques."

"While the potential for benefit with the use of RAASi and the risks from stopping them is more evident, potential harm by RAASi may also be caused by the increase in the activity of the ACE2 receptor which the SARS-CoV-2 binds and enters into the host, the doubtful protective effects of the ACE2/ANG [1–7]/Mas axis in the lungs, and the proinflammatory properties of ACE2(+) cells infected with SARS-CoV-2."

"Acknowledging the proven RAASi benefit in patients with several diseases such as hypertension, heart failure, coronary disease, and diabetic kidney disease in the non-COVID-19 era, it is a reasonable strategy in this period of uncertainty to use these agents judiciously with careful consideration to avoid the use of RAASi in select patients whenever possible, until definitive evidence becomes available."

Future Perspective

"Studies evaluating the pharmacological properties of the different drugs focused on their pharmacokinetic and pharmacodynamic effects."

"The possibility that a viral infection may alter drug effects and consequently the final disease outcome was not taken into consideration."

"This is a new area of research in which pharmacologists, virologists, epidemiologists, and clinicians should be involved."

[Section 9]

"Amos Bronson Alcott Coronavirus disease 2019 (COVID-19) is due to severe acute respiratory syndrome coronavirus (SARS-CoV)-2 which binds and enters the host cells through the angiotensin-converting enzyme (ACE)2."

"Therapy with renin-angiotensin-aldosterone system (RAAS) inhibitors (ACE inhibitors [ACEi], angiotensin [ANG] II receptor blockers [ARB], and mineralocorticoid receptor antagonists [MRA]) may increase ACE2 [92]."

"The concern, therefore, has been raised that a potential increase in ACE2 by these agents may facilitate development and increase severity of COVID-19."

"In this brief review, we contend that a potential harmful effect of RAAS inhibitors cannot be excluded in the COVID-19 era and thus, caution required when prescribing these agents."

Ethnic Prevalence of Angiotensin-Converting Enzyme Deletion (D) Polymorphism and COVID-19 Risk: Rationale for Use of Angiotensin-Converting Enzyme Inhibitors/Angiotensin Receptor Blockers [114]

This is a machine-generated summary of:

Sarangarajan, Rangaprasad; Winn, Robert; Kiebish, Michael A.; Bountra, Chas; Granger, Elder; Narain, Niven R.: Ethnic Prevalence of Angiotensin-Converting Enzyme Deletion (D) Polymorphism and COVID-19 Risk: Rationale for Use of Angiotensin-Converting Enzyme Inhibitors/Angiotensin Receptor Blockers [114].

Published in: Journal of Racial and Ethnic Health Disparities (2020).

Link to original: https://doi.org/10.1007/s40615-020-00853-0

If you want to cite the papers, please refer to the original.

For technical reasons we could not place the page where the original quote is coming from.

Abstract-Summary "Regression analysis correlated presence of ACE insertion/deletion (I/D) polymorphism to COVID-19 incidence and mortality."

"COVID-19 prevalence correlated to allele frequency of angiotensin-converting enzyme (ACE) deletion (D) polymorphism within the European population."

"Homozygous ACE deletion polymorphism is associated with increase in ACE and angiotensin II (Ang-II), sustained levels can result in inflammation, fibrosis and organ damage."

"The ACE DD polymorphism is also associated with hypertension, acute respiratory distress and diabetic nephropathy, all considered high risk for COVID-19 infection and outcomes."

"The study objective was to describe a biological framework associating ethnic prevalence of ACE deletion polymorphism to COVID-19 comorbidities providing rationale for therapeutic utility of ACE-I/ARBs to improve outcomes."

"The presence of ACE DD polymorphism with COVID-19 infection likely augments ACE/Ang-II activities, increasing severity of COVID-19 morbidities and impacts outcomes."

"Ethnic prevalence of ACE DD polymorphism can explain in part the severity of COVID-19 morbidity providing rationale for the use of ACE-I/ARBs to improve outcomes."

Introduction

"Hypertension, obesity, and diabetes were identified as the most common comorbidities associated with COVID-19 infection; higher severity of disease and mortality was generally reported in the elderly (>50 years) population."

"Angiotensin-converting enzyme 2 (ACE2) is the predominant receptor for SARS-CoV viral entry and infection, resulting in the reduction of expression of ACE2 [89, 115]."

"The deleterious activities of RAS within the COVID-19-infected cohorts can be further amplified by the presence of genetic polymorphism in the angiotensin-converting enzyme (ACE)."

"Increased prevalence in frequency of the ACE polymorphism within ethnic groups, in part, is likely responsible for the observed severity of COVID-19 comorbidities and mortality in this population."

"This is substantiated by recent regression analysis linking presence of ACE-1 I/D (insertion/deletion) polymorphism with incidence and mortality with COVID-19 infection [116]."

Renin-Angiotensin System: ACE, Ang-II, and Inflammation

"Activation of AT-1 receptors is associated with the well-characterized physiological actions of Ang-II in various organs including the lung, heart, kidney, and the vascular system [117]."

"To its hemodynamic effect, Ang-II has significant pro-inflammatory effects, promoting generation of reactive oxygen species (ROS), cell proliferation, extracellular matrix remodelling, and regulation of gene expression via signalling pathways leading to tissue injury [118, 119]."

"Ang-II promotes expression of pro-inflammatory chemokines in the kidneys, heart, and vasculature to induce inflammation [120]."

"Several studies have characterized key inflammatory processes influenced by Ang-II on macrophages, dendritic cells, and mesangial cells resulting in mobilization and activation of cytokines, chemokines, and pro-inflammatory factors resulting in tissue damage and progressive organ failure [121]."

"The pro-inflammatory effects of ACE/Ang-II axis are balanced by activation of anti-inflammatory pathways by ACE2 and other systems."

ACE Insertion/Deletion (ID) Polymorphisms: Prevalence

"It is reported that the deletion (D) allele occurs in 55% of the population and associated with increased ACE activity, implicating the presence of D allele with disease pathologies associated with RAS activity [122]."

"To Europe, among the African population, the frequency of D allele was almost twice compared with the I allele among 2126 population samples with highest levels observed in Pygmies, Ethiopian Jews, Moroccan, Nigerian and Tunisian populations."

"These are consistent with other studies reporting significant increase in the frequency of deletion polymorphism of ACE observed in individuals of African descent and associated with disease pathology [123]."

"The frequency of the D allele was increased compared with the I allele within the Middle Eastern population with higher values observed in both Arab and Saudi Arabia sample populations."

ACE Deletion (D) Polymorphism and Disease: Increased Susceptibility and Severity to Co-morbidities Associated with COVID-19

"Presence of ACE insertion/deletion (I/D) polymorphism is associated with susceptibility and is an independent risk factor for mortality in patients with acute respiratory distress syndrome (ARDS) [124, 125]."

"Further, the DD genotype is usually associated with higher ACE levels relative to other genotypes and with increased mortality in acute lung injury (ALI)/ARDS patients [126, 127]."

"ACE insertion/deletion polymorphism is also associated with diabetic kidney disease, the frequency of DD and ID genotype distribution being higher compared with non-diabetic kidney disease cohorts, leading to functional decline [128, 129]."

"The above observations suggest that presence of the DD genotype of ACE in patients with COVID-19 infection may be associated with severe respiratory distress compared with the other genotypes."

"Multiple studies have reported on the prevalence of ACE I/D polymorphism, specifically the ID and DD polymorphism in increasing levels of ACE and Ang-II, which could in part influence susceptibility to underlying pathologies considered high risk for COVID-19 infections, progressive organ dysfunction and poor outcomes."

ACE-2 Inhibition by COVID-19: Increased RAS Activity

"In patients with active COVID-19 infections, decrease in ACE2 expression/activity should most likely lead to sustained ACE-mediated generation of Ang-II and downstream signalling deleterious to organ functions including that of lung, kidney and heart [130]."

"Although the status of circulating and lung ACE levels in COVID-19 patients is unclear, the ability of SARS-CoV-2 binding specifically to ACE2 decreases its expression and activity suggesting upregulation of ACE/Ang-II-mediated activities."

"In a pilot clinical investigation, administration of recombinant human ACE2 (APN311) in patients with acute respiratory distress was associated with rapid decrease in Ang-II level and did not significantly influence oxygenation indices in the treated population compared with placebo-controlled group [90]."

"The recombinant human ACE2 is undergoing renewed clinical testing in the COVID-19 patient population to investigate clinical outcomes [130]."

ACE2 Inhibition by COVID-19 Plus ACE D Polymorphism: Synergized RAS—Rationale for Use of ACE-I and ARBs in Clinical Management

"Based on the described biological consequence of COVID-19 infections on the RAS system, treatment with ACE-I and ARBs should be associated with improved outcomes within the overall COVID-19 patient cohorts."

"Several meta-analyses provide preliminary support for the potential benefits of the use of ACE-I/ARBs in management of COVID-19 infections."

"In a multicenter study of 1128 adult patients with hypertension with positive COVID-19 diagnosis, in-patient use of ACE-I/ARB was associated with reduced risk of mortality from all causes when compared with patients not treated with the medications [33]."

"These studies provide rationale for investigation into the utility of ACE-I/ARBs in the ethnic population with known prevalence of ACE deletion polymorphisms in an effort to mitigate severity and improve outcomes in response to COVID-19 infections."

Use of ACE-I/ARBs in Ethnic Population with Increased Prevalence of ACE D Polymorphism for Management of COVID-19

"The specificity of hypertension and cardiovascular disease as underlying causes for severity of COVID-19 infection, the inherent role of ACE-mediated generation of Ang-II and downstream signalling to potentially exacerbate inflammation and organ damage along with genotypic impact on ACE status provide compelling support of the use of ACE-I and ARBs in the clinical management of patient with positive diagnosis of COVID-19."

"The significant genetic, scientific and clinical data supporting a potential role for increased ACE levels and associated Ang-II effect in target organs provides compelling argument for use of ACE-I and ARBs in the clinical management of patients with COVID-19 infections to improve outcomes."

"This study describes the biological relevance of genetic polymorphism of ACE deletion with higher prevalence in certain ethnic populations including African Americans in context of COVID-19 infection and rationale for the use of ACE-I/ARBs for therapeutic management of severity of morbidity and improving outcomes associated with COVID-19."

Role of Angiotensin-Converting Enzyme 2 (ACE2) in COVID-19 [131]

This is a machine-generated summary of:

Ni, Wentao; Yang, Xiuwen; Yang, Deqing; Bao, Jing; Li, Ran; Xiao, Yongjiu; Hou, Chang; Wang, Haibin; Liu, Jie; Yang, Donghong; Xu, Yu; Cao, Zhaolong; Gao, Zhancheng: Role of angiotensin-converting enzyme 2 (ACE2) in COVID-19 [131].

Published in: Critical Care (2020).

Link to original: https://doi.org/10.1186/s13054-020-03120-0

If you want to cite the papers, please refer to the original.

For technical reasons we could not place the page where the original quote is coming from.

Abstract-Summary "Both SARS-CoV-2 and SARS-CoV enter host cells via the angiotensin-converting enzyme 2 (ACE2) receptor, which is expressed in various human organs."

"To the direct viral effects and inflammatory and immune factors associated with COVID-19 pathogenesis, ACE2 downregulation and the imbalance between the RAS and ACE2/angiotensin-(1–7)/MAS after infection may also contribute to multiple organ injury in COVID-19."

"Restoring the balance between the RAS and ACE2/angiotensin-(1–7)/MAS may help attenuate organ injuries."

"SARS-CoV-2 enters lung cells via the ACE2 receptor."

"The cell-free and macrophage-phagocytosed virus can spread to other organs and infect ACE2-expressing cells at local sites, causing multi-organ injury."

Background

"Autopsy studies of SARS patients further found that PICs and MCP-1 were highly expressed in SARS-CoV-infected ACE2+ cells, but not in tissues without infected ACE2+ cells, suggesting virus-induced local immune-mediated damage [132]."

"To acting as the receptor for SARS-CoV and SARS-CoV-2, ACE2 hydrolyzes Ang-II to angiotensin-(1–7), and the ACE2/angiotensin-(1–7)/MAS counteracts the negative effects of the RAS and exerts anti-inflammatory effects [133, 134]."

"Several studies have shown that SARS-CoV infection can downregulate ACE2 expression on cells, thereby disrupting the physiological balance between ACE/ACE2 and Ang-II/angiotensin-(1–7) and subsequently causing severe organ injury [135–138]."

"SARS-CoV-2 is a species of SARS-related coronaviruses and uses ACE2 as its receptor, the downregulation of ACE2 expression may be involved in multiple organ injury in COVID-19."

"In both SARS-CoV-infected mice and humans, ACE2 expression in myocardial cells is markedly downregulated in the heart [138]."

Conclusions

"The RAS and ACE2/angiotensin-(1–7)/MAS axis play important roles in various physiological and pathophysiological contexts."

"Because ACE2 is highly expressed in various organs and tissues, SARS-CoV-2 not only invades the lungs but also attacks other organs with high ACE2 expression."

"To the direct viral effects and inflammatory and immune factors, the downregulation of ACE2 and imbalance between the RAS and ACE2/angiotensin-(1–7)/MAS axis may also contribute to the multiple organ injuries in COVID-19."

"Restoring the balance between the RAS and ACE2/angiotensin-(1–7)/MAS may help attenuate organ injuries in COVID-19."

Treatment Options Available for COVID-19 and an Analysis on Possible Role of Combination of rhACE2, Angiotensin (1–7) and Angiotensin (1–9) as Effective Therapeutic Measure [139]

This is a machine-generated summary of:
Muslim, Shahnawaz; Nasrin, Nasrin; Alotaibi, Faisal Obaid; Prasad, Geeta; Singh, Shambhu Kumar; Alam, Izhar; Mustafa, Gulam: Treatment Options Available for COVID-19 and an Analysis on Possible Role of Combination of rhACE2, Angiotensin (1–7) and Angiotensin (1–9) as Effective Therapeutic Measure [139].
Published in: SN Comprehensive Clinical Medicine (2020).
Link to original: https://doi.org/10.1007/s42399-020-00407-9

If you want to cite the papers, please refer to the original.
For technical reasons we could not place the page where the original quote is coming from.

Abstract-Summary "Since SARS-CoV-2 is a novel virus, little is known about it and no effective drug is available for its treatment."

"SARS-CoV-2 like SARS-CoV binds with angiotensin-converting enzyme 2 (ACE2) present on human cells."

"SARS-CoV has been found to downregulate ACE2 and SARS-CoV-2 infection has been found to be associated with increased level of Angiotensin II."

"Based on these facts, we presume that SARS-CoV-2 like SARS-CoV down-regulates ACE2, and in absence/reduced activity of ACE2, level of angiotensin (1–7) and angiotensin (1–9) is decreased while that of angiotensin II is increased and increased level of angiotensin II has been found to correlate with lung injury and viral load."

Introduction

"Cause of this disease was attributed to a new corona virus."

"The WHO named this virus as novel corona virus (nCoV) and the disease as corona virus disease 19 (COVID-19)."

"On, the International Committee on Taxonomy of Viruses renamed the virus as severe acute respiratory syndrome corona virus 2 (SARS-CoV-2) due to its genomic similarity with SARS-CoV [80]."

"To describe the available treatment options and to find a new and effective therapeutic measure, we present a review of drugs available and an analysis on possible role of combination of recombinant human angiotensin-converting enzyme 2 (rhACE2), angiotensin (1–7) and angiotensin (1–9) (AAA) for treatment of COVID-19."

Chloroquine

"Chloroquine is a known anti-malarial drug which also possesses immunomodulatory property and recently has been found to have antiviral activity."

"In vitro study has shown that it has activity against SARS-CoV-2 in Vero E6 cells infected with virus."

"Wang and others demonstrated that chloroquine acts at both entry and post entry stage of SARS-CoV-2 infection in Vero E6 cells and EC50 of chloroquine in Vero E6 cells against SARS-CoV-2 is 1.13 μM [140, 141]."

"Clinical data also support benefit of chloroquine in patients suffering from SARS-CoV-2 infection."

Hydroxychloroquine

"Like chloroquine, hydroxychloroquine also exhibits antiviral activity against SARS-CoV-2 and mechanism of action is also similar, i.e. alteration of endosomal ph, blockage of virus entry and post entry events."

"This drug has been found to be more potent than chloroquine as far as the antiviral activity against SARS-CoV-2 is concerned."

"Yao and others demonstrated that in Vero cells, EC50 for chloroquine was 5.47 μM and EC50 for hydroxychloroquine was 0.72 μM against SARS-CoV-2 [142]."

"Gauter and others evaluated the role of hydroxychloroquine on respiratory viral load of SARS-CoV-2 and demonstrated that treatment with hydroxychloroquine was significantly associated with viral load reduction [143]."

Remdesivir

"Remdesivir is a phosphoramidate prodrug of an adenosine C–nucleoside, developed by Gilead Science Inc. [144]."

"It is metabolized to active nucleoside triphosphate and acts at RNA-dependent RNA polymerase (RdRp) to cause RNA chain termination."

"Clinical experience with first case of COVID-19 from the USA showed that treatment with remdesivir was associated with decreased viral load and improved outcome [145]."

Fapiravir

"Fapiravir is broad-spectrum antiviral drug and an RNA-dependent RNA polymerase inhibitor which causes inhibition of viral RNA synthesis."

"One Chinese trial evaluated the role of fapiravir in COVID-19 cases and demonstrated that fapiravir treatment group was associated with greater clinical recovery rate [146]."

"Very limited data is available for its use in COVID-19 patients."

Lopinavir/Ritonavir

"Lopinavir/ritonavir combination previously has been found to be effective against SARS-CoV and MERS-CoV [147]."

"Young and others from Singapore in a report on 18 patients of COVID-19 described that 5 patients who required oxygen supplementation were treated with lopinavir/ritonavir therapy."

"An open-label randomized trial comparing lopinavir/ritonavir with standard therapy in admitted patients with COVID-19 demonstrated no advantage of lopinavir/ritonavir over standard care [148]."

"There is limited data to support role of lopinavir/ritonavir for COVID-19 treatment."

Tocilizumab

"IL-6 receptors are present in two forms, soluble IL-6 receptor (sIL-6R) and membrane-bound IL-6 receptor (mIL-6R)."

"IL-6 binds with sIL-6R to form a complex and then binds with gp130 on cell membrane to start inflammatory signal."

"Tociluzumab binds with both sIL-6R and mIL-6R and causes inhibition of inflammatory response."

"Preliminary data from a Chinese study showed that treatment of severely ill COVID-19 patients with tocilizumab in addition to routine therapy was associated with reduction in oxygen requirement, improvement in CT findings of lung, improvement in peripheral blood picture and reduction in C-reactive protein level, leading to conclusion that tocilizumab is an effective treatment for severely ill COVID-19 patients [149]."

Azithromycin

"Azithromycin is a macrolide antibiotic which has been found to have some in vitro activity against viruses like influenza virus and Zika virus; however, there is no in vitro study to suggest its direct action against SARS-CoV-2."

"It is used in viral infection to prevent super added bacterial infection."

"One study with small sample size evaluating the role of hydroxychloroquine on viral load in COVID-19 patient demonstrated that hydroxycloroquine treatment leads to significant viral load reduction and this effect is enhanced by azithromycin [143]."

"Limited data is available to support its role in COVID-19 treatment."

Convalescent Plasma

"Plasma derived from the body of a person who has recovered from a disease is called convalescent plasma."

"When plasma is derived from the body of a person who has recovered from an infectious disease, it is supposed that the plasma contains antibody against that particular pathogen from which the recovered person was suffering."

"This antibody-containing plasma can be transferred to another person suffering from the same pathogen in order to target the pathogen."

Heparin

"The International Society on Thrombosis and Haemostasis (ISTH) interim guidance recommends the use of prophylactic low molecular weight heparin (LMWH) in severe COVID-19 patients [150]."

"The therapeutic effect of LMWH showed a signficant reduction ($p = 0.029$) in martality (40%) in the treatment group with coagulopathy and treated with heparin compared to the treatment group without it (64.2%) [151]."

"Increasing levels of d-dimer were related to increasing mortality in non-heparin-treated patients."

Anti-platelet Therapies

"Patient debilitation from severe COVID-19 may pose challenges in administering routine cardiovascular medications, ranging from anti-platelet therapy to beta-blockers, and may put patients with or at risk of ischemic heart disease or heart failure at risk of further deterioration of their clinical condition."

"The global reports indicate that hospitalized critical patients with COVID-19 often develop abnormalities compatible with hypercoagulability and a clinically elevated prevalence of thromboembolic [152]."

"Zhang and co-worker reported deep vein thrombosis (DVT) and pulmonary embolism (PE), thrombosis in extracorporeal circuits and arterial thrombosis associated with COVID-19 [153]."

Corticosteroids

"Role of corticosteroids is controversial because at one end it may inhibit the inflammatory response and have an overall beneficial effect while at other end it may predispose to secondary infection and delayed viral clearance."

"One study from China reported that treatment of COVID-19 patients with ARDS on treatment with methyl prednisolone showed a decrease in risk of death."

"Authors also suggested a double-blind randomized trial to validate the result [42]."

"Since corticosteroid is a double-edged sword, its use should be individualized."

Nitazoxanide

"Its active metabolite 'tizoxanide' has activity against wide range of viruses like influenza virus, parainfluenza virus, corona viruses, hepatitis B and C viruses and many other viruses."

"Broad range of its antiviral activity is probably because of the fact that, in place of direct action against virus, it acts on host-regulated pathways of viral replication which may include interferon or mTORC1 signalling pathway [154, 155]."

"As far as its role against SARS-CoV-2 is concerned, in vitro study has demonstrated a potent antiviral activity against SARS-CoV-2 (EC50 = 2.12 μM in Vero E6 cells) [141]."

Leronlimab

"Leronlimab is humanized monoclonal antibody which inhibits chemokine receptor CCR5."

"It is an investigational agent in treatment of COVID-19."

"In a clinical study involving eight critically ill COVID-19 patients, treatment with leronlimab was associated with improvement of immunological markers and trends towards normalization of CD4/CD8 ratio [156]."

"Further research is being carried out to establish its role in treatment of COVID-19 patients."

Ribavirin

"In vitro study has demonstrated that ribavirin has antiviral activity against SARS-COV-2 (EC50 of 109.5 μM) and is several times less potent than remdesivir [141]."

"Dose required for treatment of SARS was associated with significant toxicity [157]."

"Because of its low potency against SARS-CoV-2 and significant associated toxicity, it is not a good choice for consideration in cases of COVID-19."

Analysis on Possible Role of Combination of Soluble rhACE2, Angiotensin (1–7) and Angiotensin (1–9) for Treatment of COVID-19

"We presume that binding of viral S-protein with ACE2 present on cell leads to downregulation of ACE2, as a result of which ACE2 activity decreases and an imbalance in renin-angiotensin system takes place."

"In absence/reduced level of activity of ACE2, angiotensin 1 is predominantly converted into angiotensin II while conversion of angiotensin 1 to angiotensin (1–9) and angiotensin II to angiotensin (1–7) is impaired."

"Of this change, level of pro-inflammatory angiotensin II rises and that of anti-inflammatory angiotensin (1–7) and angiotensin (1–9) decreases [158]."

"Increased level of angiotensin II has been found to correlate with lung injury and viral load [159]."

"Administration of rhACE2 may help to restore the function of downregulated ACE2 and administration of angiotensin 1–7 and angiotensin 1–9 may further help in restoration of normal functioning of renin-angiotensin system by antagonizing the effect of abnormally increased angiotensin II."

Conclusion

"Until date, there is no effective treatment against COVID-19."

"Research is on and multiple drugs are being evaluated."

"Since downregulation of ACE2 and imbalance of RAS plays an important role in pathogenesis of COVID-19, we feel that restoration of RAS with the use of combination of rhACE2, angiotensin (1–7) and angiotensin (1–9) may be an effective therapeutic measure."

ACE2: The Major Cell Entry Receptor for SARS-CoV-2 [160]

This is a machine-generated summary of:

Scialo, Filippo; Daniele, Aurora; Amato, Felice; Pastore, Lucio; Matera, Maria Gabriella; Cazzola, Mario; Castaldo, Giuseppe; Bianco, Andrea: ACE2: The Major Cell Entry Receptor for SARS-CoV-2 [160].

Published in: Lung (2020).

Link to original: https://doi.org/10.1007/s00408-020-00408-4

If you want to cite the papers, please refer to the original.

For technical reasons we could not place the page where the original quote is coming from.

Abstract-Summary "We focus our attention on ACE2, a primary receptor of SARS-CoV-2."

"We will discuss its biology, tissue expression, and post-translational regulation that determine its potential to be employed by SARS-CoV-2 for cell entry."

"We will discuss repercussions that SARS-CoV-2/ACE2 binding has on the renin–angiotensin system and beyond."

"Thorough comprehension of the role that ACE2 plays in different pathways will be the key to assess the impact that SARS-CoV-2/ACE2 binding has on organismal physiology and will help us to find better therapies and diagnostic tools."

Introduction

"A focus will be given to the metallocarboxyl peptidase angiotensin receptor (ACE)2 that is used by SARS-CoV-2 to gain entry into human cells [161]."

"There are two forms of ACE2 [162]."

"This form of ACE lacks membrane anchors and circulates in low concentrations."

"We will assess whether the level of expression of ACE2 and the ratio between mACE2 and sACE2 could explain why some people experience more severe symptoms than others."

"We believe that efforts towards the full comprehension of the intricate roles that ACE2 plays in maintaining organismal physiology will be the key to better understand the multisystemic COVID-19 disease and help us to develop better therapies and diagnostic tools."

Cell Entry Receptors: Lessons from Other Respiratory Viruses

"Cell entry receptors are undoubtedly the key factors determining the tropism and influencing the severity of infection of a specific virus."

"CoV-NL63, SARS-CoV, and SARS-CoV-2 use ACE2, but CoV-NL63 leads to mild respiratory tract illness, probably because of its low-affinity interaction with the receptor [163]."

"Coronaviruses are not the only family of viruses able to cause respiratory tract illness in humans."

"The A(H1N1)pdm09 influenza virus that caused the pandemic in 2009 shows a different tropism binding to α2-6- and α2-3-linked sialyl glycans [164] that are present on different cell types and play key roles in cellular communication and cell signaling among others."

Biology, Tissue Expression, and Post-translational Modifications of ACE2 Receptor

"Since most people present respiratory difficulties in response to SARS-CoV-2 infection, these findings were explained by the fact that the release of inflammatory cytokines, such as interferons (IFNs) caused by SARS-CoV-2, can increase the expression ACE2 and potentiate the infection [165, 166]."

"Onabajo and colleagues recently showed that IFNs stimulation upon viral treatment induced the expression of a truncated ACE2 isoform designate as δACE2, which lacks 356 N-terminal amino acids, is not able to bind SARS-CoV-2 and, therefore, does not contribute to the potentiation of the infection [167]."

"Since the beginning of the COVID-19 pandemic, hypertension and diabetes have been correlated with higher risk of mortality, and initial reports speculated that angiotensin converting enzyme inhibitors (ACEi) and angiotensin receptor blockers (ARBs), which are commonly used therapeutic agents for these conditions, would up-regulate ACE2 expression, thus increasing the risk of severe illness [22]."

ACE2 Polymorphisms and Susceptibility to SARS-CoV-2 Infection

"Previous studies have demonstrated that specific residues in the ACE2 protein are essential for binding with SARS-CoV [168]."

"Genomic variability in those specific residues could modulate the binding between ACE2 and the SARS-CoV-2 Spike protein, accounting for a broad range of symptoms exhibited by people affected by COVID-19."

"Studies that aimed to find mutations in the ACE2 sequences and allele frequency in different populations have demonstrated the existence of specific variance that could affect SARS-CoV-2 binding [169–171]."

"We do not yet know whether a specific variability in the ADAM17 sequence is associated with a high level of sACE2 and whether there is a correlation with the SARS-CoV-2 infection."

"Recent studies have shown that high levels of sACE2 could be evidence of increased ACE2 expression, elevated ADAM17 activity or both and, therefore, greater susceptibility to SARS-CoV-2 infection [172, 173]."

Physiological Functions of ACE2

"Dissecting the roles that ACE2 has in maintaining organismal physiology will help us to better comprehend why its dysregulation caused by SARS-CoV-2 can have such a devastating effect, especially in the elderly with comorbidities."

"We will describe the molecular pathways in which ACE2 plays an important role."

"We will focus on the role that ACE2 plays in counterbalancing the RAAS but also on its important function in the kinin-kallikrein system (KKS) that has been mostly neglected although it plays an essential part in regulating the inflammatory process."

ACE2 and the RAAS

"Despite having a high degree of homology with ACE, ACE2 shows a remarkable difference in substrate selection, catalyzing with high efficiency the conversion of the vasoconstrictor AngII in Ang1–7 that binds and activates its own seven-transmembrane G protein-coupled receptor (GPCR) called MAS to exert anti-inflammatory and anti-remodeling effects or, with less efficiency, the formation of Ang1–9 from AngI, which can be converted to Ang1–7 by ACE [174]."

"Excessive production of ROS upon overactivation of the AngII/AT1R/nicotinamide adenine dinucleotide phosphate (NADPH) oxidase axis has been correlated with hypertension [175], and atherosclerosis [176], and can induce apoptosis through the release of cytochrome C from damaged mitochondria, activation of caspase 3 or p38 mitogen-activated protein kinase (MAPK)/Jun N-terminal kinase (JNK) cascade."

"The activation of the immune response caused by the infection in combination with the high level of AngII could result in the hyperinflammatory state that is seen in the late phase of SARS-CoV-2-infected patients."

Angiotensin A/ACE2/Alamandine/MAS-Related GPCR D (MrgD) Axis

"Ang A differs from AngII by a single amino acid (alanine) at the N-terminal."

"As in the case of AngII, ACE2 is responsible for providing a further layer in RAAS regulation by catalyzing the conversion of AngA in alamandine."

"This conversion highlights again the key role of ACE2 in the regulation of RAAS."

ACE2 and the Kinin-Kallikrein System (KKS)

"DEABK and LDEABK act on bradykinin receptor-B1 (BRB1) and have important role in the inflammation process [177, 178]."

"DEABK and LDEABK can act as proinflammatory factors that exert their function through the BRB1 receptor."

"ACE2, which does not inactivate BK, can cleave the terminal residue in DEABK and LDEABK, rendering them unable to interact with BRB1 [179, 180]."

"ACE2 internalization due to SARS-CoV-2 infection will create an imbalance in the KKS system causing an overactivation of the DEABK/LDEABK/BRB1 axis, contributing to increased inflammation and rendering the lung environment more prone to local vascular leakage, leading to angioedema [179]."

ACE2 as a Target for a SARS-CoV-2 Therapeutic Strategy

"ACE2 can be shed from the cell and released into the circulation by ADAM17 while maintaining its catalytic activity and ability to bind SARS-CoV-2."

"It has been suggested to use human recombinant ACE-2 (hrACE2) protein to saturate the viral S-protein and thus prevent cellular entry of SARS-Cov-2 [162]."

"Differently from antiviral or anti-inflammatory therapies, shrACE2 can act upstream by decreasing the binding between SARS-CoV-2/mACE2, thus reducing infectivity [181]."

"Monteil and colleagues demonstrated that shrACE2 can decrease SARS-CoV-2 infection in vitro [182], and clinical trials are already underway (Clinicaltrials.gov #NCT04335136)."

"Other potential therapeutic approaches include a SARS-CoV-2 spike protein-based vaccine, a TMPRSS inhibitor to block the priming of the spike protein, and blockage of the surface ACE2 receptor by using anti-ACE2 antibody or peptides [183]."

"Camostat mesylate, approved in Japan to treat pancreatic inflammation, has been shown to block TMPRSS2 activity and prevent cellular infection by SARS-Cov-2 [89]."

Conclusion

"Although the scientific world is making an extraordinary effort, we are still far from fully understanding whether the overactivation of the immune system and the state of hyperinflammation due to SARS-CoV-2 infection can be controlled [184]."

"It is likely, even if not yet fully ascertained, that when these pathological states combine with the viral infection, the dysregulation of both the RAAS and the KKS due to ACE2 internalization mediated by SARS-CoV-2 could create the conditions for severe illness and a fatal outcome."

"As already discussed, contrasting hypotheses have been formulated concerning the effect of therapies taken by millions of people that might increase ACE2 expression and susceptibility to SARS-CoV-2 infection."

"This may shed light on factors that modulate cell surface ACE2 receptor affecting viral cell entry and consequently susceptibility to SARS-CoV-2 infection."

Understanding the Pivotal Roles of ACE2 in SARS-CoV-2 Infection: From Structure/Function to Therapeutic Implication [185]

This is a machine-generated summary of:

Pouremamali, Amir; Babaei, Abouzar; Malekshahi, Somayeh Shatizadeh; Abbasi, Ardeshir; Rafiee, Nastaran: Understanding the pivotal roles of ACE2 in SARS-CoV-2 infection: from structure/function to therapeutic implication [185].

Published in: Egyptian Journal of Medical Human Genetics (2022).

Link to original: https://doi.org/10.1186/s43042-022-00314-9

If you want to cite the papers, please refer to the original.

For technical reasons we could not place the page where the original quote is coming from.

Abstract-Summary "The S glycoprotein is a crucial viral protein for binding, fusion, and entry into the target cells."

"Binding the receptor-binding domain (RBD) of S protein to angiotensin-converting enzyme 2 (ACE 2), a cell-surface receptor, mediates virus entry into cells; thus, understanding the basics of ACE2 and S protein, their interactions, and ACE2 targeting could be a potent priority for inhibition of virus infection."

"It highlights ACE2 targeting by recombinant ACE2 (rACE2), ACE2 activators, ACE inhibitor, and angiotensin II (Ang II) receptor blocker to control the SARS-CoV-2 infection."

Background

"The coronavirus genus Beta includes highly pathogenic viruses such as severe acute respiratory syndrome coronavirus (SARS-CoV), Middle East respiratory syndrome coronavirus (MERS-CoV), and the novel SARS-CoV-2 and low pathogenic viruses including HCoV-OC43 and HCoV-HKU."

"The SARS-CoV-2 infection starts by binding of viral receptors to angiotensin-converting enzyme 2 (ACE2) in the surface of alveolar epithelial cells [186–188]."

"Due to recombination of SARS-CoV-2 RNA sequences and involvement of host enzymes in viral RNA editing, the SARS-CoV-2 spike protein has undergone many mutations that led to emergence of different variants including alpha, beta, gamma, delta, omicron, etc., with increased reproduction number (R) and transmission potential [189–191]."

"Since worldwide administration of different SARS-CoV-2 vaccine platforms, including mRNA, viral vector, inactivated virus, and live attenuated virus vaccines, the elevated neutralizing antibodies in vaccinated individuals raised hope for reducing the risk of infection; however, the appearance of delta and omicron variants has challenged vaccines efficacy [190, 192]."

SARS-CoV-2 and Cellular Receptors

"The S protein [1273 amino acids], presented on the surface of mature CoVs in homotrimer form, is the main viral mediator in virus entry into host cells [193]."

"This viral protein consists of two functional subunits: (i) the S1 subunit, containing a receptor-binding domain (RBD) which mediates virus binding to host cells, and (ii) the S2 subunit that fuses membranes of virus and host cell [194, 195]."

"Some reports confirmed that little but functionally important differences at residues 331–524 of SARS-CoV-2-RBD, enable this virus to bind to cellular receptors with higher affinity than SARS-CoV [196–199]."

"All these data indicate that viral S protein and human ACE2 play important roles in establishing SARS-CoV-2 infection and are required for virus entry [200–203]."

ACE2 Structure and Function

"ACE has 2 active catalytic sites while ACE2 possesses only a single active site in the N-terminal domain, and also there is no similarity between the C-terminal domain of ACE2 with ACE [204, 205]."

"In ACE2, the protease domain (PD) in the N-terminal portion performs all peptidase activities and the C-terminal domain, as a strong anchor, connects the C-terminal domain to the cell membrane and regulates the amino acid transporters trafficking [130]."

"ACE2 has only one single catalytic site that acts as a simple carboxypeptidase while its ACE isoform contains two active domains that cleave amino acids, located in the carboxyl end of peptides [206]."

"In RAAS, angiotensinogen, a precursor peptide secreted from the liver, is cleaved by renin and converted to angiotensin I (Ang I) decapeptide, then ACE cleaves 2 amino acids from Ang I to produce an angiotensin II (Ang II) octapeptide, while ACE2 converts Ang I to angiotensin (1–9) [Ang (1–9)] by cleaving one amino acid of that."

Organ Distribution of ACE2

"ACE2 proteins are active and extensively expressed in a wide range of organs and tissues of the human body."

"In the respiratory tract, ACE2 widely presents in the epithelium of basal and oral mucosa, nasopharynx, and alveolar epithelial cells of lungs and bronchial and also exerts protective effects on lung [17]."

"It has been shown that acute lung injury and inflammatory lesions in the respiratory tract markedly increased in the ACE2 knockout mice and these implications disappeared after injection of recombinant ACE2 [84]."

"Different organs of the gastrointestinal tract including, the stomach, colon, duodenum, jejunum, and ileum are strongly capable to express ACE2."

ACE2 and SARS-CoV-2 Pathogenesis

"Respiratory tract cells are the first target for starting SARS-CoV-2 infection because of high expression level of ACE2 [207]."

"The local and innate immune cells including dendritic cells and macrophages which serve as sentinel cells present the SARS-CoV-2-infected destroyed cells to adaptive cells [208]."

"It has been shown that the presence of ACE2 on the surface of gut cells makes them susceptible to SARS-CoV-2 infection and causes symptoms including loss of appetite, anorexia, diarrhea, vomiting, and abdominal pain [209, 210]."

"In the cardiovascular system, ACE2 as a part of the RAAS system has a protective role, but SARS-CoV-2, when binds to this cellular receptor, may facilitate targeting of myocardial cells for the viral infection [208]."

"The mild-to-moderate proteinuria is the most common kidney complication in COVID-19 patients while acute kidney injury (AKI) is detectable in the severe form of SARS-CoV-2 infection [211]."

ACE2 and Respiratory Infections

"An observational study in Wuhan, China, showed that 67–85% of COVID-19 patients were admitted to the intensive care unit (ICU), indicated severe ARDS, and the mortality rate in patients with ARDS was up to 61.5% [212]."

"The clinical outcomes in patients with COVID-19 correlated with the severity of ARDS, and the mortality of patients with moderate and severe ARDS was higher than mild ARDS."

"Seven studies showed that COPD patients were also at higher risk of severe COVID-19 compared to patients without COPD (33.4%) [213]."

"In mice models, ACE2 has been shown to protect animals from severe lung damage, caused by aspiration and sepsis [84]."

"Relatively low ACE2 expression levels in the bronchial epithelium are associated with more severe lung injury [214, 215]."

ACE2 Regulation

"ANG II considerably reduces ACE2 activity and downregulates mRNA levels of ACE2 in cardiac myocytes [216]."

"Another study showed that inhibition of Ang II synthesis altered ACE2 expression in mRNA levels [217]."

"Evidence suggests that there is a link between Ang II levels and the expression of ACE2 [218]."

"The effects of all trans-retinoic acid on gene and protein expression of ACE2 have been investigated in rats, and a significant upregulation of ACE2 expression in mRNA and protein levels was observed in the heart and kidney [219]."

"This difference could be derived from increased ACE2 expression in male that plasma levels of ACE2 were higher in males than in females and also this difference could be related to a genetic polymorphism in ACE2 [220]."

"17β-estradiol-treated cells expressed lower levels of ACE2 mRNA compared to controls."

ACE2 Targeting for Treatment

"It has been suggested that inhibiting the interaction of SARS-CoV-2 with ACE2 might be used as a therapeutic method in the treatment of patients with COVID-19 [221]."

"Decrease in pulmonary ACE2 activity is associated with pneumonia; in contrast, its activation can inhibit hyperoxia-induced lung injury by inhibiting the inflammatory response and oxidative stress [222]."

"Since upregulation of ACE2 has a protective role against severe lung injury, including ARDS and COPD, the development of an ACE2 activator could be a potential therapeutic strategy against COVID-19."

"Lei Fang and others suggested that patients with cardiac diseases, hypertension, and/or diabetes, who were treated with ACE2 activating drugs, would be at risk for severe COVID-19 infection, because treatment with ACEIs and ARBs may upregulate ACE2 expression [8]."

"Data from clinical studies suggest that ACEI/ARB administration does not increase ACE2 expression and the risk of COVID-19 complications [100, 223]."

Conclusion

"This difference may be derived from increased ACE2 plasma levels expression in men than in women, while higher tissue expression of this receptor seems to be beneficial for preventing exacerbated inflammatory response during infection."

"As, based on findings, the severity of COVID 19 symptoms can be related to ACE2 genetic polymorphisms in different populations."

"As new variants have relatively reduced vaccine's potency in increasing neutralizing antibodies, the requisite of ACE2 inhibitory drugs, discussed in this review, becomes more of interest and can be much more effective in curing patients than those which do not target ACE2."

"Prescribing drugs that may affect ACE2, such as ACEI, ARB, or ACE2 activators and targeting ACE2 by using hrsACE2 can be a potential therapeutic strategy for COVID-19; however, more clinical studies are needed to confirm the effectiveness of these methods."

Relationship Between ACE2 and Other Components of the Renin-Angiotensin System [224]

This is a machine-generated summary of:

Cohen, Jordana B.; Hanff, Thomas C.; Bress, Adam P.; South, Andrew M.: Relationship Between ACE2 and Other Components of the Renin-Angiotensin System [224].

Published in: Current Hypertension Reports (2020).

Link to original: https://doi.org/10.1007/s11906-020-01048-y

If you want to cite the papers, please refer to the original.

For technical reasons we could not place the page where the original quote is coming from.

Abstract-Summary "ACE2 converts angiotensin (Ang) II to Ang-(1–7), which directly opposes the vasoconstrictive, proinflammatory, and prothrombotic effects of Ang II."

"Drugs that interact with the renin-angiotensin system may impact ACE2 expression and COVID-19 pathogenesis; however, the magnitude and direction of these effects are unknown at this time."

"High quality research is needed to improve our understanding of how agents that act on the renin-angiotensin system impact ACE2 and COVID-19-related disease outcomes."

Introduction

"The severe acute respiratory syndrome coronavirus 2 (SARS-CoV-2), the virus responsible for the coronavirus disease 2019 (COVID-19) pandemic, is associated with a high risk of acute respiratory distress syndrome and mortality [6, 225–227]."

"Angiotensin-converting enzyme 2 (ACE2) facilitates SARS-CoV-2 entry into host cells in the respiratory tract, and altered ACE2 regulation is speculated to play a role in the pathogenesis of COVID-19 [228]."

"In the setting of the COVID-19 pandemic, there has been increasing interest in the physiologic and pathophysiologic function of ACE2 [229]."

"We briefly review the role of ACE2 in the renin-angiotensin system, the therapeutic potential of ACE2, and potential interactions of ACE2 with SARS-CoV-2 and its role in COVID-19 pathophysiology."

Counter-Regulatory Effects of ACE2 in the Renin-Angiotensin System

"ACE converts angiotensin I (Ang I) to Ang II, which acts on the Ang II type 1 receptor (AT_1R), resulting in vasoconstriction, sodium and fluid retention by the kidney, oxidative stress, inflammation, fibrosis, and impaired fibrinolysis [230, 231]."

"In direct opposition to the cascade of physiological effects of the ACE/Ang II pathway, the net effect of the ACE2/Ang-(1–7) pathway is vasodilation and anti-inflammation."

"The conversion of Ang II to Ang-(1–7) diminishes the availability of Ang II to bind AT_1R, forestalling the vasoconstrictive, proinflammatory, and prothrombotic effects of AT_1R activation [230–234]."

"ACE2 also cleaves several other peptides, including converting Ang I to Ang-(1–9), which is a less-bioactive peptide [235]."

Systemic Effects of ACE2

"ACE2 plays an important role in the development of several pathologic conditions, including hypertension, cardiac hypertrophy, and kidney disease."

"In human kidney tissue, the ratio of ACE to ACE2 expression is higher in subjects with hypertension compared with those without hypertension [236]."

"Several experimental and human studies have also demonstrated a reduction in glomerular ACE2 expression in diabetic and non-diabetic kidney disease [237]."

"Human data suggest that ACE2 may be upregulated in individuals with existing cardiovascular disease, which is speculated to be a compensatory response to counteract the deleterious effects of Ang II [238]."

ACE2 as a Therapeutic Target

"Given its vasodilatory, natriuretic, anti-inflammatory, and anti-fibrotic effects via increased Ang-(1–7) and decreased Ang II, soluble ACE2 has been proposed as a potential therapeutic target in hypertension, chronic kidney disease, cardiovascular disease, and viral respiratory disease."

"In experimental studies, chronic administration of soluble ACE2 has been associated with degradation of Ang II and an increase in Ang-(1–7) [239–241]."

"Recombinant ACE2 reduces acute lung injury and acute respiratory distress syndrome in mice with viral pneumonia [58]."

"Children infected with respiratory syncytial virus have higher plasma Ang II concentration compared with healthy controls, suggesting upregulation of ACE/Ang II and downregulation of ACE2/Ang-(1–7), and supporting ACE2 as a potential therapy in respiratory syncytial viral lung disease in humans."

"In humans, ACE inhibitors and Ang II receptor blockers have not been associated with increased kidney ACE2 expression or circulating ACE2 activity [242, 243]."

The Relationship Between ACE2 and COVID-19

"There has been recent speculation that ACE inhibitors and Ang II receptor blockers may increase the risk of development and severity of COVID-19 due to potential upregulation of ACE2 by these medications [244]."

"SARS-CoV-2 facilitates ACE2 endocytosis, downregulates ACE2 expression, and promotes ACE2 shedding from the cell surface, leading to an increase in Ang II concentration and a decrease in Ang-(1–7)."

"Extrapolating from SARS-CoV animal models, increased Ang II in patients with COVID-19 due to loss of ACE2 could mediate acute lung injury and acute respiratory distress syndrome [59]."

"ACE inhibitors and Ang II receptor blockers may have a therapeutic benefit in COVID-19 by reducing Ang II concentration and AT_1R activation."

"It remains unclear if ACE inhibitors or Ang II receptor blockers have a beneficial or harmful effect in SARS-CoV-2 infection and COVID-19."

Conclusions

"ACE2 has important counter-regulatory effects on the renin-angiotensin system and has been implicated in COVID-19 pathogenesis."

"Medications that act on the renin-angiotensin system, including ACE inhibitors and Ang II receptor blockers, may impact COVID-19 infection and severity via potential interactions with ACE2; however, the direction and magnitude of these effects are unknown at this time."

"Several international societies have released statements discouraging discontinuation of ACE inhibitors and Ang II receptor blockers in patients who are treated with these medications for hypertension, heart failure, and chronic kidney disease amidst the COVID-19 pandemic [229]."

"Given the clear benefits of these agents in hypertension, chronic kidney disease, coronary heart disease, and diabetes, there is an urgent need for further research to improve our understanding of the relationship between agents that act on the renin-angiotensin system and outcomes among individuals with COVID-19, with several studies currently underway [229]."

The Renin-Angiotensin System, Hypertension, and SARS-CoV-2 Infection: A Review [245]

This is a machine-generated summary of:

Gathiram, Premjith; Mackraj, Irene; Moodley, Jagidesa: The Renin-Angiotensin System, Hypertension, and SARS-CoV-2 Infection: a Review [245].

Published in: Current Hypertension Reports (2021).

Link to original: https://doi.org/10.1007/s11906-021-01134-9

If you want to cite the papers, please refer to the original.

For technical reasons we could not place the page where the original quote is coming from.

Abstract-Summary "There is currently no data in support of the concerns raised with the use of ACEIs/ARBs."

"Many researchers have voiced concerns that the use of ACEIs and ARBs may increase tissue ACE2 levels."

"These researchers therefore recommend that individuals on ACEIs/ARB's medications withhold such antihypertensive drugs, unless advised by their physicians to do so."

"SARS-CoV-2 uses ACE2 receptors as the port of entry to human hosts."

"The use of ARB's or ACEIs should not be discontinued if an individual is infected by SARS-CoV-2."

"Further studies are required to investigate the effect of ACEIs and ARBs on ACE2 expression and COVID-19."

Introduction

"The causative agent for COVID-19 disease which causes severe acute respiratory syndrome is the coronavirus-2 (SARS-CoV-2) [246]."

"The SARS-CoV-2, like all other coronavirus (SARS-CoV-1 and Middle East Respiratory syndrome (MERS-CoV)), enters the human body and binds to angiotensin-converting enzyme-2 (ACE2) receptors [247, 248]."

"The elderly and those with comorbid conditions, such as asthma or respiratory problems, cardiovascular abnormalities, diabetes mellitus, liver and kidney problems, are more likely to have pneumonia, either bilateral or unilateral, as a result of infection of the lower respiratory tract [249–259]."

"Reverse-transcriptase polymerase chain reaction (R-T PCR) is recognized as the gold standard for the identification of COVID-19 disease, despite having a low sensitivity compared to chest computerized tomography (CT) scan which in most cases, show positive results of lung infection as indicated by a picture of ground-glass opacities or nodules or bilateral reticular nodular opacities [252–256]."

Classical Renin-Angiotensin System

"The SARS-CoV-2 virus uses ACE2 receptors for cell entry into the human body but physiologically the main function of ACE2 enzyme is for maturation of Ang I or Ang II in blood pressure regulation [247, 260]."

"The ATIR are the main receptors of Ang II, which causes vasoconstriction of the vascular smooth muscles, increasing the total peripheral resistance, excitation of the vasomotor centers to increase the heart rate and cardiac contractility, and increasing salt and water reabsorption by the kidneys, as they are a major site for blood pressure regulation [261]."

"ACE2 only has renal effects if the systemic arterial blood pressure rises above normal (brought about by Ang II) or it is below normal levels, which will require absorption of sodium and water by the kidneys."

"While ACE generates Ang II, ACE2 is responsible for hypotensive effects by generating Ang (1–7) which act through Mas receptors found mainly on the blood vessels causing vasodilation."

SARS-CoV-2: Virus Entry into a Given Human Cell

"The SARS-CoV-2 viruses use the ACE2 receptors in the lung parenchyma and in other organs and the cellular protease, TMPRSST, to enter a given cell [262, 263]."

"ACE2 receptors and the protease enzyme TMPRSST are both essential for the viral entry into a given cell [263]."

"There is no direct evidence showing that ACE2 receptors are used for entry into the human body in all COVID-19 patients."

Development of a Vaccine for SARS-CoV-2

"Gurwitz is of the view that the development of a vaccine is time consuming and it may be developed too late for its effective use, because the SARS-CoV-2 virus may have mutated [264]."

"Gurwitz states that AT1 receptor blockers,which do not depend on mutations, should be used as therapeutic agents for reducing the aggressiveness and high mortality of the SARS-CoV-2 virus infection [264]."

The Use of ACEIs and ARBs in COVID-19 Disease

"The most common pharmaceutical drugs used for hypertension, and other cardiovascular diseases (CVDs), are (ACEIs) (such as lisinopril, enalapril) or ARBs (such as losartan)."

"In order to test the effects of using ACEIs and ARBs, Ferrario and others used the ACEI (lisinopril) or ARB (losartan) in experimental animals (normal rats) and measured, besides other parameters, ACE2 mRNA expression levels in plasma and cardiac muscle tissue."

"These researchers found that the administration of ACEI or ARB caused an increase in ACE2 mRNA expression levels [265]."

Effects of Animal Models on SARS-COV-2 Infection in Humans

"We observed that some researchers interpreted that the use of ACEI/ARB in COVID-19 disease, and the upregulation ACE2 mRNA expression (using ACEI/ARB) levels found by Ferrario and others [265], attributed a protective role that could reduce lung injury by leading away from Ang II (which is responsible for lung injury) to the pathway ACE2-Ang (1–7) [266, 267]."

"Regarding tissue expression, a few researchers are of the view that the use of ACEIs/ARBs increases ACE2 levels in the heart and the kidney but not in the lungs [268]."

"While some researchers are of the view that the use of ACEIs/ARBs does more harm than good to SARS-CoV-2 patients by increasing ACE2 receptor expression levels [268, 269], other researchers are of the view that perhaps ACEIs/ARBs should be replaced with calcium channel blockers [8]."

"We would like to offer an advice of caution to those unsure of ACEI or ARB usage or that they should reflect on the findings of Ferrario and others on the notion that ACE2 receptors would cause more SARS-CoV-2 binding, as normal rats were used in their findings of the increased mRNA expression levels of ACE2 in cardiac cells."

Recent Comments/Reviews on the Use of Angiotensin-Converting Enzyme Inhibitors and Angiotensin Receptor Blockers

"Vaduganathan and others believe that both ACEIs and ARBs are prescribed medications worldwide and as such guidance on the use of these drugs in COVID-19 patients is urgently required; however, they are hopeful that a clinical trial is underway to resolve the anomaly [48]."

"Kai and Kai also believe that administration of ACEIs/ARBs to SARS-CoV-2 patients could increase the infectivity of the virus, and could also increase the expression of ACE2 in the cardiovascular and renal system, and aggravate the morbidity and mortality of SARS-CoV and the severity of the infection in hypertensive and other CVD patients [270]."

"between those on either ACEIs or ARBs and hypertensive patients not on either medications, and supported continued ACEIs or ARBs prescriptions [271, 272]."

"According to Kuster and others, neither the withdrawal nor replacement of ACEIs or ARBs in patients with hypertension COVID-19 disease is advisable [266]."

Retrospective Studies Showing No Harm in Using ACEIs or ARBs in COVID-19

"The researchers compared 188 patients on ACEIs/ARBs (ACEIs/ARBs group) with 198 without using ACEIs/ARBs (non-ACEIs/ARBs) group (taking other anti-hypertensive medications)."

"Yang and others observed that hypertensive patients, taking ACEIs or ARBs or without taking these drugs, had a non-significant difference in the death rates between the two groups [273]."

"In an outpatients study using a large sample size, in the USA, the use of ACEIs/ARBs compared with the use of other hypertensive medications in patients with COVID-19 disease requiring hospitalization."

"The study found that the use of ACEIs on their own and the use of ARBs alone compared with the use of other medications in individuals with hypertension and COVID-19 did not show the need for hospitalization in outpatients [274]."

"In a retrospective study of 362 hospitalized hypertensive patients with COVID-19 disease, Li and others investigated 115 patients who were taking ACEIs or ARBs and compared them to those not taking these medications."

Case Control Study Showing No Harm in Using ACEIs/ARBs in COVID-19

"These researchers observed that the use of ACEIs and ARBs was more common among the case group than the control group and case group had a worse clinical profile than the control group because the case group had higher prevalence of cardiovascular diseases [275]."

"The Board members and the Director of the Italian Society of Hypertension has made the following direct statement on the use of RAAS Inhibitors (including ACEIs and ARBs) in COVID-19 disease [276]: iThe experiments were done only on animal models and not on human beings, and to date, there is no evidence that individuals with hypertension are over-represented in COVID-19 disease."

"iiThere is no clinical evidence in humans that associates the intake of ACEIs/ARBs with COVID-19 disease."

"iiiThere is no clinical evidence in SARS-CoVo-2 coronavirus patients that confirms the harmful effects of ACEIs/ARBs or protective effects in the context of COVID-19 epidemic [276]."

Conclusion

"In normal individuals, ACE2 is a homolog of ACE and it has hypotensive effects."

"Entry of SARS-CoV-2 into the cells is by binding to ACE2 receptors."

"Further studies are required to investigate if the use of ACEIs or ARBs does not upregulate ACE2 in COVID-19, and in fact, there is no data supporting evidence available the claim that this medications allows more virus entry into the any cell."

COVID-19: Zinc and Angiotensin-Converting Enzyme 2 (ACE2) Deficiencies as Determinants of Risk and Severity of Disease: A Narrative Review [277]

This is a machine-generated summary of:

Salgo, Miklos P.: COVID-19: Zinc and Angiotensin-Converting Enzyme 2 (ACE2) Deficiencies as Determinants of Risk and Severity of Disease: A Narrative Review [277].

Published in: Infectious Diseases and Therapy (2021).

Link to original: https://doi.org/10.1007/s40121-021-00478-8

If you want to cite the papers, please refer to the original.

For technical reasons we could not place the page where the original quote is coming from.

Abstract-Summary "A growing body of evidence supports the premise that deficiencies of zinc and angiotensin-converting enzyme 2 (ACE2, a zinc enzyme) determine severity of coronavirus disease 2019 (COVID-19)."

"ACE2 is part of the renin–angiotensin system (RAS) and acts as a feedback control system moderating blood pressure, keeping blood pressure within normal limits."

"The virus that causes COVID-19 uses ACE2 to get into the cell."

"The RAS is composed of two feedback loops: the ACE loop provides amplification, increasing pro-inflammatory cytokines and blood pressure; the ACE2 loop provides fine control and mitigates the vasoconstrictive, pro-inflammatory, and thrombotic actions of the ACE loop."

"There is balance, but in the setting of COVID-19, underlying deficiencies of zinc and ACE2 can lead to an imbalance."

"Exacerbated by the severe downregulation of ACE2 seen with viral entry, a "tipping point" is reached with loss of control of the RAS system resulting in increased angiotensin II (Ang II) causing downstream vasoconstriction, inflammation, and thromboses."

"This model suggests that supplemental zinc could replenish zinc in ACE2, stabilize the ACE2 axis, and prevent disruption of the RAS."

"This would prevent the vasoconstrictive, inflammatory, and thrombotic actions of Ang II, thus preventing the severe COVID-19 complications which cause the high morbidity and mortality seen in high-risk patients with underlying zinc deficiency."

"Randomized clinical trials are needed to confirm safety and efficacy of zinc supplementation to decrease severity of and morality from COVID-19 in high-risk patients."

"Since replenishment of zinc and active ACE2 in patients in whom these are deficient may take weeks, supplementation in high-risk populations prior to COVID infection may be required."

Introduction

"This is a narrative review focusing on the role of zinc and the zinc enzyme angiotensin-converting enzyme 2 (ACE2) in the renin–angiotensin system (RAS)."

"Review of the literature has revealed an emerging consistent narrative that explains much that we see in risk factors, symptoms, and course of disease in COVID-19."

"The true value of this approach will be if therapeutic interventions based on this framework are safe and effective in decreasing severity and mortality of COVID-19."

Symptoms and Demographics

"Individuals age older than 65, of male sex, and minority race or ethnicity are at high risk of contracting COVID-19 and once infected are at a higher risk of disease progression and death [278–281]."

"These same groups also have been shown to have higher rates of ACE2 deficiency [282], suggesting that ACE2 deficiency plays a role in the response to COVID and in development of hypertension."

"Risk groups for COVID-19 and zinc deficiency largely overlap [283]."

Chronic Conditions of Risk for COVID-19

"The Centers for Disease Control and Prevention (CDC) has noted risk of severe COVID-19 including rehospitalization in patients with any of five chronic conditions: chronic obstructive pulmonary disease (COPD), heart failure, diabetes with chronic complications, chronic kidney disease, and obesity [284]."

"Zinc deficiency has been implicated in COPD [285], heart failure [286], diabetes [287], and chronic kidney disease and obesity [288]."

Socioeconomics

"Patients at high risk of SARS-CoV-2 infection, disease progression, and death include racial and ethnic minorities [279]."

"These increased risks have been attributed to societal and racial inequities [289]."

"Baseline ACE2/zinc deficiency is hypothesized as a biochemical mediator of the socioeconomic conditions and diet to which high-risk individuals have been subject and also provides a logical mechanism as to how socioeconomic factors can impact individual risk."

ACE2 and RAS

"ACE and ACE2 are homologous zinc metalloenzymes, each with an N-terminal signal sequence, a hydrophobic transmembrane section, and a cytoplasmic section [290]."

"Zinc is required to catalyze peptide hydrolysis [291; for ACE, prior to discovery of ACE2]."

"Activity of ACE is dependent on adequate dietary zinc."

"Adding zinc to the serum from zinc-deficient animals restored ACE activity and adding EDTA inhibited activity, reversible with zinc but not copper [292]."

Viral Entry

"SARS-CoV-2 utilizes epithelial cell ACE2 as a cellular entry receptor [282]."

"The viral spike glycoprotein S binds to the host cell ACE2 receptor [8, 293]."

"This is followed by release of the viral genome into the cell, accompanied by severe downregulation of the ACE2 receptor [282]."

ACE "Adverse" Vs. ACE2 "Protective" Axes of RAS

"The major difference between ACE and ACE2 is the specificity of their carboxypeptidases—the ACE carboxypeptidase removes a single amino acid from inactive angiotensin (Ang) to yield active angiotensin II (Ang II)."

"The major substrate of ACE2 is Ang II; ACE2 degrades (active) Ang II to generate (vasodilatory) Ang 1–7 and Ang 1–9."

"In normal functioning, the ACE positive feedback loop leads to amplification of Ang II and increased BP, inflammation, and thrombosis."

"With zinc deficiency ACE2 activity is decreased which can lead to decrease of the "preventive" Ang 1–7 and Ang 1–9 and predominance of the ACE "adverse" Ang II."

Hypothesis: Deficiencies of Zinc and ACE2, Dysregulation, and the Tipping Point

"Building on work of others [282, 290, 294] a hypothesis has emerged that deficiencies of ACE2 and zinc can explain the high-risk groups for COVID-19."

"This loss of control and predominance of the ACE "adverse" axis [295] is signaled downstream by Ang II acting via the AT1 receptor to increase vasoconstriction, inflammation, and thromboses, In the lung, Ang II hyperactivity could result in multifocal pneumonia, acute respiratory distress syndrome (ARDS), thromboses, or (systemically) cytokine storm [282, 295–297]."

"Others [298] have stressed the cytokine actions with little mention of the failed RAS."

"Loss of control in feedback systems occurs when perturbations or delays exceed the limits of the system [299]."

Zinc and ACE2 Deficiency in Patients with COVID-19

"In one series of hospitalized patients with COVID-19, 57.4% were zinc deficient at the time of hospitalization compared to healthy controls [300]."

"Patients with COVID-19 who were zinc deficient at time of hospitalization were compared with those with normal zinc levels at hospitalization."

"Those showing zinc deficiency had increased complications (OR 5.54), ARDS (18.5% vs. 0%, $p = 0.06$), and mortality (18.5% vs. 0%, $p = 0.06$)."

"Verdecchia and colleagues [282] noted that the groups with higher rates of disease progression with COVID-19 (advanced age, male sex) have higher rates of ACE2 deficiency."

Time Course of COVID-19: Acute Exacerbation and Complications

"Many patients with COVID-19 do relatively well in the first week after onset but then (especially high-risk patients) may experience an acute exacerbation, often with ARDS or other sequelae in the second week."

"They noted clinical exacerbation (defined as moving from the general ward to the intensive care unit) at 8.8 days after disease onset."

"With exacerbation, patients had more clinical symptoms, and an increase in number of lung lobes involved, with multifocal lesions in 100%."

"Berlin and others [301] have reviewed this "severe COVID-19″ starting approximately 1 week after onset of illness."

Time Course of COVID-19 Disease: Right Drug at the Right Phase of Disease

"Cantini and Goletti [302, 303] also raised an important concept regarding treatments for COVID-19: we have to use the right drug at the right phase of disease."

"Remdesivir and other antivirals are expected to be active early during active viral replication while dexamethasone or baricitinib act later dampening the SARS-CoV-2-mediated immune response."

"Zinc supplementation for replenishment of zinc deficiency would be expected to be most beneficial if administered early, to maintain or replenish ACE2 and the ACE2 axis."

"Late administration, after the acute exacerbation of the "tipping point", would likely have diminished chance of success, as the pro-inflammatory Ang II "horse" would already be "out of the proverbial barn."".

Kawasaki Disease and MIS-C

"Late onset inflammatory disease resembling Kawasaki disease has been reported with COVID-19."

"Because it effects children older than usually seen with Kawasaki disease, it has now been renamed as multisystem inflammatory syndrome in children (MIS-C)."

"Decreased plasma zinc levels have been reported in children with Kawasaki disease [304]."

"This zinc deficiency resolved after treatment with intravenous immunoglobulins."

COVID-19 Long-Term Complications

"Zinc supplementation for those found to be deficient may be of benefit."

"Overt zinc deficiency is not common [283, 305]; however, in a study of older adults (>60 years old), 20–25% had insufficient zinc intake [305]."

"Zinc deficiency in hypertensives can be corrected with supplemental zinc."

"Excess zinc supplementation 150–450 mg/day has been associated with disruption of iron and immune function."

"Zinc replacement for zinc deficiency with 30 mg/day zinc is generally considered safe."

"The AREDS studies for delaying progression of macular degeneration have provided long-term safety data on zinc supplementation; 3640 patients were randomized to (1) antioxidants plus zinc 80 mg/day and copper daily 2 mg/day, (2) zinc and copper without antioxidants, (3) antioxidants alone, and (4) inactive placebo."

"Optimal dosing and duration for treatment of zinc deficiency in COVID-19 has not been established; 30 mg/day is considered safe while 80 mg/day zinc with 2 mg/day copper while monitoring for genitourinary events might be appropriate for clinical trials."

Recent Studies

"They summarized that direct evidence of benefit of zinc for prevention or treatment of SARS-CoV-2 infection is not yet available; however, indirect evidence from the literature suggests that zinc supplementation may be useful to reduce the "risk, duration, and severity" of SARS-CoV-2 in older patients and those with chronic conditions known to be associated with zinc deficiency."

"Those found to have low or borderline zinc levels or those with evidence of insufficient intake or excess loss of zinc should be considered for zinc supplementation."

"Thomas and others [306] randomized 214 newly diagnosed ambulatory patients to open-label zinc (50 mg zinc gluconate daily), ascorbic acid, both, or neither for 10 days of treatment."

"The study was limited to ambulatory patients; this may have led inadvertently to underrepresentation of zinc-deficient patients most likely to benefit from zinc supplementation [307]."

Proposal: Randomized Clinical Trials

"The accumulating evidence above and the fact that zinc supplements are available, easy to use, well studied, and relatively safe suggests that randomized clinical trials for high-risk groups could be initiated now."

"Zinc supplementation should not be a substitute for COVID-19 vaccination."

"Zinc assessment and supplementation for those found to be zinc deficient may be of benefit for those unable or unwilling to access vaccination or those who may be at increased risk from viral variants that are insufficiently covered by currently available vaccines."

Limitations

"This manuscript presents an internally consistent narrative to explain a number of observations of COVID-19, especially those occurring in high-risk patients."

"The optimal duration of zinc supplementation to replenish ACE2 in the setting of COVID has not been established."

"If supplementation longer than a week is required, initiation after COVID infection may be too late; zinc deficient patients at risk of COVID may have to be identified and zinc supplementation initiated prior to infection."

"Other models of pathophysiology of COVID-19 have been proposed [308]."

Conclusions

"A growing body of evidence supports the premise that deficiencies of zinc and the zinc enzyme ACE2 are determinants of risk and severity of COVID-19."

"Anosmia, demographics of high-risk groups, and the actions of the RAS point to deficiencies of zinc and ACE2 playing a role in COVID-19 exacerbation in high-risk individuals."

"This in turn results in downstream increases in vasoconstriction, inflammation, and thromboses, leading to clinical sequelae of COVID-19 such as ARDs, thromboses, MIS-C, cytokine storm, etc RCTs are needed to confirm safety and efficacy of zinc supplementation to decrease incidence and severity of COVID-19 in high-risk patients."

"If RCTs confirm the proposed benefit of zinc replacement therapy in high-risk zinc-deficient patients, this would open a new window of attack to prevent the increased vasoconstriction, inflammation and thromboses seen in severe COVID."

The Role of Angiotensin-Converting Enzyme 2 (ACE2) Genetic Variations in COVID-19 Infection: A Literature Review [309]

This is a machine-generated summary of:

Fawzy, Manal S.; Ashour, Hend; Shafie, Aya Allah Ashraf; Dahman, Nesrine Ben Hadj; Fares, Abdelhamid M.; Antar, Sarah; Elnoby, Ahmed S.; Fouad, Fatma Mohamed: The role of angiotensin-converting enzyme 2 (ACE2) genetic variations in COVID-19 infection: a literature review [309].

Published in: Egyptian Journal of Medical Human Genetics (2022).

Link to original: https://doi.org/10.1186/s43042-022-00309-6

If you want to cite the papers, please refer to the original.

For technical reasons we could not place the page where the original quote is coming from.

Abstract-Summary "Emerging studies tried to determine whether the ACE2 variants and/or expression could be associated with SARS-CoV/SARS-CoV2 have conflicting results."

"Some studies use data mining to predict several ACE2 variants that could enhance or decline susceptibility to SARS-CoV. On the other hand, fewer studies revealed an association of ACE2 expression with COVID-19 outcome reporting higher expression levels of ACE2 in East Asians."

"ACE2 gene variants and expression may modify the deleterious consequences of SARS-CoV2 to the host cells."

"Apart from the differences in gene expression and the genetic variations of ACE2, many other environmental and/or genetic factors could modify the disease outcome, including the genes for the innate and the adaptive immune response."

Background

"ACE2 is reported to be the fundamental entry point of SARS-CoV [59]."

"Rather than the pulmonary expression, ACE2 is reported to be also distributed in the heart, the renal and luminal surface of intestinal epithelial cells, among others [310], explaining the SARS-CoV2 entry site in Wuhan patients and the multi-organ dysfunction observed in infected patients [311]."

"By using normal lung tissues, Zhao and others have detected that about 83% of the lung ACE2 expression is situated in the alveolar epithelial cells type II, which may facilitate coronaviral invasion and harbor the virus for replication [312]."

"Accumulating evidence indicates that ACE2 genetic polymorphisms among populations and racial considerations may correlate with cellular susceptibility to SARS-CoV2 infection with controversial findings [6, 8, 48, 170–184, 186–223, 225–244, 246–276, 278–308, 310–314]."

"This review aimed to explore some basics related to ACE2-SARS-CoV2 interaction and cell entry and the relation of different ACE2 variants to disease risk, severity, and progression among different populations worldwide."

Main Text

"The identified records evaluated against the following inclusion criteria: studies are exploring the association of COVID-19 with ACE2 genetic variations, all types of studies, and the studies published in both peer-reviewed journals and as a preprint."

"Different databases were applied to explore the structural and functional characteristics of the ACE2 gene."

"Protter (http://wlab.ethz.ch/protter/), a web application to visualize the sequence, annotations, and topology of the individual proteins, has been applied to visualize the amino acid residues of ACE2 and domains [315]."

COVID-19 Cell Entry

"The infectivity assays on HeLa cells with or without ACE2 proteins extracted from bats, civets, pigs, mice, and humans, revealed that SARS-CoV-2 uses ACE2 to promote its entry into ACE2-expressing cells, but not from mouse species."

"It cannot enter those cells without ACE2, which can be considered specific receptors for this virus resembling SARS-CoV [316]."

"Tai and his research team discovered the presence of RBD in the SARS-CoV-2 S1 subunit and observed a robust binding ability to ACE2; moreover, they showed a significantly higher binding affinity than that to SARS-CoV, which may explain the higher infectious rate of SARS-CoV-2 over SARS-CoV [199, 317]."

"Such structural similarity and succession unequivocally contend for the evolution between the SARS-CoV-2 and SARS-CoV RBDs to improve the binding ability to ACE2 receptors [318]."

Angiotensin-Converting Enzyme 2 (ACE2): The Hottest Target of SARS-CoV-2 Invasion

"Like ACE, ACE2 has two domains: an amino-terminal catalytic domain and another carboxy-terminal domain."

"ACE2 can also be trimmed by "a disintegrin and metalloproteinase domain-containing protein 17 (ADAM 17)," which releases an extracellular fragment called soluble ACE2 (sACE2) and is measured as sACE2 plasma activity [319]."

"Kornilov and colleagues have observed that COVID-19-related regulatory pathways may induce ACE2 shedding, and the sACE2 concentrations may correlate with the level of systemic inflammation associated with COVID-19 [172]."

"The calmodulin–calcium signaling pathway which contributes to ACE2 release has been suggested to add new insights for clinical/therapeutic applications of ACE2 for COVID-19 [320]."

[Section 5]

"A recent study by Fujikura and Uesaka REF has identified 349 single nucleotide variants (SNVs) in the coding regions and splice sites."

"The residual 2% of SNVs, stop-gained (n = 2), splice site variants (n = 2), start-loss (n = 1), and indels (n = 3) were recorded."

"The majority of these SNVs were rare or quite rare, with allele frequency < 1% or < 0.001%, respectively."

"The frequency of deleterious SNVs is higher for rare SNVs than for SNVs with a high allele frequency [321]."

[Section 6]

"Although an earlier report demonstrated no association between ACE2 variants and SARS-CoV susceptibility or outcomes with no difference related to sex [313], Gemmati and others reported a higher incidence of COVID-19 infection in males with more severe representations."

"The genetic analysis by Cao and co-workers did not find any mutation difference in ACE2 that would influence SARS-CoV2/S-protein binding [314]."

"Using data mining in several data sets and applying "structural predictions," Suryamohan and others could predict several ACE2 variants (i.e., "E23K, S19P, I21V, K26R, T27A, N64K, T92I, K26E, H378R, Q102P, and M383T") which have the potential to increase the sensitivity of the host to SARS-CoV. Alternatively, "N33I, K31R, D38V, H34R, E35K, E37K, N51S, K68E, Y50F, F72V, G326E, G352V, Y83H, D355N and Q388L" variants were predicted to decrease S-protein-ACE2 binding affinity with a subsequent decline in infection susceptibility [322]."

[Section 7]

"The mechanisms by which ACE2 gene variants could impact the structural and/or the catalytic activity of the gene product could be at the transcriptional (mRNA expression), post-transcriptional modifications (such as N-glycosylation), or ACE2 protein levels that influence the outcome of COVID-19 by acting on blood pressure through the RAS and possible impact on lung/heart damages through the Ang II-triggered oxidative stress [323]."

"The ACE insertion/deletion (I/D) variant, which influences enzyme levels with subsequent change in the "ACE/Ang II/AT1R axis" function, also showed many correlations with SARS-CoV-2 infection and appeared to impact the outcome of COVID-19 disease [324]."

"It has been observed that the (II) genotype (that is associated with the least ACE plasma levels compared to the ID/DD variants) is the most prevalent genotype among asymptomatic COVID-19 cases."

[Section 8]

"Higher ACE2 expression was reported in men's lungs more than women, while serum activities appear higher in females than males, supporting the hypothesis related to the observed gender-related differences in disease severity/outcome [325–327]."

"The putative role of estrogen in upregulating the ACE2 expression/plasma activity was suggested as a possible cause for relative female protection against COVID-19 infection compared to males [328]."

"Osman and others reported a decrease in the expression of circulating ACE2 mRNA and cell surface ACE2 during COVID-19, and prolonged viral shedders of COVID-19 were associated with low sACE2 plasma concentrations [329]."

"Wooster and others have suggested in their preprint article that five ACE2-related variants "rs4240157, rs6632680, rs4830965, rs1476524, and rs2048683" might be associated with higher ACE2 tissue-specific expression, resulting in hospitalization, whereas the "rs1548474" variant showed association with low tissue expression and lesser severity [330]."

ACE2 Role in Emerging COVID-19-Related Treatment

"In seeking a suitable treatment for COVID-19, recently, the RBD of SARS-CoV-2 spike glycoprotein (S-protein) was modeled in 242 structural models with variations of human ACE2 binding [331]."

"One of the proposed strategies for COVID-19 treatment was the soluble ACE2 and ACE2-Fc fusion protein that work as decoy receptors to SARS-CoV2 [332]."

"El-Shennawy and others reported "an increase about 135-fold higher potency in blocking the binding of the viral spike protein RBD, and a 60- to 80-fold higher efficacy in preventing infections by SARS-CoV-2" for their newly identified circulating extracellular vesicles that express ACE2 (evACE2) compared to vesicle-free rhACE2 [333]."

"Another emerging proposal for COVID-19 treatment has been assumed by Bakry and others, in which they suggested the use of the mesenchymal stem cells that are coated with anti-ACE2 antibodies to help in the achievement of better cell attachment to SARS-CoV2-infected cells and competing with the virus for the same receptor [334]."

Conclusions

"Apart from the differences in ACE2 genetic variations and gene expression, many other genetic and/or environmental factors, including, for example, the genes related to the innate and adaptive immunity, the viral load, the preventive precautions that are taken at the level of the individuals and the countries, among others, could influence COVID-19 virulence and modify disease outcome."

"Most of the studies mentioned above have limitations, including the non-reproducibility of genetic variant studies among different ethnic groups [319]."

Angiotensin-Converting-Enzyme 2 and Renin-Angiotensin System Inhibitors in COVID-19: An Update [335]

This is a machine-generated summary of:

Shukla, Ashwin Kumar; Banerjee, Monisha: Angiotensin-Converting-Enzyme 2 and Renin-Angiotensin System Inhibitors in COVID-19: An Update [335].

Published in: High Blood Pressure & Cardiovascular Prevention (2021).

Link to original: https://doi.org/10.1007/s40292-021-00439-9

If you want to cite the papers, please refer to the original.

For technical reasons we could not place the page where the original quote is coming from.

Abstract-Summary "There are several treatment strategies for controlling diabetes, hypertension, etc; like ACE2 gene therapies, endogenous ACE2 activators, human recombinant ACE2 (hrACE2), Angiotensin-II receptor blockers (ARBs) and ACE inhibitors (ACEi) medications."

"ACE2, the receptors for SARS-CoV2, facilitates virus entry inside host cell."

"Clinicians are using two classes of medications for the treatment of COVID-19; one targets the SARS-CoV-2-ACE2 interaction, while other targets human immune system."

"The aim of this review is to discuss the role of ACE2 in diabetes and in COVID-19 and to provide an analysis of data proposing harm and benefit of RAS inhibitor treatment in COVID-19 infection as well as showing no association whatsoever."

Introduction

"Although the mortality rate of COVID-19 is low, patients with diabetes mellitus (DM) and hypertension have shown more severe disease and increased fatality [8, 336]."

"One of the initial studies done in Wuhan before 2 January, 2020, reported that out of 41 patients infected and identified with COVID-19, 8 were diabetes patients (20%), 6 were hypertensive (15%) and 6 had cardiovascular diseases (15%) [337]."

"Another study including 26 deceased COVID-19 infected patients reported that, 53.8% were hypertensive, 42.3% diabetes patients, and 19.2% had coronary heart disease."

"The present knowledge lacks any clinical data to support the hypothesis that use of ARBs/ACEi increases patients' susceptibility to COVID-19 infection and suggests both benefit as well as harm."

"We have discussed the role of ACE2 in diabetes and in COVID-19 and analysed the data proposing harm and benefit of RAS inhibitor treatment in COVID-19 infection as well as showing no association whatsoever."

ACE2: Overview and Function

"ACE2 is a component of RAS which maintains blood pressure, fluid and electrolyte balance and reabsorption of sodium in kidney [338] by controlling vasoconstriction."

"As a usual physiological feedback to low renal blood flow, juxtaglomerular cells convert inactive prorenin to active renin, which is secreted directly into the circulation."

"ACE2 counterbalances the whole mechanism by targeting Ang-II and converting it to Ang 1–7, which is a vasodilator [338]."

ACE2: Role in Diabetes

"ACE2 can be considered as a protective agent, as it increases and decreases the levels of Ang-(1–7) and Ang-II respectively, which prevents the harmful effects of overactive RAS."

"Ang-II prevents elevated insulin secretion from pancreatic islets in hyperglycemic condition by disrupting β-cell function, and ACE2 gene therapy reduces this damaging effect of Ang-II and insulin is released accordingly from β-cells during hyperglycemic condition [339]."

"Some studies have reported role of ACE2 in reducing Ang-II-mediated oxidative stress [339], thus improving pancreatic dysfunction."

"Although, ACE2 therapy in Ang-II treated mice models exhibited no increase in pancreatic blood flow [339], but ACE2 as a vasodilator may affect insulin secretion [339] by increasing the blood flow in islets suggesting that further studies should be done."

"In diabetes models, upregulation of RAS leads to Ang-II pathway activation and subsequently increase oxidative stress, fibrosis, inflammation, cell proliferation and even apoptosis."

ACE2: Role in COVID-19

"The host when exposed to the virus, CoVs by the help of spike protein bind to the cells expressing specific ACE2 receptors."

"As the expression of ACE2 is down-regulated with the onset of infection, its role in developing lung injury in patients with SARS-CoV infection was disputable [340]."

"Few experimental data demonstrate that severe lung injury and fibrosis in SARS-CoV animal models is mainly mediated by Ang-II inflammation [341, 342]."

"The decrease in ACE2 expression prior to SARS-CoV-2 infection increases local concentration of Ang-II in the lungs and causes severe lung injury."

"SARS-CoV epidemic data also suggested that ACE2 dependent SARS-CoV-2 infection may decrease ACE2 expression in heart, promoting severe heart injury [16]."

"ARBs and ACEi could increase the expression of ACE2 in lungs, which increases the risk of COVID-19 infection [343]."

RAS Inhibitor Drugs: Role in COVID-19

"An early study considered the use of RAS inhibitor medications to increase lethal COVID-19 infection [344]."

"Fang and others [8] hypothesised that patients with diabetes and hypertension, who are treated with RAS modulators are at increased risk of COVID-19 as it elevates the ACE2 concentration."

"Several retrospective studies done on patients with hypertension and COVID-19, showed decreased mortality rate in patients receiving RAS inhibitors when compared with patients receiving other hypertensive medications [345, 346]."

"Improved clinical outcomes in hypertension patients with COVID-19 was found related with medications including RAS inhibitors [347]."

"A study done on patients in Italy, included 6272 cases compared with 30,759 controls and found no association of RAS antagonist risk and severity of COVID-19 infection [348]."

"There are several other studies which have reported no association between RAS inhibitor medication and increased severity and mortality of COVID-19 patients [99, 349, 350]."

Future Perspectives

"SARS-CoV and SARS-CoV-2 enters the host-cell by the help of a protein termed as SPIKE (S-protein), expressed on the viral coat."

"These S-proteins have receptor binding regions which binds to ACE2's extra cellular domain [351]."

"SARS-CoV-2 entry into the host cell also depends on the priming between S-protein and TMPRSS2 (a transmembrane protease serine 2) [352]."

"It is also important to note that camostat mesylate, a serine protease inhibitor, has been proved to block the activity of TMPRSS2 [352–354], and in Japan they have been approved for human use."

Conclusion

"Time, no data supports the hypothesis that use of ARBs/ACEi increases patients' susceptibility to COVID-19 infection, its severity and mortality."

"In the joint statement, American Heart Association (AHA), American College of Cardiology (ACC) and Heart Failure Society of America (HFSA) have recommended physicians not to begin or discontinue the usual RAS related medications (ARBs/ACEi) in COVID-19 patients."

"Research done on RAS expression, especially ACE2/Ang-(1–7) pathway in COVID-19 cases can fill the knowledge gaps and may significantly affect the treatment guidelines of the patients on ACEi/ARBs medications."

Bibliography

1. Mehta N, Kalra A, Nowacki AS, Anjewierden S, Han Z, Bhat P, Carmona-Rubio AE, Jacob M, Procop GW, Harrington S, Milinovich A, Svensson LG, Jehi L, Young JB, Chung MK (2020) Association of use of angiotensin-converting enzyme inhibitors and angiotensin II receptor blockers with testing positive for coronavirus disease 2019 (COVID-19). JAMA Cardiol 5:1020–1026. https://doi.org/10.1001/jamacardio.2020.1855
2. Shukla AK, Banerjee M (2021) Angiotensin-converting-enzyme 2 and renin-angiotensin system inhibitors in COVID-19: an update. High Blood Press Cardiovasc Prev 28:129–139
3. Ishiyama Y et al (2004) Upregulation of angiotensin-converting enzyme 2 after myocardial infarction by blockade of angiotensin II receptors. Hypertension 43:970–976
4. Ferrario CM et al (2005) Effect of angiotensin-converting enzyme inhibition and angiotensin II receptor blockers on cardiac angiotensin-converting enzyme 2. Circulation 111:2605–2610
5. Vaduganathan M et al (2020) Renin–angiotensin–aldosterone system inhibitors in patients with Covid-19. N Engl J Med 382:1653–1659
6. Wu Z, McGoogan JM (2020) Characteristics of and important lessons from the coronavirus disease 2019 (COVID-19) outbreak in China: summary of a report of 72314 cases from the Chinese Center for Disease Control and Prevention. JAMA 323(13):1239–1242. https://doi.org/10.1001/jama.2020.2648
7. Biswas M, Rahaman S, Biswas TK, Haque Z, Ibrahim B (2020) Association of sex, age, and comorbidities with mortality in COVID-19 patients: a systematic review and meta-analysis. Intervirology 9:1–12. https://doi.org/10.1159/000512592
8. Fang L, Karakiulakis G, Roth M (2020) Are patients with hypertension and diabetes mellitus at increased risk for COVID-19 infection? Lancet Respir Med 8:e21. https://doi.org/10.1016/S2213-2600(20)30116-8
9. Gurwitz D (2020) Angiotensin receptor blockers as tentative SARS-CoV-2 therapeutics. Drug Dev Res 81:537–540. https://doi.org/10.1002/ddr.21656

10. Biswas M, Kali MSK (2021) Association of angiotensin-converting enzyme inhibitors and angiotensin-receptor blockers with risk of mortality, severity or SARS-CoV-2 test positivity in COVID-19 patients: meta-analysis. Sci Rep 11:5012. https://doi.org/10.1038/s41598-021-84678-9
11. Mackey K et al (2020) Risks and impact of angiotensin-converting enzyme inhibitors or angiotensin-receptor blockers on SARS-CoV-2 infection in adults. Ann Intern Med 173:195–203. https://doi.org/10.7326/m20-1515
12. de Vries AAF (2020) Renin-angiotensin system inhibition in COVID-19 patients. Neth Heart J 28:396–405. https://doi.org/10.1007/s12471-020-01439-5
13. Xu J, Huang C, Fan G, Liu Z, Shang L, Zhou F, Wang Y, Yu J, Yang L, Xie K, Huang Z, Huang L, Gu X, Li H, Zhang Y, Wang Y, Hayden FG, Horby PW, Cao B, Wang C (2020) Use of angiotensin-converting enzyme inhibitors and angiotensin II receptor blockers in context of COVID-19 outbreak: a retrospective analysis. Front Med 14:601–612. https://doi.org/10.1007/s11684-020-0800-y
14. Rico-Mesa JS, White A, Anderson AS (2020) Outcomes in patients with COVID-19 infection taking ACEI/ARB. Curr Cardiol Rep 22:31. https://doi.org/10.1007/s11886-020-01291-4
15. Liu J, Zheng X, Tong Q, Li W, Wang B, Sutter K, Trilling M, Lu M, Dittmer U, Yang D (2020) Overlapping and discrete aspects of the pathology and pathogenesis of the emerging human pathogenic coronaviruses SARSCoV, MERS-CoV, and 2019-nCoV. J Med Virol 92(5):491–494
16. Sparks MA, Crowley SD, Gurley SB, Mirotsou M, Coffman TM (2014) Classical renin-angiotensin system in kidney physiology. Compr Physiol 4(3):1201–1228
17. Kuba K, Imai Y, Ohto-Nakanishi T, Penninger JM (2010) Trilogy of ACE2: a peptidase in the renin- angiotensin system, a SARS receptor, and a partner for amino acid transporters. Pharmacol Ther 128(1):119–128
18. Yang X, Yu Y, Xu J, Shu H, Xia J, Liu H, Wu Y, Zhang L, Yu Z, Fang M, Yu T, Wang Y, Pan S, Zou X, Yuan S (2020) Clinical course and outcomes of critically ill patients with SARS-CoV-2 pneumonia in Wuhan, China: a single-centered, retrospective, observational study. Lancet Respir Med. 8(5):475–481
19. Guan WJ, Ni ZY, Hu Y, Liang WH, Ou CQ, He JX, Liu L, Shan H, Lei CL, Hui DS, Du B, Li LJ, Zeng G, Yuen KY, Chen R, Tang CL, Wang T, Chen PY, Xiang J, Li SY, Wang JL, Liang ZJ, Peng YX, Wei L, Liu Y, Hu YH, Peng P, Wang JM, Liu JY, Chen Z, Li G, Zheng ZJ, Qiu SQ, Luo J, Ye CJ, Zhu SY, Zhong NS (2020) Clinical characteristics of coronavirus disease 2019 in China. N Engl J Med. 382:1708–1720
20. Zhang JJ, Dong X, Cao YY, Yuan YD, Yang YB, Yan YQ, Akdis CA, Gao YD (2020) Clinical characteristics of 140 patients infected with SARS-CoV-2 in Wuhan, China. Allergy 75(7):1730–1741
21. Li XC, Zhang J, Zhuo JL (2017) The vasoprotective axes of the renin-angiotensin system: physiological relevance and therapeutic implications in cardiovascular, hypertensive and kidney diseases. Pharmacol Res 125(Pt A):21–38. https://doi.org/10.1016/j.phrs.2017.06.005. Epub 2017 Jun 12. PMID: 28619367; PMCID: PMC5607101
22. Furuhashi MMN, Mita T, Fuseya T, Ishimura S, Ohno K, Shibata S, Tanaka M, Watanabe Y, Akasaka H, Ohnishi H, Yoshida H, Takizawa H, Saitoh S, Ura N, Shimamoto K, Miura T (2015) Urinary angiotensin-converting enzyme 2 in hypertensive patients may be increased by olmesartan, an angiotensin II receptor blocker. Am J Hypertens 28(1):15–21. https://doi.org/10.1093/ajh/hpu086. Epub 2014 May 18. PMID: 24842388
23. Patients taking ACE-i and ARBs who contract COVID-19 should continue treatment, unless otherwise advised by their physician [press release]. heart.org. 17 Mar 2020
24. Landolfo M, Maino A, Di Salvo E, Fiorini G, Peterlana D, Borghi C (2022) Renin–angiotensin system modulation and outcomes in patients hospitalized for interstitial SARS-CoV2 pneumonia: a cohort study. Intern Emerg Med 17:1335–1341. https://doi.org/10.1007/s11739-022-02929-7

25. Koka V, Huang XR, Chung AC, Wang W, Truong LD, Lan HY (2008) Angiotensin II up-regulates angiotensin I-converting enzyme (ACE), but down-regulates ACE2 via the AT1-ERK/p38 MAP kinase pathway. Am J Pathol 172:1174–1183. https://doi.org/10.2353/ajpath.2008.070762
26. Deshotels MR, Xia H, Sriramula S, Lazartigues E, Filipeanu CM (2014) Angiotensin II mediates angiotensin converting enzyme type 2 internalization and degradation through an angiotensin ii type i receptor–dependent mechanism. Hypertension 64(6):1368–1375
27. Zhou F, Liu YM, Xie J, Li H, Lei F, Yang H et al (2020) Comparative impacts of ACE (angiotensin-converting enzyme) inhibitors versus angiotensin II receptor blockers on the risk of COVID-19 mortality. Hypertension 76(2):e15–e17
28. Italia L, Tomasoni D, Bisegna S, Pancaldi E, Stretti L, Adamo M et al (2021) COVID-19 and heart failure: from epidemiology during the pandemic to myocardial injury, myocarditis, and heart failure sequelae. Front Cardiovasc Med 8:713560. https://doi.org/10.3389/fcvm.2021.713560
29. Tomasoni D, Inciardi RM, Lombardi CM, Tedino C, Agostoni P, Ameri P et al (2020) Impact of heart failure on the clinical course and outcomes of patients hospitalized for COVID-19. Results of the Cardio-COVID-Italy multicentre study. Eur J Heart Fail 22(12):2238–2247
30. Xu K, He W, Yu B, Zhong K, Zhou D, Wang DW (2023) Beneficial effects of angiotensin II receptor blockers on mortality in patients with COVID-19: a retrospective study from 2019 to 2020 in China. Cardiovasc Drugs Ther. https://doi.org/10.1007/s10557-023-07494-5
31. Zheng Z, Peng F, Xu B et al (2020) Risk factors of critical & mortal COVID-19 cases: a systematic literature review and meta-analysis. J Infect 81(2):e16–e25
32. Li J, Huang DQ, Zou B et al (2021) Epidemiology of COVID-19: a systematic review and meta-analysis of clinical characteristics, risk factors, and outcomes. J Med Virol 93(3):1449–1458
33. Zhang P, Zhu L, Cai J, Lei F, Qin JJ, Xie J, Liu YM, Zhao YC, Huang X, Lin L et al (2020) Association of inpatient use of angiotensin-converting enzyme inhibitors and Angiotensin II receptor blockers with mortality among patients with hypertension hospitalized with COVID-19. Circ Res 126(12):1671–1681
34. Cannata F, Chiarito M, Reimers B, Azzolini E, Ferrante G, My I et al (2020) Continuation versus discontinuation of ACE inhibitors or angiotensin II receptor blockers in COVID-19: effects on blood pressure control and mortality. Eur Heart J Cardiovasc Pharmacother 6(6):412–414
35. Semenzato L, Botton J, Drouin J et al (2021) Antihypertensive drugs and COVID-19 risk: a cohort study of 2 million hypertensive patients. Hypertension 77(3):833–842
36. Gallo G, Calvez V, Savoia C (2022) Hypertension and COVID-19: current evidence and perspectives. High Blood Press Cardiovasc Prev 29(2):115–123
37. Task Force for the management of COVID-19 of the European Society of Cardiology (2022) ESC guidance for the diagnosis and management of cardiovascular disease during the COVID-19 pandemic: part 2-care pathways, treatment, and follow-up. Eur Heart J 43(11):1059–1103
38. Anzola GP, Bartolaminelli C, Gregorini GA, Coazzoli C, Gatti F, Mora A, Charalampakis D, Palmigiano A, De Simone M, Comini A, Dellaglio E, Cassetti S, Chiesa M, Spedini F, d'Ottavi P, Savio MC (2020) Neither ACEIs nor ARBs are associated with respiratory distress or mortality in COVID-19 results of a prospective study on a hospital-based cohort. Intern Emerg Med 15:1477–1484. https://doi.org/10.1007/s11739-020-02500-2
39. Guan WJ, Ni ZY, Hu Y, Liang WH, Ou CQ, He JX, Liu L et al (2020) Clinical characteristics of coronavirus disease 2019 in China. N Engl J Med 382(18):1708–1720. https://doi.org/10.1056/NEJMoa2002032
40. Donnelly CA, Ghani AC, Leung GM et al (2003) Epidemiological determinants of spread of causal agent of severe acute respiratory syndrome in Hong Kong. Lancet 361:1761–1766
41. Zhou F, Yu T, Du R, Fan G, Liu Y, Liu Z, Xiang J, Wang Y, Song B, Gu X, Guan L, Wei Y, Li H, Wu X, Xu J, Tu S, Zhang Y, Chen H, Cao B (2020) Clinical course and risk factors for

mortality of adult inpatients with COVID-19 in Wuhan, China: a retrospective cohort study. Lancet 395:1054–1062. https://doi.org/10.1016/s0140-6736(20)30566-3
42. Wu C et al (2020) Risk factors associated with acute respiratory distress syndrome and death in patients with coronavirus disease 2019 pneumonia in Wuhan, China. JAMA Intern Med 180:934–943. https://doi.org/10.1001/jamainternmed.2020.0994
43. Wan S, Xiang Y, Fang W et al (2020) Clinical features and treatment of COVID-19 patients in northeast Chongqing. J Med Virol 92:797–806. https://doi.org/10.1002/jmv.25783
44. Zhang JJ, Dong X, Cao YY, Yuan YD, Yang YB, Yan YQ, Akdis CA, Gao YD (2020) Clinical characteristics of 140 patients infected with SARS-CoV-2 in Wuhan, China. Allergy. https://doi.org/10.1111/all.14238
45. Wang L, He W, Yu X et al (2020) Coronavirus disease 2019 in elderly patients: characteristics and prognostic factors based on 4-week follow-up. J Infect 80:639–645. https://doi.org/10.1016/j.jinf.2020.03.019
46. Zheng YY, Ma YT, Zhang JY, Xie X (2020) COVID-19 and the cardiovascular system. Nat Rev Cardiol 17:259–260. https://doi.org/10.1038/s41569-020-0360-5
47. Yahyavi A, Hemmati N, Derakhshan P, Banivaheb B, Karimi Behnagh A, Tofighi R, TehraniYazdi A, Kabir A (2020) Angiotensin enzyme inhibitors and angiotensin receptor blockers as protective factors in COVID-19 mortality: a retrospective cohort study. Intern Emerg Med 16:883–893. https://doi.org/10.1007/s11739-020-02523-9
48. Vaduganathan M, Vardeny O, Michel T, McMurray JJV, Pfeffer MA, Solomon SD (2020) Renin–angiotensin–aldosterone system inhibitors in patients with Covid-19. N Engl J Med 382(17):1653–1659
49. Li LQ, Huang T (2020) COVID-19 patients' clinical characteristics, discharge rate, and fatality rate of meta-analysis. J Med Virol 92(6):577–583. https://doi.org/10.1002/jmv.25757
50. Chen C, Zhou Y, Wang DW (2020) SARS-CoV-2: a potential novel etiology of fulminant myocarditis. Herz 45(3):230–232. https://doi.org/10.1007/s00059-020-04909-z
51. Moon JY (2013) Recent update of renin-angiotensin-aldosterone system in the pathogenesis of hypertension. Elect Blood Press E BP 11(2):41–45. https://doi.org/10.5049/ebp.2013.11.2.41
52. World Health Organization (2020) Clinical management of severe acute respiratory infection (SARI) when COVID-19 disease is suspected: interim guidance, 13 March 2020. World Health Organization. https://www.who.int/docs/default-source/coronaviruse/situation-reports/20200921-weekly-epi-update-6.pdf?sfvrsn=d9cf9496_6. Accessed 4 Apr 2020
53. Singh AK, Gupta R, Misra A (2020) Comorbidities in COVID-19: outcomes in hypertensive cohort and controversies with renin angiotensin system blockers. Diabetes Metab Syndr 14(4):283–287. https://doi.org/10.1016/j.dsx.2020.03.016
54. Yang G, Tan Z, Zhou L, Yang M, Peng L, Liu J, Cai J et al (2020) Effects of ARBs and ACEIs on virus infection, inflammatory status and clinical outcomes in COVID-19 patients with hypertension: a single center retrospective study. Hypertension 76:51–58. https://doi.org/10.1161/HYPERTENSIONAHA.120.15143
55. Najafi N, Davoudi A, Izadyar H, Alishahi A, Mokhtariani A, Soleimanpourian B, Tabarrayi M, Moosazadeh M, Daftarian Z, Ahangarkani F (2022) The effect of ACE inhibitors and ARBs on outcomes in hospitalized patients with COVID-19. Ir J Med Sci 192:1517–1523. https://doi.org/10.1007/s11845-022-03096-6
56. Yang G, Tan Z, Zhou L et al (2020) Effects of angiotensin II receptor blockers and ACE (angiotensin-converting enzyme) inhibitors on virus infection, inflammatory status, and clinical outcomes in patients with COVID-19 and hypertension: a single-center retrospective study. Hypertension 76(1):51–58
57. Li S, Sarangarajan R, Jun T et al (2021) In-hospital use of ACE inhibitors/angiotensin receptor blockers associates with COVID-19 outcomes in African American patients. J Clin Invest 131(19):e151418
58. Gu H, Xie Z, Li T et al (2016) Angiotensin-converting enzyme 2 inhibits lung injury induced by respiratory syncytial virus. Sci Rep 6:19840

59. Kuba K et al (2005) A crucial role of angiotensin converting enzyme 2 (ACE2) in SARS coronavirus-induced lung injury. Nat Med 11:875–879. https://doi.org/10.1038/nm1267
60. Yehualashet AS, Belachew TF (2020) ACEIs and ARBs and their correlation with COVID-19: a review. Infect Drug Resist 13:3217–3224
61. Bozkurt B, Kovacs R, Harrington B (2020) Joint HFSA/ACC/AHA statement addresses concerns re: using RAAS antagonists in COVID-19. J Cardiac Fail 26(5):370
62. Manga P (2020) Should ACE inhibitors and angiotensin receptor blockers be withdrawn in the current setting of COVID-19 infection? 2(Si):25–28
63. Oori MJ, Mohammadi F, Norozi K et al (2019) Prevalence of HTN in Iran: meta-analysis of published studies in 2004–2018. Curr Hypertens Rev 15(2):113–122
64. Braude P, Carter B, Short R et al (2020) The influence of ACE inhibitors and ARBs on hospital length of stay and survival in people with COVID-19. IJC Heart Vasc 31:100660
65. Reynolds HR, Adhikari S, Pulgarin C, Troxel AB, Iturrate E, Johnson SB, Hausvater A et al (2020) Renin-angiotensin-aldosterone system inhibitors and risk of Covid-19. N Engl J Med 382:2441–2448. https://doi.org/10.1056/NEJMoa2008975
66. Singh R, Rathore SS, Khan H et al (2021) Mortality and severity in COVID-19 patients on ACEIs & ARBs-a meta-regression analysis. medRxiv
67. Kouhpayeh HR, Tabasi F, Dehvari M, Naderi M, Bahari G, Khalili T, Clark C, Ghavami S, Taheri M (2021) Association between angiotensinogen (AGT), angiotensin-converting enzyme (ACE) and angiotensin-II receptor 1 (AGTR1) polymorphisms and COVID-19 infection in the southeast of Iran: a preliminary case-control study. Transl Med Commun 6(1):26. https://doi.org/10.1186/s41231-021-00106-0
68. Nabavi SF et al (2021) Rationale for effective prophylaxis against COVID-19 through simultaneous blockade of both endosomal and non-endosomal SARS-CoV-2 entry into host cell. Clin Transl Sci 14(2):431–433
69. Darbeheshti F et al (2021) Coronavirus: pure infectious disease or genetic predisposition. Adv Exp Med Biol 1318:91–107
70. Shang J et al (2020) Structural basis of receptor recognition by SARS-CoV-2. Nature 581(7807):221–224
71. Haga S et al (2008) Modulation of TNF-α-converting enzyme by the spike protein of SARS-CoV and ACE2 induces TNF-α production and facilitates viral entry. Proc Natl Acad Sci U S A 105(22):7809–7814
72. Sriram K, Insel PA (2020) A hypothesis for pathobiology and treatment of COVID-19: the centrality of ACE1/ACE2 imbalance. Br J Pharmacol 177(21):4825–4844
73. Sriram K, Loomba R, Insel PA (2020) Targeting the renin–angiotensin signaling pathway in COVID-19: unanswered questions, opportunities, and challenges. Proc Natl Acad Sci U S A 117(47):29274–29282
74. Drozdzal S et al (2020) FDA approved drugs with pharmacotherapeutic potential for SARS-CoV-2 (COVID-19) therapy. Drug Resist Updat 53:100719
75. Di Raimondo D et al (2012) Effects of ACE-inhibitors and angiotensin receptor blockers on inflammation. Curr Pharm Des 18(28):4385–4413
76. Wang W, Zhao X, Wei W, Fan W, Gao K, He S, Zhuang X (2021) Angiotensin-converting enzyme inhibitors (ACEI) or angiotensin receptor blockers (ARBs) may be safe for COVID-19 patients. BMC Infect Dis 21:114. https://doi.org/10.1186/s12879-021-05821-5
77. Wu F, Zhao S, Yu B, Chen Y, Wang W, Hu Y et al (2020) Complete genome characterisation of a novel coronavirus associated with severe human respiratory disease in Wuhan, China. bioRxiv. https://doi.org/10.1101/2020.01.24.919183
78. Zhou P, Yang X, Wang X, Hu B, Zhang L, Zhang W et al (2020) Discovery of a novel coronavirus associated with the recent pneumonia outbreak in humans and its potential bat origin. bioRxiv. https://doi.org/10.1101/2020.01.22.914952
79. Lu R, Zhao X, Li J, Niu P, Yang B, Wu H, Wang W, Song H, Huang B, Zhu N, Bi Y (2020) Genomic characterisation and epidemiology of 2019 novel coronavirus: implications for virus origins and receptor binding. Lancet 395(10224):565–574

80. Gorbalenya AE, Baker SC, Baric RS et al (2020) Severe acute respiratory syndrome-related coronavirus: the species and its viruses -a statement of the coronavirus study group. bioRxiv. https://doi.org/10.1101/2020.02.07.937862
81. World Health Organization (2020) WHO Director-General's remarks at the media briefing on 2019-nCoV on 11 February 2020. https://www.who.int/dg/speeches/detail/who-director-general-s-remarks-at-the-media-briefing-on-2019-ncov-on-11-february-2020. Accessed 15 Apr 2020
82. Du L, He Y, Zhou Y, Liu S, Zheng BJ, Jiang S (2009) The spike protein of SARS-CoV—a target for vaccine and therapeutic development. Nat Rev Microbiol 7(3):226–236. https://doi.org/10.1038/nrmicro2090
83. Xu X, Chen P, Wang J, Feng J, Zhou H, Li X et al (2020) Evolution of the novel coronavirus from the ongoing Wuhan outbreak and modeling of its spike protein for risk of human transmission. Sci China Life Sci 63(3):457–460. https://doi.org/10.1007/s11427-020-1637-5
84. Imai Y et al (2005) Angiotensin-converting enzyme 2 protects from severe acute lung failure. Nature 436:112–116. https://doi.org/10.1038/nature03712
85. Writing Group of 2018 Chinese Guidelines for the Management of Hypertension, Chinese Hypertension League, Chinese Society of Cardiology, Chinese Medical Doctor Association Hypertension Committee, Hypertension Branch of China International Exchange and Promotive Association for Medical and Health Care, Hypertension Branch of Chinese Geriatric Medical Associarion (2018) 2018 Chinese guidelines for the management of hypertension. Chin J Cardiovasc Med 24(1):24–56. https://doi.org/10.3969/j.issn.1007-5410.2019.01.002
86. Ferrario CM, Jessup J, Chappell MC, Averill DB, Brosnihan KB, Tallant EA et al (2005) Effect of angiotensin-converting enzyme inhibition and angiotensin II receptor blockers on cardiac angiotensin-converting enzyme 2. Circulation 111(20):2605–2610
87. Wu Y (2020) Compensation of ACE2 function for possible clinical management of 2019-nCoV-induced acute lung injury. Virol Sin 35(3):256–258. https://doi.org/10.1007/s12250-020-00205-6
88. Rossi L, Malagoli A, Biagi A, Zanni A, Sticozzi C, Comastri G, Pannone L, Gandolfi S, Vergara P, Villani GQ (2020) Renin–angiotensin system inhibitors and mortality in patients with COVID-19. Infection 49:287–294. https://doi.org/10.1007/s15010-020-01550-0
89. Hoffmann M, Kleine-Weber H, Schroeder S, Kruger N, Herrler T, Erichsen S, Schiergens TS, Herrler G, Wu NH, Nitsche A, Muller MA, Drosten C, Pohlmann S (2020) SARS-CoV-2 cell entry depends on ACE2 and TMPRSS2 and is blocked by a clinically proven protease inhibitor. Cell 181:271–280. https://doi.org/10.1016/j.cell.2020.02.052
90. Khan A, Benthin C, Zeno B, Albertson TE, Boyd J, Christie JD, Hall R et al (2017) A pilot clinical trial of recombinant human angiotensin-converting enzyme 2 in acute respiratory distress syndrome. Crit Care 21(1):234. https://doi.org/10.1186/s13054-017-1823-x
91. Ishiyama Y, Gallagher PE, Averill DB, Tallant EA, Brosnihan KB, Ferrario CM (2004) Upregulation of angiotensin-converting enzyme 2 after myocardial infarction by blockade of angiotensin II receptors. Hypertension 43:970–976
92. Sommerstein R, Kochen MM, Messerli FH, Grani C (2020) Coronavirus disease 2019 (COVID-19): do angiotensin-converting enzyme inhibitors/angiotensin receptor blockers have a biphasic effect? J Am Heart Assoc 9:e016509
93. Lopes RD, Macedo AVS, de Barros ESPGM, Moll-Bernardes RJ, Feldman A, Arruda GDS et al (2020) Continuing versus suspending angiotensin-converting enzyme inhibitors and angiotensin receptor blockers: impact on adverse outcomes in hospitalized patients with severe acute respiratory syndrome coronavirus 2 (SARS-CoV-2). The BRACE CORONA trial. Am Heart J 226:49–59
94. ClinicalTrials.gov. Coronavirus (COVID-19) ACEi/ARB investigation (CORONACION). ClinicalTrials.gov identifier: NCT04330300. https://clinicaltrials.gov/ct2/show/NCT04330300. Accessed 10 Jun 2020
95. ClinicalTrials.gov. ACE inhibitors or ARBs discontinuation in context of SARS-CoV-2 pandemic (ACORES-2). ClinicalTrials.gov identifier: NCT04329195. https://clinicaltrials.gov/ct2/show/. Accessed 10 Jun 2020

96. ClinicalTrials.gov. Losartan for patients with COVID-19 not requiring hospitalization. ClinicalTrials.gov identifier: NCT04311177. https://clinicaltrials.gov/ct2/show/NCT04311177. Accessed 10 Jun 2020
97. de Abajo FJ, Rodríguez-Miguel A, Rodríguez-Martín S, Lerma V, García-Lledó A (2021) Impact of in-hospital discontinuation with angiotensin receptor blockers or converting enzyme inhibitors on mortality of COVID-19 patients: a retrospective cohort study. BMC Med 19(1):118. https://doi.org/10.1186/s12916-021-01992-9
98. Mancia G, Rea F, Ludergnani M, Apolone G, Corrao G (2020) Renin-angiotensin-aldosterone system blockers and the risk of Covid-19. N Engl J Med 382:2431–2440. https://doi.org/10.1056/NEJMoa2006923
99. de Abajo FJ, Rodríguez-Martín S, Lerma V et al (2020) Use of renin-angiotensin-aldosterone system inhibitors and risk of COVID-19 requiring admission to hospital: a case-population study. Lancet 395(10238):1705–1714
100. Lam KW, Chow KW, Vo J, Hou W, Li H, Richman PS et al (2020) Continued in-hospital angiotensin converting enzyme inhibitor and angiotensin II receptor blocker use in hypertensive COVID-19 patients is associated with positive clinical outcome. J Infect Dis 222(8):1256–1264. https://doi.org/10.1093/infdis/jiaa447
101. Chaudhri I, Koraishy FM, Bolotova O, Yoo J, Marcos LA, Taub E et al (2020) Outcomes associated with the use of renin-angiotensin-aldosterone system blockade in hospitalized patients with SARS-CoV-2 infection. Kidney360 1(8):801–809
102. Austin PS (2011) An introduction to propensity score methods for reducing the effects of confounding in observational studies. Multivar Behav Res 46(3):399–424. https://doi.org/10.1080/00273171.2011.568786
103. Vittinghof E, Gludden DV, Shiboski SC, McCulloch CE (2012) Survival analysis. In: Survival analysis, in regression methods in biostatistics, 2nd edn. Springer, New York, pp 203–259
104. Lopes RD, Macedo AVS, de Barros ESPGM et al (2021) Effect of discontinuing vs continuing angiotensin-converting enzyme inhibitors and angiotensin II receptor blockers on days alive and out of the hospital in patients admitted with COVID-19: a randomized clinical trial. JAMA 325(3):254–264
105. Cohen JB, Hanff TC, William P, Sweitzer N, Rosado-Santander NR, Medina C et al (2021) Continuation versus discontinuation of renin-angiotensin system inhibitors in patients admitted to hospital with COVID-19: a prospective, randomised, open-label trial. Lancet Respir Med 9(3):275–284
106. Triposkiadis F, Starling RC, Xanthopoulos A, Butler J, Boudoulas H (2020) Renin-angiotensin-system inhibition in the context of corona virus disease-19: experimental evidence, observational studies, and clinical implications. Heart Fail Rev 26:381–389. https://doi.org/10.1007/s10741-020-10022-4
107. Santos RAS, Sampaio WO, Alzamora AC et al (2018) The ACE2/angiotensin-(1–7)/MAS axis of the renin-angiotensin system: focus on angiotensin-(1–7). Physiol Rev 98(1):505–553
108. Serfozo P, Wysocki J, Gulua G, Schulze A, Ye M, Liu P, Jin J, Bader M, Myohanen T, Garcia-Horsman JA, Batlle D (2020) Ang II (angiotensin II) conversion to angiotensin-(1-7) in the circulation is POP (prolyloligopeptidase)-dependent and ACE2 (angiotensin-converting enzyme 2)-independent. Hypertension 75(1):173–182. https://doi.org/10.1161/HYPERTENSIONAHA.119.14071
109. Jia HP, Look DC, Shi L, Hickey M, Pewe L, Netland J, Farzan M, Wohlford-Lenane C, Perlman S, McCray PB Jr (2005) ACE2 receptor expression and severe acute respiratory syndrome coronavirus infection depend on differentiation of human airway epithelia. J Virol 79(23):14614–14621. https://doi.org/10.1128/JVI.79.23.14614-14621.2005
110. Heurich A, Hofmann-Winkler H, Gierer S, Liepold T, Jahn O, Pohlmann S (2014) TMPRSS2 and ADAM17 cleave ACE2 differentially and only proteolysis by TMPRSS2 augments entry driven by the severe acute respiratory syndrome coronavirus spike protein. J Virol 88:1293–1307. https://doi.org/10.1128/JVI.02202-13
111. He L, Ding Y, Zhang Q, Che X, He Y, Shen H, Wang H, Li Z, Zhao L, Geng J, Deng Y, Yang L, Li J, Cai J, Qiu L, Wen K, Xu X, Jiang S (2006) Expression of elevated levels of

pro-inflammatory cytokines in SARS-CoV-infected ACE2+ cells in SARS patients: relation to the acute lung injury and pathogenesis of SARS. J Pathol 210(3):288–297. https://doi.org/10.1002/path.2067
112. Li G, He X, Zhang L, Ran Q, Wang J, Xiong A, Wu D, Chen F, Sun J, Chang C (2020) Assessing ACE2 expression patterns in lung tissues in the pathogenesis of COVID-19. J Autoimmun 112:102463. https://doi.org/10.1016/j.jaut.2020.102463
113. Sackett DL, Rosenberg WM, Gray JA, Haynes RB, Richardson WS (1996) Evidence based medicine: what it is and what it isn't. BMJ 312(7023):71–72. https://doi.org/10.1136/bmj.312.7023.71
114. Sarangarajan R, Winn R, Kiebish MA, Bountra C, Granger E, Narain NR (2020) Ethnic prevalence of angiotensin-converting enzyme deletion (D) polymorphism and COVID-19 risk: rationale for use of angiotensin-converting enzyme inhibitors/angiotensin receptor blockers. J Racial Ethn Health Disparities 8:973–980. https://doi.org/10.1007/s40615-020-00853-0
115. Hamming I, Timens W, Bulthuis ML, Lely AT, Navis G, van Goor H (2004) Tissue distribution of ACE2 protein, the functional receptor for SARS coronavirus. A first step in understanding SARS pathogenesis. J Pathol 203:631–637. https://doi.org/10.1002/path.1570
116. Kenyon C. ACE-1 I/D polymorphism associated with COVID-19 incidence and mortality: an ecological study. https://doi.org/10.20944/preprints202004.0262.v1
117. Goodfriend TL, Elliott ME, Catt KJ (1996) Angiotensin receptors and their antagonists. N Engl J Med 334(25):1649–1654
118. Fyhrquist F, Saijonmaa O (2008) Renin-angiotensin system revisited. J Intern Med 264(3):224–236. https://doi.org/10.1111/j.1365-2796.2008.01981.x
119. Ruster C, Wolf G (2006) Renin-angiotensin-aldosterone system and progression of renal disease. J Am Soc Nephrol 17:2985–2991
120. Suzuki Y, Ruiz-Ortega M, Lorenzo O, Ruperez M, Esteban V, Egido J (2003) Inflammation and angiotensin II. Int J Biochem Cell Biol 35:881–900. https://doi.org/10.1016/s1357-2725(02)00271-6
121. Benigni A, Paola C, Remuzzi G (2010) Angiotensin II revisited: new roles in inflammation, immunology and aging. EMBO Mol Med 2:247–257
122. Gard PR (2010) Implications of the angiotensin converting enzyme gene insertion/deletion polymorphism in health and disease: a snapshot review. Int J Mol Epidemiol Genet 1(2):145–157
123. Staessen JA, Ginocchio G, Wang JG, Saavedra AP et al (1997) Genetic variability in the renin-angiotensin system: prevalence of alleles and genotypes. J Cardiovasc Risk 4:401–422
124. Deng X, Zhang S, Jin K, Li L, Gu W, Liu M et al (2015) Angiotensin converting enzyme I/D polymorphism and acute respiratory syndrome. J Renin-Angiotensin-Aldosterone Syst 16(4):780–786
125. Adamzik M, Frey U, Sixt S, Knemeyer L, Beiderlinden M, Peters J et al (2007) ACE I/D but not AGT (−6) A/G polymorphism is a risk factor for mortality in ARDS. Eur Respir J 29:482–488
126. Tsantes AE, Kopterides P, Bonovas S, Bagos PG, Antonakos G, Nikolopoulos GK et al (2013) Effect of angiotensin converting enzyme gene I/D polymorphism and its expression on clinical outcome in acute respiratory distress syndrome. Minerva Anestesiol 79:861–870
127. Burgts JJ, Den Uil CA (2008) ACE insertion/deletion polymorphism in sepsis and acute respiratory distress syndrome. Intensive Care Med 34:1733
128. Wang Y, Peng W, Zhang Z, Qiao H et al (2016) The association of ACE gene polymorphism with diabetic kidney disease and renoprotective efficacy of valsartan. J Renin-Angiotensin-Aldosterone Syst 17(3):1–6
129. Fava S, Ellard S, Azzopardi J, Hattersley AT (2001) ACE gene polymorphism as a prognostic indicator in patients with type 2 diabetes and established renal disease. Diabetes Care 24:2115–2120
130. Gheblawi M, Wang K, Viveiros A, Nguyen Q, Zhong JC, Turner AJ, Raizada MK, Grant MB, Oudit GY (2020) Angiotensin-converting enzyme 2: SARS-CoV-2 receptor and regulator of

the renin-angiotensin system: celebrating the 20th anniversary of the discovery of ACE2. Circ Res 126:1456–1474. https://doi.org/10.1161/circresaha.120.317015
131. Ni W, Yang X, Yang D, Bao J, Li R, Xiao Y, Hou C, Wang H, Liu J, Yang D, Xu Y, Cao Z, Gao Z (2020) Role of angiotensin-converting enzyme 2 (ACE2) in COVID-19. Crit Care 24(1):422. https://doi.org/10.1186/s13054-020-03120-0
132. He L, Ding Y, Zhang Q, Che X, He Y, Shen H et al (2006) Expression of elevated levels of pro-inflammatory cytokines in SARS-CoV-infected ACE2+ cells in SARS patients: relation to the acute lung injury and pathogenesis of SARS. J Pathol 210:288–297
133. Santos R, Sampaio W, Alzamora A, Motta-Santos D, Alenina N, Bader M et al (2018) The ACE2/angiotensin-(1-7)/MAS axis of the renin-angiotensin system: focus on angiotensin-(1-7). Physiol Rev 98:505–553
134. Rodrigues Prestes TR, Rocha NP, Miranda AS, Teixeira AL, Simoes-E-Silva AC (2017) The anti-inflammatory potential of ACE2/angiotensin-(1-7)/Mas receptor axis: evidence from basic and clinical research. Curr Drug Targets 18:1301–1313
135. Haga S, Yamamoto N, Nakai-Murakami C, Osawa Y, Tokunaga K, Sata T et al (2008) Modulation of TNF-alpha-converting enzyme by the spike protein of SARS-CoV and ACE2 induces TNF-alpha production and facilitates viral entry. Proc Natl Acad Sci U S A 105:7809–7814
136. Glowacka I, Bertram S, Herzog P, Pfefferle S, Steffen I, Muench MO et al (2010) Differential downregulation of ACE2 by the spike proteins of severe acute respiratory syndrome coronavirus and human coronavirus NL63. J Virol 84:1198–1205
137. Kuba K, Imai Y, Rao S, Gao H, Guo F, Guan B et al (2005) A crucial role of angiotensin converting enzyme 2 (ACE2) in SARS coronavirus-induced lung injury. Nat Med 11:875–879
138. Oudit GY, Kassiri Z, Jiang C, Liu PP, Poutanen SM, Penninger JM et al (2009) SARS-coronavirus modulation of myocardial ACE2 expression and inflammation in patients with SARS. Eur J Clin Investig 39:618–625
139. Muslim S, Nasrin N, Alotaibi FO, Prasad G, Singh SK, Alam I, Mustafa G (2020) Treatment options available for COVID-19 and an analysis on possible role of combination of rhACE2, angiotensin (1-7) and angiotensin (1-9) as effective therapeutic measure. SN Comprehen Clin Med 2:1761–1766. https://doi.org/10.1007/s42399-020-00407-9
140. Vincent MJ, Bergeron E, Benjannet S, Erickson BR, Rollin PE, Ksiazek TG et al (2005) Chloroquine is a potent inhibitor of SARS coronavirus infection and spread. Virol J 2:69. https://doi.org/10.1186/1743-422X-2-69
141. Wang M, Cao R, Zhang L, Yang X, Liu J, Xu M et al (2020) Remdesivir and chloroquine effectively inhibit the recently emerged novel coronavirus (2019-nCoV) in vitro. Cell Res 30:269–271. https://doi.org/10.1038/s41422-020-0282-0
142. Yao X, Ye F, Zhang M et al (2020) In vitro antiviral activity and projection of optimized dosing design of hydroxychloroquine for the treatment of severe acute respiratory syndrome coronavirus 2 (SARS-CoV-2). Clin Infect Dis 71:732–739. https://doi.org/10.1093/cid/ciaa237
143. Gautret P, Lagier JC, Parola P, Hoang VT, Meddeb L, Mailhe M, Doudier B et al (2020) Hydroxychloroquine and azithromycin as a treatment of COVID-19: results of an open-label non-randomized clinical trial. Int J Antimicrob Agent 56:105949. https://doi.org/10.1016/j.ijantimicag.2020.105949
144. Siegel D, Hui HC, Doerffler E, Clarke MO, Chun K, Zhang L et al (2017) Discovery and synthesis of a phosphoramidate prodrug of a pyrrolo[2,1-f] [triazin-4-amino] adenine c-nucleoside (GS-5734) for the treatment of Ebola and emergingviruses. J Med Chem 60:1648–1661. https://doi.org/10.1021/acs.jmedchem.6b01594
145. Holshue ML, DeBolt C, Lindquist S, Lofy KH, Wiesman J, Bruce H et al (2020) First case of 2019 novel coronavirus in the United States. N Engl J Med 382:929–936. https://doi.org/10.1056/NEJMoa2001191
146. Chen C, Huang J, Cheng Z et al (2020) Favipiravir versus arbidol for COVID-19: a randomized clinical trial. medRxiv. https://doi.org/10.1101/2020.03.17.20037432

147. Ratia K, Pegan S, Takayama J, Sleeman K, Coughlin M, Baliji S et al (2008) A noncovalent class of papain-like protease/deubiquitinase inhibitors blocks SARS virus replication. Proc Natl Acad Sci U S A 105(42):16119–16124. https://doi.org/10.1073/pnas.0805240105
148. Cao B, Wang Y, Wen D, Liu W, Wang J, Fan G, Ruan L et al (2020) A trial of lopinavir-ritonavir in adults hospitalized with severe covid-19. N Engl J Med 382(19):1787–1799. https://doi.org/10.1056/NEJMoa2001282
149. Xu X, Han M, Li T, Sun W, Wang D, Fu B et al (2020) Effective treatment of severe COVID-19 patients with tocilizumab. Proc Natl Acad Sci U S A 17(20):10970–10975. https://doi.org/10.1073/pnas.2005615117
150. Thachil J, Wada H, Gando S et al (2020) ISTH interim guidance on recognition and management of coagulopathy in COVID-19. J Thromb Haemost 18:1023–1026. https://doi.org/10.1111/jth.14810
151. Tang N, Bai H, Chen X, Gong J, Li D, Sun Z (2020) Anticoagulant treatment is associated with decreased mortality in severe coronavirus disease 2019 patients with coagulopathy. J Thromb Haemost 18(5):1094–1099. https://doi.org/10.1111/jth.14817
152. Danzi GB, Loffi M, Galeazzi G, Gherbesi E (2020) Acute pulmonary embolism and COVID-19 pneumonia: a random association? Eur Heart J 41:1858
153. Zhang Y, Xiao M, Zhang S, Xia P, Cao W, Jiang W et al (2020) Coagulopathy and antiphospholipid antibodies in patients with Covid-19. N Engl J Med 382:e38
154. Rossignol JF (2014) Nitazoxanide: a first-in-class broad-spectrum antiviral agent. Antivir Res 110:94–103
155. Lam KKY, Zheng X, Forestieri R, Balgi AD, Nodwell M, Volett S et al (2012) Nitazoxanide stimulates autophagy and inhibits mTORC1 signaling and intracellular proliferation of Mycobacterium tuberculosis. PLoS Pathog 8:e1002691. https://doi.org/10.1371/journal.ppat.1002691
156. CytoDyn, Press release (2020) Treatment with CytoDyn's leronlimab indicates significant trend toward immunological restoration in severely ill COVID-19 patients. CytoDyn Inc.
157. Tan EL, Ooi EE, Lin CY et al (2004) Inhibition of SARS coronavirus infection in vitro with clinically approved antiviral drugs. Emerg Infect Dis 10(4):581–586
158. Mancini E, Fürst J (2020) View: "Scorched Earth" strategy: the RAS as possible target for treating COVID-19 patients with a combination of three approved pharmaceutical agents. Baseline. https://doi.org/10.13140/RG.2.2.35010.94400
159. Liu Y et al (2020) Clinical and biochemical indexes from 2019-nCoV infected patients linked to viral loads and lung injury. Sci China Life Sci 63:364–374. https://doi.org/10.1007/s11427-020-1643-8
160. Scialo F, Daniele A, Amato F, Pastore L, Matera MG, Cazzola M, Castaldo G, Bianco A (2020) ACE2: the major cell entry receptor for SARS-CoV-2. Lung 198:867–877. https://doi.org/10.1007/s00408-020-00408-4
161. Samavati L, Uhal BD (2020) ACE2, much more than just a receptor for SARS-COV-2. Front Cell Infect Microbiol 10:317. https://doi.org/10.3389/fcimb.2020.00317
162. Batlle D, Wysocki J, Satchell K (2020) Soluble angiotensin-converting enzyme 2: a potential approach for coronavirus infection therapy? Clin Sci (Lond) 134:543–545. https://doi.org/10.1042/CS20200163
163. Mathewson AC, Bishop A, Yao Y, Kemp F, Ren J, Chen H, Xu X, Berkhout B, van der Hoek L, Jones IM (2008) Interaction of severe acute respiratory syndrome-coronavirus and NL63 coronavirus spike proteins with angiotensin converting enzyme-2. J Gen Virol 89(Pt 11):2741–2745. https://doi.org/10.1099/vir.0.2008/003962-0
164. Childs RA, Palma AS, Wharton S, Matrosovich T, Liu Y, Chai W, Campanero-Rhodes MA, Zhang Y, Eickmann M, Kiso M, Hay A, Matrosovich M, Feizi T (2009) Receptor-binding specificity of pandemic influenza A (H1N1) 2009 virus determined by carbohydrate microarray. Nat Biotechnol 27(9):797–799. https://doi.org/10.1038/nbt0909-797
165. Zhuang MW, Cheng Y, Zhang J, Jiang XM, Wang L, Deng J, Wang PH (2020) Increasing host cellular receptor-angiotensin-converting enzyme 2 expression by coronavirus may facilitate

2019-nCoV (or SARS-CoV-2) infection. J Med Virol 92:2693–2701. https://doi.org/10.1002/jmv.26139

166. Ziegler CGK, Allon SJ, Nyquist SK, Mbano IM, Miao VN, Tzouanas CN, Cao Y et al (2020) SARS-CoV-2 receptor ACE2 is an interferon-stimulated gene in human airway epithelial cells and is detected in specific cell subsets across tissues. Cell 181:1016–1035.e19. https://doi.org/10.1016/j.cell.2020.04.035
167. Onabajo OO, Banday AR, Stanifer ML, Yan W, Obajemu A, Santer DM, Florez-Vargas O, Piontkivska H, Vargas JM, Ring TJ, Kee C, Doldan P, Tyrrell DL, Mendoza JL, Boulant S, Prokunina-Olsson L (2020) Interferons and viruses induce a novel truncated ACE2 isoform and not the full-length SARS-CoV-2 receptor. Nat Genet 52:1283–1293. https://doi.org/10.1038/s41588-020-00731-9
168. Li W, Zhang C, Sui J, Kuhn JH, Moore MJ, Luo S, Wong SK, Huang IC, Xu K, Vasilieva N, Murakami A, He Y, Marasco WA, Guan Y, Choe H, Farzan M (2005) Receptor and viral determinants of SARS-coronavirus adaptation to human ACE2. EMBO J 24(8):1634–1643. https://doi.org/10.1038/sj.emboj.7600640
169. Li Q, Cao Z, Rahman P (2020) Genetic variability of human angiotensin-converting enzyme 2 (hACE2) among various ethnic populations. Mol Genet Genomic Med 8(8):e1344. https://doi.org/10.1002/mgg3.1344
170. Benetti E, Tita R, Spiga O, Ciolfi A, Birolo G, Bruselles A, Doddato G, Giliberti A, Marconi C, Musacchia F, Pippucci T, Torella A, Trezza A, Valentino F, Baldassarri M, Brusco A, Asselta R, Bruttini M, Furini S, Seri M, Nigro V, Matullo G, Tartaglia M, Mari F, GEN-COVID Multicenter Study, Renieri A, Pinto AM (2020) ACE2 gene variants may underlie interindividual variability and susceptibility to COVID-19 in the Italian population. Eur J Hum Genet 28(11):1602–1614
171. Guo X, Chen Z, Xia Y, Lin W, Li H (2020) Investigation of the genetic variation in ACE2 on the structural recognition by the novel coronavirus (SARS-CoV-2). J Transl Med 18(1):321. https://doi.org/10.1186/s12967-020-02486-7
172. Kornilov SA, Lucas I, Jade K, Dai CL, Lovejoy JC, Magis AT (2020) Plasma levels of soluble ACE2 are associated with sex, metabolic syndrome, and its biomarkers in a large cohort, pointing to a possible mechanism for increased severity in COVID-19. Crit Care 24(1):452. https://doi.org/10.1186/s13054-020-03141-9
173. Swärd P, Edsfeldt A, Reepalu A, Jehpsson L, Rosengren BE, Karlsson MK (2020) Age and sex differences in soluble ACE2 may give insights for COVID-19. Crit Care 24:221. https://doi.org/10.1186/s13054-020-02942-2
174. Lumpuy-Castillo J, Lorenzo-Almorós A, Pello-Lázaro AM, Sánchez-Ferrer C, Egido J, Tuñón J, Peiró C, Lorenzo Ó (2020) Cardiovascular damage in COVID-19: therapeutic approaches targeting the renin-angiotensin-aldosterone system. Int J Mol Sci 21(18):6471. https://doi.org/10.3390/ijms21186471
175. Dikalova A, Clempus R, Lassègue B, Cheng G, McCoy J, Dikalov S, San Martin A, Lyle A, Weber DS, Weiss D, Taylor WR, Schmidt HH, Owens GK, Lambeth JD, Griendling KK (2005) Nox1 overexpression potentiates angiotensin II-induced hypertension and vascular smooth muscle hypertrophy in transgenic mice. Circulation 112(17):2668–2676. https://doi.org/10.1161/CIRCULATIONAHA.105.538934
176. Jones ES, Vinh A, McCarthy CA, Gaspari TA, Widdop RE (2008) AT2 receptors: functional relevance in cardiovascular disease. Pharmacol Ther 120(3):292–316. https://doi.org/10.1016/j.pharmthera.2008.08.009
177. Qadri F, Bader M (2018) Kinin B1 receptors as a therapeutic target for inflammation. Expert Opin Ther Targets 22(1):31–44. https://doi.org/10.1080/14728222.2018.1409724
178. Murugesan P, Jung B, Lee D, Khang G, Doods H, Wu D (2016) Kinin B1 receptor inhibition with BI113823 reduces inflammatory response, mitigates organ injury, and improves survival among rats with severe sepsis. J Infect Dis 213(4):532–540. https://doi.org/10.1093/infdis/jiv426

179. van de Veerdonk FL, Netea MG, van Deuren M, van der Meer JW, de Mast Q, Brüggemann RJ, van der Hoeven H (2020) Kallikrein-kinin blockade in patients with COVID-19 to prevent acute respiratory distress syndrome. elife 9:e57555. https://doi.org/10.7554/eLife.57555
180. Ingraham NE, Barakat AG, Reilkoff R, Bezdicek T, Schacker T, Chipman JG, Tignanelli CJ, Puskarich MA (2020) Understanding the renin-angiotensin-aldosterone-SARS-CoV axis: a comprehensive review. Eur Respir J 56(1):2000912. https://doi.org/10.1183/13993003.00912-2020
181. Davidson AM, Wysocki J, Batlle D (2020) Interaction of SARS-CoV-2 and other Coronavirus with ACE (Angiotensin-Converting Enzyme)-2 as their main receptor: therapeutic implications. Hypertension 76(5):1339–1349. https://doi.org/10.1161/HYPERTENSIONAHA.120.15256
182. Monteil V, Kwon H, Prado P, Hagelkruys A, Wimmer RA, Stahl M, Leopoldi A et al (2020) Inhibition of SARS-CoV-2 infections in engineered human tissues using clinical-grade soluble human ACE2. Cell 181:905–913.e7. https://doi.org/10.1016/j.cell.2020.04.004
183. Haschke M, Schuster M, Poglitsch M, Loibner H, Salzberg M, Bruggisser M, Penninger J, Krähenbühl S (2013) Pharmacokinetics and pharmacodynamics of recombinant human angiotensin-converting enzyme 2 in healthy human subjects. Clin Pharmacokinet 52(9):783–792. https://doi.org/10.1007/s40262-013-0072-7
184. Perrotta F, Matera MG, Cazzola M, Bianco A (2020) Severe respiratory SARS-CoV2 infection: does ACE2 receptor matter? Respir Med 168:105996. https://doi.org/10.1016/j.rmed.2020.105996
185. Pouremamali A, Babaei A, Malekshahi SS, Abbasi A, Rafiee N (2022) Understanding the pivotal roles of ACE2 in SARS-CoV-2 infection: from structure/function to therapeutic implication. Egypt J Med Hum Genet 23:103. https://doi.org/10.1186/s43042-022-00314-9
186. Kai H, Kai M (2020) Interactions of coronaviruses with ACE2, angiotensin II, and RAS inhibitors—lessons from available evidence and insights into COVID-19. Hypertens Res 43:1–7
187. Leung JM, Yang CX, Tam A, Shaipanich T, Hackett T-L, Singhera GK et al (2020) ACE-2 expression in the small airway epithelia of smokers and COPD patients: implications for COVID-19. Eur Respir J 55(5):2000688
188. Dalan R, Bornstein SR, El-Armouche A, Rodionov RN, Markov A, Wielockx B et al (2020) The ACE-2 in COVID-19: foe or friend? Horm Metab Res 52(5):257–263
189. Deb P, Molla M, Ahmed M, Saif-Ur-Rahman K, Das MC, Das D (2021) A review of epidemiology, clinical features and disease course, transmission dynamics, and neutralization efficacy of SARS-CoV-2 variants. Egypt J Bronchol 15(1):1–14
190. Ferré VM, Peiffer-Smadja N, Visseaux B, Descamps D, Ghosn J, Charpentier C (2022) Omicron SARS-CoV-2 variant: what we know and what we don't. Anaesth Crit Care Pain Med 41(1):100998
191. Tao K, Tzou PL, Nouhin J, Gupta RK, de Oliveira T, Kosakovsky Pond SL et al (2021) The biological and clinical significance of emerging SARS-CoV-2 variants. Nat Rev Genet 22(12):757–773
192. Tregoning JS, Flight KE, Higham SL, Wang Z, Pierce BF (2021) Progress of the COVID-19 vaccine effort: viruses, vaccines and variants versus efficacy, effectiveness and escape. Nat Rev Immunol 21(10):626–636
193. Muniyappa R, Gubbi S (2020) COVID-19 pandemic, coronaviruses, and diabetes mellitus. Am J Physiol-Endocrinol Metab 318(5):E736–E741
194. Li F (2015) Receptor recognition mechanisms of coronaviruses: a decade of structural studies. J Virol 89(4):1954–1964
195. Saha P, Banerjee AK, Tripathi PP, Srivastava AK, Ray U (2020) A virus that has gone viral: amino acid mutation in S protein of Indian isolate of Coronavirus COVID-19 might impact receptor binding, and thus, infectivity. Biosci Rep 40(5):BSR20201312
196. Walls AC, Park Y-J, Tortorici MA, Wall A, McGuire AT, Veesler D (2020) Structure, function, and antigenicity of the SARS-CoV-2 spike glycoprotein. Cell 181:281–292.e6
197. Ou X, Liu Y, Lei X, Li P, Mi D, Ren L et al (2020) Characterization of spike glycoprotein of SARS-CoV-2 on virus entry and its immune cross-reactivity with SARS-CoV. Nat Commun 11(1):1–12

198. Shang J, Ye G, Shi K, Wan Y, Luo C, Aihara H, Geng Q, Auerbach A, Li F (2020) Structural basis of receptor recognition by SARS-CoV-2. Nature 581(7807):221–224. https://doi.org/10.1038/s41586-020-2179-y. Epub PMID: 32225175; PMCID: PMC7328981
199. Tai W, He L, Zhang X, Pu J, Voronin D, Jiang S et al (2020) Characterization of the receptor-binding domain (RBD) of 2019 novel coronavirus: implication for development of RBD protein as a viral attachment inhibitor and vaccine. Cell Mol Immunol 17(6):613–620
200. Lukassen S, Chua RL, Trefzer T, Kahn NC, Schneider MA, Muley T et al (2020) SARS-CoV-2 receptor ACE 2 and TMPRSS 2 are primarily expressed in bronchial transient secretory cells. EMBO J 39(10):e105114
201. Hoffmann M, Kleine-Weber H, Schroeder S, Krüger N, Herrler T, Erichsen S et al (2020) SARS-CoV-2 cell entry depends on ACE2 and TMPRSS2 and is blocked by a clinically proven protease inhibitor. Cell 181:271–280.e8
202. Yang G (2020) H2S as a potential defence against COVID-19? Am J Physiol-Cell Physiol. 319(2):C244–C249
203. Zhang H, Penninger JM, Li Y, Zhong N, Slutsky AS (2020) Angiotensin-converting enzyme 2 (ACE2) as a SARS-CoV-2 receptor: molecular mechanisms and potential therapeutic target. Intensive Care Med 46:586–590. https://doi.org/10.1007/s00134-020-05985-9
204. Rice GI, Thomas DA, Grant PJ et al (2004) Evaluation of angiotensin-converting enzyme (ACE), its homologue ACE2 and neprilysin in angiotensin peptide metabolism. Biochem J 383(1):45–51. https://doi.org/10.1042/BJ20040634
205. Tipnis SR, Hooper NM, Hyde R, Karran E, Christie G, Turner AJ (2000) A human homolog of angiotensin-converting enzyme. Cloning and functional expression as a captopril-insensitive carboxypeptidase. J Biol Chem 275:33238–33243
206. Klhůfek J (2020) The role of angiotensin-converting enzyme 2 in the pathogenesis of COVID-19: the villain or the hero? Acta Clin Belg 77(1):211–218
207. Gan R, Rosoman NP, Henshaw DJ, Noble EP, Georgius P, Sommerfeld N (2020) COVID-19 as a viral functional ACE2 deficiency disorder with ACE2 related multi-organ disease. Med Hypotheses 144:110024
208. Gavriatopoulou M, Korompoki E, Fotiou D, Ntanasis-Stathopoulos I, Psaltopoulou T, Kastritis E et al (2020) Organ-specific manifestations of COVID-19 infection. Clin Exp Med 20:1–14
209. Pan L, Mu M, Yang P, Sun Y, Wang R, Yan J et al (2020) Clinical characteristics of COVID-19 patients with digestive symptoms in Hubei, China: a descriptive, cross-sectional, multicenter study. Am J Gastroenterol 115:766–773
210. Chen L, Lou J, Bai Y, Wang M (2020) COVID-19 disease with positive fecal and negative pharyngeal and sputum viral tests. Am J Gastroenterol 115:790
211. Cheng Y, Luo R, Wang K, Zhang M, Wang Z, Dong L et al (2020) Kidney disease is associated with in-hospital death of patients with COVID-19. Kidney Int 97:829–838
212. Xiao K, Hou F, Huang X, Li B, Qian ZR, Xie L (2020) Mesenchymal stem cells: current clinical progress in ARDS and COVID-19. Stem Cell Res Ther 11(1):1–7
213. Alqahtani JS, Oyelade T, Aldhahir AM, Alghamdi SM, Almehmadi M, Alqahtani AS et al (2020) Prevalence, severity and mortality associated with COPD and smoking in patients with COVID-19: a rapid systematic review and meta-analysis. PLoS One 15(5):e0233147
214. Leung JM, Niikura M, Yang CWT, Sin DD (2020) COVID-19 and COPD. Eur Respiratory Soc 56:2002108
215. Sungnak W, Huang N, Becavin C, Berg M, Queen R, Litvinukova M, Talavera-Lopez C et al (2020) SARS-CoV-2 entry factors are highly expressed in nasal epithelial cells together with innate immune genes. Nat Med 26(5):681–687. https://doi.org/10.1038/s41591-020-0868-6
216. Razeghian-Jahromi I, Zibaeenezhad MJ, Lu Z, Zahra E, Mahboobeh R, Lionetti V (2020) Angiotensin-converting enzyme 2: a double-edged sword in COVID-19 patients with an increased risk of heart failure. Heart Fail Rev 26(2):371–380
217. Iyer SN, Chappell MC, Averill DB, Diz DI, Ferrario CM (1998) Vasodepressor actions of angiotensin-(1–7) unmasked during combined treatment with lisinopril and losartan. Hypertension 31(2):699–705

218. Ferreira AJ, Santos RA, Raizada MK (2012) Angiotensin-(1–7)/angiotensin-converting enzyme 2/mas receptor axis and related mechanisms. Int J Hypertens 2012:1–2
219. Zhong J-C, Huang D-Y, Yang Y-M, Li Y-F, Liu G-F, Song X-H et al (2004) Upregulation of angiotensin-converting enzyme 2 by all-trans retinoic acid in spontaneously hypertensive rats. Hypertension 44(6):907–912
220. Patel S, Rauf A, Khan H, Abu-Izneid T (2017) Renin-angiotensin-aldosterone (RAAS): the ubiquitous system for homeostasis and pathologies. Biomed Pharmacother 94:317–325
221. Monteil V, Kwon H, Prado P, Hagelkrüys A, Wimmer RA, Stahl M et al (2020) Inhibition of SARS-CoV-2 infections in engineered human tissues using clinical-grade soluble human ACE2. Cell 181:905–913.e7
222. Fang Y, Gao F, Liu Z (2019) Angiotensin-converting enzyme 2 attenuates inflammatory response and oxidative stress in hyperoxic lung injury by regulating NF-κB and Nrf2 pathways. QJM Int J Med 112(12):914–924
223. Sriram K, Insel PA (2020) Risks of ACE inhibitor and ARB usage in COVID-19: evaluating the evidence. Clin Pharmacol Ther 108(2):236–241
224. Cohen JB, Hanff TC, Bress AP, South AM (2020) Relationship between ACE2 and other components of the renin-angiotensin system. Curr Hypertens Rep 22:44. https://doi.org/10.1007/s11906-020-01048-y
225. Guan WJ, Ni ZY, Hu Y, Liang WH, Ou CQ, He JX et al (2020) Clinical characteristics of coronavirus disease 2019 in China. N Engl J Med 382:1708–1720
226. Wang D, Hu B, Hu C, Zhu F, Liu X, Zhang J et al (2020) Clinical characteristics of 138 hospitalized patients with 2019 novel coronavirus-infected pneumonia in Wuhan, China. JAMA 323:1061–1069
227. Wu C, Chen X, Cai Y, Xia J, Zhou X, Xu S et al (2020) Risk factors associated with acute respiratory distress syndrome and death in patients with coronavirus disease 2019 pneumonia in Wuhan, China. JAMA Intern Med 180:934–943
228. Sparks MA, South A, Welling P, Luther JM, Cohen J, Byrd JB et al (2020) Sound science before quick judgement regarding RAS blockade in COVID-19. Clin J Am Soc Nephrol 15:714–716
229. Sparks MA, Hiremath S, South A, Welling P, Luther JM, Cohen JB et al (2020) The coronavirus conundrum: ACE2 and hypertension edition. NephJC. http://www.nephjc.com/news/covidace2. Accessed 13 Apr 2020. This is a multidiscplinary free open access medical education document by several physician scientists whose research focuses on the renin-angiotensin system, which provides a comprehensive overview of research related to ACE2 and COVID-19, including live updates as new research emerges. The site had >260,000 page views within its first three weeks of launching
230. Sparks MA, Crowley SD, Gurley SB, Mirotsou M, Coffman TM (2014) Classical renin-angiotensin system in kidney physiology. Compr Physiol 4(3):1201–1228. https://doi.org/10.1002/cphy.c130040
231. Vaughan DE (2002) Angiotensin and vascular fibrinolytic balance. Am J Hypertens 15(1 Pt 2):3S–8S
232. South AM, Shaltout HA, Washburn LK, Hendricks AS et al (2019) Fetal programming and the angiotensin-(1-7) axis: a review of the experimental and clinical data. Clin Sci 133:55–74. https://doi.org/10.1042/CS20171550
233. Donoghue M, Hsieh F, Baronas E, Godbout K, Gosselin M, Stagliano N et al (2000) A novel angiotensin-converting enzyme-related carboxypeptidase (ACE2) converts angiotensin I to angiotensin 1-9. Circ Res 87(5):E1–E9
234. Gromotowicz-Poplawska A, Stankiewicz A, Kramkowski K, Gradzka A, Wojewodzka-Zelezniakowicz M, Dzieciol J et al (2016) The acute prothrombotic effect of aldosterone in rats is partially mediated via angiotensin II receptor type 1. Thromb Res 138:114–120
235. Flores-Munoz M, Work LM, Douglas K, Denby L, Dominiczak AF, Graham D et al (2012) Angiotensin-(1-9) attenuates cardiac fibrosis in the stroke-prone spontaneously hypertensive rat via the angiotensin type 2 receptor. Hypertension 59(2):300–307

236. Wakahara S, Konoshita T, Mizuno S, Motomura M, Aoyama C, Makino Y et al (2007) Synergistic expression of angiotensin-converting enzyme (ACE) and ACE2 in human renal tissue and confounding effects of hypertension on the ACE to ACE2 ratio. Endocrinology 148:2453–2457
237. Soler MJ, Wysocki J, Batlle D (2013) ACE2 alterations in kidney disease. Nephrol Dial Transplant 28:2687–2269
238. Rice GI, Jones AL, Grant PJ et al (2006) Circulating activities of angiotensin-converting enzyme, its homolog, angiotensin-converting enzyme 2, and neprilysin in a family study. Hypertension 48(5):914–920. https://doi.org/10.1161/01.HYP.0000244543.91937.79
239. Oudit GY, Liu GC, Zhong J, Basu R, Chow FL, Zhou J, Loibner H, Janzek E, Schuster M, Penninger JM, Herzenberg AM, Kassiri Z, Scholey JW (2010) Human recombinant ACE2 reduces the progression of diabetic nephropathy. Diabetes 59:529–538. https://doi.org/10.2337/db09-1218
240. Wysocki J, Ye M, Rodriguez E, González-Pacheco FR, Barrios C, Evora K, Schuster M, Loibner H, Brosnihan KB, Ferrario CM, Penninger JM, Batlle D (2009) Targeting the degradation of angiotensin II with recombinant angiotensin-converting enzyme 2: prevention of angiotensin II-dependent hypertension. Hypertension 55:90–98
241. Zhong J, Basu R, Guo D, Chow FL, Byrns S, Schuster M, Loibner H, Wang XH, Penninger JM, Kassiri Z, Oudit GY (2010) Angiotensin converting enzyme 2 suppresses pathological hypertrophy, myocardial fibrosis and cardiac dysfunction. Circulation 122:717–728
242. Walters TE, Kalman JM, Patel SK, Mearns M, Velkoska E, Burrell LM (2017) Angiotensin converting enzyme 2 activity and human atrial fibrillation: increased plasma angiotensin converting enzyme 2 activity is associated with atrial fibrillation and more advanced left atrial structural remodelling. Europace 19(8):1280–1287
243. Ramchand J, Patel SK, Srivastava PM, Farouque O, Burrell LM (2018) Elevated plasma angiotensin converting enzyme 2 activity is an independent predictor of major adverse cardiac events in patients with obstructive coronary artery disease. PLoS One 13(6):e0198144. This prospective observational study of 79 patients with obstructive coronary artery disease demonstrated that elevated ACE2 activity was independently associated with major adverse cardiovascular events over a median follow up of 10.5 years. The authors also observed that the frequency of elevated ACE2 activity was similar across users and non-users of ACE inhibitors and Ang II receptor blockers
244. Roth M (2020) Are patients with hypertension and diabetes mellitus at increased risk for COVID-19 infection? Lancet 8:e21
245. Gathiram P, Mackraj I, Moodley J (2021) The renin-angiotensin system, hypertension, and SARS-CoV-2 infection: a review. Curr Hypertens Rep 23:17. https://doi.org/10.1007/s11906-021-01134-9
246. World Health Organization. Clinical management of severe acute respiratory infection when COVID-19 is suspected 2020. https://www.who.int/publications-detail/clinical-management-of-severe-acute-respiratory-infection-when-novel-coronavirus-(ncov)-infection-is-suspected
247. Li W, Moore MJ, Vasilieva N, Sui J, Wong SK, Berne MA et al (2003) Angiotensin-converting enzyme 2 is a functional receptor for the SARS coronavirus. Nature 426(6965):450–454
248. Li MY, Li L, Zhang Y, Wang XS (2020) Expression of the SARS-CoV-2 cell receptor gene ACE2 in a wide variety of human tissues. Infect Dis Poverty 9(1):45
249. Chen H, Guo J, Wang C, Luo F, Yu X, Zhang W et al (2020) Clinical characteristics and intrauterine vertical transmission potential of COVID-19 infection in nine pregnant women: a retrospective review of medical records. Lancet 395(10226):809–815
250. World Health Organization. Coronavirus 2020 [cited 18 Apr 2020]. https://www.who.int/health-topics/coronavirus#tab=tab_1
251. Zhu H, Rhee JW, Cheng P, Waliany S, Chang A, Witteles RM et al (2020) Cardiovascular complications in patients with COVID-19: consequences of viral toxicities and host immune response. Curr Cardiol Rep 22(5):32

252. Ai T, Yang Z, Hou H, Zhan C, Chen C, Lv W et al (2020) Correlation of chest CT and RT-PCR testing in coronavirus disease 2019 (COVID-19) in China: a report of 1014 cases. Radiology 2020:200642
253. An P, Song P, Lian K, Wang Y (2020) CT manifestations of novel coronavirus pneumonia: a case report. Balkan Med J 37(3):163–165
254. Araujo-Filho JAB, Sawamura MVY, Costa AN, Cerri GG, Nomura CH (2020) COVID-19 pneumonia: what is the role of imaging in diagnosis? J Bras Pneumol 46(2):e20200114
255. Zhou Z, Guo D, Li C, Fang Z, Chen L, Yang R et al (2020) Coronavirus disease 2019: initial chest CT findings. Eur Radiol 30:4398–4406
256. Zheng F, Tang W, Li H, Huang YX, Xie YL, Zhou ZG (2020) Clinical characteristics of 161 cases of corona virus disease 2019 (COVID-19) in Changsha. Eur Rev Med Pharmacol Sci 24(6):3404–3410
257. Carey RM, Siragy HM (2003) Newly recognized components of the renin-angiotensin system: potential roles in cardiovascular and renal regulation. Endocr Rev 24(3):261–271. This article focuses on the actions of RAS in circulation and in tissues
258. Kurtz A (2012) Control of renin synthesis and secretion. Am J Hypertens 25(8):839–847
259. D'Ardes D, Boccatonda A, Rossi I, Guagnano MT, Santilli F, Cipollone F et al (2020) COVID-19 and RAS: unravelling an unclear relationship. Int J Mol Sci 21(8):3003
260. Yan R, Zhang Y, Li Y, Xia L, Guo Y, Zhou Q (2020) Structural basis for the recognition of SARS-CoV-2 by full-length human ACE2. Science 367(6485):1444–1448
261. Crackower MA, Sarao R, Oudit GY, Yagil C, Kozieradzki I, Scanga SE et al (2002) Angiotensin-converting enzyme 2 is an essential regulator of heart function. Nature 417(6891):822–828. This study indicates that a mutation on the X chromosome of ACE2 is associted with severe heart defects in Rat models
262. Busse LW, Chow JH, McCurdy MT, Khanna AK (2020) COVID-19 and the RAAS-a potential role for angiotensin II? Crit Care 24(1):136
263. Aronson JK, Ferner RE (2020) Drugs and the renin-angiotensin system in covid-19. BMJ 369:m1313
264. Gurwitz D (2020) Angiotensin receptor blockers as tentative SARS-CoV-2 therapeutics. Drug Dev Res 81:537–540
265. Ferrario CM, Jessup J, Chappell MC, Averill DB, Brosnihan KB, Tallant EA et al (2005) Effect of angiotensin-converting enzyme inhibition and angiotensin II receptor blockers on cardiac angiotensin-converting enzyme 2. Circulation 111(20):2605– 2610. This study discusses the effects of ACE2 inhibitors and Ang II blockers on the the ACE2 gene activity, blood pressure regulation, and Ang (1-7)
266. Kuster GM, Pfister O, Burkard T, Zhou Q, Twerenbold R, Haaf P et al (2020) SARS-CoV2: should inhibitors of the renin-angiotensin system be withdrawn in patients with COVID-19? Eur Heart J 41(19):1801–1803
267. John TJ, John K (2020) Renin-angiotensin-aldosterone system dysregulation and severe acute respiratory syndrome coronavirus 2 (SARS-CoV-2) infection. Eur Heart J 41(22):2126–2127
268. Cure E, Cumhur CM (2020) Angiotensin-converting enzyme inhibitors and angiotensin receptor blockers may be harmful in patients with diabetes during COVID-19 pandemic. Diabetes Metab Syndr 14(4):349–350
269. Diaz JH (2020) Hypothesis: angiotensin-converting enzyme inhibitors and angiotensin receptor blockers may increase the risk of severe COVID-19. J Travel Med 27(3):taaa041
270. Kai H, Kai M (2020) Interactions of coronaviruses with ACE2, angiotensin II, and RAS inhibitors-lessons from available evidence and insights into COVID-19. Hypertens Res 43(7):648–654
271. Mehta N, Kalra A, Nowacki AS, Anjewierden S, Han Z, Bhat P et al (2020) Association of use of angiotensin-converting enzyme inhibitors and angiotensin ii receptor blockers with testing positive for coronavirus disease 2019 (COVID-19). JAMA Cardiol 5:1020–1026
272. Felice C, Nardin C, Di Tanna GL, Grossi U, Bernardi E, Scaldaferri L et al (2020) Use of RAAS inhibitors and risk of clinical deterioration in COVID-19: results from an Italian cohort of 133 hypertensives. Am J Hypertens 33:944–948

273. Yang G, Tan Z, Zhou L, Yang M, Peng L, Liu J et al (2020) Effects of ARBs and ACEIs on virus infection, inflammatory status and clinical outcomes in COVID-19 patients with hypertension: a single center retrospective study. Hypertension 76:51–58
274. Khera R, Clark C, Lu Y, Guo Y, Ren S, Truax B et al (2020) Association of angiotensin-converting enzyme inhibitors and angiotensin receptor blockers with the risk of hospitalization and death in hypertensive patients with coronavirus disease-19. medRxiv
275. Mancia G, Rea F, Ludergnani M, Apolone G, Corrao G (2020) Renin-angiotensin-aldosterone system blockers and the risk of Covid-19. N Engl J Med 382:2431–2440
276. Iaccarino G, Borghi C, Cicero AFG, Ferri C, Minuz P, Muiesan ML et al (2020) Renin-angiotensin system inhibition in cardiovascular patients at the time of COVID19: much ado for nothing? A statement of activity from the Directors of the Board and the Scientific Directors of the Italian Society of Hypertension. High Blood Press Cardiovasc Prev 27(2):105–108
277. Salgo MP (2021) COVID-19: zinc and angiotensin-converting enzyme 2 (ACE2) deficiencies as determinants of risk and severity of disease: a narrative review. Infect Dis Ther 10:1215–1225. https://doi.org/10.1007/s40121-021-00478-8
278. Conti S, Cassis P, Benigni A (2012) Aging and the renin-angiotensin system. Hypertension 60(4):878–883. https://doi.org/10.1161/HYPERTENSIONAHA.110.155895
279. Centers for Disease Control and Prevention. Coronavirus disease 2019 (COVID-19): COVID-19 hospitalization and death by race/ethnicity. Updated 18 Aug 2020. https://www.cdc.gov/coronavirus/2019-ncov/covid-data/investigations-discovery/hospitalizationdeath-by-race-ethnicity.html. Accessed 29 Sept 2020
280. Centers for Disease Control and Prevention. Coronavirus disease 2019 (COVID-19): older adults. Updated 11 Sept 2020. https://www.cdc.gov/coronavirus/2019-ncov/need--extraprecautions/older-adults.html. Accessed 29 Sept 2020
281. Picheta R (2020) Black people in the UK four times more likely to die from Covid19 than white people, new data shows. CNN. https://www.cnn.com/2020/05/07/uk/uk--coronavirusethnicity-deaths-ons-scli-gbr-intl/index.html. Accessed 29 Sept 2020
282. Verdecchia P, Cavallini C, Spanevello A, Angeli F (2020) The pivotal link between ACE2 deficiency and SARS-CoV-2 infection. Eur J Intern Med 76:14–20. https://doi.org/10.1016/j.ejim.2020.04.037
283. Wessels I, Rolles B, Rink L (2020) The potential impact of zinc supplementation on COVID-19 pathogenesis. Front Immunol 11:1712. https://doi.org/10.3389/fimmu.2020.01712
284. Lavery AM, Preston LE, Ko JY et al (2020) Characteristics of of hospitalized COVID-19 patients discharged and experiencing same-hospital readmission—United States, March–August 2020. MMWR Morb Mortal Wkly Rep 69:1695–1699. https://doi.org/10.15585/mmwr.mm6945e2
285. Roscioli E, Jersmann HP, Lester S et al (2017) Zinc deficiency as a codeterminant for airway epithelial barrier dysfunction in an ex vivo model of COPD. Int J Chron Obstruct Pulmon Dis 12:3503–3510. https://doi.org/10.2147/COPD.S149589
286. Rosenblum H, Wessler JD, Gupta A, Maurer MS, Bikdeli B (2020) Zinc deficiency and heart failure: a systematic review of the current literature. J Card Fail 26(2):180–189. https://doi.org/10.1016/j.cardfail.2020.01.005
287. Farooq DM, Alamri AF, Alwhahabi BK, Metwally AM, Kareem KA (2020) The status of zinc in type 2 diabetic patients and its association with glycemic control. J Family Community Med. 27(1):29–36. https://doi.org/10.4103/jfcm.JFCM_113_19
288. Lobo JC, Torres JP, Fouque D, Mafra D (2010) Zinc deficiency in chronic kidney disease: is there a relationship with adipose tissue and atherosclerosis? Biol Trace Elem Res 135(1–3):16–21. https://doi.org/10.1007/s12011-009-8504-9
289. Bouie J (2020) Why coronavirus is killing African-Americans more than others. NY Times Sunday Rev
290. Turner AJ, Hooper NM (2004) Angiotensin-converting enzyme 2. In: Barrett AJ, Rawlings ND, Woessner JF (eds) Handbook of proteolytic enzymes, vol 1, 2nd edn. Elsevier, Amsterdam, pp 349–351. https://doi.org/10.1016/B978-0-12-079611-3.50092-6

291. Būnning P, Riordan JF (1985) The functional role of zinc in angiotensin converting enzyme: implications for the enzyme mechanics. J Inorg Biochem 24(3):183–198. https://doi.org/10.1016/0162-0134(85)85002-9
292. Reeves PG, O'Delll BL (1986) Effect of dietary zinc deprivation on the activity of angiotensin-converting enzyme in serum of rats and Guinea pigs. J Nutr 116(1):128–134. https://doi.org/10.1093/jn/116.1.128
293. Baden LR, Rubin EJ (2020) Covid-19: the search for effective therapy. N Engl J Med 382(19):1851–1852. https://doi.org/10.1056/NEJMe2005477
294. Zamai L (2020) The yin and yang of ACE/ACE2 pathways: the rationale for the use of renin-angiotensin system inhibitors in COVID-19 patients. Cells 9(7):E1704. https://doi.org/10.3390/cells9071704
295. Thomas MC, Tikellis C (2009) Losing control: positive and negative feedback in the renin angiotensin system. Curr Hypertens Rev 5(3):222–226. https://doi.org/10.2174/157340209788921194
296. Oyagbemi AA, Ajibade TO, Aboua YG et al (2021) Potential health benefits of zinc supplementation for the management of COVID-19 pandemic. J Food Biochem 00:e13604. https://doi.org/10.1111/jfbc.13604
297. Fajgenbaum DC, June CH (2020) Cytokine storm. N Engl J Med 383:2255–2273. https://doi.org/10.1056/NEJMra2026131
298. Goldin CJ, Vázquez R, Polack FP, Alvarez-Paggi D (2020) Identifying pathophysiological bases of disease in COVID-19. Transl Med Commun 5:15. https://doi.org/10.1186/s41231-020-00067-w
299. Salgo MP (2020) Angiotensin-converting enzyme 2, feedback systems, and COVID-19. Consultant 61(4):e1–e11. https://doi.org/10.25270/con.2020.10.00006
300. Jothimani D, Kailasam E, Danielraj S et al (2020) COVID-19: poor outcomes in patients with zinc deficiency. Int J Infect Dis 100:343–349. https://doi.org/10.1016/j.ijid.2020.09.014
301. Berlin DA, Gulick RM, Martinez FJ (2020) Severe Covid-19. N Engl J Med 383:2451–2460. https://doi.org/10.1056/NEJMcp2009575
302. Cantini F, Goletti D, Petrone L et al (2020) Immune therapy, antiviral therapy, or both for COVID-19. Drugs 80:11929–11946
303. Goletti D, Cantini F (2021) Baricitinib therapy in COVID-19 pneumonia: an unmet need fulfilled. N Engl J Med 384:9
304. Lebranchu Y, Malvy D, Richard MJ et al (1990) Kawasaki disease and oxidative metabolism. Clin Chim Acta 187(3):193–198. https://doi.org/10.1016/0009-8981(90)90104-z
305. National Institute of Health (2021) Zinc fact sheet for health professionals. https://ods.od.nih.gov/factsheets/Zinc-HealthProfessional/. Accessed 20 Feb 2021
306. Thomas S, Patel D, Bittel B et al (2021) Effect of high-dose zinc and ascorbic acid supplementation vs usual care on symptom length and reduction among ambulatory patients with SARS-CoV-2 infection: the COVID A to Z randomized clinical trial. JAMA Netw Open 4(2):e210369. https://doi.org/10.1001/jamanetworkopen.2021.0369. (ClinicalTrials.govIdentifier: NCT04342728)
307. Salgo M (2021) Study population selection likely excluded high-risk patients most likely to benefit. JAMA Netw Open 87:570–574
308. Bohn MK, Hall A, Sepiashvili L et al (2020) Pathophysiology of COVID-19: mechanisms underlying disease severity and progression. Physiology 35(5):288–301. https://doi.org/10.1152/physiol.00019.2020
309. Fawzy MS, Ashour H, Shafie AAA, Dahman NBH, Fares AM, Antar S, Elnoby AS, Fouad FM (2022) The role of angiotensin-converting enzyme 2 (ACE2) genetic variations in COVID-19 infection: a literature review. Egypt J Med Hum Genet 23(1):97. https://doi.org/10.1186/s43042-022-00309-6
310. Hashimoto T, Perlot T, Rehman A, Trichereau J, Ishiguro H, Paolino M, Sigl V, Hanada T, Hanada R, Lipinski S, Wild B, Camargo SM, Singer D, Richter A, Kuba K, Fukamizu A, Schreiber S, Clevers H, Verrey F, Rosenstiel P, Penninger JM (2012) ACE2 links amino acid

malnutrition to microbial ecology and intestinal inflammation. Nature 487(7408):477–481. https://doi.org/10.1038/nature11228. PMID: 22837003; PMCID: PMC7095315
311. Wang D, Hu B, Hu C, Zhu F, Liu X, Zhang J, Wang B et al (2020) Clinical characteristics of 138 hospitalized patients with 2019 novel coronavirus-infected pneumonia in Wuhan, China. JAMA 323:1061–1069. https://doi.org/10.1001/jama.2020.1585
312. Zhao Y, Zhao Z, Wang Y, Zhou Y, Ma Y, Zuo W (2020) Single-cell RNA expression profiling of ACE2, the receptor of SARS-CoV-2. Am J Respir Crit Care Med 202(5):756–759. https://doi.org/10.1164/rccm.202001-0179LE
313. Chiu RW, Tang NL, Hui DS, Chung GT, Chim SS, Chan KC et al (2004) ACE2 gene polymorphisms do not affect outcome of severe acute respiratory syndrome. Clin Chem 50(9):1683–1686. https://doi.org/10.1373/clinchem.2004.035436
314. Cao Y, Li L, Feng Z, Wan S, Huang P, Sun X et al (2020) Comparative genetic analysis of the novel coronavirus (2019-nCoV/SARS-CoV-2) receptor ACE2 in different populations. Cell Discov 6:11. https://doi.org/10.1038/s41421-020-0147-1
315. Omasits U, Ahrens CH, Müller S, Wollscheid B (2014) Protter: interactive protein feature visualization and integration with experimental proteomic data. Bioinformatics 30(6):884–886. https://doi.org/10.1093/bioinformatics/btt607
316. Zhou P, Yang XL, Wang XG, Hu B, Zhang L, Zhang W, Si HR et al (2020) A pneumonia outbreak associated with a new coronavirus of probable bat origin. Nature 579(7798):270–273. https://doi.org/10.1038/s41586-020-2012-7
317. He J, Tao H, Yan Y, Huang SY, Xiao Y (2020) Molecular mechanism of evolution and human infection with SARS-CoV-2. Viruses 12:428. https://doi.org/10.3390/v12040428
318. Lan J, Ge J, Yu J, Shan S, Zhou H, Fan S et al (2020) Structure of the SARS-CoV-2 spike receptor-binding domain bound to the ACE2 receptor. Nature 581(7807):215–220
319. Chaudhary M (2020) COVID-19 susceptibility: potential of ACE2 polymorphisms. Egypt J Med Hum Genet 21(1):54. https://doi.org/10.1186/s43042-020-00099-9
320. García-Escobar A, Vera-Vera S, Jurado-Román A, Jiménez-Valero S, Galeote G, Moreno R (2022) Calcium signaling pathway is involved in the shedding of ACE2 catalytic ectodomain: new insights for clinical and therapeutic applications of ACE2 for COVID-19. Biomol Ther 12(1):76. https://doi.org/10.3390/biom12010076
321. Fujikura K, Uesaka K (2021) Genetic variations in the human severe acute respiratory syndrome coronavirus receptor. J Clin Pathol 74(5):307–313. https://doi.org/10.1136/jclinpath-2020-206867
322. Suryamohan K, Diwanji D, Stawiski EW, Gupta R, Miersch S, Liu J et al (2021) Human ACE2 receptor polymorphisms and altered susceptibility to SARS-CoV-2. Commun Biol 4(1):475. https://doi.org/10.1038/s42003-021-02030-3
323. Devaux CA, Rolain JM, Raoult D (2020) ACE2 receptor polymorphism: susceptibility to SARS-CoV-2, hypertension, multi-organ failure, and COVID-19 disease outcome. J Microbiol Immunol Infect 53(3):425–435. https://doi.org/10.1016/j.jmii.2020.04.015
324. Gintoni I, Adamopoulou M, Yapijakis C (2022) The impact of ACE and ACE2 gene polymorphisms in pulmonary diseases including COVID-19. In Vivo 36(1):13–29. https://doi.org/10.21873/invivo.12672
325. Gwathmey TM, Shaltout HA, Nixon PA, O'Shea TM, Rose JC, Washburn LK et al (2008) Gender differences in urinary ACE and ACE2 activities in adolescents. Wiley Online Library
326. Sama IE, Ravera A, Santema BT, van Goor H, Ter Maaten JM, Cleland JGF et al (2020) Circulating plasma concentrations of angiotensin-converting enzyme 2 in men and women with heart failure and effects of renin-angiotensin-aldosterone inhibitors. Eur Heart J 41(19):1810–1817
327. Sahu S, Patil CR, Kumar S, Apparsundaram S, Goyal RK (2022) Role of ACE2-Ang (1–7)-Mas axis in post-COVID-19 complications and its dietary modulation. Mol Cell Biochem 477(1):225–240. https://doi.org/10.1007/s11010-021-04275-2
328. Ciaglia E, Vecchione C, Puca AA (2020) COVID-19 infection and circulating ACE2 levels: protective role in women and children. Front Pediatr 8:206. https://doi.org/10.3389/fped.2020.00206

329. Osman IO, Melenotte C, Brouqui P, Million M, Lagier JC, Parola P et al (2021) Expression of ACE2, soluble ACE2, angiotensin I, angiotensin II and angiotensin-(1–7) is modulated in COVID-19 patients. Front Immunol 12:625732. https://doi.org/10.3389/fimmu.2021.625732
330. Wooster L, Nicholson C, Sigurslid H, Lino Cardenas C, Malhotra R (2020) Polymorphisms in the ACE2 locus associate with severity of COVID-19 infection. medRxiv. https://doi.org/10.1101/2020.06.18.20135152
331. Sorokina M, Teixeira JMC, Barrera-Vilarmau S, Paschke R, Papasotiriou I, Rodrigues JPGL et al (2020) Structural models of human ACE2 variants with SARS-CoV-2 Spike protein for structure-based drug design. Sci Data 7(1):309. https://doi.org/10.1038/s41597-020-00652-6
332. Li G, De Clercq E (2020) Therapeutic options for the 2019 novel coronavirus (2019-nCoV). Nat Rev Drug Discov 19(3):149–150. https://doi.org/10.1038/d41573-020-00016-0
333. El-Shennawy L, Hoffmann AD, Dashzeveg NK, McAndrews KM, Mehl PJ, Cornish D et al (2022) Circulating ACE2-expressing extracellular vesicles block broad strains of SARS-CoV-2. Nat Commun 13(1):405. https://doi.org/10.1038/s41467-021-27893-2
334. Bakry NS, Abdelgawad M, Abdel-Latif A, Lotfy A (2022) Mesenchymal stromal cells coated with anti-ACE2 antibodies might improve efficacy against COVID-19. Hum Cell 35(1):418–420. https://doi.org/10.1007/s13577-021-00620-1
335. Shukla AK, Banerjee M (2021) Angiotensin-converting-enzyme 2 and renin-angiotensin system inhibitors in COVID-19: An update. High Blood Press Cardiovas Prev 28:129–139. https://doi.org/10.1007/s40292-021-00439-9
336. Guan W, Ni Z, Hu Y et al (2020) Clinical characteristics of coronavirus disease 2019 in China. N Engl J Med 382:1708–1720
337. Huang C, Wang Y, Li X et al (2020) Clinical features of patients infected with 2019 novel coronavirus in Wuhan, China. Lancet 395:497–506
338. Song Z, Xu Y, Bao L et al (2019) From SARS to MERS, thrusting coronaviruses into the spotlight. Viruses 11(1):59
339. Chhabra KH, Xia H, Pedersen KB et al (2013) Pancreatic angiotensin-converting enzyme 2 (ACE2) improves glycemia in angiotensin II-infused mice. Am J Physiol Endocrinol Metab 304:874–884
340. Zhang H, Penninger JM, Li Y et al (2020) Angiotensin-converting enzyme 2 (ACE2) as a SARS-CoV-2 receptor: molecular mechanisms and potential therapeutic target. Intensive Care Med 46:586–590
341. Kuba K, Imai Y, Rao S et al (2005) A crucial role of angiotensin converting enzyme 2 (ACE2) in SARS coronavirus-induced lung injury. Nat Med 11:875–879
342. Li X, Molina-Molina M, Abdul-Hafez A et al (2008) Angiotensin converting enzyme-2 is protective but downregulated in human and experimental lung fibrosis. Am J Physiol Lung Cell Mol Physiol 295:178–185
343. Watkins J (2020) Preventing a covid-19 pandemic. BMJ 368:m810
344. Zheng YY, Ma YT, Zhang JY et al (2020) COVID-19 and the cardiovascular system. Nat Rev Cardiol 17(5):259–260
345. Zhang P, Zhu L, Cai J et al (2020) Association of inpatient use of angiotensin converting enzyme inhibitors and angiotensin II receptor blockers with mortality among patients with hypertension hospitalized with COVID-19. Circ Res 126(12):1671–1681
346. Gao C, Cai Y, Zhang K et al (2020) Association of hypertension and antihypertensive treatment with COVID-19 mortality: a retrospective observational study. Eur Heart J 41(22):2058–2066
347. Meng J, Xiao G, Zhang J et al (2020) Renin-angiotensin system inhibitors improve the clinical outcomes of COVID-19 patients with hypertension. Emerg Microbes Infect 9(1):757–760
348. Fosbøl EL, Butt JH, Østergaard L et al (2020) Association of angiotensin-converting enzyme inhibitor or angiotensin receptor blocker use with COVID-19 diagnosis and mortality. JAMA 324(2):168–177
349. Iaccarino G, Grassi G, Borghi C et al (2020) Age and multimorbidity predict death among COVID-19 patients: results of the SARS-RAS study of the italian society of hypertension. Hypertension 76(2):366–372

350. Jung SY, Choi JC, You SH et al (2020) Association of renin-angiotensin-aldosterone system inhibitors with COVID-19-related outcomes in Korea: a nationwide population-based cohort study. Clin Infect Dis 71:2121–2128. https://doi.org/10.1093/cid/ciaa624
351. South AM, Diz D, Chappell MC (2020) COVID-19, ACE2 and the cardiovascular consequences. Am J Physiol Heart Circ Physiol 318:1084–1090
352. Hoffmann M, Kleine-Weber H, Krüger N et al (2020) The novel coronavirus 2019 (2019-nCoV) uses the SARS-coronavirus receptor ACE2 and the cellular protease TMPRSS2 for entry into target cells. bioRxiv. https://doi.org/10.1101/2020.01.31.929042
353. Kawase M, Shirato K, van der Hoek L et al (2012) Simultaneous treatment of human bronchial epithelial cells with serine and cysteine protease inhibitors prevents severe acute respiratory syndrome coronavirus entry. J Virol 86:6537–6545
354. Zhou Y, Vedantham P, Lu K et al (2015) Protease inhibitors targeting coronavirus and filovirus entry. Antivir Res 116:76–84
355. Hashimoto T, Perlot T, Rehman A, Trichereau J, Ishiguro H, Paolino M et al (2012) ACE2 links amino acid malnutrition to microbial ecology and intestinal inflammation. Nature 487:477–481
356. Oudit GY, Kassiri Z, Jiang C et al (2009) SARS-coronavirus modulation of myocardial ACE2 expression and inflammation in patients with SARS. Eur J Clin Investig 39:618–625

Chapter 10
Recent Trends in Management of Hypertension Through RAAS Inhibition

Mukesh Nandave

Introduction by the Editor

Globally, cardiovascular diseases are associated with more than 17 million deaths per year, of which hypertension complications lead to 9.4 million deaths globally. Early diagnosis and hypertension management can prevent expensive treatment, including cardiac surgery and dialysis. Non-pharmacological strategies for hypertension management includes lifestyle changes, involving exercise and diet management such as minimizing salt and fluid intake; however, most of the patients will ultimately need antihypertensive medications. In 2020, the International Society of Hypertension published global guidelines to reduce the worldwide cases of high blood pressure in adults aged 18 years or over. Currently, several classes of therapies are used for hypertension management, either as mono- or combination therapy based on the disease severity. These classes of drugs include that target the renin-angiotensin-aldosterone system (RAAS), adrenergic receptors, diuretics, calcium channel blockers, and vasodilators. Despite of significant effect showed by these drug classes in blood pressure regulation and cardiovascular mortality, the prevalence of hypertension remains high.

Several efforts have been made in developing new drug classes for BP regulation; these therapies show their therapeutic effects via different pathways and mechanisms. With several of these emerging classes undergoing phase III clinical trials, it is hoped that the development of novel therapeutic avenues will aid in reducing the global burden of hypertension [1].

Angiotensin converting enzyme (ACE) inhibitors and angiotensin receptor blockers (ARBs) are well known for blood pressure regulation and they recommended as first line therapy in the management of hypertension. European Society

M. Nandave (✉)
Department of Pharmacology, Delhi Pharmaceutical Sciences and Research University, New Delhi, Delhi, India

M. Nandave (ed.), *Angiotensin-converting Enzyme Inhibitors vs. Angiotensin Receptor Blockers*, https://doi.org/10.1007/978-981-97-7380-0_10

of Cardiology/European Society of hypertension and American College of Cardiology/American Heart Institute guidelines strongly recommend the use of ACE inhibitors and ARBs as the first line treatment for initiating the hypertension treated supported by several evidence these classes of anti-hypertensive agents are considered as class I [2, 3]. ALLHAT (Antihypertensive and Lipid-Lowering Treatment to Prevent Heart Attack Trial), HOPE (Heart Outcomes Prevention Evaluation), meta-analysis, and systemic review based on research data suggests that blood pressure regulation using ACE inhibitors and ARBs also reduces the risk of cardiovascular events [4]. There are limited extensive direct extensive comparisons between ARBs and ACE inhibitors thus leading to the conflicted conclusion [4]. Some high-quality meta-analysis and systematic reviews have reported that ARBs have comparable efficacy with fewer side effects in comparison to ACE inhibitors. However, the conclusion of these meta-analysis and systematic reviews are limited because they have studied few numbers of randomized controlled trial (RCT) to draw the comparisons. Each trial has involved less than 500 patients and studied less than 10 events in each cohort thus limiting the evidence to conclude the results [5–11]. Some of the RCT conducted on high-risk patient with pre-existing health condition such as vascular disease, diabetes, or elder age. These RCT presented conflicting data like REACH (Reduction of Atherothrombosis for Continued Health) registry reported that ARBs therapy reduces the risk of cardiovascular events by 10% however other study reported that ARBs may increase the risk of myocardial infarction [12, 13]. A study analyzed and compared 51 secondary and safety events, such as cough, angioedema, electrolyte abnormalities, and syncope in patients taking ACE inhibitors with patients taking ARBs. Researchers observed that patients who are taking ACE inhibitors are more likely to develop pancreatitis, cough, angioedema and gastrointestinal bleeding in comparison to patients who are taking ARBs. The risk of angioedema development in ACE inhibitors therapy was found to be more than three times compared to ARBs. However, the absolute risk was found to be low. Meta-analysis involving 74,857 patients who were prescribed with ACE inhibitors, around 394 patients had developed angioedema in an average duration of 129 weeks. This ACE inhibitors associated adverse event was found to be common among the African American leading to number of fatalities each year [14]. Another most common side effect of ACE inhibitors is dry cough which is found to be more common in female especially among Chinese population [15].

Despite these controversial data ACE inhibitors and ARBs are recommended as first line therapy in the management of hypertension. Globally, ACE inhibitors specifically lisinopril is prescribed more frequently in the hypertension than ARBs [16, 17] (Fig. 10.1).

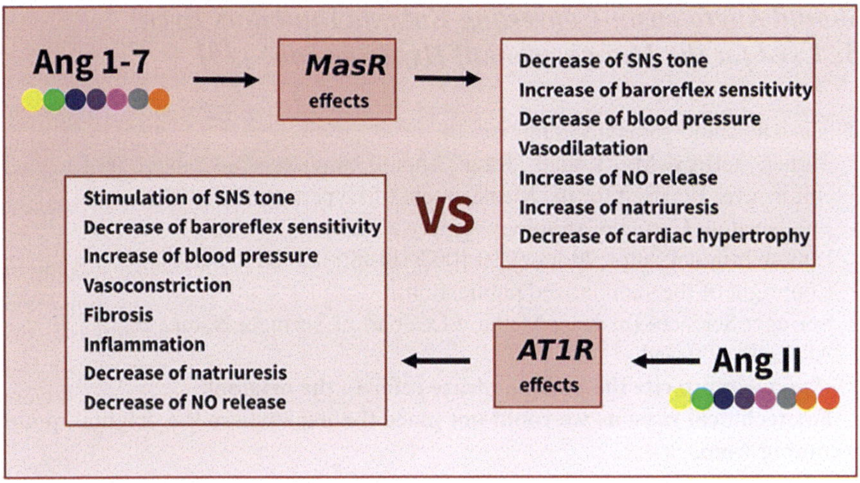

Fig. 10.1 Opposite actions of classical and alternative RAS axes. Legend: Ang II binds to AT1 receptors and produces the traditional actions of RAS classical axis, including stimulation of SNS tone, of vasoconstriction, of inflammation, and of fibrosis and decrease of baroreflex sensitivity, of natriuresis, and of NO release. The alternative axis, however, is activated mostly due to Ang-(1–7) binding to Mas receptors, promoting counter-regulatory actions, including decrease of SNS tone, of blood pressure, and of cardiac hypertrophy; increase of baroreflex sensitivity, of NO release, and of natriuresis; and stimulation of vasodilatation. *Ang 1–7* angiotensin 1–7, *Ang II* angiotensin II, *MasR* Mas receptor, *AT1R* AT1 receptor, *SNS* sympathetic nervous system, *NO* nitric oxide. (Source: Simões e Silva et al. [18])

Machine Generated Summaries

Disclaimer: The summaries in this chapter were generated from Springer Nature publications using extractive AI auto-summarization: An extraction-based summarizer aims to identify the most important sentences of a text using an algorithm and uses those original sentences to create the auto-summary (unlike generative AI). As the constituted sentences are machine selected, they may not fully reflect the body of the work, so we strongly advise that the original content is read and cited. The auto generated summaries were curated by the editor to meet Springer Nature publication standards. To cite this content, please refer to the original papers.

Machine generated keywords: combination, hypertensive, cost, hypertensive patient, adherence, ccb, achieve, arb, health, efficacy, people, amlodipine, achieve control, antihypertensive medication, tolerability.

Should Angiotensin-Converting Enzyme Inhibitors Ever Be Used for the Management of Hypertension? [19]

This is a machine-generated summary of:

Turner, Jeffrey M.; Kodali, Ravi: Should Angiotensin-Converting Enzyme Inhibitors ever Be Used for the Management of Hypertension? [19].

Published in: Current Cardiology Reports (2020).

Link to original: https://doi.org/10.1007/s11886-020-01352-8

If you want to cite the papers, please refer to the original.

For technical reasons we could not place the page where the original quote is coming from.

Abstract-Summary "We review the literature to evaluate for any differences in efficacy between the two classes in order to determine if the greater side effects associated with angiotensin-converting enzyme inhibitors are offset by any advantageous effects on outcomes to warrant their use over angiotensin receptor blockers."

"In many clinical scenarios, the data supports similar efficacy between ACE inhibitors and ARBs, while in a minority of others, there are murky signals from previous trials that suggest ACE inhibitors may be better."

"When reviewing the literature in its entirety, and taking into account recently published pooled analysis and head to head trials, it is reasonable to conclude that ACE inhibitors and ARBs have similar efficacy."

"From the available data, it is reasonable to conclude that ACE inhibitors and ARBs have equal efficacy yet unequal adverse effects."

Introduction

"The first of the RAAS inhibitors to be introduced for widespread human use for hypertension were angiotensin-converting enzyme (ACE) inhibitors."

"Several ACE inhibitors have since been synthesized and are in clinical use currently."

"Regarding side effects, the results disfavor ACE inhibitor use, because although the overall incidence is rare, angioedema-related deaths from these agents are significantly more frequent as compared to ARBs."

"It is in this context that if we conclude the benefits on outcomes are equivalent between ACE inhibitors and ARBs, then agents from these two classes should definitely not be considered interchangeable."

"The question therefore being posed is, should ACE inhibitors ever be used to treat hypertension?"

Mechanisms of Action

"Angiotensin II acts via the AT1 receptor to directly promote vasoconstriction as well as sodium reabsorption in the proximal tubule of the kidney and via the AT2 receptor to stimulate aldosterone release from the adrenal cortex."

"ACE inhibitors block the activity of angiotensin-converting enzyme, thereby preventing the conversion of angiotensin I to angiotensin II."

"ARBs directly inhibit the binding of angiotensin II to AT1 receptors."

"Unlike ACE inhibitors, ARBs do not significantly affect bradykinin levels, and therefore, cough and angioedema are much less common."

ACE Inhibitor Versus ARB Efficacy for BP Lowering

"Given the mechanisms by which ACE inhibitors and ARBs reduce blood pressure are unique for each class, significant research efforts have focused on understanding their differences."

"In another head to head study, fixed dose olmesartan 40 mg in combination with amlodipine 10 mg demonstrated superior central systolic blood pressure lowering and 24 h ambulatory blood pressure lowering effects when compared to fixed dose perindopril 8 mg in combination with amlodipine 10 mg [20]."

"The newer ARB agent azilsartan was shown to be superior to ramipril for blood pressure lowering efficacy [21]."

"In elderly individuals (65–89 years old), olmesartan had a greater effect on lowering 24 h ambulatory blood pressure than did ramipril [22]."

"In a systematic review of 47 head to head studies that reported comparative blood pressure effects between ACE inhibitors and ARBs, 37 demonstrated no difference, 2 favored ACE inhibitors, and 8 favored ARBs [23]."

ACE Inhibitor Versus ARB on Clinical Outcomes Areas of More Controversy

"A number of indirect comparisons with pooled analysis of several randomized placebo control trials have been done to further elucidate whether ACE inhibitors and ARBs have differing effects on the risk of myocardial infarction [24–27]."

"We now have well-designed head to head randomized trials comparing the effects of myocardial infarction and cardiovascular death from ACE inhibitors and ARBs."

"In the previously mentioned Bangalore paper, a separate meta-analysis of the only head to head trials between ACE inhibitors and ARBs also showed no difference in the risk for myocardial infarction or cardiovascular death between the two classes [24]."

"In randomized trials designed to compare ACE inhibitors and ARBs head to head in patients with HFrEF, the impact on all-cause mortality, as well as cardiovascular mortality and morbidity, was similar [28, 29]."

ACE Inhibitors Versus ARBs on Clinical Outcomes Areas of More Consensus

"Robust data support the benefit of using either ACE inhibitors or ARBs on improving renal outcomes in patients with chronic kidney disease with proteinuria."

"In non-diabetics with CKD and proteinuria, improvement in renal outcomes has been demonstrated with ACE inhibitors; however, studies with ARBs in this population are notably lacking [30, 31]."

"In head to head studies, ACE inhibitors and ARBs had a similar benefit on renal outcomes in those with CKD [32, 33]."

"There is a dearth of data available to directly compare the impact of ACE inhibitors versus ARBs on secondary stroke prevention, but overall, the consensus based on extrapolation from previous trials is that ACE inhibitors and ARBs are equal in this regard."

ACE Inhibitors Versus ARBs Adverse Events

"A meta-analysis by Matchar and others showed that among randomized controlled trials in the analysis, the rate of cough in ACE inhibitors group was 9.9% while ARBs group had a rate of 3.2% (absolute risk difference of 6.7%) [23]."

"In a meta-analysis by Makani and others, the incidence of angioedema with ACE inhibitors was 0.3% (95% CI 0.28–0.32), while the incidence with ARBs was 0.13% (95% CI 0.08–0.19) [34]."

"The risk of angioedema was twice as high in ACE inhibitors as compared to ARBs (RR 2.2, 95% CI 1.5–3.34, $p < 0.0001$)."

"Although the prices vary quite significantly even within ACE inhibitors and ARBs, and whether they are generic or branded, the most used generic preparations are comparable in price between these groups and are equally affordable."

ACE Inhibitor and ARB Use During the Current COVID-19 Pandemic: Where Do We Stand?

"It is now well established that angiotensin-converting enzyme 2 (ACE2) acts a receptor for SARS-COV2, the virus responsible for COVID-19, and enables its entry into cells [35]."

"Given what is known about viral entry into cells, an indirect conclusion was drawn that RAAS inhibitors can increase susceptibility to COVID-19 infection by increasing ACE2 levels."

"Based on data from a non-COVID-related lung injury, it is postulated that elevated ACE2 levels during COVID-19 infection could be protective of the lung parenchyma, thus preventing more serious illness [36–38]."

"This has led various organizations including AHA to recommend against discontinuation of ACE inhibitors or ARBs when diagnosed with COVID-19."

Conclusion

"It appears we may now be at a critical point in which enough data has amassed to allow us to conclude that the impact on clinical outcomes between ACE inhibitors and ARBs are equivalent, but the risk associated with these agents clearly favors using ARBs."

"When the data is critically reviewed in the context of the different event rates that existed due to the generational gap between placebo control ACE inhibitor and ARB trials, in addition to looking at more contemporary data from head to head studies, these arguments do not hold."

"Regarding outcomes in HFrEF, there are similar gaps between trials conducted with ACE inhibitors versus ARBs."

"We therefore conclude that the use of ARBs for RAAS inhibition is a superior therapeutic strategy over the use of ACE inhibitors, and clinical practice patterns should shift in this direction."

The Role of Angiotensin Receptor Blocker and Calcium Channel Blocker Combination Therapy in Treating Hypertension [39]

This is a machine-generated summary of:

Chrysant, Steven G.: The Role of Angiotensin Receptor Blocker and Calcium Channel Blocker Combination Therapy in Treating Hypertension [39].

Published in: American Journal of Cardiovascular Drugs (2010).

Link to original: https://doi.org/10.2165/11538850-000000000-00000

If you want to cite the papers, please refer to the original.

For technical reasons we could not place the page where the original quote is coming from.

Abstract-Summary "Of these, only 36.8% have BP controlled to recommended levels of <140/90 mmHg for uncomplicated hypertension and <130/80 mmHg for patients with diabetes mellitus or renal disease."

"For those with uncontrolled hypertension, the risk of diabetes, renal disease, stroke, and cardiovascular disease is increased."

"Therapeutic options for the treatment of hypertension include several major classes of drugs: diuretics, ß-adrenoceptor antagonists (ß-blockers), ACE inhibitors, angiotensin II type 1 receptor antagonists (angiotensin receptor blockers [ARBs]), renin inhibitors, calcium channel blockers, and central sympatholytics, alone or in combination."

"Drugs that block the renin-angiotensin-aldosterone system not only provide BP control but may also provide vascular protection and are metabolically neutral."

"This is a concise review of the safety and efficacy of ARBs in combination with amlodipine for the treatment of hypertension, with focus on the telmisartan-amlodipine combination."

"A MEDLINE search of the English literature from 2006 to 2009 of amlodipine in combination with ARBs revealed six publications, which are included in this review."

Introduction

"The relationship between BP and risk of cardiovascular events is continuous, consistent, and independent of other risk factors [40]. Hypertension is a major risk factor for heart failure and atherosclerotic cardiovascular events [41]. In addition, with every 20 mmHg increase in systolic BP or 10 mmHg increase in diastolic BP, the risk of cardiovascular disease is doubled [42, 43]. Because uncontrolled hypertension increases the risk of vascular events, it is imperative to increase the percentage of individuals who achieve BP control, and the challenge in achieving this goal is the need for multiple-drug combination therapy in most patients."

"Fixed-dose drug formulations that contain two classes of agents with complementary mechanisms of action are increasingly available."

"We discuss fixed-dose therapy with the calcium channel blocker (CCB) amlodipine combined with different angiotensin II type 1 receptor antagonists (angiotensin receptor blockers [ARBs]), two drug classes that have been shown to be effective in the treatment of hypertension, and are safe and well tolerated."

Rationale for Fixed-Dose Combination Therapy

"The fixed-dose combination of two complementary drugs was slow in gaining acceptance."

"Because the goal of antihypertensive treatment is to maximize therapeutic efficacy without significant adverse effects, the combination of two low-dose complementary drugs was a reasonable choice."

"Such low-dose combination therapy has resulted in better BP control, fewer adverse effects, prolonged duration of the antihypertensive effect due to different half-lives of component drugs, lower cost of care, and increased patient compliance

[44, 45]. Because several dose strengths of fixed-dose combinations are available, the dosing flexibility is not lost [45]. Concerning the combination of dihydropyridine CCBs with ARBs, their complementary action results from arteriolar dilation and natriuresis by the CCB and counteraction on the effects of stimulated angiotensin II by the ARBs [46]. Another benefit of this combination is the alleviation of pedal edema associated with dihydropyridine CCB monotherapy [46, 47]. The pedal edema produced mostly by the dihydropyridine CCBs is due to their preferential arteriolar vasodilation, which creates a pressure gradient between the arteriolar and venular capillaries, leading to fluid exudation in the interstitial tissue."

Angiotensin Receptor Blocker/Calcium Channel Blocker Fixed-Dose Combination Therapy: Results from Factorial Design Studies

"Response rates as reflected by proportions of responders (MSDBP <90 mmHg or a ≥ 10 mmHg reduction from baseline) ranged from 81.1% to 91.3% [48]. In addition, this study found that the incidence of peripheral edema associated with amlodipine monotherapy was reduced by the addition of an ARB (8.7% vs 5.4%, $p = 0.014$)."

"Mean changes (also reported as LSM) from baseline in MSDBP and MSSBP ranged from reductions of 14.3 to 19.4 mmHg and 22.6 to 28.5 mmHg, respectively, across currently available doses (amlodipine 5 mg/olmesartan medoxomil 20 mg, amlodipine 5 mg/olmesartan medoxomil 40 mg, amlodipine 10 mg/olmesartan medoxomil 20 mg, and amlodipine 10 mg/olmesartan medoxomil 40 mg) [49]. Response rates, defined as those who achieved a seated diastolic BP <90 mmHg, were as high as 77.6% for patients taking the amlodipine 10 mg/olmesartan medoxomil 40 mg combination."

Discussion

"Blood pressure control is very important, as a large meta-analysis of one million hypertensive patients showed that a 2 mmHg reduction in systolic BP is associated with 7% and 10% reductions in the risk for cardiovascular and stroke deaths, respectively [43]. Therapeutic options include several different classes of antihypertensive drugs, such as diuretics, β-blockers, ACEIs, ARBs, direct renin inhibitors, CCBs, and central sympatholytics, alone or in combination."

"These drug combinations include the combinations of ARBs with CCBs, among others, and have been shown to be very effective and safe in the treatment of hypertension, as is presented in this review."

"Although the BP effects of ARB/CCB combinations are similar to those of ACEI/CCB combinations, they may be a better choice for the treatment of hypertension based on their efficacy and safety profiles."

Management of Hypertension and Renin-Angiotensin-Aldosterone System Blockade in Adults with Diabetic Kidney Disease: Association of British Clinical Diabetologists and the Renal Association UK Guideline Update 2021 [50]

This is a machine-generated summary of:

Banerjee, D.; Winocour, P.; Chowdhury, T. A.; De, P.; Wahba, M.; Montero, R.; Fogarty, D.; Frankel, A. H.; Karalliedde, J.; Mark, P. B.; Patel, D. C.; Pokrajac, A.; Sharif, A.; Zac-Varghese, S.; Bain, S.; Dasgupta, I.: Management of hypertension and renin-angiotensin-aldosterone system blockade in adults with diabetic kidney disease: Association of British Clinical Diabetologists and the Renal Association UK guideline update 2021 [50].

Published in: BMC Nephrology (2022).

Link to original: https://doi.org/10.1186/s12882-021-02587-5

If you want to cite the papers, please refer to the original.

For technical reasons we could not place the page where the original quote is coming from.

Abstract-Summary "People with type 1 and type 2 diabetes are at risk of developing progressive chronic kidney disease (CKD) and end-stage kidney failure."

"Blood pressure control has been shown to be beneficial in people with diabetes in slowing progression of kidney disease and reducing cardiovascular events."

"Randomised trials demonstrate that RAAS blockade is effective in preventing/slowing progression of CKD and reducing cardiovascular events in people with type 1 and type 2 diabetes, albeit differently according to the stage of CKD."

"Emerging therapy with sodium glucose cotransporter-2 (SGLT-2) inhibitors, non-steroidal selective mineralocorticoid antagonists and endothelin-A receptor antagonists have been shown in randomised trials to lower blood pressure and further reduce the risk of progression of CKD and cardiovascular disease in people with type 2 diabetes."

Introduction

"Analysis of 1441 people with type 1 diabetes in the Diabetes Control and Complications Trial (DCCT) cohorts suggests that systolic blood pressure levels below 120 mmHg are associated with a 41% reduction in macroalbuminuria (95% confidence interval [CI] 5 to 63%) and a 68% reduction in CKD stage 3 (95% CI 25 to 84%) [51]."

"The use of RAAS blockade has significant benefits on cardiovascular and renal end points in people with diabetes, independent of their blood pressure lowering effect, as shown in the Heart Outcomes Prevention Evaluation (HOPE) trial and the European trial on reduction of cardiac events with perindopril in stable coronary artery disease [52, 53]."

"A multicentre trial in people with type 2 diabetes and nephropathy suggested that adding a non-dihydropyridine calcium channel blocker to an ACEI-based regime can be effective at lowering residual albuminuria with or without a significant reduction in systolic blood pressure [54]."

Conclusion

"People with diabetes and CKD have increased risk of morbidity and mortality."

"Tight control of blood pressure and the use RAAS inhibitors are associated with improved outcomes, particularly in the presence of proteinuria."

"Guideline-based therapy such as mentioned here can prolong life, lower risk of cardiovascular events and hospital admissions, and prevent end-stage kidney failure requiring renal replacement therapy."

Hypertensive Mediated Organ Damage and Hypertension Management. How to Assess Beneficial Effects of Antihypertensive Treatments? [55]

This is a machine-generated summary of:

Piskorz, Daniel: Hypertensive Mediated Organ Damage and Hypertension Management. How to Assess Beneficial Effects of Antihypertensive Treatments? [55].

Published in: High Blood Pressure & Cardiovascular Prevention (2020).

Link to original: https://doi.org/10.1007/s40292-020-00361-6

If you want to cite the papers, please refer to the original.
For technical reasons we could not place the page where the original quote is coming from.

Abstract-Summary "In old adult hypertensive patients the therapeutic target should be to prevent major cardiovascular events, but in young hypertensive subjects the focus should be pointed on preventing the development of hypertensive mediated organ damage, since most of the hard events are preceded by functional and structural tissues injury."

"Hypertension Guidelines of the European Society of Cardiology and European Society of Hypertension recognizes that some variables like electrocardiographic or echocardiographic left ventricle hypertrophy, chronic kidney disease or advance retinopathy, all considered as hypertensive mediated organ damage, may be modifiers of cardiovascular risk estimated by the SCORE system, and for that reason they should be screened in hypertensive patients."

"Some questions remained unanswered: the screening generalization of hypertensive mediated organ damage should modify the cardiovascular risk score of the patients, if its presence could modify the therapeutic approach, and as a consequence, if the treatment adjustment should prolong life expectancy and ameliorate the quality of life."

Introduction

"The effects of impaired renal function measured as an estimated glomerular filtration rate lower than 60 ml/min/1.73 m^2, albuminuria (albumin/creatinine-ratio in men over 2.5 mg/mmol and 3.5 mg/mmol in women), and left-ventricular hypertrophy evaluated by the ECG criteria could identify patients at a mortality very high risk as it has been shown in a cohort of patients with vascular diseases, in which after a median follow-up of 4.4 years the hazard ratio of having a vascular event after adjustment for age and sex was 1.5 (95% confidence interval 1.2–1.9) in the presence of one hypertensive mediated organ damage and increased to 3.8 times (95% CI 2.3–6.3) when three were present; at the same time, the hazard ratio for mortality was 1.4 (95% CI 1.1–1.7) and 3.2 (95% CI 1.9–5.2), respectively [56]."

Hypertensive Mediated Vascular Damage

"In 868 Japanese men between 40 and 74 years of age without a history of cardiovascular disease randomly selected to the Shiga Epidemiological Study of Subclinical Atherosclerosis (SESSA), the intima media thickness and plaque number from the common to internal carotid arteries were investigated by ultrasonography to examine whether subclinical atherosclerosis of the carotid arteries is concordant with the estimated categories 10-year absolute risk of coronary artery disease death of the NIPPON DATA 80 Risk Assessment Chart, proposed by the Japan Atherosclerosis Society in 2012 Atherosclerosis Prevention Guidelines."

"Although the Guidelines recognized that the presence of carotid plaques or an increased pulse wave velocity reclassify hypertensive patients beyond traditional risk factors, they do not recommend these methods for routine clinical practice unless a specific indications is detected, since the available evidence is weak about the predictive prognostic value of a treatment supported on the presence of carotid plaques, intima-media thickness or pulse wave velocity and a reduction of cardiovascular events [57]."

Hypertensive Mediated Kidney Disease

"In the HOPE study (Heart Outcomes Prevention Evaluation), applying cut-off points of 1.4 mg/dl for serum creatinine and 65 ml/min for calculated glomerular filtration rate, it was observed again that kidney function not only impacts on noncardiovascular events, but also predicts higher cardiovascular mortality and higher incidence of stroke."

"The 2018 European Hypertension Guidelines recommends as therapeutic strategies for treatment of hypertension in chronic kidney disease renin-angiotensin-system blockers since they are more effective at reducing albuminuria than other antihypertensive agents, and are recommended as part of the treatment strategy in hypertensive patients in the presence of microalbuminuria or proteinuria, with a class of recommendation I and level of evidence A, but a combination of this family of drugs with calcium channel blockers or diuretics is recommended as initial therapy, probably due to the severity of the hypertension and the difficulties to lower blood pressure to the targets."

Hypertensive Cardiopathy

"This has not been confirmed by other authors like Fagard and others who compared the effects of all families of antihypertensive drugs on left ventricular mass regression in patients with hypertension in a meta-analysis that included prospective, randomized comparative studies, and involved pooled pairwise comparisons of drug classes and of each class versus the others statistically combined."

"The regression of left ventricular mass was significantly lower with beta-blockers (9.8%) than with angiotensin receptor blockers (12.5%), but none of the other comparisons between drug classes revealed significant differences."

"A Bayesian network meta-analysis that included 41 randomized clinical trials involving 2566 hypertensive patients with left ventricular hypertrophy aimed to compare the efficacy of fat-soluble β1-receptor blockers with ACE inhibitors,

ARBs, calcium channel blockers, and diuretics on regression of left ventricular hypertrophy."

Conclusions

"In patients with grade 2 or 3 hypertension it is recommended that blood pressure lowering drug treatment should be initiated alongside lifestyle interventions, independently of the presence of hypertensive mediated organ damage."

"In patients with grade 1 hypertension at high risk drug treatment should also be initiated simultaneously with lifestyle interventions."

"An international expert position paper suggested that the support for an earlier pharmacologic treatment in low to moderate cardiovascular risk grade 1 hypertensive patients should be evaluated considering the patient lifestyle and behavior, the global cardiovascular risk, the medical management resources, the country health system status and social-economic politic."

"Three main questions should be answer in this scenario: the screening of hypertensive mediated organ damage should modify the cardiovascular risk score of the patient?"

The Combination of Amlodipine and Angiotensin Receptor Blocker or Diuretics in High-Risk Hypertensive Patients: Rationale, Design and Baseline Characteristics [58]

This is a machine-generated summary of:

Wang, W; Ma, L; Zhang, Y; Deng, Q; Liu, M; Liu, L: The combination of amlodipine and angiotensin receptor blocker or diuretics in high-risk hypertensive patients: rationale, design and baseline characteristics [58].

Published in: Journal of Human Hypertension (2010).

Link to original: https://doi.org/10.1038/jhh.2010.45

If you want to cite the papers, please refer to the original.

For technical reasons we could not place the page where the original quote is coming from.

Abstract-Summary "The Chinese Hypertension Intervention Efficacy Study (CHIEF) is a multi-centre randomized controlled clinical trial comparing the effects of amlodipine + angiotensin II receptor blocker and amlodipine + diuretics on the incidence of cardiovascular events, represented as a composite of non-fatal stroke, non-fatal myocardial infarction and cardiovascular death events in high-risk Chinese hypertensive patients."

"From October 2007 to October 2008, 13,542 patients were enrolled into the study in 180 centres in China."

Introduction

"[59] Therefore, an important key to reducing the burden of hypertension-related cardiovascular disease (CVD) is to increase the proportion of patients who achieve optimal BP control."

"Despite the availability of a large number of antihypertensive agents, the majority of patients with hypertension do not achieve the recommended target BP of <140/90 mm Hg (or <130/80 mm Hg for patients with certain comorbid conditions that increase the risk, that is, diabetes mellitus and chronic kidney disease) with antihypertensive monotherapy."

"The rationale for the CHIEF study is to try to intervene the overall risk factors of hypertension, and answer the following issues related to hypertension management: whether a newer combination of antihypertensive agents, CCB and ARB, can produce greater benefits in terms of reducing cardiovascular events than the combination of CCB and diuretics; whether lipid lowering with a statin provides additional beneficial effects in those hypertensive patients with a high–normal level of serum total cholesterol."

Materials and Methods

"Hypertension patients aged 50–79 years were eligible if their BP was 140–179/90–109 mm Hg at randomization after a 2-weeks run-in period."

"Patients with any of the following conditions were excluded from this study: secondary hypertension; history of cerebrovascular events or MI within 3 months before registration; severe cardiomyopathy or significant valvular disease; unstable angina; severe liver disease or nephropathy (alanine aminotransferase (ALT) elevation >2 × ULN or serum creatinine >2.5 mg per 100 ml); malignant tumor; gout; pregnancy or women not using contraceptives; uncontrolled diabetes (fasting plasma glucose >10 mmol l^{-1}, despite therapy); known allergies or contraindications to study drugs; considered to be unsuitable for participation in the clinical trial according to the investigator's opinion."

"All patients with a systolic BP (SBP) of 140–179 mm Hg and/or a diastolic BP (DBP) of 90–109 mm Hg were randomized to treatment."

Results

"Patient recruitment ended in October 2008, by which time 13,542 patients had been randomized to the two antihypertensive treatment regimens."

"Of these, 9913 patients were further randomized to lipid-lowering treatment or to the standard management group."

"The average BP at screening and randomization was 149/89 and 157/93 mm Hg, respectively."

"About 92% patients were taking antihypertensive drugs before randomization."

Discussion

"CHIEF will help to define the place of the two different treatment strategies for the lowering of BP, both alone and in combination with lipid-lowering therapy and lifestyle intervention, in the prevention of cardiovascular outcomes."

"The CHIEF study was designed to manage the hypertensive patients on the basis of an extensive intervention of the overall risk, including an initial low dose of combined antihypertensive therapy, low-dose statin-based lipid-lowering treatment and lifestyle intervention."

"There were a number of large-scale randomized clinical trials involving combination treatment, such as ACCOMPLISH (Avoiding Cardiovascular events through COMbination therapy in Patients LIving with Systolic Hypertension), [60, 61] ONTARGET (Ongoing Telmisartan Alone and in combination with Ramipril Global Endpoint Trial) [62] and ASCOT."

"Lipid-lowering treatment in hypertensive patients could exert additional effects on the prevention of cardiovascular disease."

"Combination therapy is a key treatment strategy, and the management of patients with hypertension is moving towards integrated intervention."

ARB-Based Single-Pill Platform to Guide a Practical Therapeutic Approach to Hypertensive Patients [63]

This is a machine-generated summary of:

Volpe, Massimo; de la Sierra, Alejandro; Kreutz, Reinhold; Laurent, Stéphane; Manolis, Athanasios J.: ARB-Based Single-Pill Platform to Guide a Practical Therapeutic Approach to Hypertensive Patients [63].

Published in: High Blood Pressure & Cardiovascular Prevention (2014).

Link to original: https://doi.org/10.1007/s40292-014-0043-6

If you want to cite the papers, please refer to the original.

For technical reasons we could not place the page where the original quote is coming from.

Abstract-Summary "Effective treatment of high blood pressure is an important strategy for reducing disease burden; however, in spite of the availability of numerous effective therapies only 30–40% of patients with hypertension achieve the recommended blood pressure goals of <140/90 mmHg."

"Adherence is closely related to the tolerability, effectiveness and complexity of therapy."

"Therapeutic inertia may be influenced by concerns over tolerability, as well as the lack of clear preferences for therapies when managing patients with risk factors and comorbidities."

"Effective and well-tolerated single pill combination therapies are now available that improve adherence and simplify treatment."

"The combination of a renin-angiotensin system blocker with a calcium channel blocker and a diuretic improves adherence to therapy."

"We have devised a practical tool for orienting the application of well-tolerated single pill 2/3 drug fixed dose combination therapies in clinical situations commonly encountered when treating hypertensive patients."

Introduction

"Less than one third of patients achieve control on monotherapy and most hypertensive patients who do achieve BP targets require a combination of at least two antihypertensive drugs."

"Rational and effective single pill 2/3 drug fixed dose combination therapy represents an excellent strategy for improving blood pressure control and is one of the key elements in a successful large-scale hypertension program that achieved an 80% BP control rate in over half a million patients [64]."

"We propose a platform approach for orienting single-pill 2/3 drug fixed dose combination therapies that considers risk factors and organ damage, as well as the grade of hypertension."

"It is a way to apply the guidelines to clinical practice by matching the appropriate single pill 2/3 drug fixed dose combinations with the various situations encountered when treating hypertensive patients."

Platform Organisation

"The platform is organised to match a suggested therapy intensity range with the corresponding level of CV risk."

"Achieving BP control is more urgent in patients with higher CV risk and such patients may benefit from higher dosages and/or combination therapy."

"After assessing a patient for the presence of risk factors, clinical or subclinical organ damage and BP, the appropriate intensity of therapy can be identified from the table."

"Therapy intensity, in terms of dosage range and combination, increases from left to right, in correspondence with increasing hypertension grade."

"Patients with additional risk factors such as smoking, family history of premature cardiovascular disease or age >55 for men (>65 for women) may benefit from more intense therapy, if appropriate, and a lower threshold for stepping up therapy."

Hypertensive Patients with Cardiovascular Risk Factors or Subclinical Organ Damage

"A pooled analysis of two randomised clinical trials comparing OM and the ACE inhibitor ramipril in 1,435 elderly hypertensive patients age 65–89 revealed that OM was more effective at reducing BP."

"The randomised ROADMAP study investigated the effect of OM 40 mg/day on the development of microalbuminuria, an early marker for kidney disease, in 4,000 hypertensive and normotensive diabetic patients who were at high risk of developing kidney disease."

"A subgroup analysis of the Triple Therapy with Olmesartan Medoxomil, Amlodipine, and Hydrochlorothiazide in Hypertensive Patients Study (TRINITY) revealed that diabetic patients responded as well as non-diabetic patients to triple therapy with OM/AML/HCTZ, with significantly more patients reaching the target BP (in this study <130/80 mmHg), while the frequency of adverse events was similar in both groups [65]."

"A subgroup analysis of the PB-CRUSH study also assessed the efficacy and safety of step-up fixed-dose combination therapy with OM/AML ± HCTZ assessed at 4-weekly intervals and intensified if needed in hypertensive patients with type 2 diabetes [66]."

Hypertensive Patients with Clinically Overt Organ Damage

"A subgroup analysis of the Avoiding Cardiovascular events through COMbination therapy in Patients LIving with Systolic Hypertension (ACCOMPLISH) study reveals that the combination of a RAS blocker and a CCB was more effective than a RAS blocker-diuretic combination at slowing the progression of nephropathy [67]."

"Controlling hypertension may prevent the development of heart failure or atrial fibrillation. The platform envisions starting low dose therapy with OM for grade 1 hypertension and stepping up therapy to an intermediate intensity by increasing OM dosage or switching to a fixed dose combination with OM/AML."

"Patients who have had a stroke or transient ischaemic attack are likely to be receiving antithrombotic therapy, which makes BP control very important for the prevention of bleeding."

"Controlling BP is important because many of these patients will be receiving antithrombotic therapy and hypertension is a risk factor for bleeding."

Conclusions

"Effective and well-tolerated single pill 2/3 drug fixed dose combination therapies have the potential to greatly improve BP control and close the gap between the promising results from interventional trials and the disappointing signs from routine clinical practice."

"Their success depends on how well they are applied."

"With this exercise, we have attempted to match the appropriate therapeutic intensity range to cardiovascular risk in situations commonly encountered when treating hypertensive patients."

"We believe it will increase the percentage of hypertensive patients who achieve blood pressure control and ultimately reduce the burden of cardiovascular, cerebrovascular and renal diseases when applied as part of a comprehensive approach that includes regular follow-up and timely therapy intensification as needed."

The Comparative Efficacy and Safety of the Angiotensin Receptor Blockers in the Management of Hypertension and Other Cardiovascular Diseases [68]

This is a machine-generated summary of:

Abraham, Hazel Mae A.; White, C. Michael; White, William B.: The Comparative Efficacy and Safety of the Angiotensin Receptor Blockers in the Management of Hypertension and Other Cardiovascular Diseases [68].

Published in: Drug Safety (2014).

Link to original: https://doi.org/10.1007/s40264-014-0239-7

If you want to cite the papers, please refer to the original.

For technical reasons we could not place the page where the original quote is coming from.

Abstract-Summary "All national guidelines for the management of hypertension recommend angiotensin receptor blockers (ARBs) as an initial or add-on antihypertensive therapy."

"Additive blood pressure-lowering effects have been demonstrated when ARBs are combined with thiazide diuretics or dihydropyridine calcium channel blockers, augmenting hypertension control."

"ARBs are very well tolerated as monotherapy, as well as in combination with other antihypertensive medications, which improve adherence to therapy and have become a mainstay in the treatment of stage 1 and stage 2 hypertension."

Introduction

"Recent hypertension guidelines recommend that diuretics, calcium channel blockers (CCBs), angiotensin receptor blockers (ARBs) and angiotensin-converting enzyme (ACE) inhibitors are all appropriate initial antihypertensive therapies for most people."

"ACE inhibitors or ARBs are advocated for people with stage I–II hypertension and type 1 or 2 diabetes [69]."

"ARBs have been in clinical use since 1995 and are known to be effective antihypertensive agents with excellent tolerability profiles."

"We also present pertinent research trials comparing the antihypertensive effects and cardiovascular benefits of ARBs, including the safety and tolerability issues encountered."

Pharmacology of Angiotensin Receptor Blockers

"The four classes of medications that are involved in this pathway include ACE inhibitors, angiotensin II receptor blockers (ARBs), aldosterone antagonists and direct renin inhibitors."

"The interest in this pathway is due to the action of angiotensin II on the vascular system, renal sodium and water handling, and cellular proliferation [70]."

"Inhibition of ACE only partially inhibits formation of angiotensin II."

"Angiotensin II activates two types of angiotensin II receptors (ATR): ATR_1 and ATR_2."

"Animal studies show that ATR_2 stimulation improves cardiac function and prevents cardiac remodelling post-myocardial infarction [71]."

"ARBs have more affinity for ATR_1 than for ATR_2 and can block the activities of angiotensin II on ATR_1 regardless of whether it was created from ACE or other enzymes such as cardiac chymase."

"Higher concentrations of angiotensin II cannot overcome the effect of an insurmountable ARB, but the impact of surmountability of ATR_1 blockade on final health outcomes has not been established [72]."

Pharmacokinetic Considerations

"Losartan undergoes first-pass metabolism in the liver via the CYP system to form its active metabolite EXP-3174, which is 10–40 times more potent than losartan when given intravenously [73]."

"Fluconazole, a CYP2C9 inhibitor, increases the half-life of EXP-3174 but reduces its biological creation from losartan to a greater extent, decreasing its area under the curve (AUC) and C_{max} by 47 and 30%, respectively."

"Three ARBs (candesartan cilexetil, olmesartan medoxomil and azilsartan medoxomil) are prodrugs and require activation in the gastrointestinal tract and liver to their active forms (candesartan, olmesartan and azilsartan, respectively) [74, 75]."

"The C_{max} of olmesartan is increased by 14% in elderly patients, but this is not clinically significant."

"The mean AUC of olmesartan is also significantly increased in patients with severe renal impairment (creatinine clearance <20 mL/min) and, while caution is advised, dose adjustment is not recommended [76]."

Efficacy of Angiotensin Receptor Blockers

"In the nine trials assessing the impact of adding a thiazide diuretic to an ARB versus the diuretic alone, combination therapy reduced the systolic and diastolic BP values significantly more than diuretic monotherapy (at equivalent doses) after 6–12 weeks [77–79]."

"Trials have shown that the addition of amlodipine to an ARB resulted in greater BP reductions than each component at similar doses."

"Calhoun and others [80] published the first large-scale randomized controlled trial involving patients with stage I–II hypertension (entry BP ≥145/100 mmHg), assessing the efficacy of triple therapy with valsartan, amlodipine and hydrochlorothiazide versus dual therapy with its components."

"The TRINITY trial involved 2,492 randomized patients and showed that triple therapy with olmesartan/amlodipine/hydrochlorothiazide at 40/10/25 mg/day resulted in a 37/22 mmHg reduction in mean BP, compared with 27.5/15, 30/17 and 30/18 mmHg BP reductions with amlodipine/hydrochlorothiazide 10/25 mg/day, olmesartan/hydrochlorothiazide 40/25 mg/day and olmesartan/amlodipine 40/10 mg/day dual therapies, respectively (all $p < 0.001$)."

Use of Multiple Renin–Angiotensin Blockers

"A meta-analysis comprising 38 randomized controlled trials showed no mortality benefit associated with dual ARB and ACE inhibitor therapy, and did reveal an increase in nonfatal adverse events, including hyperkalaemia (potassium level ≥6.0 mmol/L; relative risk [RR] 1.66 [95% confidence interval (CI) 1.38–1.98], $p < 0.001$), hypotension (RR 1.66 [95% CI 1.38–1.98], $p < 0.001$) and increased risk of a decline in renal function (creatinine >2.0 mg/dL; RR 1.41 [95% CI 1.09–1.84], p = 0.01) versus ARB or ACE inhibitor therapy alone [81]."

"The trial was terminated prematurely because of a lack of benefit and an increase in hyperkalaemia (potassium level ≥6.0 mm/L; 11.2% in the aliskiren arm versus 7.2% in the placebo arm, p < 0.001) and reported hypotension (12.1% in the aliskiren arm versus 8.3% in the placebo arm, p < 0.001) [82]."

[Section 6]

"In the Losartan Intervention for Endpoint Reduction in Hypertension (LIFE) trial, losartan was found to reduce cardiovascular morbidity and death by 13%, compared with the beta blocker atenolol (p = 0.021), despite similar reductions in BP among hypertensive patients with left ventricular hypertrophy [83]."

"In the Study on Cognition and Prognosis in the Elderly (SCOPE) [84], involving 4,964 participants aged 70–89 years with hypertension, candesartan (versus placebo) did not result in a significant risk reduction in major cardiovascular events, including myocardial infarction and cardiovascular mortality, but nonfatal stroke was reduced by 27.8% (95% CI 1.3–47.2, p = 0.04)."

"After 56 months of follow-up, telmisartan resulted in fewer major cardiovascular events compared with placebo (15.7 versus 17.0%), but the result was not statistically significant (HR 0.92 [95% CI 0.81–1.05], p = 0.216)."

Angiotensin Receptor Blockers in Diabetes and Kidney Disease

"The Irbesartan in Patients with Type 2 Diabetes and Microalbuminuria (IRMA 2) trial showed that over 1 year in patients with hypertension, type 2 diabetes mellitus and microalbuminuria, fewer participants progressed to macroalbuminuria among patients treated with irbesartan compared with placebo, with hazard ratios (HRs) of 0.30 in the irbesartan 300 mg/day group (95% CI 0.14–0.61, p < 0.001) and 0.61 in the irbesartan 150 mg/day group (95% CI 0.34–1.08, p = 0.08) [85]."

"In the Irbesartan Diabetic Nephropathy Trial (IDNT) involving hypertensive patients with diabetic nephropathy, the irbesartan arm had a 37% lower risk of doubling serum creatinine versus the amlodipine arm (p < 0.001) and 33% lower than the placebo group (p = 0.003)."

Angiotensin Receptor Blockers in Post-myocardial Infarction and Heart Failure Patients

"In the Losartan Heart Failure Survival Study (ELITE II), losartan 50 mg/day was not found to be superior to captopril 150 mg/day (given in three doses) in reducing all-cause mortality in patients with New York Heart Association (NYHA) class II–IV heart failure and a left ventricular ejection fraction (LVEF) ≤40%."

"The Optimal Trial in Myocardial Infarction with the Angiotensin II Antagonist Losartan (OPTIMAAL) Study demonstrated that another ARB, losartan, was comparable to captopril in reducing overall mortality in patients with a history of myocardial infarction and heart failure with left ventricular dysfunction (LVEF <35%; RR 1.13 [95% CI 0.99–1.28], p = 0.07) [86]."

"The Candesartan in Heart Failure Assessment of Reduction in Mortality and Morbidity (CHARM) study was actually composed of three trials: CHARM-Alternative (LVEF ≤40% and ACE intolerant) versus placebo; CHARM-Added (LVEF ≤40% in patients already on ACE inhibitors); and CHARM-Preserved (LVEF >40%) and were also placebo controlled [87]."

Safety and Tolerability of ARBs in Hypertension

"The ARB eprosartan was studied by Sachse and others [77], who reported 65 out of 157 patients (41.4%) having an adverse event, of which 19 were probably treatment related in the eprosartan monotherapy group (600 mg/day), compared with 69 out of 152 patients (45.4%), of which 25 were probably treatment related in the eprosartan/hydrochlorothiazide combination group (600/12.5 mg/day)."

"In a trial involving olmesartan/hydrochlorothiazide combinations of 40/25, 20/25, 40/12.5 and 20/12.5 mg/day, no differences in adverse events by treatment group thought to be related to drug were reported."

"Fogari and others [88] reported that 3.9% of patients in an olmesartan/hydrochlorothiazide 40/12.5 mg/day group had drug-related adverse events, compared with 0.7% in the olmesartan 40 mg/day monotherapy treatment arm."

"Neldam and Edwards [89] reported comparable drug-related adverse event rates with telmisartan/hydrochlorothiazide 80/25 and 80/12.5 mg/day (5.7 versus 5.0%), resulting in discontinuation rates of 1.7 and 3.0%, respectively."

Safety of Angiotensin Receptor Blockers in Outcome Studies or Analyses

"This analysis showed an increased risk of new cancers in the ARB group [7.2 versus 6.0%, RR 1.08 (95% CI 1.01–1.15), p = 0.016] versus control therapy (placebo, ACE inhibitors or beta blockers), with an absolute risk of 1.2% over an average of 4 years."

"ARB use was not associated with an increased risk of cancer mortality, compared with ACE inhibitor use (adjusted RR 0.77 [95% CI 0.72–0.82]) [90]."

"After a mean follow-up of 4.6 years, ARB use was not found to increase the overall risk of cancer (adjusted HR 1.03 [95% CI 0.99–1.06], p = 0.10) versus ACE inhibitors."

Conclusions

"While there are theoretical benefits of combining ARBs with ACE inhibitors (e.g. proteinuria reduction), event-driven trials have not shown a benefit and in fact have demonstrated increases in adverse renal events."

"There is no clinical rationale for combining ARBs with ACE inhibitors (or direct renin inhibitors) in the management of hypertension."

"The excellent safety and tolerability profile of the ARB class has improved the adherence to antihypertensive therapy and enhanced our ability to manage hypertension in those patients with sensitivities to other antihypertensive drug classes, including ACE inhibitors."

Association Between Renin–Angiotensin–Aldosterone System Blockade and Clinical Outcomes in Patients with Hypertension: Real-World Observation from a Nationwide Hypertension Cohort [91]

This is a machine-generated summary of:

Park, Chan Soon; Kim, Bongseong; Rhee, Tae-Min; Lee, Hyun Jung; Lee, Hee-Sun; Park, Jun-Bean; Kim, Yong-Jin; Han, Kyung-Do; Kim, Hyung-Kwan: Association between renin–angiotensin–aldosterone system blockade and clinical outcomes in patients with hypertension: real-world observation from a nationwide hypertension cohort [91].

Published in: Clinical Research in Cardiology (2023).

Link to original: https://doi.org/10.1007/s00392-023-02179-3

If you want to cite the papers, please refer to the original.

For technical reasons we could not place the page where the original quote is coming from.

Abstract-Summary "Patients were allocated into ACEi, ARB, and non-RASi groups and followed until 2019."

"Patients on ACEi and ARB showed unfavorable baseline characteristics compared to those on non-RASi."

"After adjusting for covariates, the ACEi group showed lower risks of MI, AF, and all-cause deaths (HR (95% CI): 0.94 (0.89–0.99), 0.96 (0.92–1.00), and 0.93 (0.90–0.96), respectively), but similar risks of IS and HF (0.97 (0.92–1.01) and 1.03 (1.00–1.06), respectively), compared to the non-RASi group."

"The ARB group showed decreased risks of MI, IS, AF, HF, and all-cause deaths (HR (95% CI): 0.93 (0.91–0.95), 0.88 (0.86–0.90), 0.86 (0.85–0.88), 0.94 (0.93–0.96), and 0.84 (0.83–0.85)), compared to the non-RASi group."

"In the propensity score matching (PSM) cohort, the ARB group showed similar risks of MI and decreased risks of IS, AF, HF, and all-cause deaths compared to the ACEi group."

"ACEi and ARB users were associated with decreased risks of MI, IS, AF, HF, and all-cause deaths, compared to non-RASi users."

Introduction

"Hypertension is a leading global disease burden with a profound clinical impact, given its high prevalence and associated cardiovascular events [92, 93]."

"RASi showed beneficial effects on blood pressure lowering and associated cardiovascular events reduction [94–96]."

"Several studies showed similar findings, which is the so-called "ARB-MI paradox"; that is, ARB might not be as effective as ACEi in preventing MI despite other cardiovascular benefits [24, 97]."

"We investigated the association between the use of ACEi, ARB, or antihypertensive medications other than RASi (non-RASi) and incident cardiovascular events, including MI, ischemic stroke (IS), atrial fibrillation (AF), heart failure (HF), and all-cause deaths in an unselected nationwide hypertension cohort."

Methods

"Patients with hypertension were defined as follows: (1) having at least one claim per year for a prescription of antihypertensive medication under ICD-10-CM codes, that is, I10-I13 and I15, from the insurance claims data or (2) systolic blood pressure $\geq$ 140 mmHg and/or diastolic blood pressure $\geq$ 90 mmHg with the aforementioned ICD-10-CM codes [98, 99]."

"Variables that could potentially affect the clinical outcomes (such as age, sex, BMI, a previous history of diabetes mellitus, dyslipidemia, chronic kidney disease, angina pectoris, systolic blood pressure, diastolic blood pressure, smoking, alcohol consumption, physical activity, levels of total cholesterol, low-density lipoprotein cholesterol, high-density lipoprotein cholesterol, triglyceride, fasting blood glucose, glomerular filtration rates, proteinuria, aspirin use, use of statins, use of P2Y12 inhibitors, hypertension duration $\geq$ 5 years, and the proportion of patients taking a combination of $\geq$ 3 antihypertensive medications) were included in the logistic regression model to produce propensity scores for each participant."

Results

"After adjusting for covariates, the ACEi group showed lower risks of MI (HR 0.94, 95% CI 0.89–0.99), AF (HR 0.96, 95% CI 0.92–1.00), and all-cause deaths (HR 0.93, 95% CI 0.90–0.96), but similar risks of IS (HR 0.97, 95% CI 0.92–1.01) and HF (HR 1.03, 95% CI 1.00–1.06) compared to those in the non-RASi group."

"The ACEi group showed lower risks of AF (HR 0.95, 95% CI 0.90–1.00) and all-cause deaths (HR 0.92, 95% CI 0.88–0.96), and similar risks of MI (HR 0.95, 95% CI 0.89–1.01), IS (HR 0.97, 95% CI 0.92–1.03), and HF (HR 1.02, 95% CI 0.98–1.06) compared to the non-RASi group."

Discussion

"According to the sensitivity analysis performed in patients taking a single antihypertensive medication, ACEi users showed reduced risks of IS, AF, and all-cause deaths, but similar risks of MI and HF, while ARB users showed reduced risks of all analyzed endpoints compared to the non-RASi group."

"When the clinical benefits provided by ACEi and ARB were compared in the PSM cohort, ARB users showed lower risks of IS, AF, HF, and all-cause deaths and similar risks of MI compared to ACEi users."

"In this large-scale longitudinal cohort study, hypertensive patients taking ACEi or ARB were associated with reduced cardiovascular risks compared to those taking non-RASi despite their unfavorable baseline characteristics, such as a more frequent history of diabetes mellitus, dyslipidemia, chronic kidney disease, and preponderance of smoking."

Conclusion

"Despite unfavorable baseline characteristics, the use of either ACEi or ARB was associated with a decreased risk of cardiovascular events compared to non-RASi use in this large nationwide hypertension cohort."

"In the PSM cohort, patients on ARB showed similar risks of MI, but lower risks of IS, AF, HF, and all-cause deaths compared to those on ACEi."

The Impact of the 'Better Care Better Value' Prescribing Policy on the Utilisation of Angiotensin-Converting Enzyme Inhibitors and Angiotensin Receptor Blockers for Treating Hypertension in the UK Primary Care Setting: Longitudinal Quasi-Experimental Design [100]

This is a machine-generated summary of:

Baker, Amanj; Chen, Li-Chia; Elliott, Rachel A.; Godman, Brian: The impact of the 'Better Care Better Value' prescribing policy on the utilisation of angiotensin-converting enzyme inhibitors and angiotensin receptor blockers for treating hypertension in the UK primary care setting: longitudinal quasi-experimental design [100].

Published in: BMC Health Services Research (2015).

Link to original: https://doi.org/10.1186/s12913-015-1013-y

If you want to cite the papers, please refer to the original.

For technical reasons we could not place the page where the original quote is coming from.

Abstract-Summary "Little is known about the actual impact of the BCBV indicator on ACEIs/ARBs utilisation and cost-savings."

"This study aimed to evaluate the impact of BCBV policy on ACEIs/ARBs utilisation and cost-savings, including exploration of regional variations of the policy's impact."

"Segmented time-series analysis was applied to monthly ACEIs prescription proportion, adjusted number of ACEIs/ARBs prescriptions and costs."

"The proportion of ACEIs prescription decreased during the study period from 71.2% in April/2006 to 70.7% in March/2012, with a small but a statistically significant pre-policy reduction in its monthly trend of 0.02% ($p < 0.001$)."

"Instantly after its initiation, the policy was associated with a sudden reduction in the proportion of ACEIs prescription; however, it resulted in a statistically significant increase in the post-policy monthly trend of ACEIs prescription proportion of 0.013% ($p < 0.001$), resulting in an overall post-policy slope of −0.007%."

"The pre-policy trend of the adjusted number of ACEIs/ARBs prescriptions was increasing; however, their trends declined after the policy implementation."

"The policy affected neither total ACEIs/ARBs cost nor individual ACEIs or ARBs costs."

"ACEIs/ARBs utilisation was not affected by the BCBV policy."

"The small increase in post-policy ACEIs prescription proportion was not associated with any savings."

Background

"The Prescription Cost Analysis (PCA) of England-2011, issued by the Health and Social Care Information Centre of the UK, considered ACEIs/ARBs as being the second most commonly prescribed drug class in English primary care, accounting for 6% of all prescribed drugs [101]."

"Even more than a decade later, the National Audit Office (NAO) report concerning prescribing costs in primary care in the UK in 2007 [102] found that a potential cost saving of more than GB£200 million a year could be achieved, without compromising the quality of care, through efficient prescribing in four therapeutic drug classes, including RAS drugs."

"This study aimed to evaluate the impact of the BCBV prescribing policy on ACEIs/ARBs utilisation and cost-saving for treating hypertension in the UK primary care setting and to explore potential regional variations of the policy's impact."

Methods

"Data from PCA of England in June 2014 [103], the most up-to-date data available at the date of submission, which contains the number of dispensed antihypertensive drug prescriptions and their costs, were also analysed to estimate the impact of the availability of low cost generic ARBs on the potential cost-saving of BCBV policy if the 80% target had been achieved in June 2014 in England."

"To validate the study results, the quarterly trends in the number of ACEIs/ARBs prescriptions and other antihypertensive drug classes were also compared with the quarterly England dispensing data, which contains the number of antihypertensive drugs prescriptions dispensed in the primary care setting in England for treatment of all conditions, and obtained directly from the Health and Social Care Information Centre (HSCIC) [104]."

Results

"There was a significant reduction in the monthly trend of ACEIs prescription proportion (β_1: −0.02%, $p < 0.001$) before the implementation of BCBV policy, and the level of ACEIs prescription proportion further reduced when the policy was implemented (β_2: −0.3%, $p < 0.001$)."

"A potential cost-saving of 23.9% (GB£227,593) of the total ACEIs/ARBs costs would have been made in March 2012 if the ACEIs prescriptions' proportion of 80% of total RAS had been achieved, instead of the current value of 70.7%, based on the total ACEIs/ARBs costs of GB£1,178,674 and the number of ACEIs prescriptions of 174,153 and ARBs prescriptions of 72,240 in March 2012."

"Although the policy had no instant impact on the level (β_2) of ACEIs prescriptions' proportion, it resulted in a significant increase in the trend of the ACEI prescriptions' proportion thereafter (β_3: 0.1%, $p < 0.001$)."

Discussion

"It could be argued that the observed lack of policy effectiveness merely reflects the fact that the encouragement of prescribing low cost generic ACEIs against patented ARBs was the subject of health authorities (HAs) in the UK some time before the launch of this BCBV policy, as seen in Scotland [105]."

"Due to the current lack of national multiple initiatives in the UK, it would be unlikely that losartan utilisation and ARBs prescribing efficiency would be improved further until more ARBs lose their patents, This would support why achieving the proposed BCBV target of 80% ACEIs could still achieve potential cost-savings in the short term, even after years of losing the cost differential between ACEIs and ARBs."

Conclusions

"The BCBV policy did not change the overall ACEIs/ARBs utilisation patterns in patients with primary hypertension."

"Intensive and specific measures would be required to enhance the policy implementation and uptake, given the existing opportunity for potential saving by further improving the efficient prescribing of ACEIs/ARBs despite the availability of low cost generic ARBs."

"This could be a key learning point for other healthcare authorities to emphasise requirements for effective implementation strategies as well as the principle policy itself."

"Further research is needed to explore the potential factors underpinning the policy ineffectiveness, and identify the most effective strategies to improve future policy effectiveness."

Temperature, Cardiovascular Mortality, and the Role of Hypertension and Renin–Angiotensin–Aldosterone Axis in Seasonal Adversity: A Narrative Review [106]

This is a machine-generated summary of:

Goel, Harsh; Shah, Kashyap; Kumar, Ashish; Hippen, John T.; Nadar, Sunil K.: Temperature, cardiovascular mortality, and the role of hypertension and renin–angiotensin–aldosterone axis in seasonal adversity: a narrative review [106].

Published in: Journal of Human Hypertension (2022).

Link to original: https://doi.org/10.1038/s41371-022-00707-8

If you want to cite the papers, please refer to the original.

For technical reasons we could not place the page where the original quote is coming from.

Abstract-Summary "Hypertension—the most important CV risk factor—has seasonal variation such that BP is significantly higher in winter."

"Besides worsening BP control in established hypertensives, cold-induced BP increase also contributes to long-term BP variability among normotensive and prehypertensive patients, also a known CV risk factor."

"Disappointingly, despite the now well-established impact of temperature on BP and on CV mortality separately, direct linkage between seasonal BP change and CV outcomes remains preliminary."

"Proving or disproving this link is of immense clinical and public health importance because if seasonal BP variation contributes to seasonal adversity, this should be a modifiable risk."

"Existing evidence strongly suggests a central role of the sympathetic nervous system (SNS), and secondarily, the renin–angiotensin–aldosterone axis (RAAS) in mediating cold-induced BP increase."

"This review aims to summarize the current evidence linking temperature, BP and CV outcomes."

Introduction

"The most significant and direct impact of this has been on global mean temperatures, which have increased by an average of ≈1.8 °F (1.0 °C) between 1901 and 2016, making this the warmest period in the history of modern civilization [107]."

"Beyond rising average global temperatures, extreme weather events such as heat and cold waves, flooding, droughts, and extreme weather phenomena have been increasing in frequency and severity, and are anticipated to continue to do so over the coming decades [108]."

"The ultimate impact of climate change on temperature extremes, mean temperatures, and extreme weather events will vary by region, depending upon a host of local geographic and climatic characteristics."

"Among the myriad cause-effect relationships between climate variables and adverse health consequences, the impact of temperature on cardiovascular (CV) health, specifically, is important, because (1) increasing temperature is perhaps the most important aspect of climate change, and (2) cardiovascular disease (CVD) remains the top cause of mortality around the world."

Temperature, Mortality, and Cardiovascular Disease

"The relationship between temperature and mortality is U- or J-shaped, with a progressive increase in mortality above and below the MMT [109–114]. Hence, studies examining the impact of heat and cold separately have both found significant associations with adversity."

"In the context of climate change, several projections regarding temperature-attributable mortality have been made for the next century under diverse climate change scenarios, ranging from a conservative 0.5 °C to an unmitigated 5 °C global mean temperature rise [115–118]. Unsurprisingly, all but the most conservative models (i.e. models with <1 °C increase in temperature over the next century) generally project a decline in cold and increase in heat attributable deaths, though with significant spatio-temporal heterogeneity."

"Notwithstanding these projections, given that current cold-related mortality burden is 9–10 times that for heat, cold is projected to contribute significantly to temperature-attributable adversity even by the end of the century [117, 119]."

Temperature and Blood Pressure: A Link to Cardiovascular Mortality?

"Emerging evidence suggests that cold-induced increase in CV mortality is indeed significantly mediated by winter-time BP increase."

"To the now fairly well-established role of SNS, RAAS involvement in cold-induced BP increase has been somewhat contradictory, with some researchers finding elevated renin, angiotensin II (Ang-II), and/or aldosterone levels with acute cold exposure [120, 121], and others not [122–124]."

"Inhibition of SNS-mediated RAAS activation by bilateral renal denervation abolished cold-induced renin increase and attenuated cold-induced BP rise, suggesting that though SNS provides the major impetus for RAAS activation in response to cold, the latter is a significant driver of such response [125]."

"Though several metabolic, inflammatory, and endothelial perturbations have been described in response to cold in addition to a rise in BP, and likely contribute to the now well-established seasonal CV mortality increase, these perturbations do not exclude, and perhaps even are consistent with the SNS/RAAS axis being the central driving force for seasonal adversity."

Mitigating the Impact of Seasonal BP on Seasonal Mortality

"A cross-sectional study from rural China (annual temperature range −2.9 to 33.7 °C), a region lacking widespread indoor climate control, found a summer-winter SBP/DBP difference of as much as 19.2/7 mmHg, causing a 14% higher prevalence of HTN and 13% of hypertensives suffering worsening of BP control during winter [126]."

"Given the finding that those with ≥9–10 mmHg winter increase in BP do indeed suffer significantly worse outcomes than those with a lesser degree change [127, 128], such patients should be identified proactively for specific mitigation measures, whether lifestyle or pharmacologic."

"The summer-winter BP difference was significantly smaller (SBP/DBP difference ≈3.5–4/1.2–2 mmHg) among patients in whom drug therapy was titrated early during change of season, compared to those in whom titration occurred mid-season (SBP/DBP difference ≈7/3 mmHg)."

Conclusion and Areas Begging Urgent Research

"Several gaps in our knowledge remain and need urgent investigation, including (1) further elucidation of seasonal BP variability in different climate zones, not only as change in BP per °C change in temperature, as most studies so far have done, but also as to how that changes the prevalence of HTN during winter versus summer, or that of uncontrolled HTN among treated hypertensives, (2) further elucidation of impact of seasonal BP variation on outcomes, both among those that are purely seasonally hypertensive, and among established hypertensives who experience significant worsening of BP control during winter, (3) continued investigation of mechanisms underlying seasonal BP change, and most importantly (4) outcomes-based research on the efficacy of seasonal titration of drug therapy in general, and ACEI/ARB therapy in particular, with special focus on populations most vulnerable to seasonal BP change and CV events (elderly, those living in lower latitudes)."

Single-Pill Combination with Three Antihypertensive Agents to Improve Blood Pressure Control in Hypertension: Focus on Olmesartan-Based Combinations [129]

This is a machine-generated summary of:

Single-Pill Combination with Three Antihypertensive Agents to Improve Blood Pressure Control in Hypertension: Focus on Olmesartan-Based Combinations [129].

Published in: (2023).

Link to original: https://doi.org/10.1007/s40292-023-00563-8

Copyright of the summarized publication:

If you want to cite the papers, please refer to the original.

For technical reasons we could not place the page where the original quote is coming from.

Abstract-Summary "Only about half of patients achieve their blood pressure (BP) targets and of these, the majority require combination and double or triple therapies."

"Among the various angiotensin receptor blockers, olmesartan (OM) is available as a monotherapy and in dual and triple single-pill combinations (SPCs) with amlodipine (AML) and/or hydrochlorothiazide (HCTZ)."

"Several phase III and IV studies, together with real-world studies, have demonstrated the additional benefits of combining OM either with AML or with HCTZ in terms of BP control and target BP achievements both in the general population and in special subgroups of hypertensive patients, such as the elderly, diabetic, chronic kidney disease or obese patients."

"The availability of OM combined with HCTZ, AML or both at different dosages makes it a valuable option to customize therapy based on the levels of BP and the clinical characteristics of hypertensive patients."

Introduction

"Blood pressure (BP) and the prevalence of raised BP have declined substantially in high-income regions but have continued to rise in low- and middle-income countries [130]."

"Even in high income countries, BP control among treated hypertensive adults remains poor with less than 50% of them having BP values at or below recommended targets [92]."

"More worrisome are recent observations indicating a recent decline in BP control in some patient groups such as the elderly, women and non-Hispanic blacks in the US [131] or women in France [132]."

Rationale for the Use of Single Pill Combinations

"Since polypharmacy and the complexity of treatments are two determining factors of poor adherence, simplifying drug regimens by using a single pill combination (SPC) has been proposed as a therapeutic strategy in hypertension to improve drug adherence [133–135], a strategy which has now been included in the most recent guidelines as will be discussed below [2, 136, 137]."

"The use of SPCs can also be associated with cost saving over using free combinations for many reasons, including fewer follow-up visits, and fewer hospitalizations for uncontrolled hypertension and cardiovascular events [134]."

"Adverse events with CCB and thiazides are strongly dose related [138], therefore their use at low doses in combination therapies can improve their tolerability profile."

"On these bases, recent guidelines recommend as a first-line therapy for the majority of patients in uncomplicated hypertension, a single-pill dual combination therapy based on an ACEi or an ARB and a calcium channel blocker (CCB) or a diuretic [2, 136, 137]."

Olmesartan Medoxomil-Based Combinations

"Among the various angiotensin receptor blockers, olmesartan medoxomil (OM) is available as a monotherapy and in dual and triple SPCs with amlodipine (AML) and/or hydrochlorothiazide (HCTZ)."

"Numerous phase III and phase IV studies have demonstrated the additional benefits of combining OM either with AML or with HCTZ in terms of BP control and target BP achievements [139–143]."

"Studies performed using 24 h ambulatory BP monitoring have also demonstrated that dual as well as triple OM-based SPCs induce a more sustained and smoother BP reduction than placebo and monotherapies [140]."

"In a prospective, double-blind, placebo-controlled, multicenter study, Fliser and others [144] have evaluated the anti-inflammatory effect of OM, alone or in combination with pravastatin, in patients with essential hypertension and signs of microinflammation (i.e. highly-sensitivity C-reactive protein (hsCRP) > 3 mg/L)."

Olmesartan-Based Available Combinations: Focus on Triple SPCs

"In the 44-week open-label extension of the 8-week, double-blind Combination of Olmesartan Medoxomil and Amlodipine Besylate in Controlling High Blood Pressure (COACH) study conducted in 1684 patients, OM-based combination therapy was titrated as needed up to OM/AML/HCTZ 10/40/12.5 and then to 10/40/25 mg in those patients who did not reach the BP target (<140/90 mmHg or <130/80 mmHg in patients with diabetes) [145]."

"The study demonstrated that in Korean patients with uncontrolled moderate hypertension treated first-line with the double combination (OM/HCTZ 20/12.5), the triple SPC (OM/AML/HCTZ 20/5/12.5) was associated with significant blood pressure reductions and greater achievement of blood pressure goals and was well tolerated [146, 147]."

"The RESOLVE-PRO study [148] demonstrated that OM/AML/HCTZ triple SPC treatment has significant efficacy in reducing BP and achieving BP control over the 1-year observation period in 3752 Korean hypertensive patients and it was well tolerated."

Olmesartan-Based Triple SPC: Impact on Adherence and Health-Related Quality of Life

"The AMTRAC study is an open-label RCT performed in China with 145 patients randomized to receive OM/AML/HCTZ or the equivalent combination of two pills [149]."

"The observational, retrospective cohort study, RESOLVE-PRO, conducted in more than 3500 hypertensive patients treated with OM/AML/HCTZ SPC for 1 year, confirmed the finding of a high percentage of days covered by the drug over 1 year with an SPC treatment."

"The SPC of OM/AML/HCTZ contributes to the improvement of Health-related quality of life, as demonstrated by a post-hoc analysis that was performed on the data from a 54-week phase III study to measure changes in the health-related quality of life (HRQoL) of 2,690 patients with moderate-to-severe hypertension who received OM/AML/HCTZ SPC [150]."

"This study showed that triple OM/AML/HCTZ SPC reduced BP and significantly increased BP control whilst improving patients' HRQoL."

OM-Based SPCs for a Patient-Oriented Therapy

"This platform can help to identify patients that can benefit from the different available combinations, in the context of a personalized therapeutic approach."

"Patients with specific risk factors, subclinical or overt organ damage could receive the right combination on the basis of clinical trials, guidelines, best practices and clinical experience, following an approach aimed at determining the appropriate therapeutic intensity based on concomitant conditions and thereby help physicians to tailor treatment strategies on an individual basis."

"The platform is organized to match the intensity of therapy (defined as the recommended dose range and type of association) with the appropriate grade of hypertension and the overall cardiovascular risk profile of an individual patient (which is achieved by assessing risk factors, subclinical organ damage or clinical conditions)."

"Such patients may benefit from higher doses and/or from combination therapy, potentially as first-line treatment [63, 151]."

Conclusion and Future Perspective

"To reduce the complexity of therapies and thus improve therapeutic adherence, they recommend that these combinations be administered as SPCs [2, 136, 137]."

"Among RAS blockers, the evidence presented indicates ARBs, alone or in combination, as appropriate in the treatment of hypertension [152]."

"Long lasting ARBs, such as OM, are more suitable for the purpose of SPCs which need to control BP over the 24 h [153]."

"The use of these combinations in a single pill provides benefits in terms of therapeutic adherence and quality of life and should simplify the management of hypertension by physicians."

Bibliography

1. Ojha U, Ruddaraju S, Sabapathy N et al (2022) Current and emerging classes of pharmacological agents for the management of hypertension. Am J Cardiovasc Drugs 22:271–285. https://doi.org/10.1007/s40256-021-00510-9
2. Whelton PK, Carey RM, Aronow WS, Casey DE, Collins KJ, Dennison Himmelfarb C et al (2018) 2017 ACC/AHA/AAPA/ABC/ACPM/AGS/APhA/ASH/ASPC/NMA/PCNA guideline for the prevention, detection, evaluation, and management of high blood pressure in adults: a report of the American College of Cardiology/American Heart Association task force on clinical practice guidelines. J Am Coll Cardiol 71(19):e127–e248. https://doi.org/10.1016/j.jacc.2017.11.006
3. Williams B, Mancia G (2018) Ten commandments of the 2018 ESC/ESH HTN guidelines on hypertension in adults. Eur Heart J 39:3007–3008. https://doi.org/10.1093/eurheartj/ehy439
4. Chen R, Suchard MA, Krumholz HM et al (2021) Comparative first-line effectiveness and safety of ACE (angiotensin-converting enzyme) inhibitors and angiotensin receptor blockers: a multinational cohort study. Hypertension 78(3):591–603
5. Reboussin DM, Allen NB, Griswold ME, Guallar E, Hong Y, Lackland DT, Miller EPR, Polonsky T, Thompson-Paul AM, Vupputuri S (2018) Systematic review for the 2017 ACC/AHA/AAPA/ABC/ACPM/AGS/APhA/ASH/ASPC/NMA/PCNA guideline for the prevention, detection, evaluation, and management of high blood pressure in adults: a report of the American College of Cardiology/American Heart Association task force on clinical practice guidelines. Hypertension 71:e116–e135
6. The ONTARGET Investigators (2008) Telmisartan, ramipril, or both in patients at high risk for vascular events. N Engl J Med 358:1547–1559
7. Li EC, Heran BS, Wright JM (2014) Angiotensin converting enzyme (ACE) inhibitors versus angiotensin receptor blockers for primary hypertension. Cochrane Database Syst Rev 2014:CD009096
8. Sanders GD, Coeytaux R, Dolor RJ, Hasselblad V, Patel UD, Powers B et al (2011) Angiotensin-converting enzyme inhibitors (ACEIs), angiotensin II receptor antagonists (ARBs), and direct renin inhibitors for treating essential hypertension: an update. Agency for Healthcare Research and Quality (US), Rockville (MD)

9. Bremner AD, Baur M, Oddou-Stock P, Bodin F (1997) Valsartan: long-term efficacy and tolerability compared to lisinopril in elderly patients with essential hypertension. Clin Exp Hypertens 19:1263–1285
10. Barnett AH, Bain SC, Bouter P, Karlberg B, Madsbad S, Jervell J, Mustonen J, Diabetics Exposed to Telmisartan and Enalapril Study Group (2004) Angiotensin-receptor blockade versus converting–enzyme inhibition in type 2 diabetes and nephropathy. N Engl J Med 351:1952–1961
11. Špinar J, Vítovec J, Souček M, Dušek L, Pavlík T (2010) CORD: COmparison of Recommended Doses of ace inhibitors and angiotensin II receptor blockers. Int J Cardiol 144:293–294
12. Potier L, Roussel R, Elbez Y, Marre M, Zeymer U, Reid CM, Ohman M, Eagle KA, Bhatt DL, Steg PG, REACH Registry Investigators* (2017) Angiotensin-converting enzyme inhibitors and angiotensin receptor blockers in high vascular risk. Heart 103:1339–1346
13. Strauss MH, Hall AS (2006) Angiotensin receptor blockers may increase risk of myocardial infarction. Circulation 114:838–854
14. Makani H, Messerli FH, Romero J, Wever-Pinzon O, Korniyenko A, Berrios RS, Bangalore S (2012) Meta-analysis of randomized trials of angioedema as an adverse event of renin-angiotensin system inhibitors. Am J Cardiol 110:383–391
15. Tseng DS, Kwong J, Rezvani F, Coates AO (2010) Angiotensin-converting enzyme-related cough among Chinese Americans. Am J Med 123:183.e11–183.e15
16. Hripcsak G, Ryan PB, Duke JD, Shah NH, Park RW, Huser V, Suchard MA, Schuemie MJ, DeFalco FJ, Perotte A et al (2016) Characterizing treatment pathways at scale using the OHDSI network. Proc Natl Acad Sci USA 113:7329–7336
17. Gu Q, Burt VL, Dillon CF, Yoon S (2012) Trends in antihypertensive medication use and blood pressure control among United States adults with hypertension: the National Health and Nutrition Examination Survey, 2001 to 2010. Circulation 126:2105–2114
18. Simões e Silva AC, Lanza K, Palmeira VA et al (2021) 2020 update on the renin–angiotensin–aldosterone system in pediatric kidney disease and its interactions with coronavirus. Pediatr Nephrol 36:1407–1426. https://doi.org/10.1007/s00467-020-04759-1
19. Turner JM, Kodali R (2020) Should angiotensin-converting enzyme inhibitors ever be used for the management of hypertension? Curr Cardiol Rep 22(9):95. https://doi.org/10.1007/s11886-020-01352-8
20. Ruilope L, Schaefer A (2013) The fixed-dose combination of olmesartan/amlodipine was superior in central aortic blood pressure reduction compared with perindopril/amlodipine: a randomized, double-blind trial in patients with hypertension. Adv Ther 30(12):1086–1099. https://doi.org/10.1007/s12325-013-0076-6
21. Bonner G, Bakris GL, Sica D, Weber MA, White WB, Perez A et al (2013) Antihypertensive efficacy of the angiotensin receptor blocker azilsartan medoxomil compared with the angiotensin-converting enzyme inhibitor ramipril. J Hum Hypertens 27(8):479–486
22. Omboni S, Malacco E, Mallion JM, Volpe M, Zanchetti A, Group S (2012) Twenty-four hour and early morning blood pressure control of olmesartan vs. ramipril in elderly hypertensive patients: pooled individual data analysis of two randomized, double-blind, parallel-group studies. J Hypertens 30(7):1468–1477. https://doi.org/10.1097/HJH.0b013e32835466ac
23. Matchar DB, McCrory DC, Orlando LA, Patel MR, Patel UD, Patwardhan MB et al (2008) Systematic review: comparative effectiveness of angiotensin-converting enzyme inhibitors and angiotensin II receptor blockers for treating essential hypertension. Ann Intern Med 148(1):16–29. https://doi.org/10.7326/0003-4819-148-1-200801010-00189
24. Bangalore S, Fakheri R, Toklu B, Ogedegbe G, Weintraub H, Messerli FH (2016) Angiotensin-converting enzyme inhibitors or angiotensin receptor blockers in patients without heart failure? Insights from 254,301 patients from randomized trials. Mayo Clin Proc 91:51–60. https://doi.org/10.1016/J.MAYOCP.2015.10.019

25. Savarese G, Costanzo P, Cleland JG, Vassallo E, Ruggiero D, Rosano G, Perrone-Filardi P (2013) A meta-analysis reporting effects of angiotensin-converting enzyme inhibitors and angiotensin receptor blockers in patients without heart failure. J Am Coll Cardiol 61:131–142
26. Cheng J, Zhang W, Zhang X, Han F, Li X, He X, Chen J (2014) Effect of angiotensin-converting enzyme inhibitors and angiotensin II receptor blockers on all-cause mortality, cardiovascular deaths, and cardiovascular events in patients with diabetes mellitus: a meta-analysis. JAMA Intern Med 174:773–785
27. Thomopoulos C, Parati G, Zanchetti A (2015) Effects of blood pressure lowering on outcome incidence in hypertension: 4. Effects of various classes of antihypertensive drugs–overview and meta-analyses. J Hypertens 33(2):195–211
28. Pitt B, Poole-Wilson PA, Segal R, Martinez FA, Dickstein K, Camm AJ et al (2000) Effect of losartan compared with captopril on mortality in patients with symptomatic heart failure: randomised trial—the Losartan Heart Failure Survival Study ELITE II. Lancet 355(9215):1582–1587
29. Pfeffer MA, McMurray JJV, Velazquez EJ et al (2003) Valsartan, captopril, or both in myocardial infarction complicated by heart failure, left ventricular dysfunction, or both. N Engl J Med 349:1893–1906. https://doi.org/10.1056/NEJMoa032292
30. Ruggenenti P, Perna A, Gherardi G, Garini G, Zoccali C, Salvadori M et al (1999) Renoprotective properties of ACE-inhibition in non-diabetic nephropathies with non-nephrotic proteinuria. Lancet 354(9176):359–364. https://doi.org/10.1016/S0140-6736(98)10363-X
31. Wright JT, Bakris G, Greene T, Agodoa LY, Appel LJ, Charleston J et al (2002) Effect of blood pressure lowering and antihypertensive drug class on progression of hypertensive kidney disease: results from the AASK trial. JAMA 288(19):2421–2431. https://doi.org/10.1001/jama.288.19.2421
32. Barnett AH, Bain SC, Bouter P, Karlberg B, Madsbad S, Jervell J et al (2004) Angiotensin-receptor blockade versus converting-enzyme inhibition in type 2 diabetes and nephropathy. N Engl J Med 351(19):1952–1961
33. Mann JF, Schmieder RE, McQueen M, Dyal L, Schumacher H, Pogue J, Wang X, Maggioni A, Budaj A, Chaithiraphan S, Dickstein K, Keltai M, Metsarinne K, Oto A, Parkhomenko A, Piegas LS, Svendsen TL, Teo KK, Yusuf S, ONTARGET Investigators (2008) Renal outcomes with telmisartan, ramipril, or both, in people at high vascular risk (the ONTARGET study): a multicentre, randomised, double-blind, controlled trial. Lancet 372(9638):547–553. https://doi.org/10.1016/S0140-6736(08)61236-2
34. Makani H, Messerli FH, Romero J, Wever-Pinzon O, Korniyenko A, Berrios RS et al (2012) Meta-analysis of randomized trials of angioedema as an adverse event of renin–angiotensin system inhibitors. Am J Cardiol 110(3):383–391. https://doi.org/10.1016/j.amjcard.2012.03.034
35. Hoffmann M, Kleine-Weber H, Schroeder S, Kruger N, Herrler T, Erichsen S, Schiergens TS, Herrler G, Wu NH, Nitsche A, Muller MA, Drosten C, Pohlmann S (2020) SARS-CoV-2 cell entry depends on ACE2 and TMPRSS2 and is blocked by a clinically proven protease inhibitor. Cell 181:271–280. https://doi.org/10.1016/j.cell.2020.02.052
36. Khan A, Benthin C, Zeno B, Albertson TE, Boyd J, Christie JD, Hall R et al (2017) A pilot clinical trial of recombinant human angiotensin-converting enzyme 2 in acute respiratory distress syndrome. Crit Care 21(1):234. https://doi.org/10.1186/s13054-017-1823-x
37. Gu H, Xie Z, Li T et al (2016) Angiotensin-converting enzyme 2 inhibits lung injury induced by respiratory syncytial virus. Sci Rep 6:19840
38. Imai Y et al (2005) Angiotensin-converting enzyme 2 protects from severe acute lung failure. Nature 436:112–116. https://doi.org/10.1038/nature03712
39. Chrysant SG (2010) The role of angiotensin receptor blocker and calcium channel blocker combination therapy in treating hypertension: focus on recent studies. Am J Cardiovasc Drugs 10(5):315–320. https://doi.org/10.2165/11538850-000000000-00000

40. Chobanian AV, Bakris GL, Black HR et al (2003) The seventh report of the Joint National Committee on prevention, detection, evaluation, and treatment of high blood pressure: the JNC 7 report. JAMA 289:2560–2572
41. Tocci G, Sciarretta S, Volpe M (2008) Development of heart failure in recent hypertension trials. J Hypertens 26:1477–1486
42. Padwal R, Straus SE, McAlister FA (2001) Evidence based management of hypertension: cardiovascular risk factors and their effects on the decision to treat hypertension. Evidence based review. BMJ 322:977–980
43. Lewington S, Clarke R, Qizilbash N, Peto R, Collins R (2002) Age-specific relevance of usual blood pressure to vascular mortality: a meta-analysis of individual data for one million adults in 61 prospective studies. Lancet 360(9349):1903–1913
44. Chrysant SG (2008) Using fixed-dose combination therapies to achieve blood pressure goals. Clin Drug Investig 28:713–734
45. Epstein M, Bakris G (1996) Newer approaches to antihypertensive therapy: use of fixed-dose combination therapy. Arch Intern Med 156:1969–1978
46. Chrysant SG (2008) Amlodipine/ARB fixed-dose combinations for the treatment of hypertension: focus on amlodipine/olmesartan combination. Drugs Today 44:443–453
47. Messerli FH (2001) Vasodilatory edema: a common side effect of antihypertensive therapy. Am J Hypertens 14:978–979
48. Philipp T, Smith TR, Glazer R et al (2007) Two multicenter, 8-week, randomized, double-blind, placebo-controlled, parallel-group studies evaluating the efficacy and tolerability of amlodipine and valsartan in combination and as monotherapy in adult patients with mild to moderate essential hypertension. Clin Ther 29:563–580
49. Chrysant SG, Melino M, Karki S et al (2008) The combination of olmesartan medoxomil and amlodipine besylate in controlling high blood pressure: COACH, a randomized, double-blind, placebo-controlled, 8-week factorial efficacy and safety study. Clin Ther 30:587–604
50. Banerjee D, Winocour P, Chowdhury TA, De P, Wahba M, Montero R, Fogarty D, Frankel AH, Karalliedde J, Mark PB, Patel DC, Pokrajac A, Sharif A, Zac-Varghese S, Bain S, Dasgupta I, Association of British Clinical Diabetologists and The Renal Association (2022) Management of hypertension and renin-angiotensin-aldosterone system blockade in adults with diabetic kidney disease: Association of British clinical diabetologists and the Renal Association UK guideline update 2021. BMC Nephrol 23(1):9. https://doi.org/10.1186/s12882-021-02587-5
51. Ku E, McCulloch CE, Mauer M, Gitelman SE, Grimes BA, Hsu C (2016) Association between blood pressure and adverse renal events in type 1 diabetes. Diabetes Care 30:2218–2224
52. Heart Outcomes Prevention Evaluation Study Investigators (2000) Effects of ramipril on cardiovascular and microvascular outcomes in people with diabetes mellitus: results of the HOPE study and the MICRO-HOPE substudy. Lancet 355:253–259
53. (2015) Standards of medical care in diabetes—2015: summary of revisions. Diabetes Care 38(Suppl 1):S4–S4. https://doi.org/10.2337/dc15-S003
54. Toto RD, Tian M, Fakouhi K, Champion A, Bacher P (2008) Effects of calcium channel blockers on proteinuria in patients with diabetic nephropathy. J Clin Hypertens 10(10):761–769
55. Piskorz D (2020) Hypertensive mediated organ damage and hypertension management. How to assess beneficial effects of antihypertensive treatments? High Blood Press Cardiovasc Prev 27(1):9–17. https://doi.org/10.1007/s40292-020-00361-6
56. Vernooij JWP, van der Graaf Y, Nathoe HM, Bemelmans RHH, Visseren FLJ, Spiering W (2013) Hypertensive target organ damage and the risk for vascular events and all-cause mortality in patients with vascular disease. J Hypertens 31:492–500
57. Williams B, Mancia G, Spiering W, Agabiti Rosei E, Azizi M, Burnier M, Clement DL, Coca A, de Simone G, Dominiczak A, Kahan T, Mahfoud F, Redon J, Ruilope L, Zanchetti A, Kerins M, Kjeldsen SE, Kreutz R, Laurent S, Lip GYH, McManus R, Narkiewicz K, Ruschitzka F, Schmieder RE, Shlyakhto E, Tsioufis C, Aboyans V, Desormais I (2018) 2018 ESH/ESC guidelines for the management of arterial hypertension. The task force for the

management of arterial hypertension of the European Society of Hypertension (ESH) and of the European Society of Cardiology (ESC). J Hypertens 36:1953–2041
58. Wang W, Ma L, Zhang Y, Deng Q, Liu M, Liu L (2011) The combination of amlodipine and angiotensin receptor blocker or diuretics in high-risk hypertensive patients: rationale, design and baseline characteristics. J Hum Hypertens 25(4):271–277. https://doi.org/10.1038/jhh.2010.45
59. Law MR, Morris JK, Wald NJ (2009) Use of blood pressure lowering drugs in the prevention of cardiovascular disease: meta-analysis of 147 randomised trials in the context of expectations from prospective epidemiological studies. BMJ 338:b1665
60. Weber MA, Bakris GL, Dahlöf B, Pitt B, Velazquez E, Gupte J et al (2007) Baseline characteristics in the avoiding cardiovascular events through combination therapy in patients living with systolic hypertension (ACCOMPLISH) trial: a hypertensive population at high cardiovascular risk. Blood Press 16(1):13–19
61. Jamerson KA, Bakris GL, Wun CC, Dahlöf B, Lefkowitz M, Manfreda S et al (2004) Rationale and design of the avoiding cardiovascular events through combination therapy in patients living with systolic hypertension (ACCOMPLISH) trial: the first randomized controlled trial to compare the clinical outcome effects of first-line combination therapies in hypertension. Am J Hypertens 17(9):793–801
62. Teo K, Yusuf S, Sleight P, Anderson C, Mookadam F, Ramos B et al (2004) Rationale, design, and baseline characteristics of 2 large, simple, randomized trials evaluating telmisartan, ramipril, and their combination in high-risk patients: the Ongoing Telmisartan Alone and in Combination with Ramipril Global Endpoint Trial/Telmisartan Randomized Assessment Study in ACE Intolerant Subjects with Cardiovascular Disease (ONTARGET/TRANSCEND) trials. Am Heart J 148(1):52–61
63. Volpe M, de la Sierra A, Kreutz R, Laurent S, Manolis AJ (2014) ARB-based single-pill platform to guide a practical therapeutic approach to hypertensive patients. High Blood Press Cardiovasc Prev 21(2):137–147. https://doi.org/10.1007/s40292-014-0043-6
64. Jaffe MG, Lee GA, Young JD, Sidney S, Go AS (2013) Improved blood pressure control associated with a large-scale hypertension program. JAMA 310(7):699–705
65. Chrysant SG, Izzo JL Jr, Kereiakes DJ et al (2012) Efficacy and safety of triple-combination therapy with olmesartan, amlodipine, and hydrochlorothiazide in study participants with hypertension and diabetes: a subpopulation analysis of the TRINITY study. J Am Soc Hypertens 6(2):132–141
66. Nesbitt SD, Shojaee A, Maa JF et al (2013) Efficacy of an amlodipine/olmesartan treatment algorithm in patients with or without type 2 diabetes and hypertension (a secondary analysis of the BP-CRUSH study). J Hum Hypertens 27(7):445–452
67. Bakris GL, Sarafidis PA, Weir MR et al (2010) Renal outcomes with different fixed-dose combination therapies in patients with hypertension at high risk for cardiovascular events (ACCOMPLISH): a prespecified secondary analysis of a randomised controlled trial. Lancet 375(9721):1173–1181
68. Abraham HM, White CM, White WB (2015) The comparative efficacy and safety of the angiotensin receptor blockers in the management of hypertension and other cardiovascular diseases. Drug Saf 38(1):33–54. https://doi.org/10.1007/s40264-014-0239-7
69. James PA, Oparil S, Carter BL et al (2014) Evidence-based guideline for the management of high blood pressure in adults: report from the panel members appointed to the Eighth Joint National Committee (JNC 8). JAMA 311:507–520
70. Brenner GM, Stevens CW (2013) Pharmacology, 4th edn. Saunders, Philadelphia. PA
71. Lauer D, Slavic S, Sommerfeld M et al (2014) Angiotensin type 2 receptor stimulation ameliorates left ventricular fibrosis and dysfunction via regulation of tissue inhibitor of matrix metalloproteinase 1/matrix metalloproteinase 9 axis and transforming growth factor β1 in the rat heart. Hypertension 63:e60–e67
72. Burnier M (2001) Angiotensin II, type 1 receptor blockers. Circulation 103:904–912

73. Israili ZH (2000) Clinical pharmacokinetics of angiotensin II (AT1) receptor blockers in hypertension. J Hum Hypertens 14(Suppl 1):S73–S86
74. Hübner R, Högemann AM, Sunzel M et al (1997) Pharmacokinetics of candesartan after single and repeated doses of candesartan cilexetil in young and elderly healthy volunteers. J Hum Hypertens 11(Suppl 2):S19–S25
75. Derosa G, Ragonesi PD, Mugellini A, Ciccarelli L, Fogari R (2004) Effects of telmisartan compared with eprosartan on blood pressure control, glucose metabolism and lipid profile in hypertensive, type 2 diabetic patients: a randomized, double-blind, placebo-controlled 12-month study. Hypertens Res 27:457–464
76. Scott LJ, McCormack PL (2008) Olmesartan medoxomil a review of its use in the management of hypertension. Drugs 68:1239–1272
77. Sachse A, Verboom CN, Jäger B (2002) Efficacy of eprosartan in combination with HCTZ in patients with essential hypertension. J Hum Hypertens 16:169–176
78. Lacourcière Y, Tytus R, O'Keefe D et al (2001) Efficacy and tolerability of a fixed-dose combination of telmisartan plus hydrochlorothiazide in patients uncontrolled with telmisartan monotherapy. J Hum Hypertens 15:763–770
79. Rakugi H, Ogihara T, Miyata Y, Sasai K, Totsuka N (2012) Evaluation of the efficacy and tolerability of combination therapy with candesartan cilexetil and amlodipine besilate compared with candesartan cilexetil monotherapy and amlodipine besilate monotherapy in Japanese patients with mild-to-moderate essential hypertension: a multicenter, 12-week, randomized, double-blind, placebo-controlled, parallel-group study. Clin Ther 34:838–848
80. Calhoun DA, Lacourcière Y, Chiang YT, Glazer RD (2009) Triple antihypertensive therapy with amlodipine, valsartan, and hydrochlorothiazide: a randomized clinical trial. Hypertension 54:32–39
81. Makani H, Bangalore S, Desouza KA, Shah A, Messerli FH (2013) Efficacy and safety of dual blockade of the renin–angiotensin system: meta-analysis of randomised trials. BMJ 346:360
82. Parving HH, Brenner BM, McMurray JJ et al (2012) Cardiorenal end points in a trial of aliskiren for type 2 diabetes. N Engl J Med 367:2204–2213
83. Dahlöf B, Devereux RB, Kjeldsen SE, LIFE Study Group et al (2002) Cardiovascular morbidity and mortality in the Losartan Intervention For Endpoint Reduction in Hypertension study (LIFE): a randomised trial against atenolol. Lancet 359:995–1003
84. Lithell H, Hansson L, Skoog I et al (2003) The Study on Cognition and Prognosis in the Elderly (SCOPE): principal results of a randomized double-blind intervention trial. J Hypertens 21:875–886
85. Parving HH, Lehnert H, Bröchner-Mortensen J, Gomis R, Andersen S, Arner P, Irbesartan in Patients with Type 2 Diabetes and Microalbuminuria Study Group (2001) The effect of irbesartan on the development of diabetic nephropathy in patients with type 2 diabetes. N Engl J Med 345:870–878
86. Dickstein K, Kjekshus J, OPTIMAAL Steering Committee of the OPTIMAAL Study Group (2002) Effects of losartan and captopril on mortality and morbidity in high-risk patients after acute myocardial infarction: the OPTIMAAL randomised trial. Optimal Trial in Myocardial Infarction with Angiotensin II Antagonist Losartan. Lancet 360:752–760
87. Pfeffer MA, Swedberg K, Granger CB et al (2003) Effects of candesartan on mortality and morbidity in patients with chronic heart failure: the CHARM-Overall programme. Lancet 362:759–766
88. Fogari R, Taddei S, Holm-Bentzen M et al (2010) Efficacy and safety of olmesartan medoxomil 40 mg/hydrochlorothiazide 12.5 mg combination therapy versus olmesartan medoxomil 40 mg monotherapy in patients with moderate to severe hypertension. Clin Drug Investig 30:581–597
89. Neldam S, Edwards C (2008) Results of increasing doses of hydrochlorothiazide in combination with an angiotensin receptor blocker in patients with uncontrolled hypertension. J Clin Hypertens (Greenwich) 10:612–618

90. Pasternak B, Svanström H, Callréus T, Melbye M, Hviid A (2011) Use of angiotensin receptor blockers and the risk of cancer. Circulation 123:1729–1736
91. Park CS, Kim B, Rhee TM, Lee HJ, Lee HS, Park JB, Kim YJ, Han KD, Kim HK (2023) Association between renin-angiotensin-aldosterone system blockade and clinical outcomes in patients with hypertension: real-world observation from a nationwide hypertension cohort. Clin Res Cardiol 112(11):1577–1586. https://doi.org/10.1007/s00392-023-02179-3
92. Collaboration NCDRF (2021) Worldwide trends in hypertension prevalence and progress in treatment and control from 1990 to 2019: a pooled analysis of 1201 population-representative studies with 104 million participants. Lancet 398(10304):957–980
93. GBD 2017 Risk Factor Collaborators (2018) Global, regional, and national comparative risk assessment of 84 behavioural, environmental and occupational, and metabolic risks or clusters of risks for 195 countries and territories, 1990-2017: a systematic analysis for the Global Burden of Disease Study 2017. Lancet 392(10159):1923–1994
94. Heran BS, Wong MM, Heran IK, Wright JM (2008) Blood pressure lowering efficacy of angiotensin converting enzyme (ACE) inhibitors for primary hypertension. Cochrane Database Syst Rev 2008(4):CD003823. https://doi.org/10.1002/14651858.CD003823.pub2
95. Heran BS, Wong MM, Heran IK, Wright JM (2008) Blood pressure lowering efficacy of angiotensin receptor blockers for primary hypertension. Cochrane Database Syst Rev 2008(4):CD003822. https://doi.org/10.1002/14651858.CD003822.pub2
96. Li EC, Heran BS, Wright JM (2014) Angiotensin converting enzyme (ACE) inhibitors versus angiotensin receptor blockers for primary hypertension. Cochrane Database Syst Rev 8:CD009096
97. Strauss MH, Hall AS (2006) Angiotensin receptor blockers may increase risk of myocardial infarction: unraveling the ARB-MI paradox. Circulation 114(8):838–854
98. Choi EK (2020) Cardiovascular research using the Korean national health information database. Korean Circ J 50:754–772
99. Lee SR, Park CS, Choi EK, Ahn HJ, Han KD, Oh S, Lip GYH (2021) Hypertension burden and the risk of new-onset atrial fibrillation: a nationwide population-based study. Hypertension 77:919–928
100. Baker A, Chen LC, Elliott RA, Godman B (2015) The impact of the 'Better Care Better value' prescribing policy on the utilisation of angiotensin-converting enzyme inhibitors and angiotensin receptor blockers for treating hypertension in the UK primary care setting: longitudinal quasi-experimental design. BMC Health Serv Res 15:367. https://doi.org/10.1186/s12913-015-1013-y
101. Prescription Cost Analysis England 2011. http://www.hscic.gov.uk/catalogue/PUB05807/pres-cost-anal-eng-2011-rep.pdf
102. Prescribing costs in primary care. Report by the Comptroller and Auditor General (HC 454 Session 2006–2007). http://www.nao.org.uk/wp-content/uploads/2007/05/0607454es.pdf
103. Prescription Cost Analysis (PCA) data: monthly drug data. http://www.nhsbsa.nhs.uk/PrescriptionServices/3494.aspx
104. The Health and Social Care Information Centre. http://www.hscic.gov.uk
105. Martin A, Godman B, Miranda J, Tilstone J, Saleem N, Olsson E et al (2014) Measures to improve angiotensin receptor blockers prescribing efficiency in the UK: findings and implications. J Comp Eff Res 3:41–51
106. Goel H, Shah K, Kumar A, Hippen JT, Nadar SK (2022) Temperature, cardiovascular mortality, and the role of hypertension and renin-angiotensin-aldosterone axis in seasonal adversity: a narrative review. J Hum Hypertens 36(12):1035–1047. https://doi.org/10.1038/s41371-022-00707-8
107. GISTEMP team 2021 (2021) GISS Surface Temperature Analysis (GISTEMP), version 4. NASA Goddard Institute for Space Studies. https://data.giss.nasa.gov/gistemp/. Dataset Accessed 3 Jul 2021
108. Climate Change 2014: Impacts, Adaptation, and Vulnerability (2014) Part A: global and sectoral aspects. Contribution of Working Group II to the fifth assessment report of the

Intergovernmental Panel on Climate Change. Cambridge University Press and IPCC, Cambridge/New York, p 1132
109. Guo Y, Gasparrini A, Armstrong B, Li S, Tawatsupa B, Tobias A et al (2014) Global variation in the effects of ambient temperature on mortality: a systematic evaluation. Epidemiology 25:781–789
110. Gasparrini A, Guo Y, Hashizume M, Lavigne E, Zanobetti A, Schwartz J et al (2015) Mortality risk attributable to high and low ambient temperature: a multicountry observational study. Lancet 386:369–375. https://linkinghub.elsevier.com/retrieve/pii/S0140673614621140
111. Chen R, Yin P, Wang L, Liu C, Niu Y, Wang W et al (2018) Association between ambient temperature and mortality risk and burden: time series study in 272 main Chinese cities. BMJ 363:k4306. https://doi.org/10.1136/bmj.k4306
112. van Rossum CT, Shipley MJ, Hemingway H, Grobbee DE, Mackenbach JP, Marmot MG (2001) Seasonal variation in cause-specific mortality: are there high-risk groups? 25-year follow-up of civil servants from the first Whitehall study. Int J Epidemiol 30:1109–1116
113. Zhang Y, Li S, Pan X, Tong S, Jaakkola JJK, Gasparrini A et al (2014) The effects of ambient temperature on cerebrovascular mortality: an epidemiologic study in four climatic zones in China. Environ Health Glob Access Sci Source 13:24
114. Singh N, Mhawish A, Ghosh S, Banerjee T, Mall RK (2019) Attributing mortality from temperature extremes: a time series analysis in Varanasi, India. Sci Total Environ 665:453–464
115. Martínez-Solanas È, Quijal-Zamorano M, Achebak H, Petrova D, Robine JM, Herrmann FR et al (2021) Projections of temperature-attributable mortality in Europe: a time series analysis of 147 contiguous regions in 16 countries. Lancet Planet Health 5:e446–e454
116. Ballester J, Robine JM, Herrmann FR, Rodó X (2011) Long-term projections and acclimatization scenarios of temperature-related mortality in Europe. Nat Commun 2:358
117. Gasparrini A, Guo Y, Sera F, Vicedo-Cabrera AM, Huber V, Tong S et al (2017) Projections of temperature-related excess mortality under climate change scenarios. Lancet Planet Health 1:e360–e367
118. Vicedo-Cabrera AM, Guo Y, Sera F, Huber V, Schleussner CF, Mitchell D et al (2018) Temperature-related mortality impacts under and beyond Paris Agreement climate change scenarios. Clim Chang 150:391–402
119. Vardoulakis S, Dear K, Hajat S, Heaviside C, Eggen B, McMichael AJ (2015) Comparative assessment of the effects of climate change on heat- and cold-related mortality in the United Kingdom and Australia. Environ Health Perspect 122:1285–1292
120. Zhang X, Zhang S, Wang C, Wang B, Guo P (2014) Effects of moderate strength cold air exposure on blood pressure and biochemical indicators among cardiovascular and cerebrovascular patients. Int J Environ Res Public Health 11:2472–2487
121. Gasic S, Ratheiser K, Wagner O, Nowotny P, Vierhapper H, Waldhäusl W (1999) Alterations in angiotensin II release and vascular reactivity in hypertensive men: a pilot study. Am J Hypertens 12(11):1055–1062. https://doi.org/10.1016/S0895-7061(99)00137-5. https://academic.oup.com/ajh/article/12/11/1055/242236
122. Jansky L, Sramek P, Savlikova J, Ulicny B, Janakova H, Horky K (1996) Change in sympathetic activity, cardiovascular functions and plasma hormone concentrations due to cold water immersion in men. Eur J Appl Physiol 74:148–152
123. Hiramatsu K, Yamada T, Katakura M (1984) Acute effects of cold on blood pressure, renin-angiotensin-aldosterone system, catecholamines and adrenal steroids in man. Clin Exp Pharmacol Physiol 11:171–179
124. Sramek P, Simeckova M, Jansky L, Savlikova J, Vybiral S (2000) Human physiological responses to immersion into water of different temperatures. Eur J Appl Physiol 81:436–442
125. Sun Z, Fregly MJ, Cade JR (1995) Effect of renal denervation on elevation of blood pressure in cold-exposed rats. Can J Physiol Pharmacol 73:72–78
126. Su D, Du H, Zhang X, Qian Y, Chen L, Chen Y et al (2014) Season and outdoor temperature in relation to detection and control of hypertension in a large rural Chinese population. Int J Epidemiol 43:1835–1845

127. Yang L, Li L, Lewington S, Guo Y, Sherliker P, Bian Z et al (2015) Outdoor temperature, blood pressure, and cardiovascular disease mortality among 23 000 individuals with diagnosed cardiovascular diseases from China. Eur Heart J 36:1178–1185. https://academic.oup.com/eurheartj/article-lookup/doi/10.1093/eurheartj/ehv023
128. Hanazawa T, Asayama K, Watabe D, Tanabe A, Satoh M, Inoue R et al (2018) Association between amplitude of seasonal variation in self-measured home blood pressure and cardiovascular outcomes: HOMED-BP (Hypertension Objective Treatment Based on Measurement by Electrical Devices of Blood Pressure) study. J Am Heart Assoc 7:e008509
129. Burnier M, Redon J, Volpe M (2023) Single-pill combination with three antihypertensive agents to improve blood pressure control in hypertension: focus on olmesartan-based combinations. High Blood Press Cardiovasc Prev. 30(2):109–121. https://doi.org/10.1007/s40292-023-00563-8
130. Zhou B, Perel P, Mensah GA, Ezzati M (2021) Global epidemiology, health burden and effective interventions for elevated blood pressure and hypertension. Nat Rev Cardiol 18(11):785–802
131. Muntner P, Miles MA, Jaeger BC, Hannon Iii L, Hardy ST, Ostchega Y, Wozniak G, Schwartz JE (2022) Blood pressure control among US adults, 2009 to 2012 through 2017 to 2020. Hypertension 79(9):1971–1980. https://doi.org/10.1161/HYPERTENSIONAHA.122.19222
132. Perrine Al LC, Blacher J, Ollié V (2018) L'hypertension artérielle en France: prévalence, traitement et contrôle en 2015 et évolutions depuis 2006. Bull Epidemiol Hebd 10:170–179
133. Brunner HR, Ménard J, Waeber B, Burnier M, Biollaz J, Nussberger J, Bellet M (1990) Treating the individual hypertensive patient: considerations on dose, sequential monotherapy and drug combinations. J Hypertens 8(1):3–11; discussion 13-9. https://doi.org/10.1097/00004872-199001000-00002
134. Burnier M, Brown RE, Ong SH, Keskinaslan A, Khan ZM (2009) Issues in blood pressure control and the potential role of single-pill combination therapies. Int J Clin Pract 63(5):790–798. https://doi.org/10.1111/j.1742-1241.2009.01999.x
135. Gradman AH, Basile JN, Carter BL, Bakris GL, Materson BJ, Black HR, Izzo JL Jr, Oparil S, Weber MA (2010) Combination therapy in hypertension. J Am Soc Hypertens 4(2):90–98. https://doi.org/10.1016/j.jash.2010.03.001
136. Williams B, Mancia G, Spiering W, Agabiti Rosei E, Azizi M, Burnier M, Clement DL, Coca A, de Simone G, Dominiczak A, Kahan T, Mahfoud F, Redon J, Ruilope L, Zanchetti A, Kerins M, Kjeldsen SE, Kreutz R, Laurent S, Lip GYH, McManus R, Narkiewicz K, Ruschitzka F, Schmieder RE, Shlyakhto E, Tsioufis C, Aboyans V, Desormais I, Authors/Task Force Members (2018) 2018 ESC/ESH guidelines for the management of arterial hypertension: the task force for the management of arterial hypertension of the European Society of Cardiology and the European Society of Hypertension: the task force for the management of arterial hypertension of the European Society of Cardiology and the European Society of Hypertension. J Hypertens 36(10):1953–2041. https://doi.org/10.1097/HJH.0000000000001940. Erratum. In: J Hypertens. 2019 Jan;37(1):226
137. Unger T, Borghi C, Charchar F, Khan NA, Poulter NR, Prabhakaran D, Ramirez A, Schlaich M, Stergiou GS, Tomaszewski M, Wainford RD, Williams B, Schutte AE (2020) 2020 International Society of Hypertension global hypertension practice guidelines. Hypertension 75:1334–1357
138. Volpe M, Tocci G (2012) Rationale for triple fixed-dose combination therapy with an angiotensin II receptor blocker, a calcium channel blocker, and a thiazide diuretic. Vasc Health Risk Manag 8:371–380. https://doi.org/10.2147/VHRM.S28359
139. Kreutz R (2011) Olmesartan/amlodipine: a review of its use in the management of hypertension. Vasc Health Risk Manag 7:183–192. https://doi.org/10.2147/VHRM.S16852
140. Omboni S, Kario K, Bakris G, Parati G (2018) Effect of antihypertensive treatment on 24-h blood pressure variability: pooled individual data analysis of ambulatory blood pressure monitoring studies based on olmesartan mono or combination treatment. J Hypertens 36(4):720–733. https://doi.org/10.1097/HJH.0000000000001608

141. Greathouse M (2006) Olmesartan medoxomil combined with hydrochlorothiazide for the treatment of hypertension. Vasc Health Risk Manag 2(4):401–409. https://doi.org/10.2147/vhrm.2006.2.4.401
142. Deedwania P, Weber M, Reimitz PE, Bakris G (2017) Olmesartan-based monotherapy vs combination therapy in hypertension: a meta-analysis based on age and chronic kidney disease status. J Clin Hypertens (Greenwich) 19(12):1309–1318. https://doi.org/10.1111/jch.13103
143. Fogari R, Taddei S, Holm-Bentzen M, Baszak J, Melani L, Schumacher K (2010) Efficacy and safety of olmesartan medoxomil 40 mg/hydrochlorothiazide 12.5 mg combination therapy versus olmesartan medoxomil 40 mg monotherapy in patients with moderate to severe hypertension: a randomized, double-blind, parallel-group, multicentre, multinational, phase III study. Clin Drug Investig 30(9):581–597. https://doi.org/10.2165/11536710-000000000-00000
144. Fliser D, Buchholz K, Haller H, European Trial on Olmesartan and Pravastatin in Inflammation and Atherosclerosis (EUTOPIA) Investigators (2004) Antiinflammatory effects of angiotensin II subtype 1 receptor blockade in hypertensive patients with microinflammation. Circulation 110(9):1103–1107
145. Chrysant SG, Oparil S, Melino M, Karki S, Lee J, Heyrman R (2009) Efficacy and safety of long-term treatment with the combination of amlodipine besylate and olmesartan medoxomil in patients with hypertension. J Clin Hypertens (Greenwich) 11(9):475–482. https://doi.org/10.1111/j.1751-7176.2009.00159.x
146. Sohn IS, Kim CJ, Oh BH, Hong TJ, Park CG, Kim BS, Chung WB, Investigators (2016) Erratum to: Efficacy and safety study of olmesartan medoxomil, amlodipine, and hydrochlorothiazide combination therapy in patients with hypertension not controlled with olmesartan medoxomil and hydrochlorothiazide combination therapy: results of a randomized, double-blind, multicenter trial. Am J Cardiovasc Drugs 16(2):139. https://doi.org/10.1007/s40256-016-0167-2. [Erratum for: Am J Cardiovasc Drugs. 2016;16(2):129–38]
147. Sohn IS, Kim CJ, Oh BH, Hong TJ, Park CG, Kim BS, Chung WB, Investigators. (2016) Efficacy and safety study of olmesartan medoxomil, amlodipine, and hydrochlorothiazide combination therapy in patients with hypertension not controlled with olmesartan medoxomil and hydrochlorothiazide combination therapy: results of a randomized, double-blind, multicenter trial. Am J Cardiovasc Drugs 16(2):129–138. https://doi.org/10.1007/s40256-015-0156-x
148. Sohn IS, Ihm SH, Kim GH, Park SM, Hong BK, Lee CH, Lee SH, Chang DI, Joo SP, Lee SC, Lee YH, Jeon DW, Jung KT, Rhee SJ, Cho YJ, Kim CJ, Investigators. (2021) Real-world evidence on the strategy of olmesartan-based triple single-pill combination in Korean hypertensive patients: a prospective, multicenter, observational study (RESOLVE-PRO). Clin Hypertens 27(1):21. https://doi.org/10.1186/s40885-021-00177-z
149. Sung J, Ahn KT, Cho BR, Lee SY, Kim BJ, Kim DK, Park JI, Lee WS (2021) Adherence to triple-component antihypertensive regimens is higher with single-pill than equivalent two-pill regimens: a randomized controlled trial. Clin Transl Sci 14(3):1185–1192. https://doi.org/10.1111/cts.12979. Epub 2021 Feb 13
150. Marques da Silva P, Haag U, Guest JF, Brazier JE, Soro M (2015) Health-related quality of life impact of a triple combination of olmesartan medoxomil, amlodipine besylate and hydrochlorotiazide in subjects with hypertension. Health Qual Life Outcomes 13:24. https://doi.org/10.1186/s12955-015-0216-6
151. Volpe M, Tocci G, de la Sierra A, Kreutz R, Laurent S, Manolis AJ, Tsioufis K (2017) Personalised single-pill combination therapy in hypertensive patients: an update of a practical treatment platform. High Blood Press Cardiovasc Prev. 24(4):463–472. https://doi.org/10.1007/s40292-017-0239-7
152. Chen R, Suchard MA, Krumholz HM, Schuemie MJ, Shea S, Duke J, Pratt N, Reich CG, Madigan D, You SC, Ryan PB, Hripcsak G (2021) Comparative first-line effectiveness and safety of ACE (angiotensin-converting enzyme) inhibitors and angiotensin receptor

blockers: a multinational cohort study. Hypertension 78(3):591–603. https://doi.org/10.1161/HYPERTENSIONAHA.120.16667

153. Izzo JL Jr, Chrysant SG, Kereiakes DJ, Littlejohn Iii T, Oparil S, Melino M, Lee J, Fernandez V, Heyrman R (2011) 24-hour efficacy and safety of triple-combination therapy with olmesartan, amlodipine, and hydrochlorothiazide: the TRINITY ambulatory blood pressure substudy. J Clin Hypertens (Greenwich) 13(12):873–880. https://doi.org/10.1111/j.1751-7176.2011.00544.x
154. Burnier M, Egan BM (2019) Adherence in hypertension. Circ Res 124(7):1124–1140. https://doi.org/10.1161/CIRCRESAHA.118.313220
155. Egan BM, Kjeldsen SE, Narkiewicz K, Kreutz R, Burnier M (2022) Single-pill combinations, hypertension control and clinical outcomes: potential, pitfalls and solutions. Blood Press 31(1):164–168. https://doi.org/10.1080/08037051.2022.2095254

The manufacturer's authorised representative in the EU is Springer Nature Customer Service Centre GmbH, Europaplatz 3, 69115 Heidelberg, Germany. If you have any concerns regarding our products, please contact ProductSafety@springernature.com

Printed and bound by CPI Group (UK) Ltd, Croydon, CR0 4YY
01/10/2026
02225962-0019